CHURCHILL LIVINGSTONE
Nurses Dictionary

1
80

Alistair A. Brown

January 1980

CHURCHILL LIVINGSTONE

Nurses Dictionary

(Lois Oakes)

Edited by

Nancy Roper MPhil, SRN, RSCN, RNT

British Commonwealth Nurses War Memorial Fund
Research Fellow 1970
In association with the Royal College of Nursing

FIFTEENTH EDITION

CHURCHILL LIVINGSTONE
EDINBURGH LONDON AND NEW YORK 1978

CHURCHILL LIVINGSTONE
Medical Division of Longman Group Limited

Distributed in the United States of America by
Longman Inc., 19 West 44th Street, New York,
N.Y. 10036, and by associated companies,
branches and representatives throughout
the world.

First Edition 1932
Second Edition 1933
Third Edition 1934
Fourth Edition 1936
Fifth Edition 1938
Sixth Edition 1940
Seventh Edition 1941
  Reprinted 1942
Eighth Edition 1943
  Reprinted 1944
Ninth Edition 1946
Tenth Edition 1949
  Reprinted 1953, 1955, 1956, 1957, 1958, 1960
Eleventh Edition 1961
Twelfth Edition 1966
Thirteenth Edition 1969
  Reprinted 1972
Fourteenth Edition 1973
  Reprinted 1976
  Reprinted 1977
Fifteenth Edition 1978

ISBN 0 443 01637 2

British Library Cataloguing in Publication Data
Oakes, Lois
  Churchill Livingstone nurses dictionary.   15th ed.
  1. Nursing – Dictionaries
  I. Roper, Nancy   II. Livingstone dictionary for
  nurses
  III. Royal College of Nursing
  610.73'03   RT21   LC. 78-40580

Printed in Great Britain by Hazell, Watson & Viney l td., Aylesbury

Preface to the Fifteenth Edition

The 15th edition of this dictionary has been extensively revised in both content and appearance. In an effort to bring the material completely up to date, medical experts were engaged to review and check appropriate sections of the dictionary and to add new definitions where necessary. In addition, many of the illustrations have been redrawn and new illustrations have been included.

The appendices to the dictionary have also been considerably revised and expanded. A 7-page section has been added illustrating over 50 different types of surgical instruments in common use. There is a new appendix on Side-Room Testing, which includes descriptions of urine, blood, serum, plasma and faeces testing, and one on Body Fluid Tests, which gives normal ranges for each test in both traditional and SI units. A Vitamins Table has been added listing, for each vitamin, its functions, properties, deficiency, sources and daily requirement. Finally, an important section has been included on the SI or International System of Units, which gives conversion scales for certain chemical pathology tests.

The format of this edition is visably different from its predecessors. A slightly larger page size has been adopted, which should make for more comfortable reading and easier handling.

I am indebted to many people who have helped to make this major revision possible, and to them I offer my sincere thanks. I hope that the users of the dictionary will agree that the changes undertaken are a substantial improvement.

Edinburgh, 1978   NANCY ROPER

Preface to the Twelfth Edition

On the death of Lois Oakes in 1952 the royalties from, and interests in, her dictionary were bequeathed to the Royal College of Nursing. As their chosen editor, with the guidance of a sub-committee, I have attempted the formidable task, not only of bringing the text up to date, but also of including the etymology and a biographical note where appropriate, so that this twelfth edition will make history in being the first dictionary *for nurses* to appear in this style.

A capital letter has often been used when repeating the 'entry' word in the text to save space, since at the beginning of the revision it was impossible to predict the size of the book. A capital letter has also been used to differentiate proprietary drugs.

The hyphen has been omitted in compounded words, except for the separation of two vowels, unless by custom the hyphen (1) is *not* used for this purpose, e.g. preoccupation, readjust, etc.; (2) *is retained,* e.g. bedclothes, club-foot, ultra-violet, etc.

With ever-increasing specialization it has been necessary to enlist the help of many specialists, to whom I am deeply indebted, for without their help and encouragement a complete revision of the dictionary would have been impossible.

To the staff of the Cumberland Infirmary, Carlisle, I tender my grateful thanks, especially to Dr Herbert J. Bell, M.B.E., M.A., M.B., Ch.B., D.P.H., and Dr V. A. Erskine, M.R.C.P., L.R.C.S., L.R.F.P.S., D.P.M.

Others who helped and deserve special mention are Professor G.L. Montgomery, T.D., M.D., F.R.C.P.E., Ph.D., F.R.S.E., Professor of Pathology, University of Edinburgh; Dr. S. H. Davies, M.B., Ch.B., M.R.C.P., Senior Registrar, Edinburgh and South-East Scotland Blood Transfusion Service; Dr A. A. Donaldson, D.M.R.D.Ed., Consultant Radiologist, Royal Infirmary, Edinburgh; Dr J. G. Gould, M.D., B.Sc., Lecturer in Bacteriology, University of Edinburgh; Dr R. Passmore, M.A., D.M.(Oxon), Reader in Physiology, University of Edinburgh; Mr Ian S. R. Sinclair, F.R.C.S.E., Senior Lecturer in Surgery, University of Edinburgh; Dr. R. W. D. Turner, O.B.E., M.A., M.D.(Cantab), F.R.C.P.E., Senior Lecturer, Department of Medicine, University of Edinburgh; The Ames Company, London; Miss Jessie Dobson, B.A., M.Sc., Curator, Hunterian Museum, Royal College of Surgeons of England; Mr S. J. Hopkins, F.P.S., Cambridge.

To the sub-committee of the Royal College of Nursing I record my thanks for their guidance.

To the publishers, especially Mr Charles Macmillan and Mr James Parker, I offer my sincere thanks, for when the task seemed greatest they were ever ready with suggestions to lighten the load.

Now that the dictionary is complete, I hope that those who use it will derive both benefit and pleasure from it. The effort will then have been worthwhile.

Carlisle, 1961   NANCY ROPER

Contents

Guide to pronunciation: Consonants

ch (= tsh) as in   cheese (chēz),
                         stitch (stich),
                         picture (pik'chėr).
   j (dzh)   judge (juj),
                         rigid (rij'id).
      sh   dish,
                         lotion (lō'-shun).
      zh   vision (vizh'-'n).
      ng   sing,
                         think (thingk).
       g   Always hard as in good.
       r   This letter is often left unsounded or is slurred into the preceding vowel. In the combination 'er' (see Vowels) the 'r' is rarely trilled or marked. Where it receives its full consonantal value it is usually placed preceding a vowel; in most other cases its force is determined by individual taste and custom.
    th   No attempt has been made to distinguish between the breathed sound as in 'think' and the voiced sound as in 'them.'
Accent: The accented syllable is indicated by a slanting stroke at its termination, e.g. fibrositis (fī-brō-sī'-tis).

Guide to pronunciation: Vowels

a as in fat, back, tap.
ā   lame, brain (brān), vein (vān).
å   far, calf (kåf), heart (hårt), coma (kō'må).
e   flesh, deaf (def), said (sed).
ē   he, tea (tē), knee (nē), anaemia (an-ē'-mi-å).
ê   there, air (êr), area (êr'-i-å).*
i   sit, busy (biz'-i).
ī   spine, my, eye, tie.
o   hot, cough (kof).
ō   bone, moan (mōn), dough (dō).
u   gum, love (luv), tough (tuf), colour (kul'-êr).
ū   mute, due, new, you, rupture (rup'-tūr).
aw   saw, gall (gawl), caul (kawl), water (waw'têr).
oi   loin, boy.
oo   foot, womb (woom), wound (woond), rude (rood).
ow   cow, sound (sownd), gout (gowt).

*When followed by 'r', 'e' is often sounded as in 'her' or as 'u' in 'fur' (for example, 'ferment'); in '-er' as a final unaccented syllable, the 'e' is sometimes more or less elided (drawer, tower). See also consonant 'r'.

Abbreviations used in definitions

adj	Adjective
adv.	Adverb
Ar.	Arabic
A.S.	Anglo-Saxon
cf.	[L. *confer*] Compare
dim.	Diminution of
dub.	Dubious
E.	English
e.g.	[L. *exempli gratia*] For example
Etym.	Etymology
F.	French
G.	Greek
i.e.	[L. *id est*] That is
It.	Italian
L.	Latin
L.L.	Late Latin
M.E.	Middle English
n.	Noun
N.L.	New Latin
O.N.	Old Norse
Opp.	Opposite to
per se	As such
Pg.	Portuguese
pl.	Plural
q.v.	[L. *quod vide*] Which see
Sing.	Singular
Syn.	Synonym
v.	Verb
v.i.	Intransitive verb
v.t.	Transitive verb

A

abacterial (ā-bak-tē'-ri-ål) [G. *a-*, not; *bakterion*, small rod]. Without bacteria. A word used to describe a condition, for instance inflammation, not caused by bacteria.

abdomen (ab-dō'-men) [L. belly]. The largest body cavity, immediately below the thorax, from which it is separated by the diaphragm. It is enclosed largely by muscle and fascia, and is therefore capable of change in size and shape. It is lined with a serous membrane, the peritoneum, which is reflected as a covering over most of the organs. **acute a.**, pathological condition within the belly requiring immediate surgical intervention. **pendulous a.**, a relaxed condition of the anterior wall, allowing it to hang down over the pubis. **scaphoid a.** (navicular), concavity of the anterior wall—abdominal, adj.

abdominopelvic (ab-dom'-in-ō-pel'-vik) [L. *abdomen*, belly; L. *pelvis*, basin]. Pertaining to the abdomen and pelvis or pelvic cavity.

abdominoperineal (ab-dom'-in-ō-per-in-ē'-al) [L. *abdomen*, belly; G. *perineos*, space between the anus and the scrotum]. Pertaining to the abdomen and perineum **a excision of the rectum**, above a cancerous growth of the rectum, the bowel is divided and the proximal end brought out on to the abdominal wall as a permanent colostomy. The distal portion is dissected down, the growth and glands freed and these are then removed by the perineal route.

abduct (ab-dukt') [L. *abductum*, from *abducere*, to lead away]. To draw away from the median line of the body. Opp. to adduct.

abduction (ab-duk'-shun) [L. *abductum*, from *abducere*, to lead away]. The act of abducting away from the midline. Opp. to adduction.

abductor (ab-duk'-tor) [L. *abducere*, to lead away]. A muscle which, on contraction, draws a part away from the median line of the body. Opp. to adductor.

aberration (ab-er-rā'-shun) [L. *aberrare*, to wander from]. A deviation from normal. **mental a.**, a mild mental abnormality. **optical a.**, imperfect focus of light rays by a lens—aberrant, adj.

ablation (ab-lā'-shun) [L. *ablatio*, take away]. Removal. In surgery, excision or amputation—ablative, adj.

abort (ab-awrt') [L. *abortus*, premature birth]. To terminate before full development.

abortifacient (ab-awr-ti-fā'-shi-ent) [L. *abortus*, premature birth; *facere*, to make]. Causing abortion. Drug or agent inducing expulsion of a non-viable fetus.

abortion (ab-awr'-shun) [L. *abortus*, premature birth]. 1. Abrupt termination of a process. 2. Expulsion from uterus of product of conception before it is viable, i.e. before the end of the 28th week. **complete a.**, the entire contents of the uterus are expelled. **criminal a.**, intentional evacuation of uterus on any other than medical grounds. **habitual a.**; preferable syn. **recurrent a.**, term used when abortion recurs in successive pregnancies. **incomplete a.**, part of the fetus or placenta is retained within the uterus. **induced a.** (also called 'artificial'), intentional evacuation of uterus. **inevitable a.**, one which has advanced to a stage where termination of pregnancy cannot be prevented. **missed a.**, early signs and symptoms of pregnancy disappear and the fetus dies, but is not expelled for some time. See MOLE under which carneous mole is defined. **septic a.**, one associated with uterine infection and rise in body temperature. **therapeutic a.**, intentional termination of a pregnancy which is a hazard to the mother's life and health. **threatened a.**, slight blood loss per vaginam whilst cervix remains closed. **tubal a.**, a tubal pregnancy that dies and is expelled from the fimbriated end of the Fallopian tube—abortive, adj.

abortus fever. See BRUCELLOSIS.

abrasion (ab-rā'-zhun) [L. *abradere*, to scrape off]. Superficial injury to skin or mucous membrane from scraping or rubbing; excoriation—abrade, v.t.; to undergo abrasion, v.i.

abreaction (ab-rē-ak'-shun) [L. *ab*, away; *re-*, again; *agere*, to do]. An emotional reaction resulting from recall of past painful experiences relived in speech and action during psychoanalysis or under the influence of light anaesthesia, or drugs. See NARCOANALYSIS, CATHARSIS.

abscess (ab'-ses) [L. *abscessus*, a going away]. Localized collection of pus produced by pyogenic organisms. May be acute or chronic. **alveolar a.**, at the root of a tooth. **Brodie's a.**, chronic osteomyelitis (q.v.) occurring without previous acute phase. **cold a.**, one occurring in the course of such chronic inflammation as may be due to the tubercle bacillus (*Mycobacterium tuberculosis*). **psoas a.**, a cold abscess in the psoas muscle, resulting from tuberculosis of the lower dorsal or lumbar vertebrae.

Abstem (ab'-stem). Citrated calcium carbimide. Analogue of disulfiram (q.v.).

acapnia (a-kap'-ni-á) [G. *a-*, not; *kapnos*, smoke]. Absence of CO_2 in the blood, sometimes used synonymously with hypocapnia (q.v.); can be produced by hyperventilation—acapnial, adj.

acatalasia (a-kat-al-āz'-i-á) Absence of the enzyme catalase; predisposes to oral sepsis.

accommodation (ak-kom-mo-dā'-shun) [L. *accommodare*, to adapt]. Adjustment, e.g. the power of the eye to alter the convexity of the lens according to the nearness or distance of objects, so that a distinct image is always retained—accommodative, adj.

accouchement (ak-koosh'-mong) [F.]. Delivery in childbirth. Confinement.

accoucheur (ak-koo-shèr') [F.]. A man skilled in midwifery; an obstetrician.

accoucheuse (ak-koo-shèz') [F.]. A midwife; a female obstetrician.

accretion (ak-krē'-shun) [L. *accrescere*, to grow]. An increase of substance or deposit round a central object; in dentistry, an accumulation of tartar round the teeth—accrete, adj., v.t and i.; accretive, adj.

acebutolol (ac-bū'-to-lol). A β-adrenoceptor blocking agent used in cardiac dysrhythmias, angina pectoris and hypertension.

acephalous (a-kef'-a-lus) [G. *a-*, not; *kephale*, head]. Without a head.

acetabuloplasty (as-et-ab'-ūl-ō-plas-ti) [L. *acetabulum*, vinegar cup; G. *plassein*, to form]. An operation to improve the depth and shape of the hip socket (acetabulum); necessary in such conditions as congenital dislocation of the hip and osteoarthritis of the hip -acetabuloplastic, adj.

acetabulum (as-et-ab'-ūl-um) [L.]. A cup-like socket on the external surface of the innominate bone, into which the head of the femur fits to form the hip joint—acetabula, pl.

acetarsol (á-set-ár'-sol). An organic compound of arsenic, used in amoebiasis (q.v.), usually to supplement emetine.

acetate (as'-ē-tāt). A salt of acetic acid.

acetazolamide (a-set-az-ol'-a-mīd). Diuretic. Inhibits action of carbonic anhydrase, the kidney enzyme controlling excretion of bicarbonate; results in excretion of increased amount of alkaline urine. As the body has limited reserves of bicarbonate, acetazolamide is self-limiting in action. Also used in glaucoma and epilepsy.

acetic acid (as-ē'-tic as'-id). The acid present in vinegar. Three varieties are used medicinally: (1) glacial acetic acid, sometimes used as a caustic; (2) ordinary acetic acid, used in urine testing; (3) dilute acetic acid, used occasionally in cough mixtures.

acetoacetic acid (as-ē'-to as-ē'-tik as'-id). Syn., diacetic acid. A monobasic keto acid. Produced at an interim stage in the oxidation of fats in the human body. In some metabolic upsets, e.g. acidosis and diabetes mellitus, it is present in excess in the blood and escapes in the urine. (It changes to acetone if urine is left standing.) The excess acid in the blood can produce coma.

acetohexamide (as-ēt-ō-heks'-á-mīd). One of the sulphonylureas. Antidiabetic agent.

acetomenaphthone (a-sēt-o-men-af'-thōn). A synthetic form of vitamin K (q.v.). It is active orally; used in the treatment of obstructive jaundice and in prophylaxis against neonatal haemorrhage.

acetonaemia (as-ē-tō-nē'-mi-á) [L. *acetum*, vinegar: G. *haima*, blood]. Acetone bodies in the blood—acetonaemic, adj.

acetone (as'-ē-tōn). Inflammable liquid with characteristic odour; valuable as a solvent. **a. bodies**, a term which includes acetone, acetoacetic acid and β-hydroxybutyric acid. See KETOSIS.

acetonuria (as-ē-tō-nū'-ri-á) [L. *acetum*, vinegar; G. *ouron*, urine]. Excess acetone bodies in the urine causing a characteristic sweet smell—acetonuric, adj.

acetophenetidin (a-sēt-o-fen-et'-id-in). Phenacetin (q.v.).

acetylcholine (as-et-il-kō'-lēn). Chemical substance released from nerve endings to activate muscle, secretory glands and other nerve cells. The fibres releasing this chemical are termed 'cholinergic.' Hydrolysed into choline and acetic acid by the enzyme acetylcholinesterase, which is present in blood and other tissues.

acetylcysteine (as-et-il-sis'-tēn). A mucolytic agent, invaluable in mucoviscidosis (q.v.).

acetylsalicylic acid (a-set-il-sal'-is-il-ik). Aspirin; an extensively used mild analgesic. It forms the basis of a large number of proprietary analgesic tablets. Gastric irritant. Can cause haematemesis. Aspirin (q.v.) is now the official BP name.

achalasia (ak-a-lā'-zi-ā) [G. *a-*, not; *chalasis*, relaxation]. Failure to relax. **cardiac a.**, food fails to pass normally into stomach, though there is no obvious obstruction. The oesophagus does not demonstrate normal waves of contraction after swallowing; this prevents the normal relaxation of the cardiac sphincter. Associated with loss of ganglion cells within muscle layers of at least some areas of the affected oesophagus.

Achilles tendon (ak-il'-ēz ten'-don) [G. *Achilles*; L. *tendo*, tendon]. The tendinous termination of the soleus and gastrocnemius muscles inserted into the heel bone (os calcis).

achillorrhaphy (ak-il-or'-af-i) [G. *Achilles*; *rhaphe*, a seam]. The operation of stitching the Achilles tendon.

achillotomy (ak-il-ot'-om-i) [G. *Achilles*; *tome*, a cutting]. Subcutaneous division of Achilles tendon.

achlorhydria (a-klor-hi'-dri-ā) [G. *a-*, not; *chloros*, green; *hydrios*, from *hydor*, water]. The absence of free hydrochloric acid in the stomach. Found in pernicious anaemia and gastric cancer—achlorhydric, adj.

acholia (a-kōl'-i-ā) [G. *a-*, not; *chole*, bile]. Absence of bile—acholic, adj.

acholuria (a-kol-ū'-ri-ā) [G. *a-*, not; *chole*, bile; *ouron*, urine]. Absence of bile pigment from the urine. See JAUNDICE—acholuric, adj.

achondroplasia (a-kon-drō-plā'-zi-ā) [G. *a-*, not; *chondros*, cartilage; *plassein*, to form]. An inherited condition characterized by arrested growth of the long bones resulting in dwarfism. The intellect is not impaired. Syn., fetal rickets—achondroplastic, adj.

achromatopsia (a-krō-mat-op'-zi-ā) [G. *a-*, not; *chroma*, colour; *opsis*, vision]. Complete colour blindness as only monochromatic grey is visible.

Achromycin (ak-rō-mī'-sin). Tetracycline (q.v.).

achylia (a-kī'-li-ā) [G. *a-*, not; *chylos*, juice]. Absence of chyle (q.v.)—achylic, adj.

acid (as'-id) [L. *acidus*, sour]. Any substance which in solution gives rise to an excess of hydrogen ions. Identified (1) by turning blue litmus paper red; (2) by being neutralized by an alkali with the formation of a salt. (In popular jargon, any substance with a sour taste.)

acidaemia (as-id-ē'-mi-ā) [L. *acidus*, sour; G. *haima*, blood]. Abnormal acidity of the blood, giving increased hydrogen ions, and a below normal pH (q.v.). **respiratory a.**, caused by poor ventilation and increasing carbon dioxide. **metabolic a.**, caused by increased lactic acid production in muscles. See ACIDOSIS—acidaemic, adj.

acid-base balance. Equilibrium between the acid and base elements of the blood and body fluids.

acid-fast. In bacteriology, describes an organism which, when stained, does not become decolo(u)rized when subjected to dilute acids, e.g. *Mycobacterium tuberculosis*.

acid-alcohol-fast. Stained bacteria, resistant to decolo(u)rization by alcohol as well as acid.

acidity (as-id' it i) [L. *acidus*, acid]. The state of being acid or sour. The degree of acidity can be determined and interpreted on the pH scale, pH 6.9 denoting a very weak acid and pH 1 a caustic acid.

acidosis (as-id-ō'-sis) [L. *acidus*, sour; G. *-osis* condition]. Depletion of the body's alkali reserve, with resulting disturbance of the acid-base balance. Acidaemia. **renal tubular a.**, metabolic abnormality. See KETOSIS—acidotic, adj.

acid phosphatase (fos'-fa-tāz). Enzyme in seminal fluid. Secreted by prostate gland.

aciduria (as-id-ū'-ri-ā) [L. *acidus*, sour; G. *-osis* condition]. Excretion of an acid urine. Current work suggests there might be some association with mental subnormality.

acini (as'-in-ī) [L.]. Minute saccules or alveoli, lined or filled with secreting cells. Several acini combine to form a lobule—acinus, sing.; acinous, acinar, adj.

acme (ak'-mē) [G. *akme*, prime]. 1. Highest point. 2. Crisis or critical state of a disease.

acne, acne vulgaris (ak'-nē vul-gar'-is). A skin condition common in adolescence, in which blackheads (comedones) are associated with a papular and pustular eruption of the pilosebaceous follicles. Usual sites are the face, neck and upper part of chest and back. See ROSACEA.

acneiform (ak-nē'-i-form). Resembling acne.

acriflavine (ak-ri-flā'-vēn). Orange-red, soluble powder. Powerful antiseptic, used as a 1:1000 solution for wounds, and 1:4000 to 1:8000 for irrigation. Acriflavine emulsion is a bland wound dressing containing liquid paraffin. Proflavine and euflavine are similar compounds.

acroarthritis (ak-rō-árth-rī'-tis) [G. *akron*, extremity; *arthron*, joint; *-itis*, inflammation]. Inflammation of the joints of hands or feet.

acrocephalia: acrocephaly (ak-rō-kef'-ā-li-à) [G. *akron*, extremity; *kephale* head]. A congenital malformation whereby the top of the head is pointed—acrocephalic, acrocephalous, adj.

acrocephalosyndactyly (ák-rō-kef'-a-lō-sin-dak'-til-i) [G. *akron*, extremity; *kephale*, head; *syn.* with; *daktylos*, digit]. A congenital malformation consisting of a pointed top of head, with webbed hands and feet. Acrocephalosyndactylism. See SYNDACTYLY.

acrocyanosis (ak-rō-sī-an-ō'-sis) [G. *akron*, extremity; *kyanos* blue; *-osis*, condition]. Coldness and blueness of the extremities due to circulatory disorder—acrocyanotic, adj.

acrodynia (ak-rō-din'-i-à) [G. *akron*, extremity; *odyne*, pain]. Painful reddening of the extremities such as occurs in pink disease (q.v.).

acromegaly (ak-rō-meg'-a-li) [G. *akron*, extremity; *megas*, large]. Enlargement of the hands, face and feet, occurring in an adult due to disturbed function of the pituitary gland—acromegalic, adj.

acromicria (ak-rō-mik'-ri-à) [G. *akron*, extremity; *mikros*, small]. Smallness of the hands, face and feet, probably due to deficiency of growth hormone from the pituitary gland.

acromioclavicular (ak-rō-mi-ō-kla-vi'-kū-lár) [G. *akron*, extremity; *omos*, shoulder; L. *clavicula*, dim. of *clavis*, key]. Pertaining to the acromion process (of scapula) and the clavicle.

acromion (ak-rō'-mi-on) [G. *akron*, extremity; *omos*, shoulder]. The point or summit of the shoulder; the triangular process at the extreme outer end of the spine of the scapula—acromial, adj.

acronyx (ak'-rō-niks) [G. *akron*, extremity; *onyx*, nail]. Ingrowing of a nail.

acroparaesthesia (ak-rō-par-es-thē'-zi-a) [G. *akron*, extremity; *paroesthesis*, misperception]. Tingling and numbness of the hands.

acrophobia (ak-rō-fō'-bi-à) [G. *akron*, extremity; *phobos*, fear]. Morbid fear of being at a height.

acrylics (a-kril'-iks). A group of thermoplastic substances used in making prostheses—acrylic, adj.

ACTH. Corticotrophin (q.v.).

Acthar gel (ak-thá jel). Given in units to suppress disseminated sclerosis.

Actifed (ak'-ti-fed). Pseudoephedrine (q.v.) and triprolidine (q.v.).

actinic dermatoses. Skin conditions (such as xeroderma pigmentosum, summer prurigo (q.v.) and others) in which the integument is abnormally sensitive to ultraviolet light.

actinism (ak'-tin-izm) [G. *aktis*, ray]. The chemical action of spectral rays—actinic, adj.

actinobiology (ak'-tin-ō-bī-ol'-ōj-i) [G. *aktis*, ray; *bios*, life; *logos*, discourse]. The study of the effects of radiation on living organisms.

Actinomyces (ak-tin-ō-mī'-sēz) [G. *aktis*, ray; *mykes*, fungus]. A genus of parasitic fungus having a radiating mycelium. Also called 'ray fungus.' Many of the antibiotic drugs are produced from this genus.

actinomycin C (ak-tin-ō-mī'-sin). A cytostatic antibiotic useful in Hodgkin's disease and for suppression of the immune reaction in organ transplants.

actinomycin D (ak-tin-ō-mī'-sin). An intravenous cytostatic agent especially useful in Wilms' tumour. Also used in Burkitt's lymphoma. Best results obtained with doses high enough to interfere with the action of FOLIC ACID, a substance required by rapidly dividing cells, but insufficient for really deep depression of the patient's capacity to react immunologically.

actinomycosis (ak-tin-ō-kō'-sis) [G. *aktis*, ray; *mykes*, fungus; *-osis*, condition]. A disease caused by Actinomyces, the sites most affected being the lung, jaw and intestine. Granulomatous tumours form which usually suppurate, discharging a thick, oily pus containing yellowish granules ('sulphur granules')—actinomycotic, adj.

actinotherapy (ak-tin-ō-thē'-rap-i) [G. *aktis*, ray; *therapeia*, therapy]. Treatment radiations, similar to those in natural sunlight, but produced by artificial means.

action (ak'-shun) [L. *actio*, from *agere*, to do or to perform]. The activity or function of any part of the body. **antagonistic a.**, performed by those muscles which limit the movement of an opposing group. **compulsive a.**, performed by an individual at the supposed instigation of another's dominant will, but against his own. **impulsive a.**, resulting from a sudden urge rather than the will. **reflex a.**, a specific, involuntary motor or secretory response to a sensory stimulus. **sexual a.**, coitus, cohabitation, sexual intercourse. **specific a.**, that brought about by certain remedial agents in a particular disease, e.g. salicylates in acute rheumatism. **specific dynamic a.**, the stimulating effect upon the metabolism produced by the ingestion of food, especially proteins, causing the metabolic rate to rise above basal levels. **synergistic a.**, that brought about by the co-operation of two or more muscles, neither of which could bring about the action alone.

activator [L. *activus*]. A substance which renders something else active, e.g. the hormone secretin, the enzyme enterokinase. An enzyme activator is called 'co-enzyme' or 'kinase'—activate, v.

active [L. *activus*, active]. Energetic. Opp. to passive (q.v.). **a. hyperaemia**, see HYPERAEMIA. **a. immunity**, see IMMUNITY. **a. movements**, those produced by the patient using his neuromuscular mechanism. **a. principle**, an ingredient which gives a complex drug its chief therapeutic value, e.g. atropine is the active principle in belladonna.

Actrapid (ak'-tra-pid). Neutral insulin injection BP.

acuity (ak-ū'-it-i) [L. *acuere*, to sharpen]. Sharpness, clearness, keenness, distinctness. **auditory a.**, ability to hear clearly and distinctly. Tests include the use of tuning fork, whispered voice and audiometer. In infants, simple sounds, e.g. bells, rattles, cup and spoon are utilized. **visual a.**, extent of visual perception dependent on the clarity of retinal focus, integrity of nervous elements and cerebral interpretation of the stimulus. Usually tested by Snellen's test types (q.v.) at 6 metres.

acupuncture (ak-ū-punk'-tūr) [L. *acus*, needle; *punctura*, a pricking]. 1. The incision or introduction of fine, hollow tubes into oedematous tissue for the purpose of withdrawing fluid. 2. A technique of insertion of special needles into particular parts of the body for the treatment of disease, relief of pain or production of anaesthesia.

acute (a-kūt') [L. *acutus*, sharp]. Short and severe; not long drawn out or chronic. **a. defibrination syndrome**, (hypofibrinogenaemia), excessive bleeding due to maternal absorption of thromboplastins from retained blood clot or damaged placenta within the uterus. A missed abortion, placental abruption, amniotic fluid embolus, prolonged retention in utero of a dead fetus and the intravenous administration of dextran can lead to ADS. **a. dilatation of the stomach**, sudden enlargement of this organ due to paralysis of the muscular wall. See PARALYTIC ILEUS. **a. heart failure**, cessation or impairment of heart action, in previously undiagnosed heart disease, or in the course of another disease. **a. yellow atrophy**, acute diffuse necrosis of the liver; icterus gravis; malignant jaundice.

acyanosis (a-sī-an-ō'-sis) [G. *a-*, not; *kyanos*, blue; *-osis*, condition]. Without cyanosis.

acyanotic (a-sī-an-ot'-ik). Without cyanosis; term used to differentiate congenital cardiovascular defects.

acyesis (a-sī-ē'-sis) [G. *a-*, not; *kyesis*, pregnancy]. Absence of pregnancy—acyetic, adj.

acystia (a-sis'-ti-á) [G. *a-*, not; *kystis*, bladder]. Congenital absence of the bladder—acystic, adj.

Adam's apple. The laryngeal prominence in front of the neck, especially in the adult male, formed by the junction of the two wings of the thyroid cartilage.

adaptability (ad-apt'-a-bil-it-i) [L. *adaptare*, to adjust]. The ability to adjust mentally and physically to circumstances.

Adcortyl (ad-kor'-til). Triamcinalone (q.v.) **a. in orabase**, emollient dental paste for mouth ulcers.

addict (ad'-ikt) [L. *addictum,* from *addicere,* to devote]. One who is unable to resist indulgence in some habit, such as the drug (q.v.) habit—addict, v.t., v.i.; addiction, n.

Addison's disease. Deficient secretion of aldosterone and cortisol from the adrenal cortex, causing electrolytic upset, diminution of blood volume, lowered blood pressure, marked anaemia, hypoglycaemia, great muscular weakness, gastrointestinal upsets and pigmentation of skin. [Thomas Addison, English physician, diagnostician and teacher, 1793–1860.]

adduct (ad-dukt') [L. *ad,* to; *ducere,* to lead]. To draw towards the midline of the body. Opp. to abduct.

adduction (ad-duk'-shun) [L. *ad,* to; *ducere,* to lead]. The act of adducting, drawing towards the midline. Opp. to abduction.

adductor (ad-duk'-tor) [L. *ad,* to; *ducere,* to lead]. Any muscle which moves a part toward the median axis of the body. Opp. to abductor.

adenectomy (ad-en-ek'-to-mi) [G. *aden,* gland; *ektome,* excision]. Surgical removal of a gland.

adenitis (ad-en-ī-tis) [G. *aden,* gland; *-itis,* inflammation]. Inflammation of a gland or lymph node. **hilar a.,** inflammation of bronchial lymph nodes.

adenocarcinoma (ad-en-ō-kár-sin-ō'-má) [G. *aden,* gland; *karkinos,* crab; *omos,* raw flesh]. A malignant growth of glandular tissue—adenocarcinomatous, adj.; adenocarcinomata, pl.

adenofibroma (ad-en-ō-fī-brō'-má). See FIBROADENOMA.

adenoid (ad'-en-oid) [G. *aden,* gland; *eidos,* form]. Resembling a gland. See ADENOIDS.

adenoidectomy (ad-e-noid-ek'-to-mi) [G. *aden,* gland; *eidos,* form; *ektome,* excision]. Surgical removal from nasopharynx of adenoid tissue.

adenoids (ad'-en-oidz) [G. *aden,* gland; *eidos,* form]. Enlarged mass of lymphoid tissue in the nasopharynx which can obstruct breathing and interfere with hearing.

adenoma (ad-en-ō'-má) [G. *aden,* gland; *omos,* raw flesh]. A non-malignant tumour of glandular tissue—adenomatous, adj.; adenomata, pl.

adenomyoma (ad-en-ō-mī-ō'-má) [G. *aden,* gland; *mys,* muscle; *omos,* raw flesh]. A non-malignant tumour composed of muscle and glandular elements, e.g. an adenomyoma of the uterosacral ligaments is composed of smooth muscle in which islands of aberrant endometrium are found—adenomyomatous, adj.; adenomyomata, pl.

adenomyosis uteri (ad-en-ō-mī-ō'- sis ū'-te-rī) [G. *aden,* gland; *mys,* muscle; *-osis,* condition]. A general enlargement of the uterus due to overgrowth of the myometrium, in which there is a benign invasion of endometrium.

adenopathy (ad-en-op'-a-thi) [G. *aden,* gland; *pathos,* disease]. Any disease of a gland, especially a lymphatic gland—adenopathic, adj.

adenosclerosis (ad-en-ō-skle-rō'-sis) [G. *aden,* gland; *sklerosis,* a hardening]. Hardening of a gland with or without swelling, usually due to replacement by fibrous tissue or calcification—adenosclerotic, adj.

adenosine diphosphate (ad-en-ō'-sin dī-fos'-fāt) ADP. A derivative of phosphoric acid; plays a part in cellular energy currency. After release of some of its energy, ADP becomes adenosine monophosphate; with addition of energy, ADP becomes ADENOSINE TRIPHOSPHATE.

adenosine triphosphate (ad-en-o'-sin trī-fos'-fāt) ATP. A derivative of phosphoric acid. The ATP molecule carries the chemical energy released in the body by the breakdown of large molecules from food (catabolism).

adenotonsillectomy (ad-en-ō-ton-sil-ek'-to-mi) [G. *aden,* gland; L. *tonsilloe,* tonsils; G. *ektome,* excision]. Surgical removal of the adenoids and tonsils.

adenovirus (ad-en-ō-vī'-rus) [G. *aden,* gland; L. *virus,* poison]. A group of DNA-containing viruses composed of 47 serologically distinct types: 31 serotypes have been found in man, and many in various animal species. Some cause upper respiratory infection, others pneumonia, others epidemic keratoconjunctivitis.

adermin (ad'-ér-min) See PYRIDOXIN.

Adexolin (ad-eks'-o-lin). Proprietary mixture of vitamin A and D.

ADH Antidiuretic hormone (q.v.).

adhesion (ad-hē'-zhun) [L. *ad,* to; *haerere,* to stick]. Abnormal union of two parts, often after inflammation; a band of fibrous tissue which joins such parts. In the abdomen such a band may cause intestinal obstruction; in joints it restricts movement; between two surfaces of pleura it prevents complete pneumothorax—adherent, adj.; adherence, n.; adhere, v.t., v.i.

adiaphoretic (ā-dī-a-for-et'-ik) [G. *a-*, not; *diaphoretikos*, promoting perspiration]. Preventing or reducing perspiration—adiaphoresis, n.

adipose (ad'-ip-ōz) [L. *adeps*, lard]. Fat; of a fatty nature.

adiposity (ad-i-pos'-it-i) [L. *adeps*, lard; G. *-osis*, condition]. Excessive accumulation of fat in the body.

adiposuria (ad-i-pos-ū'-ri-ā) [L. *adeps*, lard; G. *ouron*, urine]. See LIPURIA.

aditus (ad'-it-us) [L.]. In anatomy, an entrance or opening.

adjustment. 1. The mechanism used in focusing a microscope. 2. In psychology, the establishment of a satisfactory relationship between the individual and his environment.

adjuvant (ad'-joo-vant) [L. *adjuvare*, to assist]. A substance included in a prescription to aid the action of other drugs. **a. therapy**, supportive measures in addition to main treatment.

Adler's theory (ád'-ler). The idea that neuroses arise from feelings of inferiority either social or physical. [Alfred Adler, Austrian psychiatrist, 1870–1937.]

adnexa (ad-neks'-á) [L. *ad*, to; *nectere*, to bind]. Structures which are in close proximity to a part. **a. oculi**, the lacrimal apparatus. **a. uteri**, the ovaries and Fallopian tubes—adnexal, adj.

adolescence (ad-o-les'-sens) [L. *adolescere*, to grow up]. The period between puberty and full maturity, youth—adolescent, adj., n.

adoral (ad-awr'-al) [L. *ad*, to; *os*, mouth]. Near the mouth.

ADP. Adenosine diphosphate (q.v.).

adrenal (ad-rē'-nal) [L. *ad*, to; *renes*, kidneys]. Near the kidney, by custom referring to the adrenal glands, one lying above each kidney. The **a. cortex** secretes mineral and glucocorticoids which control the chemical constitution of body fluids, metabolism and sexual characteristics. Functionally closely related to the pituitary and other endocrine glands. The **a. medulla** secretes noradrenaline. See ADRENALECTOMY.

adrenalectomy (ad-rē-nal-ek'-to-mi) [L. *ad*, to; *renes*, kidney; G. *ektome*, excision]. Removal of an adrenal gland, for tumour or for treatment of hypertension, malignant disease of breast, etc. If both adrenal glands are removed, replacement administration of cortical hormones is required.

adrenaline (ad-ren'-a-lin). A hormone produced by the adrenal medulla in mammals. It can be prepared synthetically. Solutions may darken in colour and lose activity if stored for long periods. Applied locally as liquor adrenaline (1:1000) in epistaxis; given by subcutaneous injection, it is invaluable in relieving serum sickness, asthmatic attacks, urticaria and other allergic states. It is added to local anaesthetic solutions to reduce diffusion and so prolong the anaesthetic effect. Also used in circulatory collapse, but only in very dilute solution (1:100 000) by slow intravenous infusion.

adrenergic (ad-ren-ér'-jik) [L. *ad*, to; *renes*, kidney; G. *ergon*, work]. Term applied to sympathetic nerves which liberate adrenaline and noradrenaline from their terminations. Opp. to cholinergic.

adrenocorticotrophic (ad-ren'-ō-kor-ti-kō-trōf'-ik) [L. *ad*, to; *renes*, kidney; *cortex*, bark; G. *trephein*, to nourish]. Having an effect on the adrenal cortex. See CORTICOTROPHIN.

adrenogenital syndrome (ad-ren-ō-jen'-it al sin'-drōm) [L. *ad*, to; *renes*, kidney; *genitalis*, genital]. 17-Hydroxycorticosteroids in a 24 hour collection of urine is high. Glucocorticoid secretion is deficient and ACTH secretion is stimulated. Steroid intermediates pile up behind the block due to enzyme deficiency and are converted via the remaining unblocked pathways to androgens. Treatment with glucocorticoids inhibits ACTH secretion, thus preventing the abnormal secretion of androgens and other steroids. Hereditary pattern not precise, determined by an autosomal recessive gene. A female child will show enlarged clitoris and possibly labial fusion, perhaps being confused with a male. The male child may show pubic hair and enlarged penis. In both male and female there is rapid growth, muscularity and advanced bone age.

adrenolytic (ad-rè-no-li'-tic) [L. *ad*, to; *renes*, kidney; G. *lysis*, dissolution]. That which antagonizes the action or secretion of adrenaline and noradrenaline.

adriamycin (ad-ri-á-mī'-sin). Antitumour antibiotic of the anthracycline group, particularly effective in childhood malignancies. Similar to daunorubicin, but has less cardiotoxic effect.

adsorbents (ad-sawrb'-ents) [L. *ad*, to; *sorbere*, to suck]. Solids which attract gases or dissolved substances, to their surfaces, as a film. Charcoal adsorbs gases and acts as a deodorant. Kaolin adsorbs bacterial and other toxins, hence used in food poisoning.

adsorption (ad-sorp'-shun) [L. *ad*, to; *sorbere*, to suck]. The property of a substance to attract and to hold to its surface a gas or a liquid—adsorptive, adj.; adsorb, v.t., v.i.

advancement. An operation to remedy squint. The muscle tendon opposite to the direction of the squint is detached and sutured to the sclera anteriorly.

adventitia (ad-ven-tish'-i-á) [L. *adventicius*, foreign]. The external coat, especially of an artery or vein—adventitious, adj.

Aëdes (á-ē'-dēz) [G. *a*-, not; *edos*, pleasure]. A genus of mosquitoes that includes *Aëdes aegypti*, the principal vector of yellow fever and dengue.

AEG. Air encephalography. See PNEUMOENCEPHALOGRAPHY.

aerobe (a'-ér-ōb) [G. *aer*, air; *bios*, life]. A micro-organism which requires O_2 to maintain life—aerobic, adj.

aerogenous (ā-ér-oj'-en-us) [G. *aer*, air; *genesis*, production]. Gas producing.

aerogram (ā'-ér-ō-gram) [G. *aer*, air; *gramma*, letter]. X-ray of tube or hollow viscus after introduction of air or gas. Especially useful after barium meal or enema, when aerogram shows the mucosa coated with a thin layer of barium.

aerophagia: aerophagy (ā-ér-ō-faj'-i-á: ā-ér-of'-á-ji) [G. *aer*, air; *phagein*, to eat]. Excessive air swallowing (as in hysteria).

aerosol (ā'-ér-o-sol). Atomized particles; can be packaged under pressure and from such a source can be used: (1) as inhalation therapy: (2) to sterilize the air; (3) in insect control; (4) as a deodorant or other skin application.

Aerosporin (ā-ér-o-spor-in). Polymyxin B sulphate (q.v.).

aetiology (ē-ti-ol'-o-ji) [G. *aitia*, cause; *logos*, discourse]. A science dealing with the causation of disease. Also spelt etiology—aetiological, adj.; aetiologically, adv.

afebrile (ā-feb'-rīl) [G. *a*-, not; L. *febris*, fever]. Without fever.

affect (af-ekt) [L. *afficere*, to affect]. Feeling; refers to the general emotional state of a person, and includes mood.

afferent (af'-er-ent) [L. *afferre*, to bring]. Conducting inward to a part or organ; used to describe nerves, blood and lymphatic vessels. Opp. to efferent.

affiliation (af-fil-i-ā'-shun). Settling of the paternity of an illegitimate child on the putative father.

affinity (af-in'-i-ti) [L. *affinis*, adjoining]. A chemical attraction between two substances, e.g. oxygen and haemoglobin.

afibrinogenaemia (ā-fi-brin'-ō-jen-ē'-mi-á) [G. *a*-, not; L. *fibra*, fibre; G. *genein*, from *gignesthai*, to be born; *haima*, blood]. More specifically fibrinogen-fibrin conversion syndrome; a serious disorder of coagulation in which it is thought that placental thromboplastin causes this conversion—afibrinogenaemic, adj.

aflatoxin (af-la-toks'-in). Carcinogenic metabolite of certain strains of *Aspergillus flavus* that infect peanuts.

afterbirth [A.S. *aefter*; M.E. *burth*]. The placenta, cord and membranes which are expelled from the uterus after childbirth.

aftercare. A term used in the NHS Act. It denotes the care given during convalescence and rehabilitation. It need not be medical or nursing.

afterimage [A.S. *aefter*; L. *imago*, image]. A visual impression of an object which persists after the object has been removed. This is called 'positive' when the image is seen in its natural bright colours; 'negative' when the bright parts become dark, while the dark parts become light.

afterpains [A.S. *aefter*; M.E. *pain*, from O.F. *peine*]. The pains felt after childbirth, due to contraction and retraction of the uterine muscle fibres.

agalactia (a-gal-ak'-ti-á) [G. *a*-, not; *gala*, milk]. Non-secretion or imperfect secretion of milk after childbirth —agalactic, adj.

agammaglobulinaemia (a-gam-a-glob'-ūl-in-ēm'-i-á). Absence of gamma-globulin in the blood, with consequent inability to produce immunity to infection. **Bruton's a.**, a congenital condition in boys, in which B-lymphocytes are absent but cellular immunity remains intact. See DYSGAMMAGLOBULIN-AEMIA — agammaglobulinaemic, adj.

aganglionosis (a-gang-li-on-ō'-sis)[G. *a-*, not; *ganglion*, swelling; *-osis*, condition]. Absence of ganglia, as those of the distant bowel. See MEGACOLON.

agar (ā'-gar). A gelatinous substance obtained from certain seaweeds. It is used as a bulk-increasing laxative, and as a solidifying agent in bacterial culture media.

age: chronological, a person's actual age in years. **mental a.**, the age of a person with regard to his mental development; this can be determined by a series of tests. If a woman of 30 can only pass the tests for a child of 12, she is said to have a mental age of 12. **physiological a.**, the term applied to age as assessed from appearance and behaviour; thus some people are old at 40, while others are young at 60.

agenesis (a-jen-ēs'-is)[G. *a-*, not; *genesis*, production]. Incomplete and imperfect development — agenetic, adj.

agglutination (a-gloo'-tin-ā'-shun) [L. *agglutinare*, to glue]. The clumping of bacteria or red blood cells as effected by the specific immune antibodies called 'agglutinins,' developed in the blood serum of a previously infected or sensitized person — agglutinable, agglutinative, adj.; agglutinate, v.t. and i.

agglutinins (a-gloo'-tin-inz) [L. *agglutinare*, to glue]. Specific factors present in sera which agglutinate or clump organisms or particulate protein matter. See ANTIBODIES.

agglutinogen (a-gloo'-tin-ō-jen) [*agglutinare*, to glue; G. *genesthai*, to be produced]. A factor which stimulates production of a specific agglutinin, used in the production of immunity, e.g. dead bacteria as in vaccine, particulate protein as in toxoid.

aggressin (a-gres'-in) [L. *aggressus*, attacked]. A metabolic substance, produced by certain bacteria to enhance their aggressive action against their host.

aggression (a-gre'-shun) [L. *aggressio*, from *aggredi*, to attack]. An attitude of animosity or hostility, usually resulting from frustration or a feeling of inferiority — aggressive, adj.

agitated depression (aj'-i-tā-ted dē-pre'-shun). Marked restlessness, continual activity, despondency and apprehension. Often associated with menopause.

aglossia (a-glos'-i-á) [G. *a-*, not; *glossa*, tongue]. Absence of the tongue — aglossic, adj.

aglutition (a-gloo-ti'-shun)[G. a-, not; L. *glutire*, to swallow]. See DYSPHAGIA.

agnosia (ag-nō'-zē-á) [G. *a-*, not; *gnosis*, recognizing]. Inability to understand sensory impressions — agnosic, adj.

agonist (ag'-on-ist) [G. *agonistes*, combatant]. Muscle that shortens to perform a movement. See ANTAGONIST.

agoraphobia (ag-or-a-fō'-bi-á) [G. *agora*, market place; *phobos*, fear]. Morbid fear of being alone in large open places — agoraphobic, adj.

agranulocytosis (ā-gran-ū-lō-sī-tō'-sis) [G. *a-*, not; L. *granulum*, a small grain; G. *kytos*, cell; *-osis*, condition]. Marked reduction in or complete absence of granulocytes or polymorphonuclear leucocytes. Usually results from bone marrow depression caused by (1) hypersensitivity to drugs, (2) cytotoxic drugs or (3) irradiation — agranulocytic adj.

agraphia (a-graf'-i-á) [G. *a-*, not; *graphein*, to write]. Inability to express the thoughts in writing — agraphic, adj

ague (ā'-gū) [F. *aigu*, sharp, from L. *acutus*]. See MALARIA.

AHG. Antihaemophilic globulin (q.v.).

AID. Artificial insemination (q.v.) of a female with donor semen.

AIH. Artificial insemination (q.v.) of a female with her husband's semen.

air [G. *aer*, air]. The gaseous mixture which makes up the atmosphere surrounding the earth. It consists of approximately 78 per cent nitrogen, 20 per cent oxygen, 0.04 per cent carbon dioxide, 1 per cent argon, and traces of ozone, neon, helium, etc. and a variable amount of water vapour. **a-bed**, a rubber mattress inflated with air. **Complemental a.**, the extra air that can be drawn into the lungs by deep inspiration. **a. hunger**, inspiratory and expiratory distress characterized by sighing and gasping; due to anoxia (q.v.) **residual a.**, that which still remains in the alveoli of the lung after forced expiration. **stationary a.**, that which remains after normal expiration. **supplemental a.**, the extra air that can be expired with effort. **a. swallowing**, see AEROPHAGIA. **tidal a.**, that which passes in and out of the lungs in normal breathing.

Airbron (ér'-bron). Acetylcysteine (q.v.).

akathisia (ak'-ath-i-zi-a) [G. a-, not; kathisis, a sitting down]. Inability to sit still. A state in which the patient feels a distressing inner restlessness.

akinetic (ā-kīn-et'-ik) [G. a-, without: kinesis, motion]. Without movement. a. epilepsy, epileptic fits where instead of a tonic and clonic phase the patient is limp, the whole body remains flaccid until consciousness returns. a. catatonia occurs in schizophrenia. a. mutism, sustained periods of unconsciousness in which the patient appears to be relaxed and asleep, but he can only be roused for a few moments; occurs in tumours of third ventricle, midbrain and thalamus—akinesia, n.

alastrim (al-as'-trim) [Pg. from alastrar, to spread, cover]. A less virulent form of smallpox known as variola minor, which may be confused with chickenpox.

Albamycin (al-ba-mī'-sin). Novobiocin (q.v.).

Albee's operation (al'-bēz). For producing ankylosis of the hip. Upper surface of head of femur is removed, and corresponding edge of acetabulum. A.'s bone graft, operation for spinal fixation. Spinous processes of diseased area are exposed and split. Graft from tibia is placed in raw area. [Fred Houdlett Albee, New York surgeon, 1876–1945.]

Albers-Schönberg disease. A spotty calcifying of the bones, which fracture spontaneously. 'Marble bones.' Syn., osteopetrosis. [Heinrich Ernst Albers-Schönberg, German surgeon, 1865–1921.]

albinism (al-biń-ism) [L. albus, white]. Failure of the tyrosine system to oxidize tyrosine through dopa to melanin, so that the skin is fair, the hair white and the eyes pink.

albino (al-bē' nō) [L. albus, white]. A male affected with albinism—albinotic, adj.; albiness, female.

Albucid (al-bū'-sid). Sulphacetamide (q.v.).

albumen (al-bū'-men) [L. albumen, albuminis, white of an egg]. Also spelt albumin. A variety of protein found in animal and vegetable matter. It is soluble in water and coagulates on heating. serum a., the chief protein of blood plasma and other serous fluids. Lactalbumen is the albumen found in milk—albuminous, albuminoid, adj.

albuminometer (al-bū-min-om'-et-er). A graduated test-tube in special stand for estimating quantity of albumen in a fluid. Esbach's (q.v.) is the most familiar pattern.

albuminuria (al-bū-min-ū'-ri-á) [L. albus, white; G. ouron, urine] The presence of albumen in the urine. The condition may be temporary and clear up completely, as in many febrile states. chronic a. leads to hypoproteinaemia (q.v.). orthostatic or postural a. is an abnormality of little importance in which albumen depends on the upright posture, and is absent in the urine secreted during sleep (the morning specimen)—albuminuric, adj.

albumose (al'-bū-mōz). An early product of proteolysis. It resembles albumen, but is not coagulated by heat.

albumosuria (al-bū-mōz-ū'-ri-á). The presence of albumose in the urine—albumosuric, adj.

alcohol (al'-ko-hol). The principal constituent of wines and spirits. Absolute alcohol is occasionally used by injection for the relief of trigeminal neuralgia and other intractable pain; rectified spirit (90 per cent alcohol) is widely used in the preparation of tinctures: methylated spirit contains 95 per cent alcohol with wood naphtha and is for external application only. Enhances the action of barbiturates and tranquillizers. Intravenous alcohol therapy has been tried in premature labour to delay birth. It is thought to prevent release of substances which stimulate uterine contraction. Alcohol inhibits the milk ejection reflex in humans. a. psychosis, see KORSAKOFF'S SYNDROME.

alcohol-fast. A bacteriological term used when alcohol fails to decolo(u)rize a stained organism.

Alcoholics Anonymous. A fellowship of people previously addicted to alcohol. Their main aim is curing others of alcoholism.

alcoholism (al'-ko-hol-izm). Alcoholic poisoning. In its chronic form it causes severe disturbances of the nervous and digestive systems.

alcoholuria (al-ko-hol-ū'-ri-á). Alcohol in the urine. Basis of one test for fitness to drive after drinking alcohol.

Alcopar (al'-kō-pár). Bephenium hydroxynaphthoate (q.v.).

Aldactone A (al-dak'-tōn). Spironolactone (q.v.).

Aldomet. Methyldopa (q.v.).

aldosterone (al-dos-tēr'-ōn). An adrenocortical steroid which, by renal control, regulates electrolyte metabolism; hence described as a 'mineralocorticoid'. Secretion is regulated by the renin-angiotensin system. It increases excretion of potassium and conserves sodium and chloride. Primary aldosteronism is a condition resulting from tumours of the adrenal cortex in which this electrolyte imbalance is marked and alkalosis and tetany may ensue.

Aleppo boil. See LEISHMANIASIS.

Aleudrin (al'-ū-drin). Isoprenaline (q.v.).

aleukaemic (ā-lū-kē'-mik) [G. a-, not; leukos, white; haima, blood]. See LEUKAEMIA.

Alevaire (al'-ē-ver). A solution of glycerine, sodium bicarbonate and a detergent which helps to liquefy tenacious sputum. The patient inhales it as a fine mist produced by passing O_2 through a nebulizer containing Alevaire.

alexia (a-leks'-i-ā) [G. a-, not; lexis, word]. Word blindness; loss of the ability to interpret the significance of the printed or written word, but without loss of visual power. Due to a brain lesion—alexic, adj.

algesia (al-jē'-zi-ā) [G. algesis, sense of pain]. Excessive sensitiveness to pain; hyperaesthesia—algesic, adj. Opp. to analgesia.

algesimeter (al-jēz-im'-ēt-er). An instrument which registers the degree of sensitivity to pain.

algid (al'-jid) [L. algidus, cold]. Cold. Description of severe attack of fever, especially malaria, with collapse, extreme coldness of the body, suggesting a fatal termination. During this stage the rectal temperature may be high.

alginates (al'-jin-ātz). Seaweed derivatives which, when applied locally, encourage the clotting of blood. They are available in solution and in specially impregnated gauze.

Alidine (a'-li-dīn). Anileridine (q.v.).

alienation (ā-li-en-ā'-shun) [L. alienatio, alienation]. In psychiatry, mental illness.

alienist (ā'-li-en-ist) [L. alienus, of another]. One skilled in treatment of mental disorders. Psychiatrist (q.v.).

alimentary (al-i-ment'-a-ri) [L. alimenta, nourishment, food]. Pertaining to food.

alimentation (al-i-men-tā'-shun) [L. alere, to nourish]. Act of nourishing with food; feeding.

aliquot (al'-i-kwat) [L. some, so many]. Part contained by the whole an integral number of times. The sample withdrawn from a 24-hour specimen.

alkalaemia (al-kal-ē'-mi-ā) [Ar. alqili, ashes of saltwort; G. haima, blood]. Alkalosis (q.v.)—alkalaemic, adj.

alkali (al'-kal-ī) [Ar. al-qili, ashes of saltwort]. A series of soluble corrosive bases analogous to and including soda, potash and ammonia which neutralize acids forming salts, and combine with fats, to form soaps. Alkaline solutions turn red litmus blue—alkalis, pl. a. reserve, a biochemical term denoting the amount of buffered alkali (normally bicarbonate) available in the blood for the neutralization of acids (normally CO_2) formed in or introduced into the body.

alkaline (al'-kal-īn) [Ar. al-qili, ashes of saltwort]. 1. Possessing the properties of or pertaining to an alkali. 2. Containing an excess of hydroxyl over hydrogen ions.

alkalinuria (al-kal-in-ūr'-i-ā) [Ar. al-qili, ashes of saltwort; G. ouron, urine]. Alkalinity of urine—alkalinuric, adj.

alkaloid (al'-kal-oid). Resembling an alkali. A name often applied to a large group of organic bases found in plants and which possess important physiological actions. Morphine, quinine, caffeine, atropine and strychnine are well-known examples of alkaloids—alkaloidal, adj.

alkalosis (al-kal-ō'-sis) [Ar. al, qili, ashes of saltwort; G. -osis, condition]. Alkalaemia. Excess of alkali or reductions of acid in the body. Develops from a variety of causes such as overdosage with alkali, excessive vomiting or diarrhoea, and hyperventilation. See HYPERPNOEA. Results in neuromuscular excitability expressed clinically as tetany (q.v.).

alkaptonuria (al-kap-ton-ūr'-i-ā). The presence of alkaptone (homogentisic acid) in the urine, resulting from only partial oxidation of phenylalanine and tyrosine. Condition usually noticed because urine goes black in the nappies, or when left to stand. Apart from this, and a tendency to arthritis in later life, there are no ill-effects from a.

Alkeran (al'-ker-an). Melphalan (q.v.).

alkylating agents. Disrupt the process of cell division by affecting DNA in nucleus, by addition of alkyl groups. Alternatively called nitrogen mustard compounds. Used as cytotoxic drugs in neoplastic disorders.

Allegron. Nortriptyline. Similar to amitriptyline (q.v.). See ANTIDEPRESSANT.

allelomorphs (a-lē'-lo-morfz) [G. *allelon,* of one another; *morphe,* form]. Inherited characteristics which are alternative and contrasting (typical of artificial selection), such as tallness or shortness. The basis of Mendel's law of dominants and recessives—allelomorphic, adj.; allelomorphism, n.

allergen (al'-ėr-jen) [G. *allos,* other; *ergon,* activity; *genesis,* production]. Any agent capable of producing a state or manifestation of allergy—allergenic, adj.; allergenicity, n.

allergy (al'-ėr-ji) [G. *allos,* other; *ergon,* work]. An altered or exaggerated susceptibility to various foreign substances or physical agents which are harmless to the great majority of individuals. It is due to an antigen-antibody reaction, though the antibody formed is not always demonstrable. Hay fever, asthma, urticaria and infantile eczema are allergic conditions and are familial in origin—allergic, adj. See ANAPHYLAXIS and SENSITIZATION.

allocheiria (a-lō-chir'-i-á) [G. *allos,* other; *cheir,* hand]. An abnormality of tactile sensibility under test, wherein patient refers a given stimulus to the other side of the body.

allograft (al'-lo-graft) [G. *allos,* other; *graphein,* to write]. Transplantation of part of one person to another. The term **non-viable a.** is used when skin (which cannot regenerate) is taken from a cadaver. See LYOPHILIZED SKIN.

Allonal (al'-on-al). Amidopyrine (q.v.).

allopurinol (al-lo-pū'-rin-ol). A substance which prevents the formation of deposits of crystals from insoluble uric acid. Diminishes tophi in gout and substantially reduces the frequency and severity of further attacks. Can cause skin rash.

aloes (al'-ōz). The dried juice from the cut leaves of a tropical plant. Powerful purgative with an intensely bitter taste.

alopecia (al-ō-pē'-si-á) [L. from G. *alopekia,* fox-mange]. Baldness which can be congenital, premature or senile. **a.**

areata, a patchy baldness, usually of a temporary nature. Cause unknown, but shock and anxiety are common precipitating factors. Exclamation mark hairs are diagnostic. **a. cicatrisata,** syn. pseudopelade, progressive alopecia of the scalp in which tufts of normal hair occur between many bald patches. Folliculitis decalvans is an alopecia of the scalp characterized by pustulation and scars.

Alophen (al'-ō-fen). Compound containing phenolphthalein (q.v.).

Aloxiprin (al-oks'-i-prin). Aluminium aspirin. Causes less gastric irritation than aspirin; broken down in small intestine to release aspirin. See ACETYLSALICYLIC ACID.

alphachymotrypsin (al-fa-kī-mō-trip'-sin). A pancreatic enzyme which dissolves the capsular ligament and allows the lens to be extracted through the pupil and out of the wound without undue physical manipulation. Anti-inflammatory agent when taken orally.

alphafetoprotein (al-fa-fē'-tō-prō'-tēn). Present in maternal serum and amniotic fluid in cases of fetal abnormality.

Alphosyl (al'-fo-sil). Colourless preparation of coal tar.

alprenolol (al-pren'-o-lol). An adrenergic blocker. Acts in angina pectoris by decreasing cardiac work; decreases heart rate, cardiac output and arterial pressure.

ALS antilymphocyte serum. Immunosuppressive, which appears to act mainly on lymphocytes in the blood stream. It appears to diminish the number of circulating lymphocytes, thereby giving a transplanted organ a better chance of survival in the recipient. It does not interfere with the body's general defence mechanism.

Althesin (al'-the-sin). Induces anaesthesia.

alum. Potassium or ammonium aluminium sulphate. Used for its astringent properties as a mouthwash (1 per cent) and as a douche (½ per cent). Also for precipitating toxoid. See APT.

aluminium hydroxide. An antacid with a prolonged action used in the treatment of peptic ulcer. It is usually given as a thin cream or gel. There is no risk of alkalosis with long treatment, as drug is not absorbed.

aluminium paste. A mixture of aluminium powder, zinc oxide and liquid paraffin, used as a skin protective in ileostomy. This paste is sometimes known as 'Baltimore paste'.

Alupent (al'-ū-pent). Orciprenaline sulphate (q.v.).

alveolar-capillary block syndrome. A rare syndrome of unknown aetiology characterized by breathlessness, cyanosis and right heart failure, due to thickening of the alveolar walls of the lungs, thus impairing diffusion of oxygen.

alveolitis (al-vē-ol-ī-tis) [L. *alveolus,* air sac; G. *-itis,* inflammation]. Inflammation of alveoli, by custom usually referring to those in the lung; when caused by inhalation of an allergen such as pollen, it is termed **extrinsic allergic a.**

alveolus (al-vē'-o-lus) [L.]. 1. An air vesicle of the lung. 2. A tooth socket. 3. A gland follicle or acinus—alveoli, pl.; alveolar, adj.

Alzheimer's disease. A form of presenile dementia caused by atrophy of the prefrontal areas of the brain.[Alois Alzheimer, German physician, 1864–1915.]

amalgam (a-mal'-gam) [G. *malagma,* emollient] An alloy of mercury. **dental a.,** used for filling teeth, contains mercury, silver and tin.

amantadine (am un'-ta-din) An antiviral agent (influenza A_2) which is now used mainly in the management of some patients with Parkinson's disease.

amastia (a-mas-'ti-á) [G. *a-,* not; *mastos,* breast]. Congenital absence of the breasts.

amaurosis (am-aw-rō'-sis) [G. *amauros,* dim]. Partial or total blindness.

amaurotic familial idiocy. A form of familial mental subnormality with spastic paralysis of the legs which commences in infancy or childhood. Later, the upper limbs are similarly affected and vision is lost. Tay-Sach's disease.

ambidextrous (am-bi-deks'-trus) [L. *ambo,* both; *dexter,* right]. Able to use both hands equally well—ambidexter, adj.; ambidexterity, n.

Ambilhar. Niridazole (q.v.).

ambivalence (am-biv'-al-ens) [L. *ambo,* both; *valere,* to be powerful]. Coexistence in one person of contradictory and opposing emotions at the same time, e.g. love and hate—ambivalent, adj.

ambivalent (am-biv'-al-ent) [L. *ambo,* both; *valere,* to be powerful]. A normal type of personality varying between introversion and extroversion (q.v.).

amblyopia (am-bli-ō'-pi-á) [G. *amblys,*

dulled; *ops.* eye]. Defective vision approaching blindness. **tobacco a.,** smoker's blindness, due to absorption of cyanide in the nicotine of the smoke. The sight gets worse, colour vision goes, the victim can go blind. Recently it was discovered that the cyanide prevents absorption of vitamin A. When this vitamin was injected the blindness was halted and cured—amblyopic, adj.

amboceptor (am-bo-sep'-tor) [L. *ambo,* both; *capere,* to take]. The antibody developed in immune serum which, in association with complement, causes lysis of the specific bacteria or other antigen to which the host has been sensitized. See ANTIBODIES.

ambulant (am'-bū-lant) [L. *ambulare,* to go about, walk]. Able to walk.

ambulatory (am'-bū-lā-tor-i) [L. *ambulare*]. Mobile. Walking about. **a. treatment,** method of treatment which insists on keeping the patient on his feet as much as possible, as in Charcot's joint (q.v.).

amelia (a-mē'-li-a) [G. *a-,* not; *melos,* a limb]. Congenital absence of a limb or limbs. **complete a.,** absence of both arms and legs.

amelioration (a-mē-li-or-ā'-shun) [L. *melius,* better]. Reduction of the severity of symptoms. Improvement in the general condition.

amenorrhoea (a-men-o-rē'-á) [G. *a-,* not; *men,* month; *rheein,* to flow]. Absence of the menses. **primary a.,** when menstruation has not been established at the time when it should first appear. **secondary a.,** absence of the menses after they have once commenced—amenorrhoeal, adj

amentia (a-men'-shi-á) [L. madness]. Mental subnormality; to be distinguished from 'dementia'.

amethocaine hydrochloride (a-meth'-o-kān). A synthetic substance with some of the properties of cocaine. Used for surface infiltration and spinal anaesthesia; more potent and more toxic than procaine. Lozenges for use before gastroscopy contain 65 mg, and this should be regarded as a maximum dose.

amethopterin (am-eth-op'-ter-in). Antifolic acid drug. Inhibits the enzyme which converts folic acid to its biologically active form, and is thus predominantly active against cells in division, having little effect in the resting stage. Used in treatment of choriocarcinoma,

Burkitt's lymphoma and acute leukaemia of childhood.

ametria (a-mēt-ri'-á) [G. *a-*, not; *metra*, womb]. Congenital absence of the uterus.

ametropia (ā-met-rō'-pi-á) [G. *a-*, not; *metron*, a measure; *ops*, eye]. Defective sight due to imperfect refractive power of the eye—ametropic, adj.; ametrope, n.

Amicar (am-ī'-kar). Epsilon aminocaproic acid (q.v.).

amidone (amīl-ē-dōn). Methadone (q.v.).

amikacin (am-ik'-a-sin). Antibiotic for especial use in serious Gram-negative gentamicin-resistant infections; a semisynthetic derivative of Ranamycin, it has been altered structurally to resist degradation by bacterial enzymes.

Amikin (am'-i-kin). Amikacin (q.v.).

amiloride (am-il-or'-īd). Less powerful diuretic, but has unusual potassium-conserving properties, and when it is used, potassium supplements are rarely required.

aminoacidopathy (am-ēn'-ō-as-id-op'-ath-i). Disease caused by imbalance of amino acids.

amino acids (am-ēn'-ō as-idz). Organic acids in which one or more of the hydrogen atoms are replaced by the amino group, NH_2. They are the end product of protein hydrolysis and from them the body resynthesizes its protein. Ten cannot be elaborated in the body and are therefore essential in the diet—arginine, histidine, isoleucine; leucine, lysine, methionine, phenylalanine, threonine, treptophane, and valine. The remainder are designated non-essential amino acids.

aminoaciduria (am-ēn'-ō-as-id-ū'-ri-á). Increase in urinary excretion of amino acids in Fanconi syndrome, in which there is a congenital defect in the metabolism of protein, and the reabsorptive functions of the kidney are abnormal—amino aciduric, adj.

aminocrine (am-ēn'-ō-crin). Non-staining acridine antiseptic similar to acriflavine, and used for similar purposes in similar strength.

aminophenazole (am-ēn'-ō-fen'-a-zol). An analeptic with a marked stimulant action on the respiratory centre.

aminophylline (am-in-of'-i-lin). Theophylline with ethylene-diamine. A soluble derivative of theophylline, widely used in the treatment of asthma, congestive heart failure, and cardiac oedema. Available as tablets 0.1 g, ampoules (intramuscular) 0.5 g, ampoules (intravenous) 0.25 g, suppositories 0.36 g.

Aminoplex 14 (am-ēn'-ō-pleks). Synthetic preparation of those amino acids normally ingested as protein in egg, meat and fish.

aminosalicylic acid (am-in-ō-sal-is-il'-ik). Has a bacteriostatic action when given in tuberculous disease. High blood levels essential; owing to rapid elimination, frequency of dose is essential. Given with other antitubercular drugs to reduce drug resistance. Has nauseating taste, therefore best given as cachets or tablets.

Aminosol (am-in'-ō-sol). A solution of amino acids that can be given orally or intravenously. Preparations containing glucose, fructose, and ethyl alcohol are available.

amiphenazole. See AMINOPHENAZOLE.

amithiozone (am-i-thī'-o-zōn). Antileprotic.

amitosis (a-mī-tō'-sis) [G. *a-*, not; *mitos*, thread; *osis*, condition]. Multiplication of a cell by direct fission—amitotic, adj.

amitriptyline (am-i-trip-ti-lēn). A tricyclic antidepressant similar to imipramine but possessing a pronounced sedative effect which is of particular value in the agitated depressive.

ammonia. See A. SOLUTION.

ammonium bicarbonate. Widely used in cough mixtures as a mild expectorant, and occasionally as a carminative in flatulent dyspepsia.

ammonium chloride. Used to increase the acidity of the urine in urinary infections, and to augment the diuretic action of mersalyl (q.v.). Occasionally given as a mild expectorant.

ammonia solution. Liq. ammon. Colourless liquid with a characteristic pungent odour. Used in urine testing—ammoniated, ammoniacal, adj.

amnesia (am-nē'-si-a) [G. *a-*, not; *mnesis*, memory]. Partial or complete loss of memory. Occurs following concussion, in dementia, hysteria and following electrotherapy (q.v.). amnesic, adj. **anterograde a.**, loss of memory for recent events since an accident, etc. **retrograde a.**, loss of memory for past events before an accident, etc.

amniocentesis (am-ni-ō-sen-tē'sis) [G. *amnio,* fetal membrane; *kentesis,* a prickling]. Aspiration of liquor amnii from its sac. The liquor contains increased haemoglobin breakdown products in rhesus incompatibility. -es, pl.

amniography (am-ni-og'-ra'fi) [G. *amnio,* fetal membrane; *graphein,* to write]. X-ray of the amniotic sac after injection of opaque medium into same: out-lines the umbilical cord and placenta—amniogram, n; amniographical, adj.; amniographically, adv.

amnion (am'-ni-on) [G.]. The innermost membrane enclosing the fetus and containing the amniotic fluid (liquor amnii). It ensheaths the umbilical cord and is connected with the fetus at the umbilicus—amnionic, amniotic, adj.

amnioscopy (am-ni-os'-ko-pi) [G. *amnio,* fetal membrane; *skopein;* to examine]. Amnioscope allows inspection of the forewaters through the intact membranes. Clear, colourless fluid is normal; yellow or green staining is due to meconium and occurs in cases of fetal hypoxia—amnioscopic, adj.; amnioscopically, adv.

amniotic fluid embolism. Formation of an embolus in the amniotic sac and its transference in the blood circulation of mother to lung or brain. A rare complication of pregnancy. May occur at any time after rupture of the membranes.

amniotic fluid infusion (am-ni-ot'-ik). Escape of amniotic fluid into the maternal circulation.

amniotome (am'-ni-ot-ōm) [G. *amnio,* fetal membrane; *tomos,* cutting]. An instrument for rupturing the fetal membranes.

amniotomy (am-ni-ot'-o-mil) [G. *amnio,* fetal membrane; *tome,* a cutting]. Artificial rupture of the fetal membranes to induce or expedite labour.

amodiaquine (a-mō-dī'-a-kwin). Potent antimalarial compound similar in action to chloroquine.

amoeba (am-ē'-bá) [G. *amoibe,* change]. A protozoon. One of the elementary, unicellular forms of life. The one cell is capable of ingestion and absorption, respiration, excretion, movement and reproduction by simple fission. One form, *Entamoeba histolytica,* is a parasitic pathogen producing amoebic dysentery (q.v.) in man—amoebae, pl.; amoebic, adj.

amoebiasis (am-ē-bī'-a-sis) [G. *amoibe,*

change; N.L.-*iasis,* condition]. Infestation of large intestine by the protozoon *Entamoeba histolytica,* where it causes ulceration by invasion of the mucosa. This results in passage per rectum of necrotic mucous membrane and blood, hence the term 'amoebic dysentery'. If the amoebae enter the portal circulation they may cause liver necrocrosis (hepatic abscess). Diagnosis is by isolating the amoeba in the stools.

amoebicide (am-ē'-bi-sīd). An agent that kills amoebae—amoebicidal, adj.

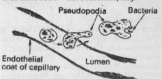

Diagram illustrating amoeboid movement of white blood cells

amoeboid (am-ē'-boid) [G. *amoibe,* change; *eidos,* form]. Resembling an amoeba in shape or in mode of movement, e.g. white blood cells.

amorphous (a-mor'-fus) [G. *a-,* not; *morphe,* form]. Having no regular shape.

amoxycillin (am-oks-i-sil'-lin). Antibiotic; penetrates bronchial secretions more readily than ampicillin independent of the level of purulence, therefore preferable in chronic lower respiratory tract infections. In acute infections the sole advantage is its greater absorption and high blood levels for an equivalent dose.

amphetamine (am-fet'-a-mēn). A sympathomimetic agent (structurally related to adrenaline) which is a potent CNS stimulant. It was formerly used as an appetite suppressant and in the treatment of depression but, because of its addictive potential and frequent abuse, is now restricted to use in narcolepsy and certain psychiatric states under specialist supervision.

Amphotericin B (am-fō-ter'-i-sēn). Antifungal agent given by i.v. infusion to treat serious systemic infections, e.g. histoplasmosis, candidiasis. It is used to eradicate Candida from mouth (lozenges), vagina (cream or pessaries) and gut (tablets).

ampicillin (am-pi-sil'-lin). Active against many, but certainly not all, strains of *E. coli,* Proteus, Salmonella and Shigella; these are bacteria against which benzylpenicillin is far less active. Ampicillin is also effective against benzylpenicillin-sensitive (but not resistant) staphylococci, streptococci and other Gram-positive bacteria. It has a wide range of activity and is a broad-spectrum antibiotic. Given orally and by injection.

Ampiclox (am'-pi-kloks). Mixture of ampicillin (q.v.) and cloxacillin (q.v.).

ampoule (am'-pool) [L. *ampulla*, bottle]. A small, hermetically sealed glass phial containing a single sterile dose of a drug.

ampulla am-pool'-á) [L. bottle]. Any flask-like dilatation. **a. of Vater**, the enlargement formed by the union of the common bile duct with the pancreatic duct where they enter the duodenum—ampullae, pl.; ampullar, ampullary, ampullate, adj. [Abraham Vater, German anatomist, 1684–1751.]

amputation (am-pū-tā'shun) [L. *amputare*, to cut away]. Removal of an appending part, e.g. breast, limb. **a. bandage**, applied to produce a cone-shaped stump.

amputee (am'-pū-tē) [L. *amputare*, to cut away]. A person who has had amputation of one or more limbs.

amylase (am'-i-lāz) [G. *amylon*, starch]. Any enzyme which converts starches into sugars. **pancreatic a.**, amylopsin (q.v.). **salivary a.**, ptyalin (q.v.).

amyl nitrite (am'-il nīt'-rīt). Volatile rapid-acting vasodilator, used by inhalation from crushed ampoules. Its action is brief, and its main use is in the treatment of angina.

amylobarbitone (am-il-ō-bár'-bit-ōn). Barbiturate of medium intensity and duration of action. The sodium salt has a more rapid but less prolonged action.

amyloid (am'-i-loid) [G. *amylon*, starch; *eidos*, form]. A starch which is wax-like in appearance. **a. disease or degeneration**, formation and deposit of amyloid in any organ, notably the liver and kidney. It can occur in the terminal phase of any prolonged toxic condition. Amyloidosis.

amylolysis (am-il-ol'-is-is) [G. *amylon*, starch; *lysis*, a loosening]. The digestion of starch—amylolytic, adj.

amylopsin (am'-i-lop-sin). A pancreatic enzyme, which in an alkaline medium, converts insoluble starch into soluble maltose.

amylum (am'-il-um) [G.]. Starch.

Amytal (am'-i-tal). Amylobarbitone (q.v.).

Anabol (an'-a-bol). Steroid preparation that increases anabolism and is a protein sparer.

anabolic compound (an-ab-ol'-ik). Chemical substance which causes a synthesis of body protein. Useful in convalescence. Many of the androgens come into this category.

anabolism (an-ab'-ol-izm) [G. *anabole*, throwing up]. The series of chemical reactions in the living body requiring energy to change simple substances into complex ones. See ADENOSINE DIPHOSPHATE and TRIPHOSPHATE, METABOLISM.

anacidity (an-as-id'-it-i) [G. *a-*, not; *acere*, to be sour]. Lack of normal acidity, especially in the gastric juice. See ACHLORHYDRIA.

anacrotism (an-ak'-rot-izm) [G. *ana*, up; *krotos*, rattling noise]. An oscillation in the ascending curve of a sphygmographic pulse tracing, occurring in aortic stenosis—anacrotic, adj.

anaemia (an-ē'-mi-á) [G. *a-*, not; *haima*, blood]. A deficiency of haemoglobin concentration in the blood due to lack of red blood cells and/or their haemoglobin content. Produces clinical manifestations arising from hypoxaemia. **Addisonian pernicious a.** results from failure to absorb food vitamin B_{12} so that erythropoiesis becomes megaloblastic. Treated with vitamin B_{12}. **haemolytic a.**, associated with excessive destruction of red blood cells and haemolytic jaundice. See ACHOLURICJAUNDICE. **iron deficiency a.**, the commonest type; due to blood loss, lack of dietary iron or poor iron absorption. Very common in pregnancy when iron requirement increased. **megaloblastic a.**, associated with diminished and abnormal production of red blood cells due to deficiency of vitamin B_{12} or folic acid. Peripheral blood shows **macrocytic a.**, i.e. large red cell picture—anaemic, adj.

anaerobe (an'ér-ōb) [G. *a-*, not; *aer*, air; *bios*, life]. A micro-organism which will not grow in the presence of molecular oxygen. When this is strictly so, it is termed an 'obligatory anaerobe'. The majority of pathogens are indifferent to atmospheric conditions and will flourish in the presence or absence of oxygen and are therefore termed 'facultative anaerobes'—anaerobic, adj.

anaesthesia (an-es-thēz'-i-á) [G. *anaisthesia*, lack of sensation]. Loss of sensation. **general a.**, loss of sensation with loss of consciousness. In **local a.** the nerve conduction is blocked and painful impulses fail to reach the brain. **spinal a.** may be caused by (1) injection of an anaesthetic into the spinal subarachnoid space; (2) a lesion of the spinal cord.

anaesthesiology (an-es-thēz-i-ol'-o-ji) [G. *anaisthesia*, lack of sensation; *logos*, discourse]. The science dealing with anaesthetics, their administration and effect.

anaesthetic (an-es-thet'-ik) [G. *anaisthesia*, lack of sensation]. 1. A drug which produces anaesthesia. 2. Causing anaesthesia. 3. Insensible to stimuli. **general a.**, a drug which produces general anaesthesia by inhalation or injection. **local a.**, a drug which injected into the tissues or applied topically causes local insensibility to pain. See SPINAL—anaesthetize, v.t.

anaesthetist (an-ēs'-the-tist) [G. *anaisthesia*, lack of sensation]. One who administers anaesthetics.

Anafranil (an-af'-ran-il). Clomipramine (q.v.).

analeptic (an-al-ep'-tik) [G. *analepsis*, restoration]. Restorative. Most analeptics stimulate the central nervous system. 'Household' analeptics include smelling salts, sal volatile, whisky and brandy.

analgesia (an-al-jē'-zi-á) [G. *a-*, not; *algos*, pain]. Loss of painful impressions without loss of tactile sense—analgesic, adj.

analgesic (an-al-jē'-zik). Insensible to pain; alleviating pain; a drug which relieves pain. Syn., anodyne.

analogous (an-al'-o-gus) [G. *analogia*, conformity]. Similar in function, but not in origin.

analysis (an-al'-i-sis) [G. a loosening]. A term used in chemistry to denote the determination of the composition of a compound substance—analyses, pl.; analytic, adj.; analytically, adv. See PSYCHOANALYSIS.

analyst (an'-a-list) [G. *analyein*, to unloose]. A person experienced in performing analyses.

anaphrodisiac (an-af-rō-diz'-i-ak) [G. *a-*, not; *aphrodisiakos*, sexual]. See ANTAPHRODISIAC.

anaphylactoid (an-a-fil-ak'-toid) [G. *ana*, up; *phylaxis*, protection]. Pertaining to or resembling anaphylaxis.

anaphylaxis (an-a-fil-aks'-is) [G. *ana*, up; *phylaxis*, protection]. A hypersensitive state of the body to a foreign protein (e.g. horse serum) so that the injection of a second dose after ten days brings about an acute reaction which may be fatal; in lesser degree it produces breathlessness, pallor and collapse—anaphylactic, adj. See ALLERGY and SENSITIZATION.

anaplasia (an-a-plāz'-i-á) [G. *anaplassein*, to remould]. Loss of the distinctive characteristics of a cell, associated with proliferative activity as in cancer—anaplastic, adj.

anasarca (an-a-sark'-á) [G. *ana*, up; *sarx*, flesh]. Serous infiltration of the cellular tissues and serous cavities; generalized oedema; dropsy—anasarcous, adj.

anastomosis (an-as-to-mō'-sis) [G. *anastomoein*, to furnish with a mouth]. 1. The intercommunication of the branches of two or more arteries or veins. 2. In surgery, the establishment of an intercommunication between two hollow organs, vessels or nerves—anastomoses, pl.; anastomotic, adj.; anastomose, v.i., v.t.

anatomy (a-nat'-o-mi) [G. *anatome*, dissection]. The science which deals with the structure of the body by means of dissection—anatomical, adj.; anatomically, adv.

Ancolan. Antihistamine useful in hyperemesis gravidarum.

ancrod (an'-krod). Anticoagulant obtained from the venom of the Malayan pit viper. It destroys fibrinogen, so depleting the blood of its essential factor for fibrin formation. Being a foreign protein it induces antibody formation so that after a few weeks, patients develop resistance to its action. Ancrod can therefore be used only for short-term effects.

Ancylostoma (ang-ki-lō-stō'-má). Human hookworm. *Ancylostoma duodenale* is predominantly found in southern Europe and the Middle and Far East. *Necator americanus* is found in the New World and tropical Africa. Mixed infections are not uncommon. Only clinically significant when infestation is moderate or heavy. As hookworms suck blood, it may be necessary to treat ensuing anaemia. Worm inhabits duodenum and upper jejunum, eggs are passed in stools, hatch in moist soil and produce larvae which can penetrate bare feet and reinfect people. Prevention is by wearing shoes and using latrines. See ANKYLOSTOMIASIS.

andria (an'-dri-ă) [G. *aner*, pseudo-male hermaphrodite (q.v.), i.e. one in whom the male characteristics predominate.

androgens (an'-dro-jens) [G. *aner*, man; *genesis*, production]. Hormones secreted by the testes and adrenal cortex or synthetic substances which control the building up of protein and the male secondary sex characteristics, e.g. distribution of hair and deepening of voice. When given to females they have a masculinizing effect—androgenic, androgenous, adj. See TESTOSTERONE.

androgyna (an-drō-gī'-nă) [G. *aner*, man; *gyne*, woman]. A pseudofemale hermaphrodite (q.v.), i.e. one in whom the female characteristics are predominant—androgynous, adj.

androphobia (an-drō-fō'-bi-ă) [G. *aner*, man; *phobos*, fear]. A morbid dislike or fear of men—androphobic, adj.

Andursil (and'-ur-sil). Aluminium hydroxide with magnesium hydroxide and carbonate. Antacid and antiflatulent.

anencephaly (an-en-kef'-a-li) [G. *a-*, not; *egkephalos*, brain]. Absence of the brain. A term used in connection with fetal monsters. The condition is incompatible with life—anencephalous, anencephalic, adj.

Anethaine (an-ē-thān'). Amethocaine (q.v.).

aneurine (an'-ū-rin). Thiamine or vitamin B_1. Concerned in carbohydrate metabolism; indicated therapeutically in aneurine deficiency disorders such as beri-beri, and some forms of neuritis; also as adjunct to oral antibiotic therapy.

aneurysm (an'-ūr-izm) [G. *aneurysma*, dilation]. Local dilatation of a blood vessel, usually artery, due to local fault in the wall through defect, disease or injury, producing a pulsating swelling over which a murmur may be heard. True aneurysms may be saccular, fusiform, or dissecting where the blood flows between the layers of the arterial wall. **false a.** follows rupture of the wall and consists of a cavity lined by blood clot surrounded by the adjacent tissues. **arteriovenous a.**, an abnormal direct connection between an artery and a vein, usually following injury and sometimes producing dilated pulsating veins, **cirsoid a.** (q.v.)—aneurysmal, adj.

angiectasis (an-ji-ek'-ta-sis) [G. *aggeion*, vessel; *ektasis*, extension]. Abnormal dilatation of blood vessels, Telangiectasis (q.v.)—angiectatic, adj.

angiitis (an-ji-ī'-tis) [G. *aggeion*, vessel; *-itis*, inflammation]. Inflammation of a blood or lymph vessel—angiitic, adj.

angina (an-jī'-nă) [L. *angere*, to strangle]. Sense of suffocation or constriction. Ludwig's **a.**, see CELLULITIS. **a. pectoris**, severe but temporary attack of cardiac pain which may radiate to the arms. Results from myocardial ischaemia. Often the attack is induced by exercise (angina of effort). Vincent's **a.** is infection of mouth or throat by a spirochaete and a bacillus in synergism—anginal, adj.

angiocardiogram (an-ji-o-kár'-di-o-gram) [G. *aggeion*, vessel; *kardia;* heart; *gramma*, letter]. Film demonstrating the heart and great vessels after injection of opaque medium.

angiocardiography (an-ji-o-kár-di-og'-raf-i) [G. *aggeion*, vessel; *kardia*, heart; *graphein*, to write]. Demonstration of heart and great vessels by means of injection of opaque medium into cardiac circulation—angiocardiographic, adj.; angiocardiographically, adv.

angiogram (an'-ji-ō-gram) [G. *aggeion*, vessel; *gramma*, letter]. Film demonstrating the arterial system after injection of opaque medium.

angiography (an-ji-og'-raf-i) [G. *aggeion*, vessel; *graphein*, to write]. Demonstration of the arterial system by means of injection of opaque medium—angiographic, adj.; angiographically, adv.

angiology (an-ji-ol'-o-ji) [G. *aggeion*, vessel; *logos*, discourse]. The science dealing with blood and lymphatic vessels—angiological, adj.; angiologically, adv.

angioma (an-ji-ō'-mă) [G. *aggeion*, vessel; *-oma*, tumour]. A non-malignant tumour formed of blood vessels, usually capillaries. **cavernous a.**, when larger spaces are occupied by blood—angiomatous, adj.; angiomata, pl.

angioneurotic oedema (an-ji-ō-nū-rot'-ik ē-dē'-mă) [G. *aggeion*, vessel; *neuron*, nerve; *-osis*, condition; *oidema*, swelling]. A severe form of urticaria which may involve the skin of the face, hands or genitals and the mucous membrane of the mouth and throat: oedema of the glottis may be fatal. Occasionally forms part of the clinical picture in anaphylaxis and penicillin sensitization. Immediate cause is an abrupt local increase in vascular permeability, as a result of which fluid escapes from blood vessels into surrounding tissues. Swelling may be due to an allergic hypersensitivity reaction to drugs, pollens or other known allergens, but in many cases no cause can be found. Runs a benign course with spontaneous remission.

angioplasty (an-ji-ō'-plast-i) [G. *aggeion*, vessel; *plassein*, to form]. Plastic surgery of blood vessels—angioplastic, adj.

angiosarcoma (an-ji-ō'-sar-kō'-mà) [G. *aggeion*, vessel; *sarkoma*, fleshy excrescence]. A malignant tumour arising from blood vessels—angiosarcomatous, adj.; angiosarcomata, pl.

angiospasm (an-ji-ō'-spazm) [G. *aggeion*, vessel; *spasmos*, spasm]. Constricting spasm of blood vessels—angiospastic, adj.

angiotensin (an-ji-ō-ten'-sin) [G. *aggeion*, vessel; *teno*, to stretch]. A polypeptide formed by the action on a plasma substrate of the enzyme renin (q.v.) found in the kidney. It is the most potent pressor substance known and has been synthesized; available commercially.

ångström unit (ang'-strom). Measure of wavelength of any radiation [A. J. Ångström, Swedish physicist, 1814–74.]

anhidrosis (an-hi-drō'-sis) [G. *a-*, not; *hidros*, sweat; *-osis*, condition]. Deficient sweat secretion—anhidrotic, adj.

anhidrotics (an-hid-rot'-iks). Agents which reduce perspiration.

anhydraemia (an-hid-rēm'-i-à) [G. *a-*, not; *hydor*, water; *haima*, blood]. Deficient fluid content of blood—anhydraemic, adj.

anhydrous (an-hid'-rus) [G. *a-*, not; *hydor*, water]. Entirely without water, dry.

anicteric (an-ik'-ter-ik) [G. *a-*, not; *icteros*, jaundice]. Without jaundice.

anileridine (an-il'-er-i-din). Analgesic that is useful pre- and post-operatively.

aniline (an'-il-ēn). An oily compound obtained from the dry distillation of coal and much used in the preparation of dyes.

aniridia (an-i-rid'-ē-à) [G. *a-*, not; *iris*,

rainbow]. Lack or defect of the iris; usually congenital.

anisocoria (an-ē-so-kor'-ē-à) [G. *anisos*, unequal; *kore*, pupil]. Inequality in diameter of the pupils.

anisocytosis (an-ē-so-sī-tō'-sis) [G. *anisos*, unequal; *kytos*, cell; *-osis*, condition]. Inequality in size of red blood cells.

anisomelia (an-ē-so-mē'-li-à) [G. *anisos*, unequal; *melos*, limb]. Unequal length of limbs—anisomelous, adj.

anisometropia (an-ē-so-me-trō'-pi-à)[G. *anisos*, unequal; *metron*, a measure; *ops*, eye]. A difference in the refraction of the two eyes—anisometropic, adj.

ankle clonus. A series of rapid muscular contractions of the calf muscle when the foot is dorsiflexed by pressure upon the sole.

ankyloblepharon (ang-ki-lō-blef'-a-ron) [G. *agkylos*, crooked; *blepharon*, eyelid]. Adhesion of the ciliary edges of the eyelids.

ankylosis (ang-ki-lō'-sis) [G. *agkyle*, a thong]. Stiffness or fixation of a joint—ankylose, v.t., vi.; ankylosed, adj.

Ankylostoma (ang-ki-lō-stō'-mà) [G. *agkylos*, crooked; *stoma*, mouth]. Ancylostoma (q.v.).

ankylostomiasis (ang-ki-los-tom-ī'-a-sis) [G. *agkylos*, crooked; *stoma*, mouth; N.L. *-iasis*, condition]. Infestation of the human intestine with Ankylostoma, giving rise to malnutrition and severe anaemia. Hookworm disease.

annular (an'-ū-lar) [L. *annulus*, ring]. Ring-shaped. **a. ligaments**, found surrounding the ankle and proximal and distal ends of radius.

anodyne (an'-ō-din) [G. *a-*, not; *odyne*, pain]. A remedy which relieves pain. Analgesic.

anogenital (ā-nō-jen'-it-al) [L. *anus*; G. *genesis*, descent]. Pertaining to the anus and the genital region.

anomaly (an-om'-a-li) [G. *anomalia*, irregularity]. That which is unusual or differs from the normal—anomalous, adj.

anomia (an-ō'-mi-à) [G. *a-*, not; *onoma*, name]. Inability to name objects or persons. Same as nominal aphasia.

anomie (an'-om-ē). Sociological term applied to a person who is lonely because he cannot relate with others, consequently he no longer identifies with them.

ANONYCHIA

anonychia (an-o-nik'-i-á) [G. *a-*, not; *onyx*, nail]. Absence of nails.

anoperineal (ā'-nō-per-in-ē'-al) [L. *anus*, anus; G. *perineos*, space between anus and scrotum]. Pertaining to the anus and perineum.

Anopheles (an-of'-i-lēz) [G. *anopheles*, harmful]. A genus of mosquito. The females are the host of the malarial parasite, and their bite is the means of transmitting the disease to man. See MALARIA.

anorchus (an-awr'-kus) [G. *a-*, not; *orchis*, testis]. Without testicles. A male with congenital absence of testes in the scrotum.

anorectal (ā-nō-rek'-tal) [L. *anus*, anus; *rectus*, straight]. Pertaining to the anus and rectum, as a fissure (q.v.).

anorectic (an-o-rek'-tik) [G. *a-*, not; *orexis*, appetite]. Appetite depressant.

anorexia (an-o-reks'-i-á) [G. *a-*, not; *orexis*, appetite]. Loss or deficiency of appetite for food. **a. nervosa**, hysterical aversion to food leading to atrophy of stomach—anorexic, anorectic, adj.

anosmia (an-oz'-mi-á) [G. *a-*, not; *osme*, smell]. Absence of the sense of smell—anosmic, anosmatic, adj.

anovular (an-ov'-ū-lar) [G. *a-*, not; L. *ovum*, egg]. **a. bleeding** is uterine bleeding which has not been preceded by ovulation, e.g. in metropathia haemorrhagica. An endometrial biopsy following an **a. cycle** shows no progestational changes.

anoxaemia (an-oks-ē'-mi-á) [G. *a-*, not; *oxys*, sharp; *haima*, blood]. Literally no oxygen in the blood. Usually used to indicate hypoxaemia (q.v.)—anoxaemic, adj.

anoxia (an-ok'-si-á) [G. *a-*, not; *oxys*, sharp]. Literally no oxygen in the tissues. Usually used to signify hypoxia (q.v.)—anoxic, adj.

Ansolysen (an'-zō-lī-sen). Pentolinium (q.v.).

Antabuse (ant'-a-būs). Disulfiram (q.v.).

antacid (ant-as'-id) [G. *anti*, against; L. *acidus*, sour]. A substance which neutralizes or counteracts acidity. Commonly used in alkaline stomach powders and mixtures.

antagonism (an-tag'-on-izm) [G. *antagonizesthai*, to struggle against]. Active opposition; a characteristic of some drugs, muscles and organisms—antagonistic, adj.

antagonist (an-tag'-on-ist) [G. *antagonistes*, adversary]. A muscle that relaxes to allow the agonist (q.v.) to perform a movement. When applied to a drug it is one which blocks, nullifies or reverses the effects of another drug.

antaphrodisiac (ant-af-rō-diz'-i-ak) [G. *anti*, against; *aphrodisiakos*, sexual]. An agent that diminishes sexual desire; absence of sexual impulse. Also ANAPHRODISIAC.

antazoline (an-ta'-zō-lin). An antihistamine with local anaesthetic properties. Mostly used locally.

anteflexion (an'-tē-flek'-shun) [L. *ante*, before; *flectere*, to bend]. The bending forward of an organ. Commonly applied to the position of the uterus. Opp. to retroflexion.

antemortem (an'-tē-mawr'-tem) [L]. Before death. Opp. to postmortem.

antenatal (an-tē-nā'-tal) [L. *ante*, before; *natus*, birth]. The period between conception and delivery of the child. The term prenatal is now preferred. Normally 40 weeks or 280 days.

Antepar (an'-tē-par). Elixir and tablets containing piperazine (q.v.).

antepartum (an'-tē-pár-tum) [L.]. Before birth. More generally confined to the three months preceding full-term delivery, i.e. the 6th to 9th month. See PLACENTA.

anterior (an-tē-ri-ér) [L. foremost, former]. In front of; the front suface of; ventral—anteriorly, adv. **a. chamber of the eye**, the space between the posterior surface of the cornea and the anterior surface of the iris. See AQUEOUS. **a. tibial syndrome**, severe pain and inflammation over anterior tibial muscle group, with inability to dorsiflex the foot.

anterograde (an'-ter-ō-grād) [L. *anterior*, foremost; *gradi*, to go]. Proceeding forward. See AMNESIA.

anteversion (an'-tē-vér'-shun) [L. *ante*, before; *vertere*, to turn]. The forward tilting or displacement forward of an organ or part. Opp. to retroversion—anteverted, adj.; antevert, v.t., v.i.

anthelmintic (an-thel-min'-tik) [G. *anti*, against; *helminus*, worm]. Any remedy for the destruction or elimination of intestinal worms.

Anthiomaline (an-thi-om'-á-lin). Antimony lithium thiomalate (q.v.).

Anthiphen (an'-thi-fen). Dichlorophen (q.v.).

Anthisan (an'-thiz-an). Mepyramine (q.v.).

anthracaemia (an-thra-sēm'-i-à) [G. *anthrax*, malignant, pustule; *haima*, blood]. Anthrax septicaemia—anthracaemic, adj.

anthracosis (an-thra-kō'-sis) [G. *anthrax*, coal; *-osis*, condition]. Black pigmentation of lungs due to inhalation of carbon particles; causes chronic inflammation. A form of pneumoconiosis (q.v.)—anthracotic, adj.

anthrax (an'-thraks) [G.]. A contagious disease of cattle, which may be transmitted to man by inoculation, inhalation and ingestion, causing malignant pustule, woolsorter's disease and gastrointestinal anthrax respectively. Causative organism is *Bacillus anthracis* (q.v.). Preventive measures include prophylactic immunization of cattle and man.

anthropology (an'-thrō-pol'-o-ji) [G. *anthropos*, a human being; *logos*, discourse]. The study of mankind. Divided into various branches, such as criminal, cultural and physical anthropology—anthropological, adj.; anthropologically, adv.

antiadrenaline (an-ti-ad-ren'-al-in). Neutralizing or lessening the effects of adrenaline, e.g. piperoxane.

antialdosterone (an-ti-al-dos-tēr'-ōn). Any substance that neutralizes or destroys aldosterone, e.g. spironolactone.

antiallergic (an-ti-al-êr'-jik) [G. *anti*, against; *allos*, other; *ergon*, activity; *genesis*, production]. Preventing or lessening allergy.

antianabolic (an-ti-an-ab-ol'-ik) [G. *anti*, against; *anabole*, throwing up]. Preventing the synthesis of body protein.

antianaemic (an-ti-an-ēm'-ik) [G. *anti*-against; *a-*, not; *haima*, blood]. An agent, e.g. vitamin K (q.v.), used to prevent haemorrhage.

antibacterial (an'-ti-bak-tēr'-i-ál) [G. *anti*, against; *bakterion*, little staff]. Any agent which destroys bacteria.

antiberi-beri (an-ti-ber'-ē-ber'-ē) [G. *anti*, against; Singhalese, *beri*, weakness]. Against beri-beri (q.v.). The aneurine portion of vitamin B complex.

antibilharzial (an-ti-bil-hár'-zē-al). Against bilharziasis. See SCHISTOSOMIASIS.

antibiosis (an-ti-bi-ōs'-is) [G. *anti*, against; *bios*, life]. An association between organisms which is harmful to one of them. Opp. to symbiosis—antibiotic, adj.

antibiotics (an-ti-bī-ot'-iks) n. Antibacterial substances derived from fungi and bacteria, exemplified by penicillin (q.v.). Later antibiotics such as tetracycline (q.v.) are active against a wider range of organisms, and are also effective orally. Others, such as neomycin and bacitracin, are rarely used internally owing to high toxicity, but are effective when applied topically, and skin sensitization is uncommon.

antibodies (an'-ti-bod-iz) [G. *anti*, against; A.S. *bodig*, body]. Specific substances produced in the blood as a reaction to an antigen. They cause agglutination, flocculation, inactivation or lysis of the antigen. See DYS-GAMMAGLOBULINAEMIA.

anticholinergic (an-ti-kōl-in-ėrj'-ik) [G. *anti*, against; *chole*, bile; *ergon*, work]. Inhibitory to the action of a cholinergic nerve (q.v.) by interfering with the action of acetylcholine, a chemical by which such a nerve transmits its impulses at neural or myoneural junctions.

anticholinesterase (an-ti-kōl-in-es'-têr-āz). Enzyme that destroys acetylcholine at nerve endings. Used for reversing the effects of muscle relaxant drugs.

anticoagulant (an-ti-kō-ag'-ūl-ant [G. *anti*, against; L. *coagulare*, to curdle]. An agent which prevents or retards clotting of blood. Small amount made in human body. Uses: (1) to obtain specimens suitable for pathological investigation and chemical analyses where whole blood or plasma is required instead of serum; the anticoagulant usually is oxalate. (2) To obtain blood suitable for transfusion, the anticoagulant usually being sodium citrate. (3) as a therapeutic agent in the treatment of coronary thrombosis; phlebothrombosis (thrombophlebitis), etc. when aspirin should not be given.

anticonvulsant (an-ti-kon-vul'-sant) [G. *anti*, against; L. *convulsus*, shaken]. An agent which stops or prevents convulsions—anticonvulsive, adj.

anti D. Anti-Rh$_0$. A gammaglobulin (q.v.).

antidepressant (an-ti-de-pres'-ant) [G. *anti*, against; L. *depressus*, from *deprimere*, to depress]. Name given to drugs that reduce depression. Divided into two categories: (1) Mainly for endogenous depression: imipramine (Tofranil) and amitriptyline (Tryptizol, Saroten, Laroxyl), desipramine (Pertofran), nortriptyline (Allegron, Aventyl), and protriptyline all have a similar action, more rapid than the MAOIs. (2) The monoamine oxidase inhibitors (Niamid, Nardil, Marplan, Actomol, Marsilid, and Parnate) prolong or increase the action of serotonin by interfering with enzyme activity; catecholamines in brain increased. Cheese potentiates these substances and must be avoided during treatment. This group are mainly for exogenous or reactive depression.

antidiabetic (an-ti-dī'-ab-et-ik) [G. *anti,* against; *dia,* through; *bainein,* to go]. Literally 'against diabetes.' Used to describe therapeutic measures in diabetes mellitus; the hormone insulin (q.v.); tolbutamide (q.v.).

antidiphtheritic (an-ti-dif-thèr-it'-ik) [G. *anti,* against; *diphthera,* leather, membrane]. Against diphtheria. Describes preventive measures such as immunization; therapeutic measures; serum used to give passive immunity.

antidiuretic (an-ti-dī-ū-ret'-ik) [G. *anti,* against; *dia,* through; *ouron,* urine]. Reducing the volume of urine. Against diuresis. **a. hormone,** secreted by the posterior pituitary gland. ADH. See DIABETES.

antidote (an'-ti-dōt) [G. *anti,* against; *didonai,* to give]. A remedy which counteracts or neutralizes the action of a poison.

antiemetic (an-ti-ē-met'-ik) [G. *anti,* against; *emetikos,* provoking sickness]. Against emesis (q.v.). Any agent which prevents nausea and vomiting.

antienzyme (an'-ti-en'-zīm) [G. *anti,* against; *en,* within; *zyme,* leaven]. A substance which exerts a specific inhibiting action on an enzyme. Antienzymes are found in the digestive tract to prevent digestion of its lining, in blood where they act as antibodies (q.v.).

antiepileptic (an-ti-ep-i-lep'-tik) [G. *anti,* against; *epilepsis,* seizure]. Name given to drugs that reduce the frequency of epileptic attacks.

antifebrile (an-ti-feb'-rīl) [G. *anti,* against; L. *febris,* fever]. Any agent which reduces or allays fever.

antifibrinolytic (an-ti-fi-brin-ō-lit'-ik) [G. *anti,* against; L. *fibra,* fibre; G. *lysis,* a loosening]. Any agent which prevents fibrinolysis (a possible cause of haemorrhage).

antifols (an'-ti-fols). A group of substances used in combination with a sulpha drug or a dapsone as an antimalarial compound.

antifungal (an-ti-fung'-al). Any agent which destroys fungi.

antigen (an'-ti-jen) [G. *anti,* against; *genos,* birth]. Any substance which, under favourable conditions, can stimulate the production of antibodies (q.v.). See D-VAC ANTIGEN—antigenic, adj.

antihaemophilic globulin (an-ti-hē-mō-fil'-ik glob'-ū-lin) (AHG). Factor VIII involved in bloodclotting, present in plasma; absent from serum; deficient in haemophilia (q.v.).

antihaemorrhagic (an-ti-hem'-or-aj-ik) [G. *anti,* against; *haima,* blood; *rhegnynai,* to burst forth]. Any agent which prevents haemorrhage. Pertaining to vitamin K (q.v.).

antihistamines (an-ti-hist'-a-mēnz) [G. *anti,* against; *histos,* tissue; *ammoniakon,* resinous gum]. Drugs which suppress some of the effects of released histamine, and are widely used in the palliative treatment of hay fever, urticaria, angioneurotic oedema and some forms of pruritus. They also have antiemetic properties, and are effective in motion and radiation sickness. Side effects include drowsiness, which is most marked with diphenhydramine, and least with phenindamine and cyclizine.

antihypertensive (an-ti-hī-per-ten'-siv) [G. *anti,* against; *hyper,* above; *tendere,* to stretch]. Any agent which reduces high blood pressure.

anti-infective [G. *anti,* against; L. *infectus,* to infect]. Any agent which prevents infection. Pertaining to vitamin A (q.v.).

anti-inflammatory (an-ti-in-flam'-at-o-ri) [G. *anti,* against; L. *inflammare,* to set on fire]Any agent which prevents inflammation.

antileprotic (an-ti-lep-rot'-ik) [G. *anti,* against; *lepros,* scaly]. Any agent which prevents or cures leprosy.

antiluetic (an-ti-loo-et'-ik) [G. *anti,* against; L. *lues,* plague]. Any agent which prevents or cures syphilis (lues).

antimalarial (an-ti-mal-ār'-i-al) [G. *anti,* against; It. *mala aria,* bad air]. Any measure taken to prevent or suppress malaria.

antimetabolite (an-ti-met-ab'-ol-ītz) [G.

anti, against; *metabole*, change]. A compound which is sufficiently similar to the chemicals needed by a cell to be incorporated into the nucleoproteins of that cell, thereby preventing its development. Examples are methotrexate, a folic acid antagonist, and mercaptopurine, a purine antagonist. They are used in the treatment of leukaemia.

antimicrobial (an-ti-mī-krō'-bi-al) [G. *anti*, against; *mikros*, small; *bios*, life]. Against microbes.

antimigraine (an-ti-mē'-gren). Against migraine, e.g. Ergodryl, methysergide.

antimitotic (an-ti-mī-tot'-ik) [G. *anti*, against; *mitos*, thread; *osis*, condition]. Any agent which prevents reproduction of a cell by mitosis.

antimony and potassium tartrate (an-tim'-on-i pot-as'-si-um tár'-trāt). Tartar emetic. An old drug, now used mainly in leishmaniasis (q.v.) and other tropical diseases—antimonial, adj.

antimony lithium thiomalate (an-tim'-on-i lith'-i-um thī-om'-al-āt) Antibilharzial, (q.v.). Administered by intramuscular injection.

antimycotic (an-ti-mī-kot'-ik) [G. *anti*, against; *mykes*, a fungus]. Any agent which destroys fungi.

antineuritic (an-ti-nū-rit'-ik) [G. *anti*, against; *neuron*, tendon; *-itis*, inflammation]. Any agent which prevents neuritis. Specially applied to vitamin B complex (q.v.).

antioxidants (an-ti-oks'-id-ants) [G. *anti*, against; *oxys*, sharp]. Any substances which delay the process of oxidation.

antiparasitic (an'-ti-par-a-sit'-ik) [G. *anti*, against; *parasitos*, parasite]. Any agent which prevents or destroys parasites.

anti-Parkinson(ism) (an-ti-par'-kin-son-izm). Name given to drugs, e.g. benzhexol, orphenadrine, that counteract the side effects of antidepressants.

antipellagra (an-ti-pel-a'-gra) [It. *pelle*, skin; *agro*, rough]. Against pellagra. Pertaining to the nicotinic acid portion of vitamin B complex.

antiperiodic (an-ti-pēr-i-od'-ik) [G. *anti*, against; *periodikos*, periodical]. Any agent which prevents the periodic return of a disease, e.g. the use of quinine in malaria.

antiperistalsis (an-ti-pe-ri-stal'-sis) [G. *anti*, against; *peri*, around; *stalsis*, constriction]. A reversal of the normal peristaltic action—antiperistaltic, adj.

Antiphlogistine (an-ti-flō-jis'-tin) [G. *anti*, against; *phlogistos*, burnt, roasted]. A proprietary preparation containing kaolin, glycerine, antiseptic and aromatic substances. It is used for poultices, acting as an antiseptic, analgesic and counterirritant in cases of deep-seated inflammation.

antiprothrombin (an-ti-prō-throm'-bin). Arrests blood clotting by preventing conversion of prothrombin into thrombin. Anticoagulant.

antipruritic (an-ti-proo-rit'-ik) [G. *anti*, against; L. *pruritus*, itching]. Any agent which relieves or prevents itching.

antipurpura (an-ti-pur'-pū-rá) [G. *anti*, against; L. purple]. Against purpura. Pertaining to vitamin P (hesperidin).

antipyretic (an-ti-pī-ret'-ik) [G. *anti*, against; *pyretos*, fever]. Any agent which allays or reduces fever.

antirabic (an-ti-rā'-bik) [G. *anti*, against; L. *rabies*, madness]. Any agent which prevents or cures rabies.

antirachitic (an-ti-rak-it'-ik) [G. *anti*, against; *rhachis*, spine]. Any agent preventing or curing rickets. Pertaining to vitamin D (q.v.).

antireflux (an-ti-rē'-fluks) [G. *anti*, against; L. *re*, back; *fluxus*, to flow]. Against backward flow. Usually refers to re-implantation of ureters into bladder in cases of chronic pyelonephritis (q.v.). See LEADBETTER-POLITANO OPERATION.

antirheumatic (an-ti-roo-mat'-ik) [G. *anti*, against; *rheuma*, flow, flux]. Any agent which prevents or lessens rheumatism.

antiscorbutic (an-ti-skawr-bū'-tik) [G. *anti*, against; L. *scorbutus*, scurvy]. Any agent which prevents or cures scurvy (q.v.). Pertaining to vitamin C (q.v.).

antisecretory (an-ti-sē-crēt'-o-ri) [G. *anti*, against; L. *secretus*, separate]. Any agent which inhibits secretion.

antisepsis (an-ti-sep'-sis) [G. *anti*, against; *sepsis*, decay]. The prevention of sepsis; introduced into surgery in 1880 by Lord Lister, who used carbolic acid.

antisera. See SERUM.

antiseptics. Substances which destroy or inhibit the growth of micro-organisms. They can be applied to living tissues.

antisialagogue (an-ti-sī'-al-a-gog) [G.

anti, against; *sialon,* saliva; *agogos,* leading]. Inhibits salivation.

antiserotonin (an-ti-sē'rō-tōn-in). Neutralizes or lessens the effect of serotonin (q.v.), e.g. methysergide given for migraine.

antisocial (an-ti-sō'-shal) [G. *anti,* against; L. *socius,* comrade]. Against society. A term used to denote a psychopathic state in which the individual cannot accept the obligations and restraints imposed on a community by its members—antisocialism, n.

antispasmodic (an-ti-spaz-mod'-ik) [G. *anti,* against; *spasmos,* spasm]. Any measure used to relieve spasm occurring in muscle.

antistatic (an-ti-stat'-ik) [G. *anti,* against; *statikos,* causing to stand]. Any measures taken to prevent or deal with the collection of static electricity.

antisterility (an-ti-ster-il'-it-i) [G. *anti,* against; L. *sterilitas,* infertile]. Pertaining to vitamin E (q.v.).

Antistin (an-tis'-tin). Antazoline, one of the milder antihistamines (q.v.).

antistreptolysin (an-ti-strep-tō-lī'sin) [G. *anti,* against; *streptos,* curved; *lysis,* a loosening]. Against streptolysin, (q.v.). A raised antistreptolysin titre in the blood is indicative of recent streptococcal infection.

antisyphilitic (an-ti-sif-il-it'-ik). Any measures taken to combat syphilis (q.v.).

antithrombin (an-ti-throm'-bin) [G. *anti,* against; *thrombos,* clot]. Antithrombin or antithrombins are substances occurring naturally in the blood, e.g. heparin. See THROMBIN.

antithrombotic (an-ti-throm-bot'-ik) [G. *anti,* against; *thrombos,* clot]. Any measures that prevent or cure thrombosis.

antithyroid (an-ti-thī'-roid) [G. *anti,* against; *thureoeides,* shield-shaped]. Any agent used to decrease the activity of the thyroid gland.

antitoxic sera (an-ti-toks'-ik sē'-rā). The serum of horses which have been immunized by injections of pathogenic bacterial toxins, such as tetanus and gas gangrene. Such serum contains antibodies or antitoxins, and after injection confers a temporary immunity against the original toxin. The therapeutic use of antitoxic sera declined after the discovery of the sulphonamides and antibiotics.

antitoxin (an-ti-toks'-in) [G. *anti,* against; *toxikon,* poison]. An agent which neutralizes a given toxin. It is elaborated in the body, in direct response to the invasion by bacteria, or the injection of a small dose of treated toxin—antitoxic, adj.

antituberculosis (an'-ti-tū-ber-kū-lō'-sis). Any measures used to prevent or cure tuberculosis—antitubercular, adj.

antitumour (an-ti-tū'-mor) [G. *anti,* against; L.]. Against tumour formation, Inhibits growth of tumour.

antitussive (an-ti-tus'-iv) [G. *anti,* against; L. *tussis,* cough]. Any measures which suppress cough.

antivenin (an-ti-ven'-in) [G. *anti,* against; L. *venenum,* poison]. A serum prepared from animals injected with the venom of snakes; used as an antidote in cases of poisoning by snakebite.

antiviral (an-ti-vī'-ral) [G. *anti,* against; L. *virus,* poison]. Acting against viruses.

antivitamin (an-ti-vīt'-a-min) [G. *anti,* against; L. *vita,* life; *ammoniacum,* resinous gum]. A substance interfering with the absorption or utilization of a vitamin, e.g. avidin.

antrectomy (an-trek'-to-mi) [G. *antron,* cave; *ektome,* excision]. Excision of pyloric antrum of stomach thus removing the source of the hormone gastrin in the treatment of duodenal ulcer.

Antrenyl (an'-tren-il). Oxyphenonium. An antispasmodic (q.v.).

antrobuccal (an-trō-buk'-al) [G. *antron,* cave; L. *bucca,* cheek]. Pertaining to the maxillary antrum and the mouth. **a. fistula** can occur after extraction of an upper molar tooth, the root of which has protruded into the floor of the antrum.

antrostomy (an-tros'-to-mi) [G. *antron,* cave; *stoma,* mouth]. An artificial opening from nasal cavity to antrum of Highmore (maxillary sinus) for the purpose of drainage.

antrum (an'-trum) [L.]. A cavity, especially in a bone, e.g. the **a. of Highmore** in the superior maxillary bone—antral, adj. [Nathaniel Highmore, English physician, 1613–85.]

Antrypol (an'-tri-pol) Suramin (q.v.).

Antuitrin (an-tū'-it-rin). Proprietary extract of the anterior pituitary gland.

Anturan (an'-tūr-an). Sulphinpyrazone (q.v.).

anuria (an-ū'-ri-á) [G. *a-*, not; *ouron*, urine]. Absence of secretion of urine by the kidneys. See SUPPRESSION—anuric, adj.

anus (ā'-nus) [L.]. The end of the alimentary canal, at the extreme termination of the rectum. It is formed of a sphincter muscle which relaxes to allow faecal matter to pass through. **artifical a.**, one produced surgically in some higher part of the bowel in cases of obstruction through any cause. **imperforate a.**, one which has no opening; atresia ani. It is often due to a congenital defect—anal, adj.

anxiety (ang-zi'-et-i) [L. *anxietas*, anxiety]. Feelings of fear, apprehension and dread. See NEUROSIS. **a. neurosis, a. state**, a neurosis characterized by recurrent acute anxiety attacks (panics). The attacks consist of all the signs and symptoms of fear, leading up to fear of impending collapse and sometimes death. **'free floating a.'** is used to indicate that the apprehension has no source in the external world.

anxiolytics (ang-zi-ō-lit'-iks) [L. *anxietas*, anxiety; G. *lysis*, a loosening]. Agents that reduce anxiety.

aorta (ā-or'-tá) [G. *aorte*, the great artery]. The main artery arising out of the left ventricle of the heart.

aortic (ā-or'-tik) [G. *aorte*, great artery]. Pertaining to the aorta. **a. aneurysm**, see ANEURYSM. **a. incompetence**, regurgitation, resulting from rheumatic or syphilitic disease and allowing reflux of blood from aorta back into the left ventricle. **a. murmur**, abnormal heart sound heard over aortic area; a systolic murmur alone is the murmur of aortic stenosis, a diastolic, the murmur of aortic incompetence. Advanced syphilitic valvular disease causes abnormality of both the first and second sounds, the so-called 'to and fro' aortic murmur. **a. stenosis**, narrowing of aortic valve found as result of rheumatic heart disease. The aortic valve can also be damaged by the presence of a congenital bicuspid valve which predisposes to the deposit of calcium; by syphilitic aortitis, ankylosing spondylitis, and in Marfan's syndrome where there is a deficiency of elastic tissue.

aortitis (ā-or-tī'-tis) [G. *aorte*, great artery; *-itis*, inflammation]. Inflammation of the aorta.

aortogram (ā-or'-to-gram). See ARTERIOGRAM.

aortography (ā-or-tog'-raf-i). See ARTERIOGRAPHY—aortographic, adj.; aortographically, adv.

apathy (a'-pa-thi) [G. *a-* without; *pathos*, feeling]. In psychiatry abnormal listlessness and lack of activity—apathetic, adj.

aperients (a-pēr'-i-ents) [L. *aperire*, to open]. Drugs which stimulate evacuation of the bowel. May be further classified as lubricants, laxatives, purgatives and drastic purgatives (q.v.).

aperistalsis (ā-per-is-tal'-sis) [G. *a-*, not; *peri*, around; *stalsis*, constriction]. Absence of peristaltic movement in the bowel. Characterizes the condition of paralytic ileus (q.v.)—aperistaltic, adj.

Apert's syndrome (ap'-ertz). Congenital craniosyntosis (q.v.) accompanied by deformities of the hands, syndactyly. [Eugene Apert, Paris paediatrician, 1868-1940.]

apex (ā'-peks) [L. the extreme end]. The summit or top of anything which is cone-shaped. **a. beat**, in a heart of normal size the a. beat (systolic impulse) can be seen or felt in the 5th left intercostal space in the mid-clavicular line. It is the lowest and most lateral point at which an impulse can be detected and provides a rough indication of the size of the heart—apical, adj.; apices, pl.

Apgar score (ap'-gár). Introduced by Dr Virginia Apgar in 1952. Used for assessing the newborn. Numerical values are given to: Appearance—colour; Pulse—heart rate; Grimace—certain reflexes; Activity—tone; Respiration—breathing.

aphagia (a-fā'-ji-á) [G, *a-*, not; *phagein*, to eat]. Inability to swallow—aphagic, adj.

aphakia (a-fā'-ki-a) [G. *a-*, not; *phakos*, lentil]. Absence of the crystalline lens—aphakic, adj.

aphasia (a-fā'-zi-á) [G. *a-*, not; *phasis*, speech]. Disorder of speech due to a brain lesion. There are many recognized varieties. **motor a.**, loss of ability to articulate. **sensory a.**, loss of power to recognize the written or spoken word. Aphasia is defined by the College of Speech Therapy as the absence of recognition and use of verbal expression due to impairment of the dominant cerebral hemisphere subserving the special intellectual functions concerned with the use of language—aphasic, adj.

aphonia (a-fō'-ni-á) [G. *a-*, not; *phone*,

voice]. Loss of voice from a cause other than a cerebral lesion—aphonic, adj.

aphrodisiac (af-rō-diz'-i-ak). An agent which stimulates sexual excitement.

aphthae (af'-thē) [G. thrush]. Small grey areas surrounded by a ring of erythema; they occur in the mouth; ulceration is inevitable.

apicectomy (āp-i-sek'-to-me) [L. apex, top; G. ektome, excision]. Excision of the root of a tooth.

apicolysis (āp-ik-ol'-i-sis) [L. apex, top; G. lysis, a loosening]. The parietal pleura is stripped from the upper chest wall to cause collapse of the lung apex when it contains a tuberculous cavity.

aplasia (ā-plā'-zi-ā) [G. a-, not; plassein, to form]. Incomplete development of tissue; absence of growth.

aplastic (ā-plás'-tik) [G. a-, not; plassein, to form]. 1. Without structure or form. 2. Incapable of forming new tissue. **a. anaemia**, the result of complete bone marrow failure.

apnoea (ap-nē'-ā) [G. a-, not; pnein, to breathe]. A transitory cessation of breathing as seen in Cheyne-Stokes respiration (q.v.). It is due to lack of the necessary CO_2 tension in the blood for stimulation of the respiratory centre—apnoeic, adj.

apocrine (ap'-o-krīn) [G. apo, from; krinein, to separate]. Modified sweat glands, especially in axillae, genital and perineal regions. Responsible after puberty for body odour.

apodia (ā-pō'-di-ā) [G. a-, not; pous, foot]. Congenital absence of the feet.

apomorphine (a-pō-mor'-fēn). Powerful emetic when injected. Effective when gastric irritant emetics are useless, as in phenol poisoning.

aponeurosis (ap-ō-nū-rō'-sis) [G. apo, from; neuron, tendon; -osis, condition]. A broad glistening sheet of tendon-like tissue which serves to invest and attach muscles to each other, and also to the parts which they move—aponeuroses, pl.; aponeurotic, adj.

aponeurositis (ap-ō-nū-rō-sī'-tis) [G. apo, from; neuron, tendon; -osis, condition; -itis, inflammation]. Inflammation of an aponeurosis.

apophysis (ap-of'-is-is) [G.]. A projection, protuberance or outgrowth. Usually used in connection with bone.

apoplexy (ap-ō-pleks'-i) [G. apoplessein, to cripple by a stroke]. Stroke. Sudden unconsciousness usually caused by cerebral embolism, haemorrhage, or thrombosis. There is stertorous breathing, incontinence of urine and faeces and a varying degree of hemiplegia (q.v.)—apoplectic, apoplectiform. adj.

appendicectomy (ap-pen-di-sek'-to-mi) [L. appendix, appendage; G. ektome, excision]. Excision of the appendix vermiformis (q.v.).

appendicitis (ap-pen-di-sī'-tis) [L. appendix, appendage; G. -itis, inflammation]. Inflammation of the appendix vermiformis (q.v.).

appendicostomy (ap-pen-di-kos'-to-mi) [L. appendix, appendage; G. stoma, mouth]. An operation in which the appendix is brought to the surface and an opening made into it. This admits a catheter via which the large bowel can be irrigated.

appendix (ap-pen'-diks) [L.]. An appendage. **a. vermiformis**, a worm-like appendage of the caecum about the thickness of a pencil and usually measuring from 50.8 to 152.4 mm in length. Its position is variable and it is apparently functionless—appendices, pl.; appendicular, adj.

apperception (ap-per-sep'-shun) [L. ad, to; percipere, to perceive]. Clear perception of a sensory stimulus, in particular where there is identification or recognition—apperceptive, adj.

applicator (ap'-li-kā-tor) [L. applicare, to apply]. An instrument for applying local remedies, e.g. radium.

apposition (ap-o-zish'-un) [L. ad, to; ponere, to place]. The approximation or bringing together of two surfaces or edges.

apraxia (ā-praks'-i-ā) [G. a-, not; prassein, to do]. Inability to deal effectively with or manipulate objects as a result of a brain lesion—apraxic, apractic, adj.

Aprinox (ap'-rin-oks). Bendrofluazide (q.v.).

Aprotinin (ā-prō'-tin-in) Concentrated extract of bovine lung tissue. Acts as a strong protease inhibitor. Useful in acute pancreatitis, hyperplasminaemia and as prophylaxis in pancreatic surgery.

APT. Alum precipitated diphtheria toxoid. A diphtheria prophylactic used mainly for children.

Aptin (ap'-tin). Alprenolol (q.v.).

aptitude (ap'-ti-tūd). Natural ability and

facility in performing tasks, either mental or physical.

apyrexia (ā-pī-reks′ĭ-ă) [G. *a-*, not; *pyretos*, fever]. Absence of fever—apyrexial, adj.

Apyrogen (ā-pī′-rō-jen). A brand of sterile distilled water in hermetically sealed ampoules. It is free from pyrogen (q.v.). Used to make up drugs supplied in powder form, when they are to be given by injection.

aqua (ak′-wă) [L.]. Water. **a. destillata,** distilled water. **a. fortis,** nitric acid. **a. menthae piperitae,** peppermint water.

Aquamephyton (ak-wa-mef′-ĭ-ton). Vitamin K. Antagonist to anticoagulants (not heparin).

Aquamox (ak′wă-mocks) Quinethazone. See CHOLOROTHIAZIDE.

aqueduct (ak′-wĭ-dukt) [L. *aqua*, water; *ducere*, to lead]. A canal. **a. of Sylvius,** the canal connecting the 3rd and 4th ventricles of the brain; aqueductus cerebri. [François Sylvius de la Boe, French anatomist, 1614–72.]

aqueous (ā′-kwi-us) [L. *aqua*, water]. Watery. **a. humor,** the fluid contained in the anterior and posterior chambers of the eye.

Ara-C. See CYTOSINE ARABINOSIDE.

arachidonic acid (ar-ak′-id-on-ik as′ id). One of the essential fatty acids. Found in small amounts in human and animal liver and organ fats. A growth factor.

arachis oil (ar′-ak-ıs). Oil expressed from groundnuts. Similar to olive oil.

arachnodactyly (a-rak-nō-dakt′-il-i) [G. *arachne*, spider; *daktylos*, finger]. Congenital abnormality resulting in spider fingers.

arachnoid (ar-ak′-noid) [G. *arachne*, spider; *eidos*, form]. Resembling a spider's web. **a. membrane,** a delicate membrane enveloping the brain and spinal cord, lying between the pia mater internally and the dura mater externally; the middle serous membrane of the meninges—arachnoidal, adj.

Aramine. Metaraminol (q.v.).

arborization (ár-bor-ī-zā′-shun) [L. *arbor*, tree]. An arrangement resembling the branching of a tree. Characterizes both ends of a neurone, i.e. the dendrons and the axon as it supplies each muscle fibre.

arboviruses (ár-bo-vī′-rus-es) [L. *arbor*, tree; L. poison]. An abbreviation for viruses transmitted by arthropods.

Members of the mosquito-borne group include yellow fever, dengue and viruses causing infections of the CNS. Sandflies transmit sandfly fever. The tick-borne viruses can cause haemorrhagic fevers.

arcus senilis (ár′-kus sen-il′-is) [L. *arcus*, an arch; L. *senilis*, aged]. An opaque ring round the edge of the cornea, seen in old people.

areola (ar-ē′-o-la) [L. *area*, area]. The pigmented area round the nipple of the breast. **secondary a.,** a dark circle of pigmentation which surrounds the primary areola in pregnancy—areolar, adj.

ARF. Acute respiratory failure. See RESPIRATORY FAILURE.

Arfonad (ar-fo-nad′). Trimetaphan (q.v.).

arginase (ár′-jin-āz). An enzyme found in the liver, kidney and spleen. It splits arginine into ornithine and urea.

arginine (ár′-jin-ēn). One of the essential amino acids (q.v.). Used in treatment of acute liver failure to tide patient over acute ammonia intoxication.

argininosuccinuria (ár-jin-ēn′-ō-suks-in-ū′-ri-ă). The presence of arginine and succinic acid in urine. Currently associated with mental subnormality.

Argyll Robertson pupil (ár-gīl′ rob′-ertson). One which reacts to accommodation, but not to light. Diagnostic sign in neurosyphilis, but not all examples are syphilitic. Other important causes include disseminated sclerosis and diabetes mellitus. In the non-syphilitic group the pupil is not small, but often dilated and unequal and is called atypical. [D.M.C.L. Argyll Robertson, Scottish physician, 1837–1909.]

ariboflavinosis (ā-rī′-bo-flāv-in-ōs′-is) [G. *a-*, not; L. *ribes*, currant; *flavus*, yellow; G. *-osis*, condition]. A deficiency state caused by lack of riboflavine and other members of the vitamin B complex. Characterized by cheilosis, seborrhoea, angular stomatitis, glossitis and photophobia.

arithmomania (ar-ith-mō-mā′-ni-ă) [G. *arithmos*, number; *mania*, madness]. A form of insanity in which there is an obsession with numbers.

Arlef (ár′-lef). Flufenamic acid (q.v.).

arrectores pilorum (ár-ek′-tor-ēz pī-lōr′-um) [L. *arrectus*, from; *arrigere*, to erect]. Internal, plain, involuntary muscles attached to hair follicles, which, by contraction, erect the follicles, causing 'gooseflesh'—arrector pili, sing.

arrhenoblastoma (a-ren-ō-blas-tō'-má) [G. *arren*, male; *blastos*, germ; *-oma*, tumour]. A masculinizing tumour of the ovary.

arrhythmia (ā-rith'-mi-á) [G. *a-*, not; *rhythmos*, rhythm]. Any deviation from the normal rhythm, e.g. of the heart. **sinus a.**, increase of the pulse rate on inspiration, decrease on expiration. Appears to be normal in some children.

Arruga suture (á-ru'-gá). Purse-string suture placed around eye in the treatment of detached retina.

arsenic (ár'-se-nik). Occasionally used with iron as a tonic. Usually prescribed as Fowler's solution or liquor arsenicalis. See NEOARSPHENAMINE.

Artane (ar'-tān). Benzhexol (q.v.).

artefact (árt'-i-fakt) [L. *ars*, art; *factus*, made]. Any artificial product resulting from a physical or chemical agency; an unnatural change in a structure or tissue.

arteralgia (ár-ter-al'-ji-á) [L. *arteria*, artery; G. *algos*, pain]. Pain in an artery.

arteriectomy (ár-tēr-i-ek'-to-mi) [L. *arteria*, artery; G. *ektome*, excision]. Excision of an artery or more usually part of an artery.

arteriogram (ár-tēr'-i-ō-gram) [L. *arteria*, artery; G. *gramma*, letter]. Film demonstrating arteries after injection of opaque medium.

arteriography (ár-tēr-i-og'-raf-i) [L. *arteria*, artery; G. *graphein*, to write]. 1. Graphic recording of the pulse. 2. Demonstration of the arterial system by means of injection of opaque medium—arteriographic, adj.; arteriographically, adv.

arteriole (ár-tēr'-i-ōl) [L. *arteriola*, small artery]. A small artery, joining an artery to a capillary.

arteriopathy (ár-tēr-i-op'-ath-i) [G. *arteria*, artery; *pathos*, disease]. Disease of any artery—arteriopathic, adj.

arterioplasty (ár-tē'-ri-ō-plas-ti) [L. *arteria*, artery; G. *plassein*, to form]. Plastic surgery applied to an artery—arterioplastic, adj.

arteriorrhaphy (ár-tē'-ri-or-raf-i) [L. *arteria*, artery; G. *rhaphe*, suture]. A plastic procedure on an artery, such as obliteration of an aneurysm.

arteriosclerosis (ár-tē-ri-ō-skler-ō'-sis) [L. *arteria*, artery; G. *sklerosis*, a hardening]. Degenerative arterial change associated with advancing age. Primarily a thickening of the media and usually associated with some degree of atheroma. **cerebral a.**, a syndrome which may include a shuffling gait, tendency to lean backwards, muscle rigidity, loss of memory, mental confusion and incontinence—arteriosclerotic, adj.

arteriotomy (ár-tē-ri-ot'-o-mi) [L. *arteria*, artery; G. *tome*, a cutting]. Incision of an artery.

arteriovenous (ár-tē'-ri-ō-vēn-us) [L. *arteria*, artery; *vena*, vein]. Pertaining to an artery and a vein.

arteritis (ár-te-rī'-tis) [L. *arteria*, artery; G. *-itis*, inflammation]. Inflammation of an artery. The cause may be infective, traumatic, chemical or metabolic. Involvement of the ophthalmic arteries, or aortic arch may lead to blindness, **cranial a.**, a collagen (q.v.) disorder. Early use of steroids may prevent blindness. **temporal a.**, inflammation with possible occlusion, most often in carotid arteries and branches; alternative name **giant cell a.** See ENDARTERITIS, PERIARTERITIS—arteritic, adj.

artery (ár'-te-ri) [L. *arteria*, artery]. A vessel carrying blood from the heart to the various tissues. The internal endothelial lining provides a smooth surface to prevent clotting of blood. The middle layer of plain muscle and elastic fibres allows for distension as blood is pumped from the heart. The outer, mainly connective tissue layer prevents overdistension. The lumen is largest nearest to the heart; it gradually decreases in size. **a. forceps**, haemostatic (q.v.) forceps—arterial, adj.

arthralgia (árth-ral'-ji-á) [G. *arthron*, joint; *algos*, pain]. Pain in a joint, used especially when there is no inflammation. Syn., articular neuralgia, arthrodynia (q.v.). **Intermittent or periodic a.** is the term used when there is pain, usually accompanied by swelling of the knee at regular intervals—arthralgic, adj.

arthrectomy (árth-rek'-to-mi) [G. *arthron*, joint; *ektome*, excision]. Excision of a joint.

arthritis (árth-rī'-tis) [G. *arthron*, joint; *-itis*, inflammation]. Inflammation of a joint. **a. deformans juvenilis**, Still's disease (q.v.). See PERTHES' DISEASE. **a. deformans neoplastica**, osteitis fibrosa (q.v.). **a. nodosa (a. uratica)** gout—arthritic, adj.

arthroclasia (árth-rō-klā'-zi-á) [G. *arthron*, joint; *klaein*, to break]. Breaking down of adhesions within the joint cavity to produce a wider range of movement. Arthroclasis.

arthrodesis (árth-rō-dē'-sis) [G. *arthron*, joint; *desis*, a binding together]. The stiffening of a joint by operative means.

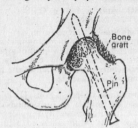

Arthrodesis of hip

arthrodynia (árth-rō-dĭn'-ĭ-á) [G. *arthron*, joint; *odyne*, pain]. Pain in a joint. See ARTHRALGIA—arthrodynic, adj.

arthroendoscopy (árth-rō-end-os'-kop-i) [G. *arthron*, joint; *endon*, within; *skopein*, to examine]. Visualization of the interior of a joint using an endoscope (q.v.).—arthroendoscopic, adj.; arthroendoscopically, adv.

arthrogram (árth'-rō-gram) [G *arthron*, joint; *gramma*, letter]. An X-ray film demonstrating a joint.

arthrography (árth-rog'-raf-i) [G. *arthron*, joint; *graphein*, to write]. X-ray of a joint, sometimes after injection of air or radio-opaque material—arthrographic, adj.; arthrographically, adv.

arthrology (árth-rol'-oj-i) [G. *arthron*, joint; *logos*, discourse]. The science which deals with joints, their diseases and treatment.

arthropathy (árth-rop'-ath-i) [G. *arthron*, joint; *pathos*, disease]. Any joint disease—arthropathic, adj.

arthroplasty (árth'-rō-plas-ti) [G. *arthron*, joint; *plassein*, to form]. The formation of an artificial joint. **cup a.**, articular surface reconstructed and covered with a vitallium cup. **excision a.**, gap is filled with fibrous tissue as in Keller's operation. **replacement a.**, insertion of an inert prosthesis of similar shape. **Girdlestone a.**, excision

arthroplasty of the hip. **McKee-Farrer a.**, stainless steel replacement of the head of femur and the acetabulum, the latter being cemented into the bone—arthroplastic, adj.

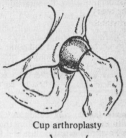

Cup arthroplasty

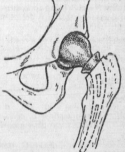

Replacement arthroplasty with metallic prothesis

arthroscope (árth'-rō-skōp) [G. *arthron*, joint; *skopein*, to examine]. An instrument used for the visualization of the interior of a joint cavity. See ENDOSCOPE—arthroscopic, adj.

arthroscopy (árth-ros'-kop-i) [G. *arthron*, joint; *skopein*, to examine]. The act of visualizing the interior of a joint—arthroscopic, adj.

arthrosis (ár-thrō'-sis) [G. *arthron*, joint; *-osis*, condition]. An articulation or joint. (Occasionally used to describe degeneration in a joint.)

arthrotomy (árth-rot'-o-mi) [G. *arthron*, joint; *tome*, a cutting]. Incision into a joint.

articular (ár-tik'-ū-lar) [L. *articulus*, joint]. Pertaining to a joint or articulation. Applied to cartilage, surface, capsule, etc.

articulation (ár-tik-ū-lā'-shun) [L. *articulus*, joint]. 1. The junction of two or more bones; a joint. 2. Enunciation of speech—articular, adj.

artificial insemination. Insertion of sperm into uterus using cannula and syringe instead of coitus.

Artosin (ár'-tos-in). Tolbutamide, (q.v.).

Arvin (ár'-vin). Ancrod (q.v.).

asbestos (as-bes'-tos) [G. unquenchable]. A fibrous, mineral substance which does not conduct heat and is incombustible. It is used in making protective clothing for industry. Industrial workers may acquire hyperkeratotic papules on their hands—asbestos corns or warts.

asbestosis (as-bes-tō'-sis) [G. asbestos, unquenchable; -osis, condition]. Fibrosis of the lungs resulting from the inhalation of fine asbestos dust and fibrils. Current research being done with radioactive gas to enable early detection. See PNEUMOCONIOSIS.

ascariasis (as-kar-ī'-a-sis) [G. ask-karis, work in the intestines; N.L. -iasis, condition]. Infestation by the ascarides. The bowel is most commonly affected, but in the case of roundworm, infestation may spread to the stomach, liver and lungs.

ascaricide (as-kar'is-īd) [G. askaris, worm in the intestine; L. caedere, to kill]. Lethal to ascarides—ascaricidal, adj.

ascarides (as-kar'-i-dēz) [G. askaris, worm in the intestines]. Nematode worms of the family Ascaridae, to which belong the roundworm (Ascaris lumbricoides) and the threadworm (Oxyuris vermicularis).

Aschoff's nodules (ash'-hofs). Nodules in the myocardium in rheumatism.

ascites (as-sī'-tēz) [G. askites, a kind of dropsy, from askos, bag]. Free fluid in the peritoneal cavity. Syn., abdominal dropsy, hydroperitoneum—ascitic, adj.

ascorbic acid (a-skor'-bik). Vitamin C. Used as dietary supplement in anaemia and to promote wound healing See VITAMIN C.

asepsis (ā-sep'-sis) [G. a-, not; sepsis, putrefaction]. The state of being free from living pathogenic organisms—aseptic, adj.

aseptic technique. A precautionary method used in any procedure where there is a possibility of introducing organisms into the patient's body. Every article used must have been sterilized.

Aserbine (as-er'-bin). A desloughing cream, useful for burns, varicose and indolent ulcers. Emollient, contains benzoic acid, which is antimycotic, and salicylic acid.

Asilone (as'-i-lōn). Polymethylsiloxane 250 mg and aluminium hydroxide 500 mg. Available in tablet, suspension and powder form to control non-specific diarrhoea and flatulent distension of abdomen.

ASO. Antistreptolysin O. See ANTI-STREPTOLYSIN.

asparaginase (as-par-a-jin'-ās) An enzyme derived from micro-organisms. Being tried in the treatment of asparagine-requiring cancers, especially the leukaemias—and especially acute lymphoblastic leukaemia.

aspergillosis (as-pér'-ji-lō-sis) [L. aspergere, to sprinkle; G. -osis, condition]. Any infection caused by any species of Aspergillus. More likely to occur in persons who handle grain or seeds. See BRONCHOMYCOSIS.

Aspergillus (as'-pér-jil'-us) [L. aspergere, to sprinkle]. A genus of fungi, found in soil, manure and on various grains.

aspermia (á-sper'-mi-á) [G. a-, without; sperma, seed]. Lack of secretion or expulsion of semen—aspermic, adj.

asphyxia (as-fiks'-i-á) [G. a-, not; sphyzein, to throb]. Suffocation; cessation of breathing. The O_2 content of the blood falls while the CO_2 rises and paralyses the respiratory centre. **blue a., a. livida,** deep blue appearance of a newborn baby. Good muscle tone. Responsive to stimuli. **white (pale) a., a. pallida,** more severe condition of newborn. Pale, flaccid, unresponsive to stimuli.

aspiration (as-pi-rā'-shun) [L. aspirare, to breathe upon]. 1. The act of drawing in the breath; inspiration. 2. The withdrawal of fluids from a body cavity by means of a suction or siphonage apparatus. **a. pneumonia,** inflammation of lung from inhalation of foreign body, usually fluid or food particles—aspirate, v.t.

aspirator (as'pi-rā-tor) [L. aspirare, to breathe upon]. A negative pressure apparatus for withdrawing fluids from cavities.

aspirin (as'pir-in). Acetylsalicylic acid (q.v.).

assimilation (as-sim-i-lā'-shun) [L. assimilatio, similarity]. The process whereby the already digested foodstuffs are absorbed and utilized by the tissues. Syn., anabolism—assimilable, adj.; assimilate, v.t., v.i.

association (as-sō-si-ā'-shun) [L. *associare*, to join to]. In psychology; **a. of ideas**, the principle by which ideas, emotions and movements are connected so that their succession in the mind occurs. **a. areas**, in the cerebral cortex the functions of which are unknown. **controlled a.**, ideas called up in consciousness in response to words spoken by the examiner. **free a.**, ideas arising spontaneously when censorship is removed.

astereognosis (a-stē-ri-og-nō'-sis) [G. *a-*, not; *stereos*, solid; *gnosis*, knowledge]. Loss of power to recognize the shape and consistency of objects.

asthenia (as-thē'-ni-á) [G. *asthenia*, want of strength]. Weakness, debility. See KRETSCHMER.—asthenic, adj.

asthenic type, Physique with small trunk and long limbs sometimes associated with schizophrenia.

asthenopia (as-thē-nō'-pi-á) [G. *a-*, not; *sthenos*, strength; *ops*, eye]. Poor vision—asthenopic, adj.; asthenope, n.

asthma (asth'-má) [G. a panting]. Paroxysmal airways obstruction due to generalized narrowing of the bronchi which reverses either spontaneously or as the result of treatment. The extrinsic classification ranges from Atopic Type I allergy (reaction on skin testing is immediate) to Non-atopic Type III allergy (delayed reaction on skin testing). The intrinsic classification implies negative skin reactions; immunology unknown. **bronchial a.**, attack of breathlessness associated with bronchial obstruction or spasm. Characterized by expiratory wheeze. **cardiac a.**, nocturnal paroxysmal dyspnoea in left ventricular failure. **status asthmaticus**, repeated attacks of asthma without any period of freedom between spasms—asthmatic, adj.

astigmatism (as-tig'-mat-izm) [G. *a-*, not; *stigma*, a point]. Defective vision caused by inequality of one or more refractive surfaces, usually the corneal, so that the light rays do not converge to a point on the retina. May be congenital or acquired—astigmatic, astigmic, adj.

astringent (as-trin'-jent) [L. *astringere*, to bind together]. An agent which contracts organic tissue, thus lessening secretion—astringency, n.

astrocytoma (as-trō-si-tō'-má) [G. *astron*, a star; *kytos*, cell; *-oma*, tumour]. A slowly growing tumour of the glial tissue of brain and cord.

asymmetry (ā-sim'-et-ri) [G. *a-*, not; *symmetria*, symmetry]. Lack of similarity of the organs or parts on each side.

asymptomatic (ā-simp-tom-at'-ik) [G. *a-*, not; *symptomatikos*, from *symptoma*, symptom]. Symptomless.

AT 10. Dihydrotachysterol (q.v.).

atactic (ā-tak'-tik). See ATAXIA.

ataractic (at-a-rak'-tik) [G. *ataraktos*, cool, steady]. Drugs that, without drowsiness, help to relieve anxiety thus providing emotional equilibrium. Syn. tranquillizer, neuroleptic. Have reduced the incidence of leucotomy.

Atarax (at'-á-raks). Hydroxazine. See ATARACTIC.

atavism (at'-a-vizm) [L. *atavas*, ancestor]. The reappearance of an hereditary trait which has skipped one or more generations—atavic, atavistic, adj.

ataxia, ataxy (ā-taks'-i-á, a-taks'-i) [G. *ataxia*, disorder]. Defective muscular control resulting in irregular and jerky movements. Staggering. **Friedreich's a.**, usually begins in childhood. Heredofamilial disease. Transmission occurs through both sexes, usually as a recessive gene, rarely a dominant one. Transmission from affected parent to child rare because adult sufferers are not as a rule able to procreate—ataxic, adj.

Atebrin (at'-e-brin). Mepacrine (q.v.).

atelectasis (at-el-ek'-ta-sis) [G. *ateles*, imperfect; *ektasis*, extension]. No air in alveoli, lung solid. **congenital a.**, air has failed to enter lung immediately after birth—atelectatic, adj.

atherogenic (ath-e-rō-jen'-ik) [G. *athere*, porridge; *genes*, producing]. Capable of producing atheroma—atherogenesis, n.

atheroma (ath-e-rō'-má) [G. *athere*, porridge; *-oma*, tumour]. Deposition of hard yellow plaques of lipoid material in the intimal layer of the arteries. May be related to high level of cholesterol in the blood, or excessive consumption of refined sugar. Of great importance in the coronary arteries in predisposing to coronary thrombosis—atheromatous, adj.

atherosclerosis (ath'-e-rō-skle-rō'-sis) [G. *athere*, porridge; *sklerosis*, a hardening]. Co-existing atheroma and arteriosclerosis—atherosclerotic, adj.

athetosis (ath-e-tō'-sis) [G. *athetos,* without position; *-osis,* condition]. A condition marked by purposeless movements of the hands and feet and generally due to a brain lesion—athetoid, athetotic, adj.

athlete's foot. See TINEA PEDIA.

Ativan (at'-i-van). Lorazepam (q.v.).

atom [G. *atomos,* uncut, indivisible]. The smallest particle of an element capable of existing individually, or in combination with one or more atoms of the same or another element. **atomic weight,** the weight of an atom compared with that of an atom of hydrogen—atomic, adj.

atomization (at'-om-īz-ā-shun). A mechanical process whereby a liquid is divided into a fine spray—atomizer, n.

atonic (a-ton'-ik) [G. *a-,* not; *tonos,* tone]. Without tone; weak—atonia, atony, atonicity, n.

atopy (at'-op-i) [G. *a-,* net; *topos,* place]. Familial allergy. Covers diseases such as hay fever, asthma, urticaria and eczema where there is a clear family history of these conditions—atopic, adj.

atresia (ā-trē'-zi-à) [G. *a-,* not; *tresis,* perforation]. Imperforation or closure of a normal opening or canal—atresic, atretic, adj.

atrial fibrillation (ā'-tri-al fib-ril-ā'-shun). Syn., auricular fibrillation. Chaotic cardiac irregularity without any semblance of order. Commonly associated with mitral stenosis and nodular toxic goitre, but also with other diseases of the heart and sometimes in general toxic states.

atrial flutter (ā'-tri-al flut'-èr). Syn., auricular flutter. Rapid regular cardiac rhythm caused by irritable focus in atrial muscle and usually associated with organic heart disease. Speed of atrial beats between 260 and 340 per minute. Ventricles usually respond to every second beat, but may be slowed by carotid sinus pressure.

atrial septal defect. Non-closure of foramen ovale at birth resulting in congenital heart defect.

atrioventricular (ā'-tri-ō-ven-trik'-ū-lar) [L. *atrium,* atrium; *ventriculus,* ventricle]. Pertaining to the atria and the ventricles of the heart. Applied to a node, tract and valves. Syn., auriculoventricular.

atrium (ā'-tri-um) [L. *atrium,* chamber].

Cavity, entrance or passage. One of the two upper cavities of the heart. Also called 'auricle'.—atria, pl.; atrial, adj.

Atromid (at'-rō-mid). Clofibrate (q.v.).

atrophy (at'-ro-fi) [G. *atrophia,* want of food]. Wasting, emaciation, diminution in size and function. **acute yellow a.,** massive necrosis of liver associated with severe infection, toxaemia of pregnancy or ingested poisons. **progressive muscular a.,** syn., motor neurone disease. Disease of the motor neurones of unknown cause, characterized by loss of power and wasting in the upper limbs. May also have upper motor neurone involvement (spasticity) in lower limbs—atrophied, atrophic, adj.

atropine (at'-ro-pēn). Principal alkaloid of belladonna. Has spasmolytic, mydriatic and central nervous system depressant properties. Given before anaesthetic to decrease secretion in bronchial and salivary systems and to prevent cardiac depression by depressing the vagus nerve thus quickening the heart beat. It can be given intravenously to produce tachycardia—*(a)* before giving Prostigmin; *(b)* when a patient has a very slow pulse. **a. methonitrate** is used in pylorospasm and in spray preparations for asthma and bronchospasm.

ATS. Antitetanus serum. Contains tetanus antibodies. Produces artificial passive immunity. A test dose must be given first. Can cause anaphylaxis.

ATT. Antitetanus toxoid. Contains treated tetanus toxins. Produces artificial active immunity. Does not cause anaphylaxis.

attenuation (at-ten-ū-ā'-shun) [L. *attenuare,* to weaken]. A bacteriological process by which organisms are rendered less virulent by exposure to an unfavourable environment. They can then be used in the preparation of vaccines—attenuant, attenuated, adj.; attenuate, v.t., v.i.

atticotomy (at-i-kot'-ō-mi). Entry into the attic of the middle ear—that portion above the tympanic membrane (epitympanum) by removal of the outer attic wall to create a wide opening of the external auditory meatus into the attic.

attitude (at'-ti-tud) [F. attitude, from L. *aptitudinem*]. A settled mode of thinking.

atypical (ā-tip'-ik-al). Not typical; unusual, irregular; not conforming to type, e.g. atypical pneumonia.

audiogram (aw'-di-ō-gram)[L. *audire*, to hear; G. *gramma*, a letter]. A chart of hearing while using an audiometer. The acuity of hearing is plotted and a visual record obtained

audiology (aw-di-ol'-o-ji) [L. *audire*, to hear; G. *logos*, discourse]. The science dealing with hearing—audiological, adj.; audiologically, adv.

audiometer (aw-di-om'-et-er) [L. *audire*, to hear; G. *metron*, a measure]. An apparatus for the clinical testing of hearing. It generates pure tones over a wide range of pitch and intensity—audiometric, adj.; audiometry, audiometrist, n.

auditory (aw'-dit-o-ri) [L. *audire*, to hear]. Pertaining to the sense of hearing. **a. area**, that portion of the temporal lobe of the cerebral cortex which interprets sound. **a. meatus**, the canal between the pinna and eardrum. **a. nerves**, the eighth pair of cranial nerves. **a. ossiscles**, the three tiny bones—malleus, incus and stapes—stretching across the cavity of the middle ear.

aura (aw'-rá)[G. breeze]. A premonition; a peculiar sensation or warning of an impending attack, such as occurs in epilepsy.

aural (awr'-al) [L. *auris*, ear]. Pertaining to the ear.

Aureomycin (aw-rē-ō-mī'-sin). Chlortetracycline. See TETRACYCLINE.

auricle (aw'-rik-l) [L. *auricula*, the external ear]. 1. The pinna of the external ear. 2. An appendage to the cardiac atrium. 3. Commonly used mistakenly for atrium (q.v.)—auricular, adj.

auricular fibrillation. See ATRIAL F.

auricular flutter. See ATRIAL F.

auriculoventricular. See ATRIOVENTRICULAR.

auriscope (aw'ris-kōp) [L. *auris* ear; G. *skopein*, to examine]. An instrument for examining the ear, usually incorporating both magnification and electric illumination.

aurothiomalate (awr-ō-thī-om'-a-lāt). Gold injection useful in chronic discoid lupus erythematosus and rheumatoid arthritis. Urine should be tested for albumen before each injection.

auscultation (aws-kul-tā'-shun) [L. *auscultare*, to listen to]. A method of listening to the body sounds for diagnostic purposes, particularly the heart, lungs and fetal circulation. It may be: (1) immediate, by placing the ear directly against the body; (2) mediate, by the use of a stethoscope—auscultatory, adj.; auscult, auscultate, v.

Australian lift. Better described as shoulder lift. A method of lifting a heavy patient, whereby his weight is taken by the upper shoulder muscles of the two lifters, and the lift is achieved by straightening the lifters' flexed hips.

autism (aw'tizm) [G. *autos*, self]. Schizophrenic (q.v.) syndrome in childhood.

autistic (aw-tis'-tik)[G.*autos*, self]. Morbidly self-centred thinking, governed by the wishes of the individual;' wishful thinking (phantasy), in contrast to reality thinking. Occurs in schizophrenia (q.v.)—autism, n.

antoantibody (aw-tō-an'ti-bod-i) [G. *autos*, self; *anti*, against; A.S. *bodig*, body]. Substance produced in a reaction, something within the body acting as the stimulus (autoantigen).

autoantigen (aw-tō-an'-ti-jen) [G. *autos*, self; *anti*, against; *genos*, birth]. Something within the body capable of initiating the production of autoantibody.

autoclave (aw'-tō-klāv)[G. *autos*, self; L. *clavis*, key]. 1. An apparatus for high-pressure steam sterilization. 2. Sterilize in an autoclave.

autodigestion (aw-tō-di-jest'-chun) [G. *autos*, self; L. *digerere*, to digest]. Self-digestion of tissues within the living body. Autolysis (q.v.).

autoeroticism (aw-tō-e-rot'-is-izm) [G. *autos*, self;*eros*, love]. Self-gratification of the sex instinct. See MASTURBATION—autoerotic, adj.

autogenous (aw-toj'-e-nus) [G. *autos*, self; *genesthai*, from *gignesthai*, to be produced]. Self-generated; endogenous. Applied to bone graft, skin graft, etc. **a. vaccine**, one prepared from bacteria obtained from the patient's own infection. Also AUTOGENETIC, AUTOGENIC.

autohaemotherapy (aw-tō-hē-mō-thēr'-a-pi)[G.*autos*, self; *haima*, blood;*therapeia*, treatment]. Intramuscular injection of a patient using his own blood, e.g. in cases of recurring urticaria.

autoimmunity (aw-tō-im-mūn'-i-ti) [G. *autos*, self; L. *immunis*, free from]. An abnormal immune reaction of unknown cause. In most cases it is directed against a constituent, often protein in nature, of the patient's own body. This constituent is regarded as a foreign body by the patient's own immune system which forms antibodies against the constituent as it would against any foreign invader.

autoimmunization (aw'-tō-im-mun-īz-ā'-shun) [G. *autos*, self; L. *immunis*, free from]. Sensitization of a person to a substance elaborated in his own body. Hashimoto's disease, myxoedema and Graves' disease are examples of autoimmune thyroid disease. Pernicious anaemia is another autoimmune disease.

autoinfection (aw-tō-in-fek'-shun) [G. *autos*, self; L. *inficere*, to infect]. Infection arising from an organism within the body or transferred from one part of the body to another by fingers, etc.

autointoxication (aw-tō-in-toks-i-kā'-shun) [G. *autos*, self; L. *in-*, in; G. *toxikon*, poison]. Poisoning from faulty metabolic products elaborated within the body.

autolysis (aw-tol'-is-is) [G. *autos*, self; *lysis*, a loosening]. Autodigestion (q.v.) which occurs if digestive ferments escape into surrounding tissues—autolytic, adj.

automatic (aw-tō-mat'-ik) [G. *automatos*, self-acting]. That which is performed without the influence of the will; spontaneous; non-volitional acts; involuntary acts.

automatism (aw-tom'-at-izm) [G. *automatos*, self-acting]. Performance of involuntary acts. Occurs in somnambulism, hysterical and epileptic states.

autonomic (aw-tō-nom'-ik) [G. *autos*, self; *nomos*, law]. Independent; self-governing. **a. nervous system** (ANS) is divided into parasympathetic and sympathetic portions. They are made up of nerve cells and fibres which cannot be controlled at will. They are concerned with reflex control of bodily functions.

autoplasty (aw-tō-plas'-ti) [G. *autos*, self; *plassein*, to form]. Replacement of tissue by a graft of tissue from the same body—autoplastic, adj.; autoplast, n.

autopsy (aw-top'-si) [G. *autopsia*, seeing with one's own eyes]. The examination of a dead body for diagnostic purposes.

autosome (aw'-tō-sōm) [G. *autos*, self; *soma*, body]. A chromosome other than a sex chromosome.

autosuggestion (aw-tō-su-jest'-yun) [G. *autos*, self; L. *suggestio*, from *sugger-*

ere, to suggest]. Self-suggestion; uncritical acceptance of ideas arising in the individual's own mind. Occurs in hysteria (q.v.).

autotransfusion (aw-tō-trans-fūzhun) [G. *autos*, self; L. *transfusio*, from *transfundere*, to pour off, transfer]. The infusion into a patient of the actual blood lost by haemorrhage, especially when it occurs into the abdominal cavity.

avascular (ā-vas'-kū-lar) [G. *a-*, not; L. *vasculum*, a small vessel].. Bloodless; not vascular, i.e. without blood vessels. **a. necrosis**, death of bone from deficient blood supply following injury or possibly through disease, often a precursor of osteoarthritis—avascularize, v.t., v.i.; avascularity, n.

Aventyl. Nortriptyline. Similar to amitriptyline (q.v.). See ANTIDEPRESSANT.

aversion (a-ver'-zhun). A method of treatment by deconditioning. Effective in some forms of addiction and abnormal behaviour.

Avertin (av'er-tin). Bromethol (q.v.).

avian (ā'-vi-an) [L. *avis*, bird]. Pertaining to birds. **a. tubercle bacillus** resembles the other types of tubercle bacilli, but rarely causes disease in man.

avidin (av'-i-din). An antivitamin which interferes with the absorption of biotin (q.v.). Found in raw egg white.

avirulent (ā-vir'-ūl-ent) [G. *a-*, not; L. *virus*, poison]. Without virulence (q.v.).

avitaminosis (ā-vīt'-a-min-ōs-is) [G. *a-*, not; L. *vita*, life; G. *-osis*, condition]. Any disease resulting from a deficiency of vitamins.

Avomine (av'-ō-mēn). An antiemetic drug with a powerful and prolonged action. Used in travel sickness, nausea and vomiting. Given 2 h before a journey, it will act for 6 to 12 h. Also has antihistamine properties, therefore useful in allergic conditions.

avulsion (a-vul'-shun) [L. *avellere*, to tear away]. A forcible wrenching away, as of a limb, nerve or polypus. **phrenic a.**, tearing of the phrenic nerve to paralyse one side of the diaphragm to rest a tuberculous base of lung.

axilla (aks-il'-á) [L.]. The armpit—axillary, adj., applied to nerves, blood and lymphatic vessels.

axis (aks'-is) [L.]. 1. The second cervical vertebra. 2. An imaginary line passing through the centre; the median line of the body—axial, adj.

axon (aks'-on) [G. *axon*, axis]. or axis cylinder. That process of a nerve cell conveying impulses away from the cell; the essential part of the nerve fibre and a direct prolongation of the nerve cell—axonal, adj.

axonotmesis (aks'-on-ot-mēs'-is) [G. *axon*, axis; *tmesis*, a cutting]. Peripheral degeneration as a result of damage to the axons of a nerve. The internal architecture is preserved and recovery depends upon regeneration of the axons, and may take many months (about 25.4 mm a month is the usual speed of regeneration). Such a lesion may result from pinching, crushing or prolonged pressure.

azacyclonal. Frenquel. Tranquillizer.

azathioprine (az-a-thī'-ō-prēn). Immunosuppressive drug.

azoospermia (ā-zō-ō-spérm'-i-ȧ) [G. *a-*, not; *zoe*, life; *sperma*, seed]. Sterility of the male through non-production of spermatozoa.

azotaemia (az-ot-ē'-mi-ȧ) [G. *a-*, not; *zotikos*, fit for preserving life; *haima*, blood]. Syn., uraemia (q.v.)—azotaemic, adj.

azathioprine (az-ȧ-thī'-ō-prēn) Antimetabolite. Works by competing against purine, an essential metabolite for cell division.

azoturia (az-ot-ūr'-ē-ȧ) [G. *a-*, not; *zotikos*, fit for preserving life; *ouron*, urine]. Pathological excretion of urea in the urine—azoturic, adj.

azygos (az'-ī-gos) [G. *a-*, not; *zygon*, yoke]. Occurring singly, not paired. **a. veins**, three unpaired veins of the abdomen and thorax which empty into the inferior vena cava—azygous, adj.

B

Babinski's reflex or **sign** (bab-in'-skē). Movement of the great toe upwards (dorsiflexion) instead of downwards (plantar flexion) on stroking the sole of the foot. It is indicative of disease or injury to upper motor neurones and is present in organic but not hysterical hemiplegia. Babies exhibit dorsiflexion, but after learning to walk they show the normal plantar flexion response. [Joseph François Felix Babinski, French neurologist, 1857-1932].

bacillaemia (bas-il-ēm'-i-ȧ) [L. *bacillum*, stick; G. *haima*, blood]. The presence of bacilli in the blood-bacillaemic, adj.

bacilluria (bas-il-ū'-ri-ȧ) [L. *bacillum*, stick; G. *ouron*, urine]. The presence of bacilli in the urine—bacilluric, adj.

Bacillus (bas-il'-us) [L. *bacillum*, stick]. A term now restricted to a genus of bacteria consisting of aerobic, Grampositive, rod-shaped cells which produce endospores and the majority are motile by means of peritrichate flagella. These organisms are saprophytes and their spores are common in soil and dust of the air. Colloquially the word is still used to describe any rod-shaped micro-organism *Bacillus anthracis* causes anthrax in man and in animals.

bacitracin (bas-ē-trā'-sin). An antibiotic (q.v.) used mainly for external application in conditions resistant to other forms of treatment. It does not cause sensitivity reactions.

bacitracin zinc. Replaced bacitracin in the British Pharmacopoeia 1973.

baclofen (bak'-lō-fen). Reduces spasticity of voluntary muscle; mode uncertain. Side effects include nausea, vomiting, diarrhoea, gastric discomfort, muscular inco-ordination, hypotonia, mental confusion, vertigo and drowsiness. Particularly useful for multiple sclerosis. Dosage needs to be 'titrated' to each individual, 100 mg being the maximum dose without hospital supervision.

bacteraemia (bak-te-rēm'-i-ȧ) [G. *bakterion*, staff; *haima*, blood]. The presence of bacteria in the blood—bacteraemic, adj.

bacteria (bak-tē'-ri-ȧ) [G. *bakterion*, staff]. A group of micro-organisms, also called the 'schizomycetes'. They are typically small cells of about 1 micron in transverse diameter. Structurally there is a protoplast, containing cytoplasmic and nuclear material (not seen by ordinary methods of microscopy) within a limiting cytoplasmic membrane, and a supporting cell wall. Other structures such as flagella, fimbriae and capsules may also be present. Individual cells may be spherical, straight or curved rods, or spirals; they may form chains or masses, and some show branching with mycelium formation. They may produce various pigments including chlorophyll. Some form endospores. Reproduction is chiefly by simple binary fission. They may be free living, saprophytic or parasitic; some are pathogenic to man, animals and plants—bacterium, sing.; bacterial, adj.

bactericide (bak-tēr'-i-sīd) G. *bakterion*, staff; L. *coedere*, to kill]. Any agent which destroys bacteria—bactericidal, adj.; bactericidally, adv.

bactericidin (bak-tēr-i-sīd'-in) [G. *bakterion*, staff; L. *coedere*, to kill]. Antibody which kills bacteria.

bacteriologist (bak-tēr-i-ol'-oj-ist) [G. *bakterion*, staff; *logos*, discourse]. One who studies and is skilled in the science of bacteriology.

bacteriology (bak-tē'-ri-ol'-oj-i) [G. *bakterion*, staff; *logos*, discourse]. The science and study of bacteria—bacteriological, adj.; bacteriologically, adv.

bacteriolysin (bak-tē-ri-ō-li'-sin) [G. *bakterion*, staff; *lysis*, a loosening]. A specific antibody (q.v.) which causes dissolution of bacteria.

bacteriolysis (bak-tēr-i-ol'-is-is) [G. *bakterion*, staff; *lysis*, a loosening]. The disintegration and dissolution of bacteria—bacteriolytic, adj.

bacteriophage (bak-tēr'-i-ō-fāj) [G. *bakterion*, staff; *phagein*, to eat]. A virus parasitic on bacteria. Some of these are used for typing staphylococci, etc.

bacteriostasis (bak-tēr-i-ō-stā'-sis) [G. *bakterion*, staff; *stasis*, a standing still]. Arrest or hindrance of bacterial growth—bacteriostatic, adj.

bacteriotherapy (bak-tēr'-i-ō-ther'-ap-i) [G. *bakterion*, staff; *therapeia*, treatment]. Treatment of disease by introduction of bacteria into the blood stream, e.g. malaria in the treatment of neurosyphilis—bacteriotherapeutic, adj.

bacteriuria (bak-tē-ri-ū'-ri-à) [G. *bakterion*, staff; *ouron*, urine]. The presence of bacteria in the urine (100 000 or more organisms per ml). Acute urinary tract infection may be preceded by, and active pyelonephritis may be associated with asymptomatic bacteriuria.

Bactrim (bak'-trim). Trimethoprim (q.v.) and · sulphamethoxazole (q.v.). Useful for urinary tract infections and gonorrhoea.

baker's itch. Contact dermatitis (q.v.) resulting from flour or sugar.

BAL (British anti-lewisite). Dimercaprol (q.v.).

balanitis (bal-an-ī'-tis) [L. *balanus*, acorn; G. *-itis*, inflammation]. Inflammation of the glans penis and prepuce.

balanoposthitis (bal-an-ō-pos-thī'-tis) [G. *balanos*, acorn; *posthe*, membrum virile; *-itis*, inflammation]. Inflammation of the glans penis and prepuce.

balantidiasis (bal-an-tid-ī-à-sis) Infection with the ciliate *Balantidium coli*; uncommon parasite of man; may cause dysentery. Treated with full course of metronidazole.

balanus (bal'-an-us) [G. *balanos*, acorn]. The glans of the penis or clitoris.

Balkan beam. Wooden beam attached to a hospital bed whereby a Thomas' bed splint can be slung up, with pulleys and weights attached, to allow movement and provide counterbalance to the weight of the splint and leg.

ballottement (bal-lot'-mon(g)) [F. a shaking about]. Testing for a floating object, especially used to diagnose pregnancy. A finger is inserted into the vagina and the uterus is pushed forward; if a fetus is present it will fall back again, bouncing in its bath of fluid—ballottable, adj.

balsam of Peru (bawl'-sam). A viscous aromatic liquid from the trunks of South American trees. Mild antiseptic used with zinc ointment for pressure sores.

balsam of Tolu (bawl'-sam of tō-loo'). Brown aromatic resin. Constituent of Friar's balsam. Used as syrup of Tolu in cough syrups.

Baltimore paste. See ALUMINIUM PASTE.

bandage (band'-āj) [F. from *bande*, a strip]. Traditionally a piece of cloth, calico, cotton, flannel. etc. of varying size and shape applied to some part of the body to retain a dressing or a splint; support, compress, immobilize; prevent or correct deformity. There are now several circular bandages that are applied with an applicator to almost any part of the body. Examples are Netalast, Tube-gauze, Tubigrip. **capelline b.** [L. *capella*, a cap] or divergent spica, bandage covering head or amputation stump. **compression b.**, function is as name implies. Specially used to give support without constriction of vessels after an ankle sprain, by applying alternate layers of wool and bandage thrice. Compression bandage also used to shrink a part, as an amputation stump. **elastic b.** belongs to the preceding group, specially useful for varicose veins, after a sprain or removal of plaster. **Esmarch's b.,** made from elastic rubber; used to obtain a bloodless field in surgery of the limbs. **many-tailed b.,** composed of five narrow strips joined in their middle third; used to cover abdomen or chest. **suspensory b.,** applied so that it supports and suspends the scrotum. **T b.,** used to hold dressings in position on the perineum. **triangular b.,** useful for arm slings, for securing splints, in first-aid work, and for inclusive dressings of a part, as a whole hand or foot. **Velpeau's b.,** the arm to chest bandage for a fractured clavicle. [Alfred Armond Louis Marie Velpeau, Parisian surgeon, 1795–1867.]

Bankhart's operation (bank'-harts). For recurrent dislocation of shoulder joint: the defect of the glenoid cavity is repaired. This is the modern procedure, augmented by reefing the joint capsule and pularissubsca muscle.

Banocide (ban'-o-sīd). Diethylcarbamazide (q.v.).

Banti's disease. Syn., splenic anaemia. Now regarded as a manifestation of portal hypertension (q.v.) with alimentary bleeding and splenomegaly causing leucopenia and thrombocytopenia. [Guido Banti, Italian physician, 1852–1925].

Barbados leg (bár-bā'-dŏz). Elephant leg. A tropical disease caused by a thread-like worm called 'Filaria'; lymphangitis, followed by sclerosis and fibrosis interferes with drainage of lymph, and oedema of the limb ensues. See ELEPHANTIASIS.

barber's itch or **rash.** See SYCOSIS.

barbiturates (bár-bit'-ū-rātz). A widely used group of sedative drugs derived from barbituric acid (a combination of malonic acid and urea). Small changes in the basic structure result in the formation of rapid-acting, medium or long-acting barbiturates and a wide range is now available. Continual use may result in addiction. Action potentiated in presence of alcohol. Allergic skin reactions may occur in some patients. See also BUTOBARBITONE, PHENOBARBITONE, etc.

barbotage (bár-bot-ázh') [F. from *harboter,* to dabble]. Method of spinal anaesthesia; small amount of solution from syringe injected into subarachnoid space, plunger partially withdrawn allowing CSF to mix with remaining solution in syringe. Part of this mixture then injected and plunger again par-

tially withdrawn. This process may be repeated several times before entire contents of syringe injected.

barium sulphate (bār-i-um). Heavy insoluble powder used as a contrast agent in X-ray visualization of alimentary tract.

Barlow's disease. Syn., infantile scurvy (q.v.). [Thomas Barlow, English physician, 1845–1945.].

barotrauma (bar-ō-traw'-má) [G. *baros,* weight; *trauma,* wound]. Injury due to a change in atmospheric or water pressure, e.g. ruptured eardrum.

barrier nursing. A method of preventing the spread of infection from an infectious patient to the others in an open ward. It is achieved by 'isolation' technique.

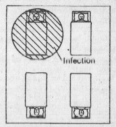

Barrier nursing

bartholinitis (bár-tol-in-ī'-tis) [after Caspar *Bartholin;* G. *-itis,* inflammation]. Inflammation of Bartholin's glands (q.v.).

Bartholin's glands (bár'-to-lin). Two small glands situated at each side of the external orifice of the vagina. Their ducts open just outside the hymen. [Caspar Bartholin, Danish anatomist, 1655–1748.]

Bartonella fever. Non-protozoal haemolytic anaemia. Syn., Oroya fever.

basal ganglia (bā'-sal-gan'-gli-á) [G. *basis,* base; G. *ganglion,* a swelling]. Grey cells at the cerebral base. The lentiform nucleus, comprising globus pallidus and putamen, together with the caudate nucleus make up the corpus striatum, which with the claustrum is called the basal ganglia. Concerned with modifying and co-ordinating voluntary muscle movement. Site of degeneration in Parkinson's disease. See PARALYSIS.

basal narcosis (nár-kō'-sis) [G. a benumbing]. The pre-anaesthetic administration of narcotic drugs which reduce fear and anxiety, induce sleep and thereby minimize postoperative shock.

base (bās) [G. *basis*, base]. 1. The lowest part. 2. The main part of a compound. 3. In chemistry, the substance which combines with an acid to form a salt—basal, basic, basilar, adj.

basilar-vertebral insufficiency. See VERTEBROBASILAR INSUFFICIENCY.

basilic (bas-il'-ik) [G. *basilikos*, royal]. Prominent. A vein on the inner side of the arm. The **median b.** at the bend of the elbow is generally chosen for venepuncture.

basophil (bā'-zo-fil) [G. *basis*, base; *philein*, to love]. Showing an affinity for basic dyes. Used in histology, e.g. basophilic; applied to some leucocytes (basophil polymorphonuclear).

basophilia (bā-zō-fil'-i-á) [G. *basis*, base; *philein*, to love]. Increase of basophils in the blood: basophilic staining of red blood corpuscles.

Batchelor plaster. A type of double abduction plaster, with the legs encased from groins to ankles, in full abduction and medial rotation. The feet are then attached to a wooden pole or 'broomstick'. Alternative to frog plaster, but the hips are free.

bath (báth) [A.S. *boeth*]. 1. The apparatus used for bathing. 2. The immersion of the body or any part of it into water or any fluid; or the application of spray, jet or vapour of such a fluid to the body. The term is modified according to (*a*) temperature, e.g. cold, contrast, hot, tepid; (*b*) medium used, e.g. mud, sand, water, wax; (*c*) medicament added, e.g. Milton, potassium permanganate, saline, sulphur; (*d*) function of medicament, e.g. astringent, disinfectant; (*e*) part bathed, e.g. arm bath, sitz bath. (*f*) environment, e.g. bed bath. See HYDROTHERAPY.

battered baby syndrome. An infant who shows clinical or radiological evidence of lesions which are frequently multiple and involve mainly the head, soft tissues, or the long bones and the thoracic cage, and which cannot be unequivocally explained by natural disease or simple accident. Described by Caffet in 1957. Widened to battered *child* syndrome by Kempe in 1961. Syn., 'abused child'; 'non-accidentally injured child'. All these terms reflect physical injuries done to child to exclusion of emotional problems of parents. 'Child mishand-

ling' therefore preferred by many people.

Bauer's operation (baw'-erz). Ligation of incompetent popliteal vein: useful when pain in calf is severe and foot is cyanosed.

Bazin's disease. Erythema induratum. A chronic recurrent disorder, involving the skin of the legs of women. There are deep-seated nodules which later ulcerate. [Antoine Pierre Ernest Bazin, French dermatologist, 1807–78.]

BCG. (Bacillus-Calmette-Guérin). A vaccine (q.v.) prepared from bovine tubercle bacilli. BCG vaccination by inhalation can be carried out using an ultrasonic nebulizer for a roomful of 500 people.

bearing-down. 1. A pseudonym for the expulsive pains in the second stage of labour. 2. A feeling of weight and descent in the pelvis associated with uterine prolapse or pelvic tumours.

beat (bēt) [A.S. *beatan*]. Pulsation of the blood in the heart and blood vessels. **apex b.**, see APEX. **dropped b.** refers to the loss of an occasional ventricular beat as occurs in extrasystoles (q.v.). **premature b.**, an extrasystole.

Beaver-breather. Intermittent positive-pressure respirator, used in respiratory paralysis for short periods of artificial respiration.

Becosym (bē-kōs'-im). Tablets, syrup and ampoules containing aneurine, riboflavine, nicotinamide and pyridoxine. Used in vitamin B deficiency.

bedbug. A blood-sucking insect belonging to the genus Cimex. *Cimex lecturlarius* is the most common species in temperate and *C. hemipterus* in tropical zones. They live and lay eggs in cracks and crevices of furniture and walls. They are nocturnal in habit and their bites leave a route for secondary infection.

bedsore. See PRESSURE SORE.

Beer's knife. Delicate instrument with triangular blade used in cataract operations for incision of cornea preparatory to removal of lens. [Georg Joseph Beer, Austrian ophthalmologist, 1763–1821.]

behaviour (bē-hā'-vūr). In general sense, conduct. As a psychological term, means response of an organism to its situation in relation to its environment. **b. therapy,** see AVERSION.

behaviourism (bē-hā'-vūr-izm). A psychological term which denotes an approach to psychology through the study of responses and reactions, i.e. behaviour.

Behçet's syndrome. Described by Behçet in 1937. Starts with ulceration of mouth and/or genitalia with eye changes such as conjunctivitis, keratitis, or hypopyon iritis. One site may be affected months or years before the others. There may also be skin nodules, thrombophlebitis and arthritis of one or more of the large joints. Pulmonary, gastrointestinal and neurological complications are being increasingly reported. Cause unknown; some favour virus, others an allergic vasculitis. No effective treatment apart from attempts to suppress worst phases with steroids. Blindness may result from ocular complications.

bejel (bej'-el). Non-venereal syphilis.

belladonna (bel-à-don'-à). Dried leaves of deadly nightshade (*Atropa belladonna*). Powerful antispasmodic. Effects mainly due to the alkaloid atropine (q.v.).

Bellergal (bel-erg'-al). Combination of phenobarbitone, belladonna alkaloids and ergotamine. Useful for menopausal syndrome, premenstrual tension and migraine.

'belle indifférence.' The incongruous lack of emotion despite incapacitating symptoms commonly shown by patients with hysteria. First noted by Janet in 1893. [Pierre Marie Félix Janet, French psychiatrist, 1859–1947.]

Bellocq's sound or cannula (bel'-oks, kan'-ū-là). A curved tube used for plugging the posterior nares.

Bell's mania. Acute delirious mania. A severe psychosis combining delirium with the gross psychomotor activity of mania. Was almost invariably fatal before the introduction of electrotherapy.

Bell's palsy. See PALSY.

bemegride (bem'-i-grīd). Analeptic. Given intravenously.

benactyzine (ben-ak'-ti-zēn). Tranquilizing drug with selective action, producing sense of detachment from environment. Used in anxiety and tension neuroses.

Benadryl (ben'-a-dril). Diphenhydramine (q.v.).

Bencard (ben'-kard). See D-VAC ANTIGENS.

Bence-Jones' protein. Protein bodies appearing in the urine of some patients with myelomatosis (q.v.). On heating the urine they are precipitated out of solution at 50° to 60° C; they redissolve on further heating to boiling point and reprecipitate on cooling. [Henry Bence-Jones, London physician. 1814–73.]

bendrofluazide (bend-rō-flū'-a-zīd). Diuretic that decreases reabsorption of sodium and chloride in kidney tubules. 10 mg daily orally, or intramuscularly on alternate days. Used with caution in renal or hepatic failure.

bends. See CAISSON DISEASE.

Benedict's solution (ben' ē dikts sol-ū'-shun). A solution of copper sulphate which is easily reduced, producing colour changes. Used to detect the presence of glucose. [Stanley R. Benedict, American chemist, 1884–1936]

Benemid (ben'-i-mid). Probenecid (q.v.).

benign (be-nīn') [L. *benigmus*, kind]. Innocent. A term used to denote the opposite of malignant.

benorylate (ben-or'-i-lāt). Esterified aspirin. Odourless. Tasteless. Well absorbed from gastrointestinal tract. Has anti-inflammatory, analgesic and antipyretic properties comparable with aspirin, and acts longer. Significantly less likely to cause hidden bleeding.

Benuride (ben'-ū-rīd) Phenylethylacetylurea (q.v.).

Benvil (ben'-vil). Tybamate (q.v.).

benzalkonium (ben-zal-kō'-ni-um). Antiseptic with detergent action. Used as 1 per cent solution for skin preparation, 1:20 000 to 1:40 000 for irrigation. Incompatible with soap, with loss of activity.

Benzedrine (ben'-zē-drin). Amphetamine (q.v.).

benzene (ben'-zēn). A colourless inflammable liquid obtained from coal tar. Extensively used as a solvent. Its chief importance in the medical sphere is in industrial toxicology. Continued exposure to it results in leucopenia, anaemia and purpura.

benzhexol (benz-heks'-ol). Antispasmodic used mainly for rigidity of Parkinsonism. Side effects include dryness of mouth, nausea and vertigo.

benzocaine (ben'-zō-kān). Relatively non-toxic surface anaesthetic. Used as dusting powder (10 per cent), ointment (10 per cent), suppositories (5 g), lozenges (1½ g). Occasionally given orally in gastric carcinoma.

benzodiazepine (ben-zō-dī-az'-e-pēn). Tranquillizer; allays acute anxiety.

benzoic acid (ben-zō'-ik as'-id). Fungistatic and antiseptic. Used with salicylic acid in Whitfield's ointment (ung. acid. benz. co.) for ringworm. Rarely given orally owing to irritant effects.

benzoin (ben'-zo-in). Natural balsamic resin from Siam and Sumatra. Widely used as Friar's balsam by steam inhalation in bronchitis and other chest conditions.

benzthiazide (bens-thī'-az-īd). Oral diuretic. See CHLOROTHIAZIDE.

benztropine methanesulphonate (benstrōp-in-mē-thān-sul'-fon-āt). Muscle relaxant. Anti-Parkinsonism.

benzyl benzoate (ben'-zil ben'-zō-āt). Aromatic liquid; has ascaricidal properties and used mainly in treatment of scabies though now replaced by Quella (q.v.). Occasionally given internally as an antispasmodic.

benzyl penicillin (ben'-zil). Penicillin (q.v.).

Beogex (bē'-o-jeks). Suppository that after insertion releases CO_2 which produces evacuation of bowel.

bephenium hydroxynaphthoate (bef-en'-i-um hī-droks-i-naf'-thō-āt). Anthelmintic, effective against hookworm and roundworm. Given on an empty stomach at least one hour before food.

beri-beri (ber'-ē-ber'-ē) [Singhalese, *beri,* weakness]. A deficiency disease caused by lack of aneurine (vitamin B_1). Occurs mainly in those countries where the staple diet is polished rice. The symptoms are pain from neuritis, paralysis, muscular wasting, progressive oedema, mental deterioration and, finally, heart failure.

berylloisis (ber-il-i-ō'-sis). Industrial disease; impaired lung function because of interstitial fibrosis from inhalation of beryllium. Steroids used in treatment.

Berkomine (berk'-ō-mēn). Imipramine (q.v.).

Berkozide (berk'-o-zīd). Bendrofluazine (q.v.).

Betadine (bet'-a-dēn). Povidoneiodine. Antibacterial. Available as aerosol spray, surgical scrub, scalp lotion and ointment.

betamethasone (bet-a-meth'-a-zōn). Slightly more potent than dexamethasone, q.v. Forty times more potent orally than cortisone. Less water-retaining effects than prednisone. Exceptionally powerful anti-inflammatory action in skin disease when applied locally. Useful in chronic ulcerative colitis and Crohn's disease.

Betaptin (bet-ap'-tin). Alprenolol (q.v.).

betazole hydrochloride (bet'-az-ol hī-drō-klor'-īd). Used to stimulate gastric juice in tests. Less reaction than histamine.

bethanecol (beth-an'-ē-kol). A compound resembling carbachol in activity, but is relatively non-toxic. Used in urinary retention, abdominal distension and myasthenia gravis.

bethanidine (beth-an'-i-dēn). Adrenergic blocking, antihypertensive drug. Interferes with transmission in sympathetic adrenergic nerves, especially sympathetically mediated vascular reflexes, thus can lead to postural and exercise hypotension.

Betnesol (bet'-nes'-ol). Betamethasone (q.v.).

Betnovate (bet'-nov-āt). Cream containing fluorocortisone. More effective than those containing hydrocortisone (see COBADEX), but it can be absorbed through the skin and can produce local or systemic side effects.

bicarbonate (bī-kár'-bon-āt). A salt of carbonic acid. **blood b.,** that in the blood indicating the alkali reserve. Also called 'plasma bicarbonate'.

bicellular (bī-sel'-ū-lár). [L. *bis,* twice; *cella,* stall, chamber]. Composed of two cells.

biconcave (bī-kon'-kāv) [L. *bis,* twice; *concavus,* hollow]. Concave or hollow on both surfaces.

biconvex (bī-kon'-veks) [L. *bis,* twice; *convexus,* convex]. Convex on both surfaces.

bicornuate (bī-korn'-ū-āt) [L. *bis,* twice; *cornutus,* horned]. Having two horns, generally applied to a double uterus or a single uterus possessing two horns.

bicuspid (bī-kus'-pid) [L. *bis,* twice *cuspis,* point]. Having two cusps or points. **b. teeth,** the premolars. **b. valve,** the mitral valve between the left atrium and ventricle of the heart.

bidet (bi'-dā). Low-set, trough-like basin in which the perineum can be immersed, whilst the legs are outside and the feet on the floor. Can have attachments for douching the vagina or rectum.

bifid (bī'-fid) [L. *bis,* twice; *findere,* to

cleave]. Divided into two parts. Cleft. Forked.

bifurcation (bī'-fur-kā-shun) [L. *bifurcus,* having two prongs]. Division into two branches—bifurcate, adj., v.t., v.i.

biguanides (bi'-gwan-īds). Oral antidiabetic agents. Useful for obese patients. Can be used with sulphonylureas. Syn., diaguanides.

bilateral (bī-lat'-er-al) æL. *bis,* twice; *lateralis,* of the side]. Pertaining to both sides—bilaterally, adv.

bile (bīl) [L. bilis]. A bitter, alkaline, viscid, greenish-yellow fluid secreted by the liver and stored in the gall-bladder. It contains water, mucin, lecithin, cholesterol, bile salts and the pigments bilirubin and biliverdin. **b. ducts,** the hepatic and cystic, which join to form the common bile duct. **b. salts,** emulsifying agents, sodium glycocholate and taurocholate—bilious, biliary, adj.

Bilharzia (bil-hár'-zē-á). Syn., Schistosoma (q.v.).

bilharziasis (bil-hár-zī'-á-sis). Syn., schistosomiasis (q.v.).

biliary (bil'-i-ar-i) [L. *bilis,* bile]. Pertaining to bile. **b. colic,** paroxysmal pain in right upper quadrant of abdomen, due to smooth muscle spasm arising in the bile passages. **b. fistula,** an abnormal track conveying bile to the surface or to some other organ.

bilious (bil'-yus) [L. *bilis,* bile]. 1. Pertaining to bile. 2. Pertaining to excess of bile. 3. A non-medical word signifying a digestive upset.

bilirubin (bī-li-roo'-bin) [L. *bilis,* bile; *ruber,* red]. A pigment largely derived from the breakdown of haemoglobin from red blood cells destroyed in the spleen. When it is released it is fat-soluble, gives an indirect reaction with Van den Bergh's test and is potentially harmful to metabolically active tissues in the body, particularly the basal nuclei of the immature brain. Indirect b. is transported to the blood attached to albumen to make it less likely to enter and damage brain cells. In the liver the enzyme glucuronyl tranferase conjugates indirect fat-soluble b. with glucuronic acid to make it water-soluble, in which state it is relatively non-toxic, reacts directly with Van den Bergh's test and can be excreted in stools and urine. See PHOTOTHERAPY.

biliuria (bī-li-ū'-ri-á) [L. *bilis,* bile; G. *ouron,* urine]. The presence of bile

pigments in the urine—biliuric, adj.

biliverdin (bī-li-ver'-din) [L. *bilis,* bile; *virens,* green]. The green pigment of bile formed by oxidation of bilirubin.

Billroth's operation. Partial gastrectomy. B.O.I. Excision of the lower part of the stomach with anastomosis of the remaining part to the duodenum. B.O.II Resection of the distal end of the stomach with closure of the lines of section and gastrojejunostomy. [Christian Theodor Billroth, Austrian surgeon, 1829–94.]

bilobate (bī-lō'-bāt) [L. *bis,* twice; G. *lobos,* rounded flap]. Having two lobes.

bilobular (bī-lob'-ū-lár) [L. *bis,* twice; G. *lobos,* lobe]. Having two little lobes or lobules.

bimanual (bī-man'-ū-al) [L. *bis,* twice; *manus,* hand]. Performed with both hands. A method used in gynaecology whereby the internal genital organs are examined between one hand on the abdomen and the other hand or finger within the vagina.

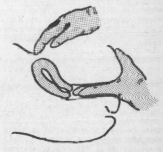

Bimanual method

binaural (bin-aw'-ral) [L. *bini,* two by two; *auris,* ear]. Pertaining to, or having two ears. Applied to a type of stethoscope (q.v.).

Binet's test (bē'-nā). Properly Binet-Simon scale. A series of graded intelligence tests in which an individual's intelligence level (mental age) is compared with his chronological age. [Alfred Binet, French psychologist, 1857–1911.]

biniodide of mercury (bin-ī'-ō-dīd of mer'-kūr-i). A solution of mercuric iodide in potassium iodide solution. It is less irritant and less toxic than mercuric chloride (perchloride, q.v.), and possibly less effective. Used as 1:2000 to

1:5000 solution for application to the skin; 1-10 000 for douches.

binocular (bin-ok'-ū-lár) [L. *bini,* two by two; *oculus,* eye]. 1. The use of both eyes in vision. 2. An optical instrument requiring both eyes for its use.

binovular (bin-ov'-ū-lár) [L. *bini,* two by two; *ovum,* egg]. Derived from two separate ova. Binovular twins may be of different sexes. See UNIOVULAR.

biochemistry (bī-ō-kem'-is-tri) [G. *bios,* life; from *chymos,* juice]. Physiological chemistry—biochemical, adj.

bioengineering   (bī'-ō-en-jin-ēr'-ing). Designing sophisticated microelectronic or mechanical equipment for external use by patients, for attachment to patients, or placement inside patients.

Biogastrone (bī-ō-gas'-trōn). Carbenoxolone sodium (q.v.).

biology (bī-ol'-oj-i) [G. *bios,* life; *logos,* discourse]. The science of life, dealing with the structure, function and organization of all living things—biological, adj; biologically, adv.

biopsy (bī-op'-si) [G. *bios,* life; *opsis,* vision]. Observation of the living. Excision of tissue from a living body for microscopic examination to establish diagnosis.

biorhythmics (bī-ō-rith'-miks) [G. *bios,* life; *rhythmos,* rhythm]. Modern study of the three main biological functions: physical, emotional and intellectual cycles.

Biotexin (bī-ō-teks'-in). Novobiocin (q.v.).

biotin (bī'-ot-in). A member of vitamin B complex; also known as vitamin H and as co-enzyme R. Probably synthesized by intestinal flora. Lack of it may cause dermatitis in human beings.

biparietal (bī-par-ī'-et-al) [L. *bis,* twice; *paries,* wall]. Pertaining to both parietal bones.

biparous (bīp'-ar-us) [L. *bis,* twice; *parere,* to bring forth]. Producing two offspring at one birth.

bipolar (bī-pō'-lár) [L. *bis,* twice; *polus,* pole]. Having two poles.

BIPP. A pasty mixture of bismuth subnitrate, iodoform, and liquid paraffin. Used as antiseptic dressing in acute osteitis.

birth. The act of expelling the young from the mother's body; delivery; being born. **b. canal,** the cavity or canal of the pelvis through which the baby passes during labour. **b. certificate.** a legal document given on registration, within 42 days of a birth. **b. control,** prevention or regulation of conception by any means; contraception. **b. injury,** any injury occurring during parturition, e.g. fracture of a bone, subluxation of a joint, injury to peripheral nerve, intracranial haemorrhage. **b. mark,** naevus (q.v.). **premature b.,** one occurring after the 7th month of pregnancy, but before term.

bisacodyl (bī-sa-kō'-dil). Dulcolax (q.v.).

bisexual (bī'-seks-ū-al) [L. *bis,* twice; *sexus,* sex]. Having the characteristics of both sexes; hermaphrodite—bisexually, adv.

bismuth (biz'-muth). A greyish metal. **b. carbonate,** a mild antacid, used with other alkalis in dyspepsia and peptic ulcer. **b. salicylate,** gastric sedative used in gastroenteritis. **b. sodium tartrate,** a soluble compound used occasionally by intramuscular injection in infective arthritis. **b. subgallate,** yellow insoluble powder. Used as dusting powder in eczema and in suppositories for haemorrhoids. Occasionally given orally as an astringent.

Bisolvin (bī-sol'-vin). Bromhexine (q.v.).

bistoury (bis'-tū-ri) [F. *bistourí*]. A long narrow knife, straight or curved, used for cutting from within outwards in the opening of a hernial sac, an abscess, sinus or fistula.

Bitot's spots (bē-tōz). Collections of dried epithelium, flaky masses and micro-organisms at the sides of the cornea. A manifestation of vitamin A deficiency. Xerosis conjunctivae. [Pierre A. Bitot, Bordeaux physician, 1822–88.]

bitters. Substances, the extracts of which are used as stomachics (q.v.).

bivalve (bī'-valv)]L. *bis,* twice; *valva,* leaf of a door]. Having two blades such as in the vaginal speculum. In orthopaedic work, to divide a plaster of Paris splint into two portions—an anterior and posterior half.

blackhead. See COMEDO.

blackwater fever. A malignant form of malaria (q.v.) occurring in the tropics, especially Africa. There is great destruction of red blood cells, and this causes a very dark coloured urine.

bladder (blad'-ár) [A.S. *blaedre*]. A membranous sac containing fluid or gas. **gall-b.,** a pear-shaped bag on the under surface of the liver; its function is to store and concentrate the bile. **ileal b.,** term used when ureters are transplanted into an isolated loop of small intestine, one end of which is made to open on the abdominal wall. See ILEO-URETEROSTOMY **neurogenic b.,** interference with nerve control gives rise to retention of urine, presenting as incontinence—or continuous dribbling without retention. Bladder emptied by manual pressure on anterior abdominal wall where necessary. **rectal b.,** term used when ureters are transplanted into the rectum in cases of severe disease of the urinary bladder. **urinary b.,** a muscular bag situated in the pelvis, a reservoir for urine.

Blalock-Hanlon operation. Failing a successful Rashkind's septostomy (q.v.), a surgical opening is made between the right and left atrium.

Blalock's operation. Anastomosis of the pulmonary artery (distal to a pulmonary stenosis) to a branch of the aorta. Most often performed for Fallot's tetralogy (q.v.). [Alfred Blalock, American surgeon, 1899–1964.]

bland. Mild, non-irritating, soothing.

Blastomyces (blas'-tō-mī-sēz) [G. *blastos,* germ; *mykes,* fungus]. A genus of yeast-like organisms—blastomycetic, adj.

blastomycosis (blas-tō-mī-kō'-sis) [G. *blastos,* germ; *mykes,* fungus; *-osis,* condition]. Granulomatous condition caused by budding, yeast-like organisms. May affect skin, viscera and bones—blastomycotic, adj.

blastula (blas'-tū-lá) An early stage in development of the fertilized ovum when the morula becomes cystic and infolds to become the gastrula.

bleb [dialect E. from *blub,* suggesting a bubbling sound]. A large blister. See BLISTER, BULLA, VESICLE.

bleeder [A.S. *bledan,* to bleed]. One who is subject to frequent loss of blood, as one suffering from haemophilia (q.v.).

'bleeding time' (blēd'-ing tīm). The time required for the spontaneous arrest of bleeding from a skin puncture: under controlled conditions this forms a clinical test.

blennophthalmia (blen-of-thal'-mi-á) [G. *blenna,* mucus; *ophthalmia,* ophthalmia]. Catarrhal conjunctivitis—blennophthalmic, adj.

blennorrhagia (blen-o-rāj'-i-á) [G. *blenna,* mucus; *rhegnynai,* to burst]. 1. A copious mucous discharge. 2. Gonorrhoea.

blennorrhoea (blen-or-ē'-á) [G. *blenna,* mucus; *rheein,* to flow]. Syn., blennorrhagia (q.v.)—blennorrhoeal, adj.

blepharitis (blef-a-rī'-tis) [G. *blepharon,* eyelid; *-itis,* inflammation]. Inflammation of the eyelids, particularly the edges—blepharitic, adj.

blepharon (blef'-ar-on) [G.]. The eyelid; palpebra—blephara, pl.

blepharoptosis (blef-ar-op-tō'-sis) [G. *blepharon,* eyelid; *ptosis,* a falling). See PTOSIS—blepharoptotic, adj.

blepharospasm (blef'-a-rō-spazm) [G. *blepharon,* eyelid; *spasmos,* spasm]. Spasm of the muscles in the eyelid. Excessive winking—blepharospastic, adj.

blind loop syndrome. Resulting from intestinal obstruction or surgical anastomosis; there is stasis in the small intestine which encourages bacterial growth thus producing diarrhoea and salt deficiencies.

blind spot. The spot at which the optic nerve leaves the retina. It is insensitive to light.

blister [O.N. *blástr,* a swelling]. Separation of the epidermis from the dermis by a collection of fluid, usually serum or blood. See VESICLE.

blistering fluid, Liquor epispasticus, a counterirritant.

Blocadren (blok'-a-dren). Timolol maleate (q.v.).

blood [A.S. *blōd*]. The red viscid fluid filling the heart and blood vessels. It consists of a colourless fluid, plasma, in which are suspended the red blood corpuscles, or erythrocytes, the white corpuscles, or leucocytes, and the platelets, or thrombocytes. The plasma (q.v.) contains a great many substances in solution including factors which enable the blood to clot. **b. bank,** a special refrigerator in which blood is kept after withdrawal from donors, until required for transfusion. **defibrinated b.,** that in which the fibrin is removed by agitation. **laked b.,** that in which the red cells are haemolysed. **occult b.,** that which is not visible. Its presence is determined by chemical tests.

blood-brain barrier. The membranes between the circulating blood and the brain. Some drugs can pass from the blood to the cerebrospinal fluid, through this barrier, others cannot, e.g. streptomycin.

blood casts. Casts of conglutinated red blood corpuscles, formed in the renal tubules and found in the urine.

blood clotting. Primary phase: constriction of damaged vessel and adhesion of platelets to site of injury and to each other. Secondary phase involves coagulation over and through the platelet mass. See table of plasma coagulation factors.

Factor Number	Synonyms
I	Fibrinogen
II	Prothrombin
III	Tissue thromboplastin
IV	Calcium ions
V	Proaccelerin
VII	Factor VII
VIII	Antihaemophilic factor (AHF)
IX	Christmas factor
X	Stuart factor, Power factor
XI	Plasma thromboplastin antecedent (PTA)
XII	Hageman factor
XIII	Fibrin-stabilizing factor

blood count. Calculation of the number of red or white cells per cubic millimetre of blood, using a haemocytometer. **differential b. c.** estimates the number of different types of white cell.

blood culture. After withdrawal of blood from a vein, it is incubated in a suitable medium, at an optimum temperature, so that any contained organisms can multiply and so be isolated and identified under the miscrocope. See BACTERAEMIA and SEPTICAEMIA.

blood formation. See HAEMOPOIESIS.

blood groups. ABO system. There are four groups, A, B, AB and O. The cells of these groups contain the corresponding antigens, A, B, AB, except group O cells, which contain neither antigen A or B. For this reason group O blood can be given to any of the other groups and it is known as the universal donor. In the plasma there are agglutinins which will cause agglutination of any cell carrying the corresponding antigen, e.g. group A plasma contains anti-B agglutinins; group B plasma contains anti-A agglutinins; group O plasma contains both anti-A and anti-B agglutinins; group AB plasma contains no agglutinins. Group AB is therefore known as the universal recipient and can receive A, B and O blood. This grouping is determined by (1) testing a suspension of red cells with anti-A and anti-B serum or (2) testing serum with known cells. Transfusion with an incompatible ABO group will cause a severe haemolytic reaction and death may occur unless the transfusion is promptly stopped. High titre agglutinins: in some persons the anti-A or anti-B content of the plasma is unusually high and their agglutinating and haemolytic effect cannot be neutralized by dilution in a recipient's blood stream. Such blood can be transfused only to a recipient of the same ABO group as the donor. Blood bottles are usually labelled to show the presence of high titre agglutinins. **rhesus b.g.**, the red cells contain four pairs of antigens which are known by the letters Cc, Dd, Ee and Ff. The letters denote allelomorphic genes which are present in all cells except the sex cells where a chromosome can carry C or c, but not both. In this way the rhesus genes and blood groups are derived equally from each parent. When the cells contain only the cde groups, then the blood is said to be rhesus negative; when the cells contain C, D or E singly or in combination with cde, then the blood is rhesus positive. These groups are antigenic, and can, under suitable conditions, produce the corresponding antibody in the serum. These antibodies are then used to detect the presence of Rh groups in cells. Antibodies to the Rh group are produced by (a) transfusion with Rh incompatible blood; (b) immunization during pregnancy by fetal cells containing the antigen entering the mother's circulation. This can cause erythroblastosis fetalis (q.v.).

blood-letting. Venesection (q.v.).

blood plasma [G. *plasma*, from plassein, to form]. Liquid portion of blood. Composed of over 90 per cent. water, the remainder being protein 6 to 8 per cent, electrolytes, foodstuffs, waste products, clotting agents, antibodies and hormones.

blood pressure. The pressure exerted by the blood on the vessel walls, measured in millimetres of mercury by the sphygmomanometer. The systolic pressure (when the heart muscle is at the maximum contraction) is recorded first, followed by the diastolic pressure (when the left ventricle is in a state of relaxation), e.g. 120 to 80 mm. See HYPERPIESIS and HYPOPIESIS.

blood sedimentation rate. BSR. see ESR.

blood serum. The fluid which exudes when blood clots; it is plasma minus the clotting agents.

blood sugar. The amount of glucose in the circulating blood; varies within the normal limits. See appendix. This level is controlled by various enzymes and hormones, the most important single factor being insulin (q.v.). See HYPERGLYCAEMIA and HYPOGLYCAEMIA.

blood transfusion. The intravenous replacement of lost or destroyed blood by compatible citrated human blood. Also used for severe anaemia with deficient blood production. Fresh blood from a donor or stored blood from a blood bank may be used. It can be given 'whole', or with some plasma removed ('packed-cell' transfusion). If incompatible blood is given severe reaction follows. See BLOOD GROUPS.

blood urea. The amount of urea (the end product of protein metabolism) in the blood; varies within the normal range. See appendix. This is virtually unaffected by the amount of protein in the diet, when the kidneys which are the main organs of urea excretion are normal. When they are diseased the blood urea quickly rises. See URAEMIA.

'blue baby'. The appearance produced by some congenital heart defects. The appearance, by contrast, of a newborn child suffering from temporary anoxia is described as 'blue asphyxia'.

blue pus. Bluish discharge from a wound infected with *Pseudomonas pyocyanea.*

blue stone. Copper sulphate (q.v.).

bluxism (bluks'-izm). Teeth clenching which can cause headache from muscle fatigue.

BMR. See METABOLIC.

body image (bo'-di im'-āj). The image in an individual's mind of his own body. Distortions of this occur as a result of affective disorders, parietal lobe tumours or trauma.

Boeck's disease (beks). A form of sarcoidosis (q.v.).

Bohn's nodules (bōnz). Tiny white nodules on the palate of the newly born.

boil [L. *bullire,* to bubble up]. A furuncle. An acute inflammatory condition, surrounding a hair follicle; caused by the *Staphylococcus aureus.* Usually attended by suppuration; it has one opening for drainage in contrast to a carbuncle (q.v.). See FURUNCULOSIS.

bolus (bo'-lus) [G. *bolos,* lump]. A soft, pulpy mass of masticated food.

bone graft [A.S. *bán,* bone; O.F. *greffe.* from G. *graphein,* to write]. The transplantation of a piece of bone from one part of the body to another, or from one person to another. Used to repair bone defects, afford support, or to supply osteogenic tissue.

Bonney's blue. Pig. tinctor, BNF. A solution of crystal violet and brilliant green in a mixture of methylated spirit and water. Used as a skin disinfectant.

borax (bor'-aks). Mild antiseptic similar to boric acid. Used in alkaline mouthwashes. Glycerin of borax, and borax with honey are used as throat paints, but should be applied sparingly.

borborygmi (bor-bor-ig'-mi) [G. *borborygmos,* intestinal rumbling]. Rumbling noises caused by the movement of flatus in the intestines.

boric acid (bor'-ik as'-id). Also known as **boracic acid.** Mild antiseptic used mainly as eye lotions and ear drops. Dusting powders and lotions should not be applied to large raw areas, as there is a danger of boric poisoning.

Bornholm disease. Named after the Danish island where it was described by Sylvest in 1934. Viral disease due to B group of Coxsackie viruses. Two to 14 days incubation. Symptoms include sudden onset of severe pain in lower chest or abdominal or lumbar muscles. Breathing may be difficult because of the pain, and fever is common. May last up to one week. There is no specific treatment.

botulism (bot'-ū-lizm) [L. *botulus,* sausage]. An intoxication with the preformed exotoxin of *Clostridium botulinum.* Vomiting, constipation, ocular and pharyngeal paralysis and sometimes aphonia manifest within 24 to 72 h of eating food contaminated with the spores which require anaerobic conditions to produce the toxin. Hence the danger of home-tinned vegetables and meat.

bougie (boo'-zhē) [F. a candle]. A cylindrical instrument made of gum elastic, metal or other material. Used in varying sizes for dilating the anus, cardiac sphincter of stomach, oesophagus, urethra, etc.

bovine (bo'-vīn) [L. *bovinus,* of an ox]. Pertaining to the cow or ox. The morphology and staining reactions of the bovine type of tubercle bacillus (*Myco-*

bacterium tuberculosis) are practically identical with those of the human type. The bovine type infects the bones, glands and joints in human beings.

bowel (bow'-el) [O.F. *boel,* from L. *botulus,* a sausage]. The intestine; the gut. See COLON.

bow-leg (bō'-leg) [A.S. *boga*; O.N. *leggr*]. Syn., genu varum (q.v.).

Boyle's anaesthetic machine. Apparatus by which chloroform, ether, nitrous oxide gas, and oxygen may be administered. Now adapted for use with cyclopropane. [Henry Edmund Gaskin Boyle, English surgeon, 1875–1941.]

Boyle's law. At any stated temperature, a given mass of gas varies in volume inversely as the pressure. [Robert Boyle, English physicist, 1627–91.]

brachial (brā'-ki-al). Pertaining to the arm. Applied to vessels in this region and a nerve plexus at the root of the neck.

brachium (brā'-ki-um) [L. *bracchium,* less correctly, *brachium,* arm]. The arm (especially from shoulder to elbow), or any arm-like appendage—brachia, pl.; brachial, adj.

Bradford frame. A stretcher type of bed used for: (1) immobilizing spine; (2) resting trunk and back muscles; (3) preventing deformity. It is a tubular steel frame fitted with two canvas slings allowing a 101.6 to 152.4 mm gap to facilitate the use of a bedpan. [Edward H. Bradford, American orthopaedic surgeon, 1848–1926.]

Bradosol (brad'-os-ol). Domiphen (q.v.).

bradycardia (bra:di-kár'-di-á) [G. *bradys,* slow; *kardia,* heart]. Slow rate of heart contraction, resulting in a slow pulse rate. In febrile states, for each degree rise in body temperature, the expected increase in pulse rate is ten beats per minute. When the latter does not occur, the term 'relative bradycardia' is used.

brain (brān). The encephalon; that part of the central nervous system contained in the cranial cavity. It consists of the cerebrum, cerebellum, pons varolii, midbrain (mesencephalon) and medulla oblongata. The last three divisions constitute the brain stem.

bran. The husk of grain. The coarse outer part of cereals, especially wheat, high in roughage and the vitamin B complex.

branchial (brang'-ki-al) [G. *bragchia,* gills]. Pertaining to the fissures or clefts which occur on each side of the neck of the human embryo, and which enter into the development of the nose, ears and mouth. **b. cyst,** a swelling in the neck arising from such embryonic remnants.

Brandt Andrews technique. Elevation of the uterus abdominally while holding the cord just taut—no traction. When the uterus is lifted the placenta will be in the cervix or upper vagina and is then expelled by suprapubic pressure directed below the fundus of the elevated uterus.

Braun's frame. A metal frame, bandaged for use, and equally useful for drying a lower leg plaster, and for applying skeletal traction (Steinmann's pin or Kirschner wire inserted through the calcaneus) to a fractured tibia, after reduction.

Braunula (brawn'-ū-lá). A plastic disposable cannula with metal needle for ease of insertion into vein.

break-bone fever. See DENGUE.

breast (brest) [A.S. *bréost*]. The anterior upper part of the thorax; the mammary gland. **b. bone,** the sternum.

Breck feeder. a graduated glass tube of 28.3 g capacity, with a rubber bulb at one end and a teat at the other. Pressure on the bulb expels fluid through the teat. Used for feeding premature and weak babies.

breech (brēch) [M.E. *brech*]. The buttocks (q.v.).

bregma (breg'-má) [G. front part of the head]. The junction of the coronal and sagittal sutures; the anterior fontanelle—bregmata, pl.; bregmatic, adj.

Bretylate (bret'-i-lāt). Acts by improving the way in which the natural electrical impulses that cause the heart to beat are conducted to the heart. In this way the heart, instead of slowing down, is actually speeded up.

bretylium (bret-il'-i-um). Adrenergic blocking, antihypertensive drug.

Brevidil (brev'-i-dil). Suxamethonium (q.v.).

Brietal (brī'-et-al). Methohexitone sodium (q.v.).

Bright's disease. Inflammation of the kidneys. Nephritis (q.v.). [Richard Bright, English physician and clinician, 1789–1858.]

brilliant green. Antiseptic aniline dye.

Used as lotion (1:1000), paint (1 per cent), and ointment (2 per cent).

Brinaldix (brin'-al-dicks). Clopamide (q.v.).

Broadbent's sign. Visible retraction of the left side and back, in the region of the 11th and 12th ribs, synchronous with each heart beat and due to adhesions between the pericardium and diaphragm. See PERICARDITIS.[William Henry Broadbent, English physician, 1835–1907.]

broad ligaments. Lateral ligaments; double fold of parietal peritoneum which hangs over the uterus and outstretched Fallopian tubes, forming a lateral partition across the pelvic cavity.

Brocadopa (brŏk-á-do'-pá). Levodopa (q.v.).

Broca's area (brok'-a). The motor centre for speech; situated at the commencement of the Sylvian fissure in the left hemisphere of the cerebrum. Injury to this centre results in inability to speak. [Pierre Paul Broca, French surgeon and anthropologist, 1824–80]

Brocillin (brō-sil'-in). Propicillin (q.v.).

Brodie's abscess. See ABSCESS.[Sir Benjamin Collins Brodie, English surgeon, 1783–1862.]

bromethol (brom'-ēth-ol). A basal anaesthetic, used occasionally in surgery, in eclampsia and obstetric amnesia, and in tetanus. It is given as a freshly prepared 2½ per cent solution per rectum.

bromhexine (brom'-hecks-ēn). Synthetic derivative of vasicine, an alkaloid derived from a plant. Mucolytic; taken orally; it loosens sputum prior to coughing. An intravenous preparation is available; useful in status asthmaticus.

bromides (brō'-mīdz). A small group of drugs, exemplified by potassium bromide, which have a mild depressant action on the central nervous system. Used extensively in epilepsy before phenobarbitone was introduced; now used in nervous insomnia and restlessness, often in association with chloral.

bromidrosis (brōm-i-drō'-sis) [G. *bromos*, stench; *hidros*, sweat]. A profuse, foetid perspiration, especially associated with the feet — bromidrotic, adj.

bromism (brō'-mizm). Chronic poisoning due to continued or excessive use of bromides.

Bromocriptine (brō-mō-krip'-tēn). A

dopamine receptor agonist useful in Parkinsonism.

bromvaletone (brom-val'-ē-tōn). Mild hypnotic and sedative similar to carbromal.

bronchi (brong'-kī) [G. *brogchos*, windpipe]. The two tubes into which the trachea divides at its lower end—bronchus, sing.; bronchial, adj.

bronchial tubes (brong'-kē-ál tūbz) [G. *brogchos*, windpipe]. Subdivisions of the bronchi after they enter the lungs.

bronchiectasis (brong-ki-ek'-tas-is) [G. *brogchos*, windpipe; *ecktasis*, extension]. Dilatation of the bronchial tubes following infection such as bronchopneumonia with lobular collapse (which may have occurred in infancy). Associated with profuse, foetid, purulent expectoration. May lead to greatly limited ventilatory capacity and recurrent infection of lungs, cerebral abscess or amyloid disease—bronchiectatic, adj.

bronchiole (brong'-ki-ōl) [G. *brogchos*, windpipe]. One of the minute subdivisions of the bronchi which terminate in the alveoli or air sacs of the lungs—bronchiolar, adj.

bronchiolitis (brong-kē-ol-īt'-is) [G. *brogchos*, windpipe; *-itis*, inflammation]. Inflammation of the bronchioles, capillary bronchitis—bronchiolitic, adj.

bronchitis (brong-kī'-tis) [G. *brogchos*, windpipe; *-itis*, inflammation]. Inflammation of the bronchi; may be primary or secondary, acute or chronic. The basic reaction in these stages is the same; excessive secretion of mucus following an overgrowth of the mucous glands, sometimes with an added infection. Symptoms are a productive cough, wheezy breathing and varying degrees of breathlessness. In **acute b.** all can return to normal but in even **simple chronic b.** the bronchial mucous glands are hypertrophied and are unlikely to return to normal. In **chronic obstructive b.** the glands have become so hypertrophied that the bronchial lumen is narrowed and this is exacerbated by the extra mucus produced. **acute b.** is currently defined as an illness with cough, sputum and wheezy breathing presenting in a patient who was previously well. **simple chronic b.** is defined as cough and sputum for at least three months of the year, and occurring in at least two years; wheezing and shortness of breath are present either constantly or intermittently. In **chronic obstructive b.** breathlessness is a more severe symptom; because of the narrowness of the bronchial airways it is more difficult both for oxygen to get into the lungs and for carbon dioxide to get out. The oxygen in the blood therefore falls and the carbon dioxide rises. Normally these two stimuli increase breathing. In the patient with chronic obstructive bronchitis and a raised blood carbon dioxide, further elevation of carbon dioxide fails to produce any response. These patients tend to respond in their breathing only to a lack of oxygen and not to excess carbon dioxide. Should such a patient be given pure oxygen to breathe, he would be robbed of his stimulus to breathing; his carbon dioxide would accumulate and cause coma and death; he may be given air enriched with oxygen but not pure oxygen. Chronic bronchitis can cause right-sided heart failure, especially when associated with gross emphysema. See COR PULMONALE—bronchitic, adj.

bronchoadenitis (brong'-kō-ad-en-ī'-is) [G. *brogchos*, windpipe; *aden*, gland; *-itis*, inflammation]. Inflammation of bronchial glands.

bronchodilator (brong'-kō-dī-lā'-tor)[G. *brogchos*, trachea; L. *dilatare*, to dilate]. Any agent which dilates the bronchi.

bronchogenic (brong-kō-jen'-ik) [G. *brogchos*, windpipe; *genesthai*, to be produced]. Arising from a bronchus.

bronchogram (brong'-kō-gram) [G. *brogchos*, windpipe; *gramma*, letter]. Radiological picture of the bronchial tree rendered radio-opaque.

bronchography (brong-kōg'-raf-i) [G. *brogchos*, windpipe; *graphein*, to write]. Preparation of X-ray film after introduction of radio-opaque substance into the bronchial tree—bronchographic, adj.; bronchographically, adv.

bronchomycosis (brong'-kō-mī-kō'-sis) [G.*brogchos*, windpipe;*mykes*, fungus; *-osis*, condition]. General term used to cover a variety of fungus infections of the bronchi and lungs, e.g. pulmonary moniliasis, aspergillosis (q.v.)—bronchomycotic, adj.

bronchophony (brong-kof'-o-ni) [G. *brogchos*, windpipe; *phone*, voice]. Abnormal transmission of voice sounds heard over consolidated lung or over a thin layer of pleural fluid.

bronchopleural fistula (brong-kō-plooʹ-rál fisʹ-tūl-á) [G. *brogchos*, windpipe; *pleura*, rib; L. tube]. Pathological communication between the pleural cavity and a bronchus.

bronchopneumonia (brong'-kō-nū-mō'-ni-á) [G. *brogchos*, windpipe; *pneumones*, the lungs]. Small areas of the lungs are consolidated and coalesce, but do not have a lobular or lobar distribution. Complication of many medical conditions, especially measles and whooping cough. Relatively more common in infancy and old age—bronchopneumonic, adj.

bronchopulmonary (brong'-kō-pul'-mon-ar-i) [G. *brogchos*, windpipe; L. *pulmo*, lung]. Pertaining to the bronchi and the lungs—bronchopulmonic, adj.

bronchorrhoea (brong-kō-rē'-á) [G. *brogchos*, windpipe; *rheein*, to flow]. An excessive discharge of mucus from the bronchial mucous membrane—bronchorrhoeal, adj.

bronchoscope (brong'-kō-skōp) [G. *brogchos*, windpipe; *skopein*, to examine]. A type of endoscope (q.v.) used for examining the interior of the bronchi, removal of a foreign body, biopsy, etc.—bronchoscopic, adj.; bronchoscopy, n.; bronchoscopically, adv.

bronchospasm (brong'-kō-spazm) [G. *brogchos*, windpipe; *spasm*, spasm]. Sudden constriction of the bronchial tubes due to contraction of involuntary plain muscle in their walls—bronchospastic, adj.

bronchospirometer (brong-kō-spī-rom'-et-er) [G. *brogchos*, windpipe; L. *spirare*, to breathe; G.*metron*, a measure]. An instrument for measuring the capacity of one lung—bronchospirometric, adj.; bronchospirometry, n.

bronchostenosis (brong-kō-sten-ōs'-is) [G. *brogchos*, windpipe; *stenos*, narrow]. Narrowing of a bronchus—bronchostenotic, adj.

bronchotracheal (brong-kō-trak-ē'-al) [G. *brogchos*, windpipe; *trachus*, rough]. Pertaining to bronchi and trachea.

brow [A.S. *brú*]. The forehead; the region of the supraorbital ridge.

Broxil (broks'-il). Phenethicillin (q.v.).

Brucella (broo-sel'-lá) [L. after David Bruce]. A genus of bacteria causing brucellosis (undulant fever in man; contagious abortion in cattle). *Brucella abortus* is the bovine strain, *B. meliten-*

sis the goat strain, both transmissible to man via infected milk. [David Bruce, British pathologist and bacteriologist, 1855–1931.]

brucellosis (broo-sel-lō′-sis) [L. *Brucella,* after David Bruce: G. *-osis,* condition]. An infective reticulosis. A generalized infection in man resulting from one of the species of Brucella. There are recurrent attacks of fever and mental depression. The condition may last for months. Prescribed as an industrial disease under the National Insurance (Industrial Injuries) Act 1965 in relation to occupations involving contact with bovine animals infected by *B. abortus,* their carcasses or untreated products, or with laboratory specimens containing *B. abortus,* by reason of employment as a farmworker, veterinary worker, slaughterhouse worker, laboratory worker or in any other work relating to the care, treatment, examination or handling of such animals, carcasses or products.

Brudzinski's sign. Immediate flexion of knees and hips on raising head from pillow. Seen in meningitis. [Josef von Brudzinski, Polish physician, 1874–1917.]

Brufen (broo′-fen). Ibuprofen (q.v.).

bruise (brooz) [A.S. *brysan,* to crush]. A discolouration of the skin due to an extravasation of blood into the underlying tissues; there is no abrasion of the skin. A contusion.

bruit (broo′-ē) [F.]. See MURMUR.

Bryant's 'gallows' traction. Skin traction (q.v.) is applied to the lower limbs, the legs are then suspended vertically (from an overhead beam), so that the buttocks are lifted just clear of the bed. Used for fractures of the femur in children up to 4 years. [Sir Thomas Bryant, English surgeon, 1828–1914.]

BSR. Blood sedimentation rate. See ESR.

bubo (bū′-bō) [G. *boubon,* groin]. Enlargement of lymphatic glands, especially in the groin. A feature of soft sore (chancroid), lymphogranuloma inguinale and plague—bubonic, adj.

buccal (buk′-ál) [L. *bucca,* cheek]. Pertaining to the cheek or mouth.

Buerger's disease (ber′-gers). Thromboangiitis obliterans. Obliterative vascular disease of peripheral vessels. In an investigation, the incidence of HLA-A9 and HLA-B5 was significantly greater in those with Buerger's disease than in the controls. **B. exercises** were designed to treat this condition. The legs are placed alternately in elevation and dependence. [Leo Buerger, American physician, 1879–1943.]

buffer 1. A chemical substance which, when present in a solution, causes resistance to pH (q.v.) change when acids or alkalis are added. **2.** Anything used to reduce shock or jarring due to contact.

bulbar [L. *bulbus,* onion]. Pertaining to the medulla oblongata. See PARALYSIS and POLIOMYELITIS.

bulbourethral (bul-bō-ūr-ēth′-ral) [L. *bulbus,* onion; G. *ourethra,* urethra]. Applied to two racemose glands (Cowper's) which open into the bulb of the male urethra.

bulimia (bū-līm′-i-á) [G. *bous,* ox; *limos,* hunger] Excessive appetite. Seen in some cerebral lesions, diabetes mellitus and psychotic states.

bulla (bool′-lá) [L.]. A large watery blister. In dermatology, bulla formation is characteristic of the pemphigus group of dermatoses, but occurs sometimes in other diseases of the skin, e.g. in impetigo, in dermatitis herpetiformis, etc.— bullae, pl., bullate, bullous, adj.

Bull's regime. A method of treating temporary uraemia by giving glucose and peanut oil via gastric drip.

Buller's shield. A watchglass enclosed within a frame of adhesive plaster, to protect one eye when the other is infected. [Frank Buller, Canadian oculist, 1844–1905.]

bumetanide (hū-met′-an-īd). Potent diuretic. See ETHACRYNIC ACID.

bunion (bun′-yun) [O.F. *bugne,* a swelling]. Syn., hallux valgus. A deformity on the head of the metatarsal bone at its junction with the great toe. Friction and pressure of shoes at this point cause a bursa to develop. The prominent bone, with its bursa, is known as a bunion.

buphthalmos (buf-thal′-mos) [G. *bous,* ox; *ophthalmos,* eye]. Oxeye. Congenital glaucoma (q.v.).

Bupivacaine (bū-piv′-a-kān). One of the longer acting local anaesthetics. Synthetic; less toxic than cocaine. Suitable for obstetric analgesia by the caudal approach.

burimamide (bū-rim′-a-mīd). A histamine H$_2$ receptor antagonist which is only

active by injection. It has been super-
seded by cimetidine for the treatment of
ulcers.

Burkitt's lymphoma. Malignant lymphoma of the jaw and other sites in
children previously infected with E B
virus (q.v.). Occurs almost exclusively
in Africa and New Guinea in areas
where malaria is endemic. [Denis Burkitt. Contemporary surgeon.]

burn. A lesion of the tissues due to
chemicals, dry heat, electricity, flame,
friction or radiation; classified in three
degrees, viz. erythema, vesiculation or
deeper destruction.

Burow's operation. A flap operation for
closing a defect in the lip. [Karl August
Burow, German surgeon, 1809–74.]

bursa (bur'-så) [L. *bursa*, purse]. A
fibrous sac lined with synovial membrane and containing a small quantity
of synovial fluid. Bursae are found
between (1) tendon and bone; (2) skin
and bone; (3) muscle and muscle. Their
function is to facilitate movement without friction between these surfaces—
bursae, pl.

bursitis (bur-sī'-tis) [L. *bursa*, purse; G.
-itis, inflammation]. Inflammation of a
bursa. **olecranon b.,** miner's or student's
elbow. **prepatellar b.,** housemaid's
knee. A blow results in haemorrhage
into the bursa. Infection may be super-
added, pyogenic, tubercular or syphilitic.

Buscopan (bus-kō-pan). Hyoscine-*N*-
butyl bromide.

busulphan (bū-sul'-fan). Cytotoxic,
alkylating drug used in chronic myeloid
leukaemia and polycythaemia. Regular
blood counts are essential, as the compound is a powerful depressant of bone
marrow.

butacaine (bū'-ta-kān). Synthetic anaesthetic similar to cocaine. Used in ophthalmology as 2 per cent solution,
which, unlike cocaine, does not dilate
the pupil.

Butazolidine (būt-az-ol'-i-dēn). Phenylbutazone (q.v.).

butobarbitone (bū-tō-bårb'-i-tōn). Hypnotic of medium rapidity and potency
of action. Soneryl.

buttock (but'-ok) [M.E.*but*, end]. One of
the two projections posterior to the hip
joints. Formed mainly of the gluteal
muscles.

butylaminobenzoate   (bū-til-am-īn-o-

ben'-zō-āt). Local anaesthetic used as
ointment (1 per cent), suppositories (1
g), or dusting powder. A constituent of
Proctocaine (q.v.).

Butyn (būt'-in). Butacaine (q.v.).

byssinosis (bis-in-ō'-sis) [G. *byssos*, flax;
-osis, condition]. Form of pneumoconiosis due to inhalation of cotton or linen
dust. Scheduled under the National
Insurance (Industrial Injuries) Act.

C

cacao (ká-kā'-ō). The seeds of *Theobroma cacao* from which chocolate,
cocoa and cacao butter are prepared.
The latter does not become rancid and
melts at body temperature. It is therefore used as a base for suppositories, in
ointments and as an emollient.

cachet (kash'-ā). A flat capsule formed of
rice paper, enclosing any bitter pow-
dered drug which is to be taken orally.

cachexia (ka-keks'-i-á) [G. *kakos*, bad;
hexis, state]. A term denoting a state of
constitutional disorder, malnutrition
and general ill-health. The chief signs of
this condition are bodily emaciation,
sallow unhealthy skin and heavy lustre-
less eyes—cachectic, adj.

caecocystoplasty (sē-kō-sis'-to-plas-ti).
See   COLOCYSTOPLASTY—caeco-
cystoplastic, adj.

caecorectostomy (sē-kō-rek-tos'-tom-i)
[L. *caecus*, blind; *rectus*, straight; G.
stoma, mouth]. Syn., caecoproctos-
tomy. Anastomosis between caecum
and rectum.

caecosigmoidostomy (sē-kō-sig-moid-
os'-to-mi) [L. *caecus*, blind; G. letter E;
stoma, mouth]. Surgical anastomosis
between caecum and sigmoid flexure of
colon.

caecostomy (sē-kos'-tom-i) [L. *caecus*,
blind; G. *stoma*, mouth]. A surgically
established fistula between the caecum
and anterior abdominal wall.

caecum (sē'-kum) [L. *caecus*, blind]. The
blind, pouch-like commencement of the
colon in the right iliac fossa. To it is
attached the vermiform appendix; it is
separated from the ileum by the ileocaecal valve—caecal, adj.

CaEDTA. Calcium disodium versanate.
Used in lead poisoning and as eyedrops
in the treatment of lime burns. Chelating agent (q.v.).

Caesarean section (sē-zār'-i-an sek'-
shun). Delivery of the fetus through an

abdominal incision. It is said to be named after Caesar, who is supposed to have been born in this way. When delivery is accomplished extra-peritoneally, the term 'low cervical c.s.' is used.

caesium 137. A radioactive substance which, when sealed in a container can be used for beam therapy instead of cobalt; when sealed in needles or tubes it can be used for local application instead of radium.

caffeine (kaf'-ē-in). The central nervous system stimulant, present in tea and coffee. It has been given as a diuretic, but its main use is in analgesic preparations.

caisson disease (kā'-son) [F. *caisse,* from L. *capsa,* a box]. 'Decompression illness'. The bends. It results from sudden reduction in atmospheric pressure, e.g. divers on return to surface, airmen ascending to great heights. Due to bubbles of nitrogen which are released from solution in the blood; symptoms vary according to the site of these. The condition is largely preventable by proper and gradual decompression technique.

Caladryl (kal'-a-dril). Lotion and cream containing calamine and diphenhydramine (q.v.).

calamine (kal'-a-min). Zinc carbonate tinted pink with ferric oxide. Widely employed in lotions and creams for its mild astringent action on the skin.

calcareous (kal-kā'-ri-us) [L. *calcarius* from *calx,* lime]. Pertaining to or containing lime or calcium; of a chalky nature.

calciferol (kal-sif'-e-rol). Synthetic vitamin D. This, or natural vitamin D, is essential for the uptake and utilization of calcium. Given in rickets and to prevent hypocalcaemia in coeliac disease, and in parathyroid deficiency and lupus vulgaris.

calcification (kal-sif-i-kā'-shun) [L. *calx,* lime; *facere,* to make]. The hardening of an organic substance by a deposit of calcium salts within it. May be normal as in bone or pathological as in arteries.

calcitonin (kal-si-tōn'-in). Hormone produced in thyroid parafollicular or 'C' cells. Does not affect general metabolic processes. Role in normal physiology as yet uncertain. May link bone breakdown under special circumstances such as pregnancy. Now being used as drug therapy in Paget's disease.

calcium chloride (kal'-si-um klōr'-īd).

Deliquescent granules, very soluble in water. Occasionally given by injection in calcium deficiency, but, owing to its irritant properties, other calcium salts are preferred. Can be given by i.v. injection for cardiac resuscitation.

calcium disodium versanate (kal'-si-um dī-sō'-di-um vėr'-san-āt). CaEDTA (q.v.).

calcium gluconate (kal'-si-um gloo'-kon-āt). A well tolerated and widely used salt of calcium. Indicated in all calcium deficiency states, in allergic conditions and in lead poisoning.

calcium lactate (kal'-si-um lak'-tāt). A soluble salt of calcium, less irritating than calcium chloride. Used orally like calcium gluconate in all calcium deficiency states.

calculus (kal'-kū-lus) [L. small stone]. An abnormal concretion composed chiefly of mineral substances and formed in the passages which transmit secretions, or in the cavities which act as reservoirs for them—calculi, pl.; calculous, adj.

Caldwell-Luc operation. An opening is made above the upper canine tooth into the anterior wall of the maxillary antrum for drainage. [George Walter Caldwell, American surgeon, 1866–1946. Henri Luc, French laryngologist, 1855–1925.]

caliper (kal'-ip-ėr) [F. *calibre,* measurement]. 1. A two-pronged instrument for measuring the diameter of a round body. Used chiefly in pelvimetry (q.v.). 2. A two-pronged instrument with sharp points which are inserted into the lower end of a fractured long bone. A weight is attached to the other end of the caliper, which maintains a steady pull on the distal end of the bone. 3. Thomas' walking caliper is similar to the Thomas' splint, but the W-shaped junction at the lower end is replaced by two small iron rods which slot into holes made in the heel of the boot. The ring should fit the groin perfectly, and all weight is then borne by the ischial tuberosity.

callosity (kal-os'-it-i) [L. *callosus,* hard-skinned]. A local hardening of the skin caused by pressure or friction. The epidermis becomes hypertrophied. Most commonly seen on the feet and palms of the hands.

callus (kal'-us) [L.]. 1. A callosity (q.v.). 2. The partly calcified tissue which forms about the ends of a broken bone, which ultimately accomplishes repair of the fracture . When this is complete the bony thickening is known as 'permanent callus'—callous, adj.

calomel (kal'-ō-mel). Mercurous chloride (q.v.).

calor kal'-or) [L.]. Heat; one of the classic local signs of inflammation.

calorie (kal'-or-ē) [L. *calor,* heat]. A unit of heat. Currently in scientific terms, energy, work, and quantity of heat are measured in the same units—the joule, (J), and it will replace calorie, the joule being approximately ¼ calorie. The **small calorie** is the amount of heat required to raise the temperature of 1 g of water 1° C; the **large calorie** used in the study of metabolism is the amount of heat required to raise the temperature of 1 kg of water 1° C, sometimes called a kilocalorie (kcal).

calorific (kal-or-if'-ik) adj. [L. *calor,* heat; *facere,* to make]. Heat producing.

calvarium (kal-vă'-ri-um) [L. *calva,* bald head]. The vault of the skull; the skull-cap.

Camcolit (kam'-kō-lit). Lithium carbonate (q.v.).

Camoquin (kam'-ō-kwin). Amodiaquine (q.v.).

camphor (kam'-for). White solid with characteristic odour. Carminative and expectorant internally, and used as paregoric (q.v.) in cough mixtures. Applied externally in the form of camphorated oil as an analgesic and rubefacient—camphorated, adj.

canaliculotomy (kan-a-lik-ūl-ot'-o-mi) [L. *canaliculus,* small channel; G. *tome,* a cutting]. Excision of posterior wall of ophthalmic canaliculus and conversion of drainage 'tube' into a channel.

canaliculus (kan-alik'-ū-lus) [L. small channel]. A minute capillary passage. Any small canal, such as the passage leading from the edge of the eyelid to the lacrimal sac, or one of the numerous small canals leading from the Haversian canals and terminating in the lacunae of bone—canaliculi, pl.; canalicular, adj.; canaliculization, n.

cancellous (kan'-sel-us) [L. *cancelli,* lattice]. Resembling latticework; light and spongy; like a honeycomb.

cancer (kan'-sèr) [L. crab]. A general term which covers many malignant growths in many parts of the body. The growth is purposeless, parasitic, and flourishes at the expense of the human host. Characteristics are the tendency to cause local destruction, to spread by metastasis, to recur after removal, and to cause toxaemia. Carcinoma refers to malignant tumours of skin or mucous membrane, sarcoma to tumours of connective tissue—cancerous, adj.

cancerocidal (kan-ser-ō-sīd'-al) [L. *cancer,* crab; *coedere,* to kill]. Lethal to cancer.

cancerophobia (kan-se-rō-fō'-bi-à) [L. *cancer,* crab; G. *phobos,* fear]. Extreme fear of cancer.

cancrum oris (kan'-krum ōr'-is). Gangrenous stomatitis of mouth in debilitated children. Often called 'noma'.

Candida (kan'-di-dà). A genus of fungi. Yeast-like cells that form some filaments. Widespread in nature. *Candida* (*Monilia*) *albicans* is a commensal of the mouth, throat, vagina, gut and skin of man. Becomes pathogenic in some physiological and pathological states. May produce infections such as thrush, vulvovaginitis, balanoposthitis and pulmonary disease. Infection can result from disturbed flora due to use of widespectrum antibiotics, steroids, contraceptive pills, immunosuppressive and/or cytotoxic drugs. Can also occur during pregnancy, secondary to debilitating general disease such as diabetes mellitus or Cushing's syndrome. Can be due to poor oral hygiene, including carious teeth and ill-fitting dentures.

candidiasis (kan-did-ī'-a-sis). Disease caused by infection with species of Candida (q.v.). Moniliasis (q.v.).

canicola fever (kan-i-kō'-là). Infection (leptospirosis) of man by species of Leptospira from rats, dogs, pigs, (*Leptospira canicola*) foxes, mice, voles and possibly cats. There is high fever, headache, conjunctival congestion, jaundice, severe muscular pains, rigors and vomiting. As the fever abates in about one week, the jaundice disappears.

canine (kān'-īn) [L. *canis,* dog]. Resembling a dog. **c. teeth,** four in all, two in each jaw, situated between the incisors and the premolars. Those in the upper jaw are popularly known as the 'eye teeth'.

cannabis indica (kan'-ab-is in'-dik-à). Indian hemp, a narcotic drug once used as a cerebral sedative in nervous disorders. Marijuana; 'pot'.

cannula (kan'-ū-là) [L. dim. *canna,* a reed]. A hollow tube for the introduction or withdrawal of fluid from the body. In some patterns the lumen is fitted with a sharp-pointed trocar to facilitate insertion. It is withdrawn when the cannula is *in situ*—cannulae, pl.

cantharides (kan-thar'-i-dēz) [G. *cantharos*, beetle]. A blistering agent prepared from the dried Spanish beetle.

canthus (kan'-thus) [G. *kanthos*, corner of the eye]. The angle formed by the junction of the eylids. The inner one is known as the 'nasal canthus' and the outer as the 'temporal canthus'—canthal, adj.; canthi, pl.

Capastat (kap'-a-stat). Capreomycin (q.v.).

capillary (kap-il'-a-ri) [L. *capillus*, hair]. Hair-like. Any tiny thin-walled vessel, forming part of a network which facilitates rapid exchange of substances between the contained fluid and the surounding tissues. **bile c.** begins in a space in the liver and joins others, eventually forming a bile duct. **blood c.** unites an arteriole and a venule. **c. fragility**, an expression of ease with which blood capillaries may rupture. **lymph c.** begins in the tissue spaces throughout the body and joins others, eventually forming a lymphatic vessel.

Caplan's syndrome. Rheumatoid pneumoconiosis. Occurs in coal or asbestos workers with pneumoconiosis, who have or may develop rheumatoid arthritis.

capreomycin (kap-rē-ō-mī'-sin). Peptide antibiotic derived from *Streptomyces capreolus*. Main indication is as a secondary drug in treating drug resistant tuberculosis.

capsicum (kap'-si-kum). African pepper, used as a carminative and rubefacient.

capsule (kap'-sūl) [L. *capsula*, small box]. 1. The ligaments which surround a joint. 2. A gelatinous or rice paper container for noxious drugs. 3. The outer membranous covering of certain organs, such as the kidney, liver, spleen, adrenals—capsular, adj.

capsulectomy (kap-sūl-ek-'to-mi) [L. *capsula*, small box; G. *ektome*, excision]. Surgical excision of a capsule. Refers to a joint or lens; less often to the kidney.

capsulitis (kap-sū-lī'-tis) [L. *capsula*, small box; G. *-itis*, inflammation]. Inflammation of a capsule. Sometimes used as a syn. for frozen shoulder (q.v.).

capsulotomy (kap-sūl-ot'-om-i) [L. *capsula*, small box; G. *tome*, a cutting]. Incision of a capsule, usually referring to that surrounding the crystalline lens of the eye.

caput succedaneum (kap'-ut-suk-sē-dā'-nē-um) [G. *caput*, head; L. *succedaneus*, following]. A serous effusion overlying the scalp periosteum on an infant's head. Due to pressure during labour.

carbachol (kâr'-ba-kol). Parasympathetic nervous system stimulant similar to acetylcholin (q.v.) but active orally, and has a sustained action by injection. Given in postoperative retention of urine and intestinal atony, and as eye drops for glaucoma. Cholinergic agent.

carbamates (kar'-bam-āts). Tranquillizers, For poisoning, see p. 337.

carbamazepine (kár-bam-az'-ē-pēn). Anticonvulsant; also relieves pain; especially useful in trigeminal neuralgia.

carbaminohaemoglobin (karb-am-in'-ō-hē-mō-glō'-bin). A compound formed between carbon dioxide and haemoglobin. Part of the carbon dioxide in the blood is carried in this form.

Carbaryl (kar'-bar-il). Useful for treatment of head lice which are resistant to DDT and gammabenzenehexachloride.

carbenicillin (kar-ben-i-sil'-in). The only semisynthetic penicillin to show any reasonable acitivity against the antibiotic-resistant *Pseudomonas aeruginosa*. Unfortunately, even carbenicillin is not highly active against this organism. High concentrations can be achieved in the urine to destroy Pseudomonas there, but much larger doses of the order of 30 to 40 g a day are required to achieve sufficient concentration in the tissues. Such large doses can only be given by intravenous infusion.

carbenoxolone (kār-ben-oks'-ō-lōn). Extracted from liquorice. A relative of the corticosteroids. Specific healing effect on gastric but not duodenal ulcers. The method needs careful observation for the occurrence of oedema and potassium depletion.

carbidopa (kar-bi-dō'-pá). When added to levodopa allows reduction of dose, decreases frequency of adverse reactions and improves control of symptoms.

carbimazole (kár-bim'-a-zōl). An anti-thyroid drug that prevents combination of iodine and tyrosine. It is more potent and less toxic than methylthiouracil, and is the drug of choice in thyrotoxicosis.

carbohydrate (kár-bō-hī'-drāt) [L. *carbo*, coal; G. *hydor*, water]. An organic compound containing carbon, hydrogen and oxygen. Formed in nature by photosynthesis in plants. Carbohydrates are heat producing; they include starches, sugars and cellulose, and are classified in three groups—monosaccharides, disaccharides and polysaccharides. See CALORIFIC.

carbolic acid (kár-bol'-ik as'-id). Phenol (q.v.).

carboluria (kár-bol-ū'-ri-á) [L. *carbo*, coal; *oleum*, oil; G. *ouron*, urine]. Green or dark coloured urine due to excretion of carbolic acid, as occurs in carbolic acid poisoning—carboluric, adj.

carbon (kár'-bon). A non-metallic element. **c. dioxide**, a gas; a waste product of many forms of combustion and metabolism, excreted via the lungs. When disolved in a fluid, carbonic acid is formed; a specific amount of this in the blood produces inspiration; in cases of insufficiency, inhalations of CO_2 act as a respiratory stimulant. In its solid form—CO_2 snow—it is used in the removal of spider naevi. **c. monoxide**, a poisonous gas which forms a stable compound with haemoglobin, thus robbing the body of its oxygen-carrying mechanism; signs and symptoms of hypoxia ensue. **c. tetrachloride**, colourless liquid with an odour similar to chloroform. Used as an anthelmintic against hookworm and tapeworm, sometimes in combination with chenopodium oil. Previous fasting and subsequent purging is necessary.

carboxyhaemoglobin (kár-boks'-i-hēm-ō-glō'-bin) [L. *carbo*, coal; G. *oxys*, sharp; *haima*, blood; L. *globus*, globe]. A stable compound formed by the union of carbon monoxide and haemoglobin; the red blood cells thus lose their respiratory function.

carboxyhaemoglobinaemia (kár-boks'-i-hēm-ō-glō-bin-ē'-mi-á). Carboxyhaemoglobin in the blood—carboxyhaemoglobinaemic, adj.

carboxyhaemoglobinuria (kár-boks'-i-hēm-ō-glō-bin-ū'-ri-á). Carboxyhaem-oglobin in the blood—carbo-xyhaemoglobinaemic, adj.

Carbrital (kár-brit-ál). Carbromal (q.v.).

carbromal (kár-brō'-mal). Mild non-barbituric sedative and hypnotic. It may cause purpuric skin reactions in sensitive patients.

carbuncle (kár'-bung-kl). An acute inflammation (usually caused by Staphylococcus) involving several hair follicles and surrounding subcutaneous tissue, forming an extensive slough with several discharging sinuses.

carcinogen (kár-sin'-ō-jen) [G. *karkinos*, crab; *genesthai*, to be produced]. Any cancer-producing substance or agent—carcinogenic, adj.; carcinogenicity, n.

carcinogenesis (kár-sin-ō-jen'-e-sis) [G-*karkinos*, crab; *genesis*, production]. The production of cancer—carcinogenetic, adj.

carcinoid syndrome. Name given to a histologically malignant but clinically benign tumour of the appendix that secretes serotonin, which stimulates smooth muscle causing diarrhoea, asthmatic spasm, flushing and other miserable symptoms.

carcinoma (kár-sin-ō'-má) [G. *karkinos*, crab; *-oma*, tumour]. Malignant growth of epidermal tissue (e.g. skin, mucous membrane) and derivatives such as glands. Cancer (q.v.). **c-in-situ**, asymptomatic condition, also called intraepithelial c. of cervix. Cells closely resembling cancer cells grow from the cervical basal layer and eventually involve the whole epithelium so that its layers can no longer be recognized. Previously called pre-invasīve c.—carcinomatous, adj.; carcinomata, pl.

carcinomatosis (kár-sin-ō-ma-tō'-sis). A condition in which cancer is widespread throughout the body.

cardia (kár'-di-á) [G. *kardia*, heart]. The oesophageal opening into the stomach.

cardiac (kár'-di-ak) [G. *kardia*, heart]. Pertaining to the heart, pertaining to the cardia. **c. arrest**, complete cessation of the heart's activity. Failure of the heart action to maintain an adequate cerebral circulation in the absence of a causative and irreversible disease (Milstein). The clinical picture of cessation of circulation in a patient who was not expected to die at the time. This naturally rules out the seriously ill patient who is dying slowly with an incurable disease. **c. asthma**, see ASTHMA. **c. bed,**

one which can be manipulated so that the patient is supported in a sitting position. **c. catheterization,** a long plastic catheter or tubing is inserted into an arm vein and passed along to the right atrium, ventricle and pulmonary artery for (1) recording pressure in these areas; (2) introducing contrast medium prior to X-ray and high speed photography. Especially useful in the diagnosis of congenital heart defects. **c. oedema,** gravitational dropsy. Such patients excrete excessive aldosterone which increases excretion of potassium and conserves sodium and chloride. Antialdosterone drugs useful, e.g. spironalactone, triamterine. Both act as diuretics. **external c. massage** done for cardiac arrest. With the patient on his back on a firm surface, the lower portion of sternum is depressed 37.2 to 50.8 mm each second. **c. tamponade,** compression of heart. Can occur in surgery and penetrating wounds or rupture of heart—from haemopericardium.

cardialgia (kar-di-al'-ji-â) [G. *kardia*, heart; *algos*, pain]. Literally pain in the heart. Often used for heartburn.

Cardiazol (kár-dĭ'-a-zol). Leptazol (q.v.).

cardiogenic (kár-di-ō-jen'-ik) [G. *kardia*, heart; *genes*, producing] Of cardiac origin, such as the shock in coronary thrombosis.

cardiogram (kár'-di-ō-gram) [G. *kardia*, heart; *gramma*, a drawing]. Recording traced by a cardiograph (q.v.).

cardiograph (kár'-di-ō-gráf) [G. *kardia*, heart; *graphein*, to write]. An instrument for recording graphically the force and form of the heart beat—cardiographic, adj.; cardiographically, adv.

cardiologist (kár-di-ol'-oj-ist) [G.*kardia*, heart; *logos*, discourse]. A specialist in the study of cardiology.

cardiology (kár-di-ol'o-ji) [G. *kardia*, heart; *logos*, discourse]. The science dealing with the heart and its functions.

cardiomegaly (kár-di-ō-meg'-ál-i) [G. *kardia*, heart; *megas*, great]. Enlargement of the heart.

cardiomyopathy (kár-di-ō-mī-op'-ath-i) [G. *kardia*, heart; *mys*, muscle; *pathos*, disease]. An acute, subacute, or chronic disorder of heart muscle, of obscure aetiology, often with associated endocardial, or sometimes with pericardial involvement, but not atherosclerotic in origin—cardiomyopathic, adj.

cardiomyotomy (kár'-di-ō-mī-ot'-om-i) [G. *kardia*, heart; *mys*, muscle; *tome*, a cutting]. Heller's operation (q.v.).

cardiopathy (kár-di-op'-ath-i) [G. *kardia*, heart; *pathos*, disease]. Heart disease—cardiopathic, adj.

cardiophone (kár'-di-ō-fōn). Microphone strapped to patient allows audible and visual signal of heart sounds. By channelling pulse through an electrocardiograph, a graphic record can be made. Can be used for the fetus.

cardioplasty (kár-di-ō-plas'-ti) [G. *kardia*, heart; *plassein*, to form]. Plastic operation to the cardiac sphincter. See HELLER'S OPERATION—cardioplastic, adj.

cardiopulmonary (kár-di-ō-pul'-mon-a-ri) [G. *kardia*, heart; L. *pulmo*, lung]. Pertaining to the heart and lungs. **c. bypass,** used in open heart surgery. The heart and lungs are excluded from the circulation and replaced by a pump oxygenator—cardiopulmonic, adj.

cardioquin (kár'-di-ō-qwin). Quinidine (q.v.).

cardiorator (kár'-di-ō-rā-tor). Apparatus for visual recording of the heart beat.

cardiorenal (kár-di-ō-rē'-nal) [G. *kardia*, heart; L. *renalis*, of the kidney]. Pertaining to the heart and kidney.

cardiorespiratory (kár-di-ō-res-pīr'-at-or-i) [G. *kardia*, heart; L. *respirare*, breathe]. Pertaining to the heart and the respiratory system.

cardiorraphy (kár-di-or'-raf-i) [G. *kardia*, heart; *rhaphe*, a suture]. Stitching of the heart wall. Usually reserved for traumatic surgery.

cardioscope (kár-di-ō-skōp) [G. *kardia*, heart; *skopein*, to examine]. An instrument fitted with a lens and illumination, for examining the inside of the heart—cardioscopic, adj.; cardioscopically, adv.

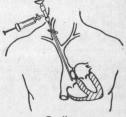

Cardioscope

cardiospasm (kár'-di-ō-spazm) [G. *kardia*, heart; *spasmos*, spasm]. Spasm of the cardiac sphincter between the oesophagus and the stomach, causing retention within the oesophagus ('achalasia of the cardia'). Usually no local pathological change is found.

cardiothoracic (kár-di-ō-thor-as'-ik) [G. *kardia*, heart; G. *thorax*]. Pertaining to the heart and thoracic cavity. A specialized branch of surgery.

cardiotocograph (kár-di-ō-tō'-kō-grof). See CARDIOGRAPH and TOCOGRAPHY.

cardiotocography (kár-di-ō-tok-og'-ra-fî). Tocography and ECG. The fetal heart rate is measured either by an external microphone or by the application of an electrode to the fetal scalp, recording the fetal ECG and from it the fetal heart rate. Using either an internal catheter which is passed into the amniotic cavity, or an external transducer placed on the mother's abdomen, the maternal contractions can also be measured. Both measurements are fed through a monitor in such a way that extraneous sounds are excluded and both measurements are recorded on heat-sensitive paper.

cardiotomy syndrome (kar-di-ot'-o-mi sin'-drōm). Pyrexia, pericarditis and pleural effusion following heart surgery.

cardiovascular (kár-di-ō-vas'-kul-ár) [G. *kardia*, heart; L. *vasculum*, a small vessel]. Pertaining to the heart and blood vessels.

cardioversion (kár-di-ō-ver'-shun). Use of electrical countershock for restoring heart rhythm to normal.

carditis (kár-dī'-tis) [G. *kardia*, heart; -*itis*, inflammation]. Inflammation of the heart. A word seldom used without the corresponding prefix, e.g. endo-, myo-, pan-, peri-.

Cardophyllin (kár-dof'-il-in). Aminophylline (q.v.).

caries (kār'-i-ēz) [L. decay]. Inflammatory decay of bone or teeth, usually associated with pus formation. spinal c. Pott's disease (q.v.)—carious, adj.

carina (kar-in'-á) [L. keel]. Any keel-like structure. Most frequently used for carina tracheae. a ridge across the base of the trachea, where the two bronchi divide—carinal. adj.

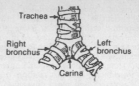

Carina

carminative (kár'-min-a-tiv) [L. *carminare*, to card; hence to cleanse]. Having the power to relieve flatulence and associated colic. The chief carminatives administered orally are aromatics, e.g. cinnamon, cloves, ginger, nutmeg, peppermint, etc.

carneous (kár'-ni-us) [L. *caro*, flesh]. Fleshy. c. mole, see MOLE.

carotene (kar'-ō-tēn) [L. *carota*, carrot]. A yellow pigment, which can be converted into vitamin A by the liver. A provitamin.

carotid (kár-ot'-id) [G. *karotides*, carotid arteries]. The principal artery on each side of the neck. At the bifurcation of the common carotid into the internal and external carotids there are: (1) the c. bodies, a collection of chemoreceptors which, being sensitive to chemical changes in the blood, protect the body against lack of O_2; (2) the c. sinus, a collection of receptors sensitive to pressure changes; increased pressure causes slowing of the heart beat and lowering of blood pressure. c. compression tonography, see TESTS.

carpal tunnel syndrome. Pain, numbness and tingling in the area of distribution of the median nerve in the hand. Due to compression as the nerve passes through the fascial band. Most common in middle-aged women. Nocturnal.

carphology (kár-fol'-o-ji) [G. *karphos*, chips; *legein*, to collect]. Involuntary picking at the bedclothes as seen in exhaustive or febrile delirium.

carpometacarpal (kár'-pō-met-a-kár'-pal) [G. *karpos*, wrist; *meta*, beyond]. Pertaining to the carpal and metacarpal bones, the joints between them and the ligaments joining them.

carpopedal (kár-pō-pē'-dal) [G. *karpos*, wrist; L. *pes*, foot]. Pertaining to the hands and feet. c. spasm, spasm of hands and feet in tetany, provoked by constriction of the limb. (Trousseau's sign.)

carrier (kar'-i-ér). A healthy animal or

human host who harbours a pathogenic or potentially pathogenic microorganism and passes it to his environment.

cartilage (kár'-til-āj) [L. *cartilago*, cartilage]. Gristle—cartilaginous, adj.

caruncle (ka-rung'-kl) [L. *caruncula*, small piece of flesh]. A red fleshy projection; that at the inner corner of eye being **lacrimal c. urethral c.** is a small bright red growth at the entrance to the urethra. It is very painful and bleeds readily on being touched. **carunculae myrtiformes**, the tag-like ends left after rupture of the hymen during coitus—caruncular, carunculate, carunculated, adj.

cascara (kas-kár'-á)· Purgative bark, used as the dry extract in tablets and as liquid extract and elixir for chronic constipation.

caseation (kā-zi-ā'-shun) [L. *caseus*, cheese]. The formation of a soft, cheese-like mass, as occurs in tuberculosis—caseous, adj.

casein (kā'-si-in) [L. *caseus*, cheese]. A protein produced when milk enters the stomach. Coagulation occurs and is due to the action of rennin upon the caseinogen in the milk, splitting it into two proteins, one being casein. The casein combines with calcium and a clot is formed. **c. hydrolysate**, predigested protein food derived from casein, easily added to other foods to increase the protein content.

caseinogen (kā-si-in'-ō-jen) [L. *caseus*, cheese; G. *genesthai*, to be produced]. The principal protein in milk. It is not soluble in water but is kept in solution in milk by inorganic salts. The proportion to lactalbumin is much higher in cows' milk than in human milk. In the presence of rennin it is converted into insoluble casein.

Casilan (kas'-ē-lan). A proprietary powder containing 90 per cent protein. Useful for maintaining adequate protein intake when patient can only take fluids.

cast. Fibrous material and exudate which has been moulded to the form of the cavity or tube in which it has collected, and this can be identified under the microscope. It is also classified according to its constitution, blood, epithelial, fatty, etc.

castor oil (kas'-tor). A purgative, of value in diarrhoea due to food poisoning.

Also used with zinc ointment for napkin rash and pressure sores.

castration (kas-trā'-shun) [L. *castrare*, to castrate]. The removal of the testicles in the male, or of the ovaries in the female—castrated, adj.; castrate, n., v.t.

catabolism (or **katabolism**) (ka-tab'-ō-lizm) [G. *kata*, down; *ballein*, to throw]. The series of chemical reactions in the living body in which complex substances, taken in as food, are broken down into simpler ones accompanied by the release of energy. This energy is needed for anabolism and the other activities of the body. See ADENOSINE DIPHOSPHATE and TRIPHOSPHATE. METABOLISM—catabolic, adj.

catalase (kat'-al-āz). An enzyme present in most human cells.

catalepsy (kat'-a-lep-si) [G. *katalepsis*, a seizing]. Term used by psychiatrists to describe sustained immobility (postural trance)—cataleptic, adj.

catalysis (kat-al'-i-sis) [G. *kata*, down; *lysis*, a loosening]. An increase in the rate at which a chemical action proceeds to equilibrium through the medium of a catalyst or catalyser. If there is retardation it is negative catalysis —catalytic, adj.

catalyst (kat'-al-ist) [G. *kata*, down; *lysis*, a loosening]. An agent which produces catalysis (q.v.). It does not undergo any change during the process. Syn., catalyser, enzyme, ferment.

cataplexy (kat'-a-pleks-i) [G. *kataplexis*, amazement]. A condition of muscular rigidity induced by severe mental shock or fear. The patient remains conscious—cataplectic, adj.

Catapres (kat'-a-pres). Clonidine (q.v.).

cataract (kat'-a-rakt) [G. *katarraktes*, cataract]. An opacity of the crystalline lens or its capsule. It may be congenital, senile, traumatic or due to diabetes mellitus. **hard c.**, contains a hard nucleus, tends to be dark in colour and occurs in older people. **soft c.**, one without a hard nucleus, occurs at any age, but particularly in the young. Cataract usually develops slowly and when mature is called a 'ripe cataract'.

catarrh (kat-ár') [G. *katarrhein*, to flow down]. Inflammation of a mucous membrane with constant flow of mucus—catarrhal, adj.

cat cry syndrome. See 'CRI DU CHAT' SYNDROME.

catecholamines   (kat-ē-kō'-la-mēns).

Adrenaline, noradrenaline and isoprenaline are the main catecholamines of pharmacological importance and they are all substances involved in the biochemical transmission of nerve impulses, particularly in the sympathetic system. Secreted by human tumours. Estimation of catecholamines in urine being carried out in research on hypertension and mental disorders. Experimental evidence suggests that catecholamines play an important role in mood regulation.

catgut (kat'-gut). A form of ligature and suture of varying thickness, strength and absorbability, prepared from sheep's intestines. After sterilization it is hermetically sealed in glass tubes in sizes 00000 to 8. The 'plain' variety is usually absorbed in 5 to 10 days. 'Chromicized' catgut and 'iodized' catgut will hold for 20 to 40 days.

catharsis (ka-thár'-sis) [G. *kathersis*, a cleansing]. In psychology, the outpouring from the patient's mind—cathartic, adj.

catheter (kath'-e-tèr) [G. *kathienai*, to send down into]. A hollow tube of variable length and bore, usually having one fluted end and a tip of varying size and shape according to function. Catheters are made of many substances including soft and hard rubber, gum elastic, glass, silver, other metals and plastic materials, some of which are now radio-opaque. They have many uses, from insufflation of hollow tubes to introduction and withdrawal of fluid from body cavities. A recent innovation is the fibre-optic cardiac catheter which, when in situ, picks up pulses of light from which the oxygen saturation of the blood can be determined.

catheterization (kath-e-te-rī-zā'-shun) [G. *kathienai*]. Insertion of a catheter, most usually into the urinary bladder. **cardiac c.**, fine polythene, or radio-opaque nylon tubing is passed via the median basilic vein at the elbow, into the heart: (1) to record pressures; (2) to introduce an opaque substance prior to X-ray; (3) to withdraw samples of blood—catheterize, v.t. See CATHETER.

cathetron (kath-e-tron). A high rate dose, remotely controlled, afterloading device for radiotherapy. Hollow steel catheters are placed in the desired position. They are then connected to a protective safe by hollow cables. The radioactive cobalt moves from the safe into the catheters. After delivery of the required dose, the cobalt returns to the safe, thus avoiding radiation hazard to staff.

Cathomycin (kath'-ō-mī'-sin). Novobiocin (q.v.).

cat scratch fever. Atypical tularaemia (q.v.). Distinguished from tularaemia by a positive LGVCFT. Probably caused by a virus.

cauda (kaw'-då) [L. *cauda*, tail]. A tail or tail-like appendage—caudal, caudate, adj.

caudal block. See EPIDURAL.

caul (kawl) [F. *cale*]. The amnion, instead of rupturing as is usual to allow the baby through, persists and covers the baby's head at birth.

cauliflower growth (kaw'-li-flour grōth). The proliferative free-growing type of cancer which forms an excrescence on the affected surface.

causalgia (kaws-al'-ji-å) [G. *kausis*, heat; *algos*, pain]. Excruciating neuralgic pain, resulting from physical trauma to a cutaneous nerve. Also known as reflex sympathetic dystrophy.

caustic (kaws'-tik) [G. *kaustos*, burnt]. Corrosive or destructive to organic tissue; the agents which produce such results. Used to destroy overgrowths of granulation tissue, warts or polypi. Carbolic acid, carbon dioxide snow and silver nitrate (lunar c.) are most commonly employed.

cautery (kaw'-tèr-i) [G. *kauterion*, a branding iron]. A caustic agent. **actual c.**, a hot iron used to apply direct heat. **galvanic c.** or electrocautery, a platinum wire maintained at red heat by an electric current. **paquelin's c.**, a form of actual cautery in which the hollow platinum point is kept at the required heat by a current of benzene vapour which is constantly pumped into it—cauterization, n.; cauterize, v.t.

caval infusion (kā'-val in-fū'-zhun). A method of treatment in acute renal failure with anuria. A radio-opaque nylon cardiac catheter is passed via the femoral vein to lie near the opening of the renal veins or at the entrance to the right atrium. A constant flow of hypertonic fluid is thus possible.

cavamesenteric shunt (kā-vå-mes-en-ter'-ik) [L. *caverna*, a hollow; G. *mesos*, middle; *enteron*; intestine]. After division of inferior vena cava the upper end is anastomosed to the superior mesenteric vein. Used in children when the portal vein is blocked.

cavernous (kav'-ėr-nus) [L. *caverna*, a hollow]. Having hollow spaces. **c. sinus**, a channel for venous blood, on either side of the sphenoid bone. It drains blood from the lips, nose and orbits. Sepsis in these areas can cause c.s thrombosis.

caved-S (kā'-ved). Liquorice compound for ulceration and inflammation of the upper intestinal tract.

cavitation (kav-i-tā'-shun)[L.*cavus*, hollow]. The formation of a cavity as in pulmonary tuberculosis.

cavity (kav'-i-ti) [L. *cavus*, hollow]. A hollow; an enclosed area. **abdominal c.**, that below the diaphragm; the abdomen. **buccal c.**, the mouth. **cerebral c.**, the ventricles of the brain. **cranial c.**, the brain box formed by the bones of the cranium. **medulary c.**, the hollow centre of a long bone, containing yellow bone marrow or medulla. **nasal c.**, that in the nose, separated into right and left halves by the nasal septum. **oral c.**, buccal cavity. **pelvic c.**, that formed by the pelvic bones, more particularly the part below the iliopectineal line. **peritoneal c.**, a potential space between the parietal and visceral layers of the peritoneum. Similarly, the **pleural c.** is the potential space between the pulmonary and parietal pleurae which in health are in contact in all phases of respiration. **synovial c.**, the potential space in a synovial joint. **uterine c.**, that of the uterus, the base extending between the orifices of the uterine tubes.

Cavodil (kav'-ō-dil). Pheniprazine.

CDH. Congenital dislocation of the hip. Recognized in the neonate by limitation of hip abduction.

Cedilanid (sed-i-lan'-id). Lanatoside C (q.v.).

Celbenin. Sodium methicillin. Antibiotic, useful in resistant staphylococcal infection.

Celevac (sel'-ē-vak). Methylcellulose. Gives bulk to intestinal contents and encourages peristalsis.

cell (sel) [L. *cella*, compartment]. A histological term for a minute mass of protoplasm containing a nucleus. Some cells, e.g. the erythrocytes, are nonnucleated; and others may be multinucleated—cellular, adj.

Cellophane (sel'-ō-fān). Trade name for a brand of a transparent, impermeable derivative of cellulose. Used in face masks; to protect, and prevent evaporation from, surgical dressings.

cellulitis (sel-ū-lī'-tis) [L. *cellula*, small cell; G. *-itis*, inflammation]. A diffuse inflammation of connective tissue, especially the loose subcutaneous tissue. When it involves the pelvic tissues in the female it is called 'parametritis.' When it occurs in the floor of the mouth it is called 'Ludwig's angina'.

cellulose (sel'-ū-lōz) [L. *cellula*, small cell]. A carbohydrate forming the outer walls of plant and vegetable cells. A polysaccharide which cannot be digested by man but supplies roughage for stimulation of peristalsis.

Celontin (sel'-on-tin). Methsuximide (q.v.).

censor (sen'-sor) [L. *censere*, to value]. Term employed by Freud to define the resistance which prevents repressed material from readily re-entering the conscious mind from the subconscious (unconscious) mind.

centigrade (sen'-ti-grād) [L. *centum*, hundred; *gradus*, a step]. Having one hundred divisions or degrees. Usually applied to the thermometric scale in which the freezing point of water is fixed at 0° and the boiling point at 100°.

centrifugal (sen-trif'-ū-gal) [G. *kentron*, centre of a circle; L. *fugere*, to flee]. Efferent. Having a tendency to move outwards from the centre as the rash in smallpox.

centrifuge (sen'-tri-fūj) [G. *kentron*, centre of a circle; L. *fugere*, to flee]. An apparatus which rotates, thereby increasing the force of gravity so that substances of different densities are separated. It is usually used to separate ('spin down') particulate material from a suspending liquid.

centripetal (sen-trip'-ct-al) [G. *kentron*, centre of a circle; L. *petere*, to seek]. Afferent. Having a tendency to move towards the centre as the rash in chickenpox.

centrosome (sen'-trō-sōm) [G. *kentron* centre of a circle; *soma*, body]. A minute spot in the cytoplasm of animal cells supposed to be concerned with division of the nucleus.

Centyl (sen'til). Bendrofluazide (q.v.).

cephalalgia (kef-al-al'-ji-á) [G. *kephale*, head; *algos*, pain]. Pain in the head. Headache.

cephalexin (kef-al-eks'-in). Cephalos-porin antibiotic, which unlike cephalor-idine, is well absorbed when given orally. Useful for urinary infections.

cephalhaematoma (kef-al-hēm-a-tō'-má) [G. *kephale,* head; *haima,* blood; *-oma,* tumour]. A collection of blood in the subperiosteal tissues of the scalp.

cephalic (kef-al'-ik) [G. *kephale,* head]. Pertaining to the head; near the head. **c. version,** an obstetric manoeuvre to change the fetal lie to a head presenta-tion.

cephalocele (kef'-al-ō-sēl) [G. *kephale,* head; *kele,* tumour]. Hernia of the brain; protrusion of part of the brain through the skull.

cephalohaematoma. See CEPHAL-HAEMATOMA.

cephalometry (kef-al-om'et-ri) [G. *kephale,* head; *metron,* a measure]. Measurement of the living human head.

cephaloridine (kef-al-or'-i-din) Semisyn-thetic antibiotic derived from cephalos-porin. Bactericidal against both penicillin sensitive and resistant strains of *Staphylococcus aureus.* Not active against *Pseudomonas pyocyanea.*

Cephalothin (kef-al-oth'-in). Antibiotic (q.v.). See CEPHALEXIN.

Ceporin. Cephaloridine (q.v.).

cerebellum (ser-i-bel'-um) [L.]. That part of the brain which lies behind and below the cerebrum. Its chief functions are the co-ordination of fine voluntary move-ments and the control of posture—cer-ebellar, adj.

cerebral (ser'-i-bral) [L. *cerebrum,* brain]. Pertaining to the cerebrum.

cerebration (ser-i-brā'-shun) [L. *cere-brum,* brain]. Mental activity.

cerebrospinal (ser'-i-bro-spī'-nal) [L. *cerebrum,* brain; *spina,* spine]. Pertain-ing to the brain and spinal cord. **c. fluid,** the clear fluid filling the ventricles of the brain and central canal of the spinal cord. Also found beneath the cranial and spinal meninges in the pia-arachnoid space. See MENINGITIS.

cerebrovascular (ser'-i-brō-vas'-kū-lár) [L. *cerebrum,* brain; *vasculum,* small vessel]. Pertaining to the blood vessels of the brain. **c. accident,** apoplexy caused by embolism, haemorrhage or thrombosis in the brain.

cerebrum (ser'-i-brum) [L.]. The largest and uppermost part of the brain; it does not include the cerebellum, pons and medulla. The longitudinal fissure divides it into two hemispheres, each containing a lateral ventricle. The inter-nal substance is white, the outer convo-luted cortex is grey—cerebral, adj.

certified (sér'-ti-fīd). A term used in rela-tion to insanity, prior to the Mental Health Act, 1960. Those patients who cannot leave a mental hospital of their own accord are now referred to as 'detained' patients.

cerumen (ser-oo'-men) [L. *cera,* wax]. A wax-like, brown secretion from special glands in the external auditory canal—ceruminous, adj.

cervical (sér-vī'-kal) [L. *cervix,* neck]. Pertaining to: (1) the neck; (2) the cervix (neck) of an organ. **c. canal,** the lumen of the cervix uteri, from the internal to the external os. **c. rib,** a supernumerary rib in cervical region, which may pres-ent no symptoms or it may press on nerves of the brachial plexus. Syn., thoracic inlet syndrome.

cervicectomy (sér-vi-sek'-to-mi) [L. *cer-vix,* neck; G. *ektome,* excision]. Ampu-tation of cervix uteri.

cervicitis (sér-vis-ī'-tis) [L. *cervix,* neck; G. *-itis,* inflammation]. Inflammation of the cervix uteri.

cervix (sér'-viks) [L.]. A neck. **c. uteri,** the neck of the uterus—cervical, adj.

cestode (ses'-tōd). Tapeworm. See TAE-NIA.

Cetiprin (set'-i-prin). Emepronium bromide (q.v.).

Cetrihex (set'-ri-heks). Mixture of cetri-mide and Physohex.

cetrimide (set'-ri-mīd) CTAB. Antiseptic with detergent properties, used as 1 per cent solution for wound, burns and skin sterilization. Cetavlon is a proprietary preparation.

CFT. Complement fixation test. See COMPLEMENT.

chalazion (kal-a'-zī-on) [G.]. A cyst on the edge of the eyelid from retained secretion of the Meibomian glands.

chalk (chawk). Native calcium carbon-ate. Used with other antacids in peptic ulcer, and with astringents in diarrhoea.

chalone (kā'-lōn). A hormone which inhibits rather than stimulates, e.g. enterogastrone inhibits gastric secre-tions and motility.

chancre (shang'-kér) [F. from L. *cancer,* crab]. The primary syphilitic ulcer asso-ciated with swelling of local lymph glands. The picture of chancre plus regional adenitis constitutes 'primary syphilis.' The chancre is painless, indurated and highly infectious.

chancroid (shang'-kroid) [L. *cancer*, crab; G. *eidos*, form]. Type of venereal disease prevalent in warmer climates. Also called 'soft sore'. Causes multiple, painful, ragged ulcers on the penis and vulva, often associated with bubo (q.v.) formation. Infection is by *Haemophilus ducreyi*.

character (ka'-rak-tér). The sum total of the known and predictable mental characteristics of an individual, particularly his conduct. **c. change**, denotes change in the form of conduct, to one foreign to the patient's natural disposition, e.g. indecent behaviour in a hitherto respectable person. Common in the psychoses.

charcoal (chár'-kōl). The residue after burning organic substances at a high temperature in an enclosed vessel. Used in medicine for its adsorptive and deodorant properties.

Charcot's joint (shár'-kōs). Complete disorganization of a joint associated with syringomyelia or advanced cases of tabes dorsalis (locomotor ataxia). Condition is painless. **c. triad**, late manifestations of disseminated sclerosis—nystagmus, intention tremor and staccato speech. [Jean Martin Charcot, French neurologist and clinician, 1825–93.]

cheilitis (kī-lī'-tis) [G. *cheilos*, lip, *-itis*, inflammation]. Inflammation of the lip.

cheiloplasty (kī-lō-plas'-ti) [G. *cheilos*, lip; *plassein*, to form]. Any plastic operation on the lip.

cheilosis (kī-lō'-sis) [G. *cheilos*, lip; *-osis*, condition]. Maceration at angles of mouth; fissures occur later. May be due to riboflavine deficiency.

cheiropompholyx (kī-rō-pom'-fo-liks) [G. *cheir*, hand; *pompholyx*, bubble]. Symmetrical eruption of skin of hands (especially fingers) characterized by the formation of tiny vesicles and associated with itching or burning. On the feet the condition is called 'podopompholyx'.

chelating agents (kē-lā'-ting). Soluble organic compounds that can fix certain metallic ions into their molecular structure. When given in cases of poisoning, the new complex so formed is excreted in the urine.

chemonucleolysis (kēm-ō-nū-klē-ol'-i-sis). Injection of an enzyme, usually into an invertebral disc, for dissolution of same—chemonucleolytic, adj.

chemopallidectomy (kem-ō-pal-id-ek'-to-mi) [Ar. *kimia*; L. *pallidus*, pale; G. *ektome*, excision]. The destruction of a predetermined section of globus pallidus by chemicals.

chemoprophylaxis (kē'-mō-prō-fil-aks'-is) [G. *prophylassein*, to guard against]. Prevention of disease (or recurrent attack) by administration of chemicals—chemoprophylactic, adj.

chemoreceptor (kēm-ō-rē-sep'-tor) [Ar. *kimia*; L. *recipere*, to receive]. 1. A chemical linkage in a living cell having an affinity for, and capable of combining with, certain other chemical substances. 2. A sensory end-organ capable of reacting to a chemical stimulus.

chemosis (kē-mō'-sis). An oedema or swelling of the bulbar conjunctiva—chemotic, adj.

chemosuppressive (kē-mō-sup-res'-iv), Syn., chemoprophylactic. See CHEM-OPROPHYLAXIS.

chemotaxis (kēm-ō-taks'-is), **chemotaxy** [Ar. *kimia*; *taxis*, arrangement]. Response of organisms to chemical stimuli; attraction towards a chemical being positive c, repulsion negative c.—chemotactic, adj.

chemotherapy (kēm-ō-ther'-ap-i) [Ar. *kimia*; *therapeia*, treatment]. Use of a specific chemical agent to arrest the progress of, or eradicate, disease in the body without causing irreversible injury to healthy tissues, e.g. employment of sulpha drugs in lobar pneumonia, of arsenic in syphilis, of nitrogen mustard in Hodgkin's disease. Chemotherapeutic agents are administered mainly by oral, intramuscular and intravenous routes, and are distributed usually by the blood stream.

Chendol (ken'-dol). Chenodeoxycholic acid, a detergent-like molecule normally present in bile. Being used to dissolve gall stones.

Cheyne-Stokes respiration. See RESPIRATION.

chiasm (kī-azm) [G. *chiasma*, cross]. An X-shaped crossing or decussation. **optic c.** or **chiasma opticum**, the meeting of the optic nerves; where the fibres from the medial or nasal half of each retina cross the middle line to join the optic tract of the opposite side. Also **chiasma**.

chickenpox. A mild, specific infection with varicella-zoster virus. Successive crops of vesicles appear first on the trunk; they scab and heal without leaving scars. Syn., varicella.

chilblain (chil'-blān). Congestion and swelling attended with severe itching and burning sensation in reaction to cold. Erythema pernio.

chimney sweep's cancer. Scrotal epithelioma (q.v.).

Chinese restaurant syndrome. Postprandial disturbance due to eating monosodium glutamate.

chiniofon (kin'-i-o-fĕn). An amoebicide used in prophylaxis, and the treatment of acute and chronic amoebiasis, often in association with emetine.

chiropodist (kī-rop'-o-dist) [G. *cheir*, hand; *pous*, foot]. One qualified in chiropody.

chiropody (kī-rop'-o-di). The treatment of callosities, corns, bunions and nail conditions.

chiropractic (kī-rō-prak'-tik). Manual movement of the vertebrae to relieve the impingement of subluxated transverse processes on the nerve roots.

chiropractor. One who believes that many diseases are due to interference with nerve flow. Skilled in vertebral manipulation.

chloasma (klō-az'-má). Patchy brown discoloration of the skin, especially the face. Can appear during pregnancy.

chloral hydrate (klor'-al hī-drāt). Rapid acting sedative and hypnotic of value in nervous insomnia.

chlorambucil (klor-am'-bū-sil). An oral alkylating agent (q.v.) used in lymphoproliferative disorders (q.v.).

chloramine (klor'-am-ēn). An organic compound that slowly liberates chlorine in solution. Has been used as a general surgical antiseptic as a 0.25 to 2 per cent solution.

chloramphenicol (klor-am-fen'-ik-ol). An orally effective wide range antibiotic. Drug of choice in typhoid and paratyphoid fevers, valuable in many infections resistant to other drugs. Used locally in eye and ear infections. Can cause aplastic anaemia.

chlorcyclizine (klor-sīk'-li-zēn). Long-acting antihistamine with few side effects. Also used in travel sickness.

chlordiazepoxide (klor-dī-az-ē-poks'-

īd). A benzodiazepine drug. Relieves anxiety and tension. Very few side effects. Useful in temporal lobe (psychomotor) epilepsy.

Chloretone (klor'-ē-tōn). Chlorbutol (q.v.).

chlorexolone (klor-eks'-ō-lōn). Thiazide diuretic. See CHLOROTHIAZIDE.

chlorhexidine (klor-heks'-i-dēn). An antiseptic effective against a wide range of bacteria. Used as 1:2000 solution as a general antiseptic, 1:5000 for douches and irrigation. Hand cream (1 per cent) is effective in reducing cross infection. (Hibitane.)

chlorine (klōr'-ēn). A greenish-yellow, irritating gaseous element. Powerful germicide, bleaching and deodorizing agent in the presence of moisture when nascent oxygen is liberated. Used chiefly as hypochlorites (eusol, Milton), chloramine or other compounds which slowly liberate active chlorine.

chlormethiazole (klor-meth-ī'-a-zol). Hypno/sedative capsules. Effective in controlling restless excitement with no Parkinsonian side effects.

chlorocresol (klor'-ō-krē'-sol). A bactericide widely used as a preservative for injections in multiple dose vials.

chlorodyne (klor'-ō-dīn). A solution of morphine, ether and chloroform in a mixture of liquorice, treacle and syrup. Widely used with kaolin as a gastric sedative as mist, kaolin et morph. BNF.

chloroform (klor'-ō-form). Heavy liquid, once used extensively as a general anaesthetic. Much used in the form of chloroform water as a flavouring and preservative in aqueous mixtures.

chloroma (klor-ō'-má) [G. *chloros*, pale green; *-oma*, tumour]. A condition in which multiple greenish-yellow growths grow on periosteum of facial and cranial bones, and vertebrae. Very rare, in association with acute myloid leukaemia.

Chloromycetin (klor'-ō-mī-sē'-tin). Chloramphenicol (q.v.).

chlorophyll (klor'-ō-fil) [G. *chloros*, pale green; *phyllon*, leaf]. The green colouring matter which assists in photosynthesis in plants. Now prepared medicinally and for external use as a deodorant.

chloroquine (klor'-ō-kwin). A potent antimalarial effective in the treatment and suppression of the disease. It is being added to the salt in some endemic areas. Also used in amoebic hepatitis and collagen diseases. Can cause ocular complications. Has a mild anti-inflammatory effect and in the long term will lower the titre of the rheumatoid factor in the serum.

chlorothiazide (klor-ō-thī'-a-zīd). Diuretic with a mild blood pressure-lowering action which does not change much with posture and rarely gives rise to symptoms of hypotension.

chlorotrianisene (klor-ō-trī-an'-i-sēn). Used as an alternative to stilboestrol. Favoured by some for menopausal symptoms, because of its prolonged oestrogenic action by slow release, but this is not an advantage if side effects occur, as the effect of the hormone cannot be immediately discontinued.

chloroxylenol (klor-oks'-i-len-ol). Antiseptic constituent of many non-caustic germicides. Less effective than phenol against some organisms.

chlorpheniramine (klor-fen-i'-rá-mēn). Short-acting antihistamine.

chlorpromazine (klor-prō'-mǎ-zēn). A drug of exceptional pharmacological action, as it is a sedative, antiemetic, antispasmodic and hypotensive. It increases the effectiveness of hypnotics, anaesthetics, alcohol and analgesics. Valuable in psychiatric conditions and management of senile patients. May cause skin sensitization, leucopenia, Parkinsonism and jaundice.

chlorpropamide (klor-prō'-pa-mīd). One of the sulphonylureas. Antidiabetic agent.

chlorprothixene (klor-prō-thicks'-ēn). Tranquillizer. Useful in acute schizophrenic conditions, but is less effective as treatment is prolonged.

chlortetracycline (klor-tet-ra-sī'-klin). Preparation of tetracycline (q.v.).

chlorthalidone (klor-thal'-i-dōn). Oral diuretic given on alternate days. Action lasts up to 48 hours.

choana (kō-ā'-ná) [G. *choane*, funnel]. Funnel-shaped opening. The posterior nasal orifices or nares (q.v.)—choanae, pl.; choanal, adj.

choked disc (or papilloedema). A blurring and obliteration of the cup or disc in the back of the eyeball (through which the optic nerve and vessels enter and leave the eye) by fluid distension, from whatever cause.

cholaemia (kol-ēm'-i-á) [G. *chole*, bile; *haima*, blood]. The presence of bile in the blood—cholaemic, adj.

cholagogue (kol'-a-gog) [G. *chole*, bile; *agogos*, leading]. A drug which causes an increased flow of bile into the intestine.

cholangiogram (kol-an'-ji-o-gram) [G. *chole*, bile; *aggeion*, vessel; *gramma*, letter]. Film demonstrating hepatic, cystic and bile ducts.

cholangiography (kol-an-ji-og'-ra-fi). [G. *chole*, bile; *aggeion*, vessel; *graphein*, to write]. Radiographic examination of hepatic, cystic and bile ducts. Can be performed: (1) after oral or intravenous administration of radio-opaque substance; (2) at operation to detect any further stones in the ducts; (3) after operation by way of a T-tube in the common bile duct; (4) by means of an injection via the skin on the anterior abdominal wall and the liver. Percutaneous transhepatic c.—cholangiographic, adj.; cholangiograph, n.; cholangiographically, adv.

cholangiohepatitis (kol-an'-ji-o-hep-a-tī-tis) [G. *chole*, bile; *aggeion*, vessel; *hepar*, liver; *-itis*, inflammation]. Inflammation of the liver and bile ducts.

cholangitis (kol-an-jī'-tis) [G. *chole*, bile; *aggeion*, vessel; *-itis*, inflammation] Inflammation of the bile ducts.

cholecystangiogram (kol-ē-sist-anj'-i-ō-gram) [G. *chole*, bile; *kystis*, bladder; *aggeion*, vessel; *gramma*, letter]. Film demonstrating gall-bladder, cystic and common bile ducts after administration of opaque medium.

cholecystangiography (kol-ē-sist-anj-i-og'-raf-i) [G. *chole*, bile; *kystis*, bladder; *aggeion*, vessel; *graphein*, to write]. Radiographic examination of the gall-bladder, cystic and common bile ducts after administration of opaque medium—cholecystangiographic, adj.; cholecystangiographically, adv.; cholecystangiograph, n.

cholecystectomy (kol-ē-sis-tek'-to-mi) [G. *chole*, bile; *kystis*, bladder; *ektome*, excision]. Surgical removal of the gall-bladder. Usually advised for stones, inflammation and occasionally for new growths.

cholecystenterostomy (kol-ē-sist-en-te-ros'-to-mi) [G. *chole*, bile; *kystis*, bladder; *enteron*, intestine; *stoma*, mouth]. Literally, the establishment of an artificial opening (anastomosis) between the gall-bladder and the small intestine.

Specific terminology more frequently used.

cholecystitis (kol-ē-sis-tī'-tis) [G. *chole*, bile; *kystis*, bladder; *-itis*, inflammation]. Inflammation of the gall-bladder.

cholecystoduodenal (kol-ē-sis'-tō-dū-ō-dēn'al) [G. *chole*, bile; *kystis*, bladder; L. *doudeni*, twelve at once]. Pertaining to the gall-bladder and duodenum as an anastomosis between them.

cholecystoduodenostomy (kol-ē-sis'-to-dū-ō-dēn-os'-to-mi) [G. *chole*, bile; *kystis*, bladder; L. *duodeni*, twelve at once; G. *stoma*, mouth]. The establishment of an anastomosis between the gall-bladder and the duodenum. Usually necessary in cases of stricture of common bile duct, which may be congenital, due to previous inflammation or operation.

cholecystogastrostomy (kol-ē-sis-tō-gas-tros'-to-mi) [G. *chole*, bile; *kystis*, bladder; *gaster*, belly; *stoma*, mouth]. The establishment of an anastomosis between the gall-bladder and the stomach; a palliative operation when the common bile duct is obstructed by an immovable growth.

cholecystogram (ko-lē-sis'-to-gram) [G. *chole*, bile; *kystis*, bladder; *gramma*, letter]. Film demonstrating gall-bladder after administration of opaque medium.

cholecystography (ko-lē-sis-tog'-raf-i) [G. *chole*, bile; *kystis*, bladder; *graphein*, to write]. Radiographic examination of the gall-bladder after administration of opaque medium—cholecystographic, adj.; cholecystographically, adv.; cholecystograph, n.

cholecystojejunostomy (kol-ē-sis-to-je-jūn-os'-tom-i) [G. *chole*, bile; *kystis*, bladder; L. *jejunus*, empty; G. *stoma*, mouth]. An anastomosis between the gall-bladder and the jejunum. Performed for obstructive jaundice due to growth in head of pancreas.

cholecystokinin (kol-ē-sis-to-kī'-nin) [G. *chole*, bile; *kystis*, bladder; *kinein*, to move]. A hormone which contracts the gall-bladder. Secreted by the upper intestinal mucosa.

cholecystolithiasis (kol-ē-sis-to-lith-ī'-as-is) [G. *chole*, bile; *kystis*, bladder; *lithos*, stone; N.L. *-iasis*, condition]. The presence of stone or stones in the gall-bladder.

cholecystostomy (kol-ē-sis-tos'-to-mi) [G. *chole*, bile; *kystis*, bladder; *stoma*, mouth]. A surgically established fistula between the gall-bladder and the abdominal surface; used to provide drainage, in empyema of the gall-bladder or after the removal of stones.

cholecystotomy (kol-ē-sis-tot'-om-i) [G. *chole*, bile; *kystis*, bladder; *tome*, a cutting]. Incision into the gall-bladder.

choledochoduodenal (kol-ē-dok-ō-dū-ō-dēn'-al) [G. *chole*, bile; *dechesthai*, to receive; L. *duodeni*, twelve]. Pertaining to the bile ducts and duodenum, e.g. c. fistula.

choledochography (kol-ē-dok-og'-ra-fi). See CHOLANGIOGRAPHY.

choledocholithiasis (kol-ē-dok-ō-lith-ī'-as-is) [G. *chole*, bile; *dechesthai*, to receive; *lithos*, stone; N.L. *-iasis*, condition]. The presence of a stone or stones in the bile ducts.

choledocholithotomy (kol-ē-dok-ō-lith-ot'-om-i) [G. *chole*, bile; *dechesthai*, to receive; *lithos*, stone; *tome*, a cutting]. Surgical removal of a stone from the common bile duct.

choledochostomy (kol-ē-dok-os'-to-mi) [G. *chole*, bile; *dechesthai*, to receive; *stoma*, mouth]. Drainage of the common bile duct, usually after exploration for a stone.

choledochotomy (kol-ē-dok-ot'-om-i) [G. *chole*, bile; *dechesthai*, to receive; *tome*, a cutting]. Incision into the common bile duct.

Choledyl (kō'-lē-dil). Choline theophyllinate (q.v.).

cholelithiasis (kol-ē-lith-ī'-a-sis) [G. *chole*, bile; *lithos*, stone; N.L. *-iasis*, condition]. The presence of stones in the gall-bladder or bile ducts.

cholera (kol'-é-rá) [G.]. An acute epidemic disease, caused by *Vibrio comma*, occurring in the East. The main symptoms are the evacuation of copious 'rice-water' stools accompanied by agonizing cramp and severe collapse. Spread mainly by contaminated water, overcrowding and insanitary conditions. High mortality.

choleric temperament (kol'-ér-ik). One of the four classical types of temperament (q.v.), hasty and prone to emotional outbursts.

cholestasis (kol-ē-stā'-sis) [G. *chole*, bile; *stasis*, a standing still]. Diminution or arrest of the flow of bile. **intrahepatic c.**, syndrome comprising jaundice of an obstructive type, itching, pale stools and dark urine, but in which the main bile ducts outside the liver are patent—cholestatic, adj.

cholesteatoma (kol-es'-te-a-tō-má) [G. *chole*, bile; *stear*, fat; *-oma*, tumour]. A benign encysted tumour containing cholesterol. Mainly occurs in the middle ear—cholesteatomatous, adj.

cholesterol (kol-es'-te-rol). [G. *chole*, bile; *sterol*, solid]. A crystalline substance of a fatty nature found in the brain, nerves, liver, blood and bile. It is not easily soluble and may crystallize in the gall-bladder and along arterial walls. When irradiated it forms vitamin D.

cholesterosis (ko-les-ter-ō'-sis) [G. *chole*, bile; *stear*, fat; *-osis*, condition]. Abnormal deposition of cholesterol.

cholestyramine (kol-es-tī'-rá-mēn). A basic ion-exchange resin which combines with bile acids in the intestine to give a product which is unabsorbed. Not only is the digestion of dietary cholesterol inhibited, but the excretion of bile acids is very much increased. Since bile acids are made from cholesterol, this leads to a pronounced loss of cholesterol from the body resulting in hypocholesterolaemia.

choline (kō'-lēn). A chemical found in animal tissues as a constituent of lecithin and acetylcholine. Thought to be part of the vitamin B complex, and is known to be a growth factor. Appears to be necessary for fat transportation in the body. Useful in preventing fat deposition in the liver in cirrhosis. Richest sources are dairy products. See CHOLEDYL.

cholinergic (kol-in-er'-jik) [G. *chole*, bile; *ergon*, work]. Applied to parasympathetic nerves which liberate acetylcholine at their terminations. See ADRENERGIC.

cholinesterase (kol-in-es'-ter-āz). An enzyme, which hydrolyses acetylcholine into choline and acetic acid, at nerve endings.

choline theophyllinate (kol'-ēn thē-of'-fil-āt). This compound resembles aminophylline in its general effects, but is less erratic in action. The incidence of gastric irritation is much less, and the response more reliable.

choluria (kol-ūr'-i-á) [G. *chole*, bile; *ouron*, urine]. The presence of bile in the urine—choluric, adj.

chondritis (kon-drī'-tis) [G. *chondros*, cartilage; *-itis*, inflammation]. Inflammation of cartilage.

chondrocostal (kon'-drō-kos'-tal) [G. *chondros*, cartilage; L. *costa*, rib]. Pertaining to the costal cartilages and ribs.

chondrodynia (kon-drō-din'-i-á) [G. *chondros*, cartilage; *odyne*, pain]. Pain in a cartilage.

chondrolysis (kon-drol'-i-sis) [G. *chondros*. cartilage; *lysis*, a loosening). Dissolution of cartilage—chondrolytic, adj.

chondroma (kon-drō'-má) [G. *chondros*, cartilage; *-oma*, tumour]. A benign tumour of cartilage. Tends to recur after removal.

chondromalacia (kon-drō-mal-ā'-si-a) [G. *chondros*, cartilage; *malakia*, softness]. Softening of cartilage.

chondrosarcoma (kon-drō-sär-kō'-má) [G. *chondros*, cartilage; *sarkoma*, fleshy overgrowth]. Malignant neoplasm of cartilage—chondrosarcomatous, adj.; chondrosarcomata, pl.

chondrosternal (kon'-drō-stēr'-nál) [G. *chondros*, cartilage; *sternon*, breast]. Pertaining to the rib cartilages and sternum.

chordee (kor-dē') [G. *corde*, string]. Painful erection of the penis due to urethritis. Common in gonorrhoea.

chorditis (kor-dī'-tis) [G. *chorde*, string; *-itis*, inflammation]. Inflammation of the spermatic or vocal cords.

chordotomy (kor-dot'-o-mi) [G. *chorde*, string; *tome*, a cutting]. Division of anterolateral nerve pathways in the spinal cord to give relief from the intense pain of advanced malignant disease. Temporary relief as for severe burns and shingles can be obtained by direct current electric c. under local anaesthesia. Also cordotomy.

chorea (kawr-ē'-á) [G. *choreia*, dance]. Disease manifested by irregular and spasmodic movements, beyond the patient's control. Even voluntary movements are rendered jerky and ungainly. The childhood disease is often called 'rheumatic chorea' or 'St. Vitus's Dance'; the adult form is part of a cerebral degenerative process called 'Huntington's chorea'—choreal, choreic, adj.

choreiform (kawr-ē'-i-form) [G. *choreia*, dance; L. *forma*, form]. Resembling chorea.

choriocarcinoma (kawr-i-ō-kár-sin-ō'-má). See CHORIONEPITHELIOMA.

chorion (kawr'-i-on) [G. outer membrane]. The outer membrane forming the embryonic sac—chorial, chorionic, adj.

chorion epithelioma (kawr-i-on-ep-i-thē-li-ō'-má)[G. *chorion*, outer membrane; *-oma*, tumour). A highly malignant tumour arising from chorionic cells, usually after a hydatiform mole, but may follow abortion or even normal pregnancy, quickly metastasizing especially to the lungs. Cytotoxic drugs have improved the prognosis.

chorionic villi (kawr-i-on'-ik-vil'-ī) [G. *chorion,* outer membrane; L. *villus,* shaggy hair]. Projections from the chorion from which the fetal part of the placenta is formed. Through the c.v. diffusion of gases, nutrient and waste products, occurs from the maternal to the fetal blood and vice versa.

chorioretinitis (kawr-i-ō-ret-in-īt'-is) [G. *chorion,* outer membrane; M.L. *retina,* from L. *rete,* net; G. *-itis,* inflammation]. Inflammation of the choroid and retina.

choroid (kawr'-oid) [G. *chorion,* outer membrane; *eidos,* form]. The middle pigmented, vascular coat of the posterior five-sixths of the eyeball, continuous with the iris in front. It lies between the sclera externally and the retina internally, and prevents the passage of light rays—choroidal, adj.

choroiditis (kawr-oid-ī'-tis) [G. *chorion,* outer membrane; *eidos,* form; *-itis,* inflammation]. Inflammation of the choroid. **Tay's c.,** degenerative change affecting the retina around the macula lutea. [Warren Tay, English physician, 1843–1927.]

choroidocyclitis (kawr-oid-ō-sīk-lī'-tis) [G. *choroeides,* choroid; *kyklos,* circle; *-itis,* inflamation]. Inflammation of the choroid and ciliary body.

choroidoretinal (kawr-oid-ō-ret'-in-al) [G. *choroeides,* choroid; L. *rete,* net]. Pertaining to the choroid and the retina.

choroidoretinitis. Syn. chorioretinitis (q.v.).

Christmas disease. Allied to haemophilia (q.v.). Caused by hereditary deficiency of clotting Factor IX (plasma thromboplastin component, PTC).

chromatogram (krō'-ma-to-gram) [G. *chroma,* colour; *gramma,* letter]. Tracing produced by chromatography.

chromatography (krō-ma-tog'-ra-fī) [G. *chroma,* colour; *graphein,* to write]. Consists of the separation of substances

on a chromatograph column. Such a column may be constructed in various ways but always consists basically of two phases. One is the stationary phase which may be solid, liquid or a mixture of both, and is finely divided and fixed in place (e.g. paper, in paper chromatography). The second is the mobile phase which may be liquid or gaseous and fills the spaces of the stationary phase through which it flows. The stationary and mobile phases are so selected that compounds which are to be separated by the chromatogram have different distribution coefficients between the phases.

chromic acid (krō'-mik as'-id). In a 5 per cent solution it is astringent, used in the preparation of chromicized catgut (q.v.); stronger solutions are caustic and can be painted on warts.

chromosome (krōm'-ō-sōm)[G.*chroma,* colour; *soma,* body]. Any one of the thread-like bodies into which the cell nucleus divides during mitosis, and which split longitudinally in that process. They carry hereditary factors (genes), the number being constant for each species—in man, 46 in each cell, except in the mature ovum and sperm where the number is halved as a result of reduction division. A set of 23 chromosomes is inherited from each parent—chromosomal, adj.

chronic (kron'-ik) [G. *chronos,* time]. Lingering, lasting, opposed to acute—chronically, adv.; chronicity, n.

Chvostek's sign (shvos'-teks). Excessive twitching of the face on tapping the facial nerve. A sign of tetany. [Franz Chvostek, Austrian surgeon, 1835–84.]

chyle (kīl) [G. *chylos,* juice]. Digested fats which, as an alkaline milky fluid, pass from the small intestine via the lymphatics to the blood stream—chylous, adj.

chylothorax (kīl-o-thaw'-raks) [G. *chylos,* juice; *thorax,* chest cavity]. Leakage of chyle from the thoracic duct into the pleural cavity.

chyluria (kīl-ūr'-i-á) [G. *chylos,* juice; *ouron,* urine]. Chyle in the urine, which can occur in some nematode infestations, when either a fistulous communication is established between a lymphatic vessel and the urinary tract, or the distension of the urinary lymphatics causes them to rupture—chyluric, adj.

Chymar (kī'-mar). Chymotrypsin (q.v.).

chyme (kīm) [G. *chymos,* juice]. Partially digested food which as an acid, creamy-yellow, thick fluid, passes from the stomach to the duodenum. Its acidity controls the pylorus so that chyme is ejected at frequent intervals—chymous, adj.

chymopapain (kī'-mō-pap-ān'). A proteolytic enzyme obtained from the latex of the pawpaw tree.

Chymoral (kī'-mor-al). Enzymes trypsin and chymotrypsin.

chymotrypsin (kī-mō-trip'-sin). Proteolytic enzyme. Useful in debridment of necrotic tissue, etc. and for loosening secretions, e.g. in respiratory tract. Also facilitates lens extraction.

Cicatrin (sik'-a-trin). Neomycin and bacitracin. Cicatrin aerosol spray is an amino acid antibiotic powder spray. It promotes healing of wounds under a light film. It is very convenient and time saving. Its best use is for superficial and shallow wounds. A two-second spray is all that is necessary at a distance of 20.32 to 30.48 cm from the wound. It has two disadvantages: if there is sensitivity to neomycin it must be stopped; it is expensive.

cicatrix (sik'-a-triks) [L. scar]. A scar; formed from connective tissue. See KELOID—cicatricial, adj.; cicatrization, n.; cicatrize, v.i.; v.t.

Cidex (sī-deks). Aqueous glutaraldehyde, a potent bactericidal agent useful for delicate surgical instruments and lenses.

Cidomycin (sīd-ō-mī'-sin). Gentamicin sulphate (q.v.).

cilia (sil'-i-a) [L.]. 1. The eyelashes. 2. Microscopic hair like projections from certain epithelial cells. Membranes containing such cells are known as ciliated membranes, e.g. those lining the trachea and Fallopian tubes—cilium, sing.; ciliary, ciliated, cilial, adj.

ciliary (sil'-i-a-ri) [L. *cilium,* eyelid]. Hair-like. c. body, a specialized structure in the eye connecting the anterior part of the choroid to the circumference of the iris; it is composed of the ciliary muscles and processes. c. muscles, fine hair-like muscle fibres arranged in a circular manner to form a greyish-white ring immediately behind the corneoscleral junction. c. processes, about 70 in number, are projections on the undersurface of the choroid which are attached to the c. muscles.

cimetidine (sim-et'-i-dīn). A histamine H_2-receptor antagonist which inhibits both resting and stimulated gastric acid secretion. Useful for active duodenal and prepyloric ulcers; should be taken after meals.

Cimex (sī'-meks). A genus of insects of the family Cimicidae. *Cimex lectularius* is the common bedbug, parasitic to man; bloodsucking.

cinchocaine (sin'-kō-kān). Powerful local anaesthetic used for surface anaesthesia (1 to 2 per cent), infiltration (0.05 to 0.2 per cent), and spinal anaesthesia. Lozenges, suppositories and ointment are available.

cinchona (sin kō'-na). The bark from which quinine (q.v.). is obtained. Occasionally used as a bitter tonic.

cinchonism (sin-kon-ism). Quininism (q.v.).

cincophen (sin'-ko-fen). Analgesic used in chronic gout and acute rheumatic fever. Toxic reactions such as nausea and jaundice may be severe.

cineangiocardiography (sin-ē-an'-ji-ō-kar-di-og'-ra-fi) Motion picture of passage of contrast medium through the heart and blood vessels.

cineangiography (sin-ē-an-ji-og'-ra-fi). Motion picture angiography (q.v.).

cineradiography (sin-ē-rā-di-og'-ra-fi) [G. *kineo,* to move; L. *radius,* ray; G. *graphein,* to write]. Moving picture radiography, e.g. showing joints or heart in action.

cineradiology (sin-ē-rā-di-ol'-o-ji). Specialist interpretation of cineradiography.

cinnamon (sin'-a-mon). An aromatic bark with carminative and mildly astringent properties. Sometimes used with chalk and other carminatives in diarrhoea.

cinnarizine (sin-á-rī'-zēn). Antihistamine drug, useful in Ménière's disease; has powerful vestibular sedative effect without concomitant hypnotic effect.

circadian rhythm. Rhythm with a periodicity of 24 hours.

circinate (sur'-sin-āt) [L. *circinare,* to make round]. In the form of a circle or segment of a circle, e.g. the skin eruptions of late syphilis, ringworm, etc.

circulation (sėr-kū-lā'-shun) [L. *circulare,* to form a circle]. Passage in a circle—circulatory, adj.; circulate, v.i. and v.t. c. of bile, the passage of bile from the liver cells where it is formed, via the gall-bladder and bile ducts to the small intestine, where its constituents are partly reabsorbed into the blood and thus return to the liver. **c. of cerebrospinal fluid**, takes place from the ventricles of the brain to the cisterna magna, from whence the fluid bathes the surface of the brain, and cord, including its central canal. It is absorbed into the blood in the cerebral venous sinuses. **collateral c.**, that established through anastomotic communication channels, when there is interference with main blood supply. **coronary c.**, that of blood through the heart walls. **extracorporeal c.**, blood is taken from the body, directed through a machine ('heart-lung,' 'artificial kidney') and returned to the general circulation. **fetal c.**, that of blood through the fetus, umbilical cord and placenta. **lymph c.**, that of lymph collected from the tissue spaces, which passes via capillaries, vessels, glands and ducts to be poured back into the blood stream. **portal c.**, that of venous blood (collected from the intestines, pancreas, spleen and stomach) to the liver before return to the heart. **pulmonary c.**, deoxygenated blood leaves the right ventricle, flows through the lungs where it becomes oxygenated and returns to the left atrium of the heart. **systemic c.**, oxygenated blood leaves the left ventricle and after flowing throughout the body, returns deoxygenated to the right atrium.

circumcision (sėr-kum-sizh'-un) [L. *circumcisus*, cut around]. Excision of the prepuce or foreskin.

circumcorneal (ser-kum-kor'-ni-al) [L. *circum*, around; *corneus*, horny]. Around the cornea.

circumoral (sėr-kum-ōr'-al) [L. *circum*, around; *os*, mouth]. Surrounding the mouth. **c. pallor**, a pale appearance of the skin around the mouth, in contrast to the flushed cheeks. A characteristic of scarlet fever—circumorally, adv.

circumvallate (sėr-kum-val'-lāt) [L. *circumvallare*, to surround with a wall]. Surrounded by a raised ring as the lingual papillae.

cirrhosis (sir-ō'-sis) [G. *kirrhos*, orange-tawny; -*osis*, condition]. Hardening of an organ. Applied almost exclusively to degenerative changes in the liver with resulting fibrosis. **c. of liver** is increasing in prosperous countries. Damage to liver cells can be by virus, microbes or toxic substances, and dietary deficiencies interfering with the nutrition of liver cells—often the result of alcoholism. Associated developments are such as ascites (q.v.), obstruction of the circulation through the portal vein with haematemesis (q.v.), jaundice and enlargement of the spleen—cirrhotic, adj.

cirsoid (sur'-soid) [G. *kirsos*, enlargement of a vein; *eidos*, form]. Resembling a tortuous, dilated vein (varix, q.v.). **c. aneurysm**, a tangled mass of pulsating blood vessels, appearing as a subcutaneous tumour, usually on the scalp.

cisterna (sis-tėr'-nä) [L. *cistern*]. Any closed space serving as a reservoir for a body fluid. **c. magna** is a subarachnoid space in the cleft between the cerebellum and medulla oblongata—cisternal, adj.

cisternal puncture. See PUNCTURE.

Citanest (sīt'-ä-nest). Prilocaine (q.v.).

citric acid (sit'-rik as'-id). The acid present in lemons. Widely used as potassium citrate; a diuretic.

citrin (sit'-rin). Syn. vitamin P. Thought to enhance the action of vitamin C in the prevention of scurvy in human beings. Capillary fragility is associated with lack of this substance. It is found in rose hips, citrus fruits and blackcurrants.

clap (klap). A slang term for gonorrhoea.

claudication (klaw-di-kā'-shun) [L. *claudicatio*, a limping]. Limping because there is interference with the blood supply to the legs. The cause may be spasm or disease of the vessels themselves. In 'intermittent claudication' patient experiences severe pain in the calves when he is walking; after a short rest he is able to continue.

claustrophobia (klaws-trō-fō'-bi-ä) [L. *claustrum*, a confined space; G. *phobos*, fear]. A form of mental disturbance in which there is a morbid fear of enclosed spaces—claustrophobic, adj.

clavicle (klav'-ikl) [L. *clavicula*, a small key]. The collar-bone—clavicular, adj.

clavus (klā'-vus) [L. nail, corn]. A corn, may be hard or soft.

claw-foot (klaw-foot). A deformity where the longitudinal arch of the foot is increased in height and associated with clawing of the toes. It may be acquired or congenital in origin. Syn., pes cavus.

claw-hand. The hand is clawed and radially deviated, due to paralysis of the flexor carpi ulnaris, ulnar half of flexor digitorum longus, affecting the small muscles of the hand.

cleft palate (pal'-it) [M.E. clift; L. pala'ium, palate]. Congenital failure of fusion between the right and left palatal processes. Often associated with harelip.

climacteric (klī-mak'-te-rik) [G. klimakter, rung of a ladder]. In the female, the menopause or 'change of life'. The end of the period of possible sexual reproduction, as evidenced by the cessation of menstrual periods. Other bodily and mental changes may occur. A corresponding period occurs in men and is called the male c.

clindamycin (klin-dá-mī'-sin). Derivative of lincomycin that is much more active than the parent compound.

clinical (klin'-ik-al) [G. kline, bed]. Pertaining to a clinic. Practical observation and treatment of sick persons as opposed to theoretical study

Clinimycin (klin-ı-mī'-sin). A brand of oxytetracycline (q.v.).

clitoridectomy (klit-or-i-dek'-to-mi) [G. kleitoris, clitoris; ektome, excision]. Surgical removal of the clitoris.

clitoriditis (klīt-or-id-ī'-tis) [G. kleitoris, clitoris; -itis, inflammation]. Inflammation of the clitoris.

clitoris (klit'-or-is) [G. kleitoris]. A small erectile organ situated just below the mons veneris at the junction anteriorly of the labia minora.

cloaca (klō-ā'-ká) [L. sewer]. 1. The common opening of the intestinal and urogenital tract in fishes and birds and reptiles. 2. In osteomyelitis, the opening through the involucrum which discharges pus —cloacal, adj.

clobetasol propionate (klō-bet'-as-ol prō-pī-on-āt). Soothing application for such skin conditions as eczema.

clofazimine (klō-faz'-i-mēn). Red dye, given orally. Controls symptoms of erythema nodosum leprosum reaction in lepromatous leprosy better than prednisolone.

clofibrate (klō-fib'-rat). Lowers blood cholesterol and is used to prevent fat embolism, particularly in patients with bone injury.

Clomid (klō'-mid). Clomiphene (q.v.).

Clomiphene (klom'-i-fēn) (MRL. 41) 'Fertility pill'. Synthetic non-steroidal compound which induces ovulation and subsequent menstruation in some otherwise anovulatory women. Consequently fertility is enhanced.

clomipramine (klom-ip'-rà-mēn). One of the tricyclic antidepressants. Effective after 3 to 15 days medication. Can be given by slow i.v. drip, in increasing dose for obsessional and phobic anxiety states.

clomocycline (klo-mō-sī'-klin). Modification of tetracycline (q.v.).

clonidine (klon'-i-dēn). Similar to methyldopa, but causes less postural hypotension though it gives some patients a very dry mouth. Early results in the prevention of migraine are promising.

clonus (klō'-nus) [G. klonos, violent]. A series of intermittent muscular contractions and relaxations. Opp. tonic (q.v.)—clonic, adj.; clonicity, n.

clopamide (klō'-pá-mīd). Thiazide diuretic. See CHLOROTHIAZIDE.

Clostridium (klos-trid'-i-um). A bacterial genus. Clostridia are large Grampositive anaerobic bacilli found as commensals of the gut of animals and man, and as saprophytes in the soil. Endospores are produced which are widely distributed. Many species are pathogenic because of the exotoxins produced e.g. Clostridium tetani (tetanus), C. botulinum (botulism); C. welchii (perfringens) (gas gangrene).

clove oil (klōv). Has antiseptic, carminative and anodyne properties. Used to relieve toothache.

cloxacillin (kloks-a-sil'-lin). Semisynthetic penicillin active against penicillin-resistant staphylococci. Acid stable. Given orally or parenterally.

clubbed fingers. Swelling of the soft tissue at the extremities. Seen in heart and lung disease.

club-foot [O.N. klubba; A.S. fot]. A congenital malformation, either unilateral or bilateral. See TALIPES.

clumping. See AGGLUTINATION.

Clutton's joints. Symmetrical swelling of joints, usually painless, the knees often being involved. Associated with congenital syphilis. [Henry Hugh Clutton, English surgeon, 1850–1909.]

clysis (klī'sis) [G. klysis, a drenching by enema]. 1. The cleansing or washing out of a cavity. 2. Term used when administering fluids by other than the oral route: subcutaneously (hypodermoclysis); intravenously (venoclysis); rectally (proctoclysis).

Clysodrast (klī'-sō-drast). Specific enema in preparation for X-ray.

coagulase (kō-ag'-ū-lās). An enzyme which clots plasma, e.g. thrombin, rennin. Produced by some bacteria (e.g. *Staphylococcus aureus*). Used to type bacteria into c. negative and positive.

coagulum (kō-ag'-ū-lum)[L.]. Any coagulated mass. Scab.

coalesce (kō-ā-les') [L. *coalescere,* to grow together]. To grow together; to unite into a mass. Often used to describe the development of a skin eruption, when discrete areas of affected skin coalesce to form sheets of a similar appearance, e.g. psoriasis, pityriasis rubra pilaris—coalescence, n.; coalescent, adj.

coal tar. The black substance obtained by the distillation of coal. Used in psoriasis and eczema. Liq. picis, carb. is an alcoholic solution of the soluble constituents of coal tar.

coarctation (kō-árk-tā'-shun) [L. *coarctare,* to press together]. Contraction, stricture, narrowing; applied to a vessel or canal.

Cobadex (kob'-ā-deks). Cream containing hydrocortisone which is not absorbed through the skin and so does not produce local or systemic side effects.

cobalt (kō'-bawlt). A mineral element considered nutritionally essential in minute traces. Thought to be linked with iron and copper in prevention of anaemia. Co 58, used as tracer in study of cobalt metabolism. Co 60 now superseding radium in radiotherapy (Co bomb), Co edetate, used in cyanide poisoning.

cocaine (kō-kān'). Powerful local anaesthetic obtained from coca leaves. It is toxic, especially to the brain. It may cause agitation, disorientation, and convulsions. It can induce addiction. It has vasoconstrictor properties, hence the blanching which occurs when it is applied to mucous membranes. It is now largely replaced by less toxic compounds such as procaine and lignocaine, but is still used as eye drops, often with homatropine.

cocainism (kō-kān'-izm). Mental and physical degeneracy caused by a morbid craving for, and excessive use of cocaine.

coccus (kok'-us) [G. *kokkos,* berry]. A spherical, or nearly spherical bacterium—cocci, pl.; coccal, coccoid, adj.

coccydynia (koks-ē-din'-i-a)[G.*kokkyx,* cuckoo; *odyne,* pain]. Pain in the region of the coccyx.

coccygectomy (kok-si-jek'-to-mi) [G. *kokkyx,* cuckoo; *ektome,* excision]. Surgical removal of the coccyx.

coccygodynia (koks-ē-go-din'-i-á). Syn. coccydynia (q.v.).

coccyx (kok'-siks) [G. *kokkyx,* cuckoo]. The last bone of the vertebral column. It is triangular in shape and curved slightly forward. It is composed of four rudimentary vertebrae, cartilaginous at birth, ossification being completed at about the 30th year—coccygeal, adj.

cochlea (kok'-lē-á) [L. snail]. A spiral canal resembling the interior of a snail shell, in the anterior part of the bony labyrinth of the ear—cochlear, adj.

Cockett's operation (kok-ots). For recurrent varicose veins or impending ulceration which has failed to respond to simple ligation and stripping. Involves deep dissection; communicating veins tied at the level of the deep fascia.

cocoa (kō'-kō). The seeds of *Theobroma cacao.* The powder is made into a nourishing pleasant beverage. Contains theobromine and caffeine. **c. butter,** obtained from the roasted seeds; is used in suppositories, ointments and as an emollient.

codeine (kō'-di-in). An alkaloid of opium. It has mild analgesic properties, and is used with aspirin and phenacetin in tab. codeine co. Valuable as a cough sedative (linctus codeine) in dry and useless cough.

cod liver oil. Contains vitamins A and D, and used on that account as a dietary supplement in mild deficiency. Can be applied as a dressing to promote healing.

coeliac (sē'-li-ak)[G.*koilia,* belly]. Relating to the abdominal cavity. Applied to arteries, veins, nerves and a plexus. **c. syndrome,** now described as a number of separate and identifiable conditions of which the most important are cystic fibrosis (fibrocystic disease of the pancreas) and **c. disease** (gluten-induced enteropathy). Cystic fibrosis is largely an abnormality of the mucus-secreting glands. There is a definite excess of mucus and it appears to be thicker and more tenacious than normal. Histologically both the glands and the mucus appear normal. It usually affects the pancreas, small intestine and lungs. The mucus blocks the digestive juices, thus halting the digestion of food. As the disease progresses the mucus-secreting glands are replaced by fibroid tissue and cysts. There is an increase of sodium and chloride in the sweat. Gluten-induced enteropathy is often called coeliac disease. It is due to intolerance to the protein gluten in wheat and rye, it being the gliadin fraction that is the harmful substance. Sensitivity occurs in the villi of the small intestine, and produces the malabsorption syndrome. Symptoms become apparent at three to six months, soon after the child is weaned on to cereals, as up to this time the digestion is not interfered with. On weaning the absorption of fats is impaired, and large amounts of split fats may be excreted in the stools. See STEATORRHOEA.

coelioscopy (sē-li-ŏs'-ko-pi) [G. koilia, belly; skopein, to view]. Syn., laparoscopy, peritoneoscopy (q.v.).

co-enzyme (ko-en'-zīm) [L. cum, with; G. en, in; zyme, leaven]. An enzyme activator; kinase. See BIOTIN.

Cogentin (kō-jen'-tin). Benztropine methanesulphonate (q.v.).

cognition (kog-ni'-shun) [L. cognitio, recognition]. Awareness; one of the three aspects of mind, the others being affection (feeling or emotion), and conation (willing or desiring). They work as a whole but any one may dominate any mental process.

coitus (kō'-it-us) [L. from coire, to come together]. The act of sexual intercourse; copulation.

colchicum (kol'-chi-kum). The dried corm of the autumn crocus. It contains colchicine, and is of value in the treatment of acute gout.

colectomy (kō-lek'-to-mi) [G. kolon; ektome, excision]. Excision of part or the whole of the colon.

colic (kol'-ik) [G. kolikos, suffering in the colon]. Severe pain resulting from periodic spasm in an abdominal organ. biliary c., spasm of smooth muscle in a bile duct caused by a gallstone. intestinal c., abnormal peristalsic movement of an irritated gut. painter's (lead) c., spasm of intestine and constriction of mesenteric vessels. renal c., spasm of ureter due to a stone. uterine c., dysmenorrhoea (q.v.)—colicky, adj.

coliform (kō'-li-form) [G. kolon, colon; forma, shape]. A word used to describe any bacterium of faecal origin which is morphologically similar to E. coli.

colistin (kol'-is-tin). An antibiotic active against many Gram-negative organisms. Useful in Pseudomonas pyocyanea infections. Less toxic than polymyxin B.

colitis (kō-lī'-tis) [G. kolon, colon; -itis, inflammation]. Inflammation of the colon. May be acute or chronic, and may be accompanied by ulcerative lesions. ulcerative c., an inflammatory and ulcerative condition of the colon. Aetiological evidence is changing from psychosomatic factors to an immunological basis for the condition. Characteristically it affects young and early middle-aged adults, producing periodic bouts of diarrhoeal stools containing mucus and blood, and it may vary in severity from a mild form with little constitutional upset to a severe, dangerous and prostrating illness.

collagen (kol'-a-jen) [G. kolla, glue; gen esthai, to be produced]. An albuminoid substance arranged in bundles. It is the main constituent of white fibrous tissue. The 'collagen diseases' are characterized by an inflammatory lesion of unknown aetiology affecting collagen and small blood vessels. c. diseases said to be due to development of a hypersensitivity state. They include dermatomyositis, lupus erythematosus, polyarteritis (periarteritis) nodosa, and scleroderma, and are almost invariably fatal collagenic, collagenous, adj.

collagen proline hydroxylase (kol'-a-jen prō'-lēn hī-droks'-i-lās). Enzyme necessary for wound healing, and vitamin C is necessary for this enzyme's maintenance and function. Research indicates that tissues which are rapidly synthesizing collagen (e.g. healing wounds) have high levels of this enzyme.

collapse (kol-aps') [L. collapsus, fallen together]. 1. Physical or nervous prostration. 2. The 'falling in' of a hollow organ or vessel, e.g. collapse of lung from change of air pressure inside or outside the organ.

collar-bone [L. collum, neck; A.S. bān]. The clavicle.

collateral (kol-lat'-ĕr-l) [L. com, with; latera, sides]. Accessory, secondary. c.

circulation established by blood flowing in vessels alternative to the direct, main one.

Colles' fracture. See FRACTURE.

Colles' law. A mother may breastfeed a syphilitic baby without herself becoming infected, the explanation being that the mother had first acquired the disease and the fetus was thereafter infected *in utero*. The mother's apparent freedom from evidence of the infection implies that she is passing through the latent (hidden) phase of syphilis. [Abraham Colles, Irish surgeon, 1773-1843.]

colliquative (kol'-i-kwāt-iv) [L. *com.* with; *liquare*, to melt]. Profuse, excessive.

collodion (ko-lō'-di-on). A solution of pyroxylin with resin and castor oil. It forms a flexible film on the skin, and is used mainly as a protective dressing.

colloid (kol'-oid) [G. *kolla*, glue; *eidos*, form]. A glue-like non-crystalline substance; diffusible but not soluble in water; unable to pass through an animal membrane. Some drugs can be prepared in their colloidal form. c. goitre, abnormal enlargement of the thyroid gland, due to the accumulation in it of viscid, iodine-containing colloid.

coloboma (kōl-o-bō'-mā) [G. *kolobos*, shortened, mutilated]. A congenital fissure or gap in the eyeball or one of its parts, e.g. c. iridis—colobomata, pl.

colocystoplasty (kol-ō-sis'-tō-plas-ti) [G. *kolon*; *kystis*, bladder; *plassein*, to form]. Operation to increase urinary bladder by using part of the colon—colocystoplastic, adj.

Colomycin. Colistin (q.v.).

colon (kō'-lon) [G. *kolon*, colon]. The large bowel extending from the caecum to the rectum. In its various parts it has appropriate names—ascending c., transverse c., descending c., sigmoid c. spasmodic c., megacolon (q.v.)—colonic, adj.

colonoscopy (kō-lon-os'-kop-i). Use of a fibreoptic colonoscope to view the inner membrane of the colon.

colony (kol'-on-i) [L. *colonia*, colony]. A mass of bacteria which is the result of multiplication of one or more organisms. A colony may contain many millions of individual organisms and become macroscopic (q.v.); its physical features are often characteristic of the species.

colostomy (kol-os'-tom-i) [G. *kolon*, colon; *stoma*, mouth]. A surgically established fistula between the colon and the surface of the abdomen; this acts as an artificial anus.

colostrum (kol-os'-trum) [L.]. The relatively clear fluid secreted in the breasts during the first three days after parturition, before the formation of true milk is established.

colotomy (kol-ot'-om-i) [G. *kolon*, colon; *tome*, a cutting]. Incision into the colon.

colour blindness. Achromatopsia (q.v.).

colour index. A term formerly used to express the amount of haemoglobin in red blood cells. Replaced by MCHC.

colovesicoplasty (kol-ō-ves'-i-kō-plas-ti) [G. *kolon*, colon; L. form]. Colocystoplasty (q.v.).

colpitis (kol-pī'-tis) [G. *kolpos*, a hollow; *-itis*, inflammation]. Inflammation of the vagina.

colpocentesis (kol-pō-sen-tē'-sis) [G. *kolpos*, a hollow; *kentesis*, puncture]. Withdrawal of fluid from the vagina, as in haematocolpos.

colpohysterectomy (kol-pō-his-ter-ek'-to-mi) [G. *kolpos*, a hollow; *hystera*, womb; *ektome*, excision]. Removal of uterus through the vagina.

colpoperineorrhaphy (kol-pō-per-in-ē-or'-af-i) [G. *kolpos*, a hollow; *perinaion*, space between the anus and scrotum; *rhaphe*, a suture]. The surgical repair of an injured vagina and deficient perineum.

colpophotography (kol-pō-fo-tog'-ra'-fi). Filming the cervix using a camera and colposcope.

colporrhaphy (kol-por'-af-i) [G. *kolpos*, a hollow; *rhaphe*, a suture]. Surgical repair of the vagina. Anterior c. for repair of cystocele (q.v.) and posterior c. for repair of a rectocele (q.v.).

colposcope (kol'-pō-skōp) [G. *kolpos*, a hollow; *skopein*, to examine]. Culdoscope (q.v.)—colposcopically, adv.; colposcopy, n.

colpotomy (kol-pot'-om-i) [G. *kolpos*, a hollow; *tome*, a cutting]. Incision of the vaginal wall. Posterior c. to drain an abscess in the pouch of Douglas through the vagina.

coma (kō'-mā) [G. *koma*, deep sleep]. Complete loss of consciousness. Seen in alcoholism, diabetes, uraemia, and following an epileptic attack, etc.

comatose (kōm'-a-tōz) [G. *koma,* deep sleep]. In a state of coma.

comedo (kom'-ē-dō) [L. a glutton]. Blackhead. A worm-like cast formed of sebum which occupies the outlet of a sebaceous gland in the skin. Comedones have a black colour because of pigmentation; a feature of acne vulgaris.

commensal (kom-en'-sál) [L. *cum,* with; *mensa,* table]. A parasitic microorganism adapted to grow on body surfaces of the host, forming part of the normal flora. Some commensals are potentially pathogenic.

communicable (kom-ūn'-ik abl) [L. *communicare,* to share, to impart]. Transmissible directly or indirectly from one person to another.

compatibility (kom-pat-ib-il'-it-i) [L. *compati,* to suffer with one]. Suitability; congruity. The power of a substance to mix with another without unfavourable results, e.g. two medicines, blood plasma and cells. See BLOOD GROUPS—compatible, adj.

compensation (kom-pen-sā'-shun) [L. *compensare,* to weigh against]. 1. A mental mechanism, employed by a person to cover up a weakness, by exaggerating a more socially acceptable quality. Used as c. neurosis in psychiatry to denote symptoms motivated by unconscious wish for monetary compensation for accident or injury. 2. The state of counterbalancing a functional or structural defect, e.g. cardiac c.

Complan (kom'-plan). Powder, 100g of which contains 31 g protein, 16 g fat, 44 g carbohydrate, and sufficient mineral salts and vitamins to maintain health. Can be taken orally or as liquid by tube.

complement (kom'-plē-ment) [L. *complere,* to complete]. A normal constituent of plasma which is of great importance in immunity mechanisms, as it combines with antigen-antibody complex (complement fixation), and this leads to the completion of reactions such as bacteriolysis and the killing of bacteria. Complement is thermolabile and non-specific and believed to consist of four fractions. c. fixation test, measures the amount of complement fixed by any given antigen-antibody complex.

complex kom'-pleks) [L. *complexus,* an encircling]. A series of emotionally charged ideas, repressed because they conflict with ideas acceptable to the individual, e.g. Oedipus c., a syndrome

attributed to suppressed sexual desire of a son for his mother; Electra c., of daughter for father.

complication (kom-plik-ā'-shun) [L. *complicare,* to fold together]. In medicine, an accident or second disease arising in the course of a primary disease; can be fatal.

compos mentis (kom'-pos men'-tis) [L.]. Of sound mind.

compound (kom'-pownd) [L. *componere,* to put together]. A substance composed of two or more elements, chemically combined in a definitive proportion to form a new substance with new properties.

comprehension (kom-pre-hen'-shun) [L. *comprehensio*]. Mental grasp of meaning and relationships.

compress (kom'-pres). Usually refers to a wet dressing of several layers of lint. cold c. on the forehead relieves headache. glycerine and ichthyol c. reduces inflammation. lead and opium c. relieves pain, swelling and bruises.

compression (kom-presh'-un) [L. *comprimere,* to press together]. The state of being compressed. The act of pressing or squeezing together. cerebral c., arises from any space-occupying, intracranial lesion. digital c., the pressure is applied by the fingers, usually to an artery to stop bleeding. c. bandage, see BANDAGE.

compromise (kom'-prom-īz) [L. *compromissum,* mutual agreement]. A mental mechanism whereby a conflict (q.v.) is evaded by disguising the repressed wish to make it acceptable in consciousness.

conation (kō-nā'-shun) [L. *conari,* to try]. Willing or desiring. The conscious tendency to action. One of the three aspects of mind, the others being cognition (awareness, understanding) and affection (feeling or emotion).

concept (kon'-sept) [L. *concipere,* to take in]. An abstract generalization resulting from the mental process of abstracting and recombining certain qualities or characteristics of a number of ideas, e.g. the individual's c. of honour, love, a rose, a house, etc.

conception (kon-sep'-shun) [L. *concipere,* to conceive]. 1. The act of becoming pregnant by the impregnation of the ovum by the spermatozoon. 2. An abstract mental idea of anything—conceptive, adj.

Concordin (kon-kor'-din). Protriptyline hydrochloride. Antidepressant (q.v.). In cases of insomnia, should not be administered later than mid-afternoon.

concretion (kon-krē'-shun) [L. *concrescere,* to grow together]. A deposit of hard material; a calculus.

concussion (kon-kush'-un) [L. *concussus* from *concutere,* to shake violently together]. A condition resulting from a violent jar or shock. **cerebral c.** characterized by loss of consciousness, pallor, coldness and usually an increase in the pulse rate. There may be incontinence of urine and faeces.

condensation (kon-dens-ā'-shun) [L. *condensare,* to condense]. The process of becoming more compact, e.g. the changing of a gas to a liquid.

condom (kon'-dom). A rubber sheath used as a male contraceptive.

conduction (kon-duk'-shun) [L. *conducere,* to conduct]. The transmission of heat, light, or sound waves through suitable media; also the passage of electrical currents and nerve impulses through body tissues—conductivity, n.

conductor (kon-duk'-tèr) [L. *conducere,* to conduct]. A substance or medium which transmits heat, light, sound, electric current, etc. **bad, good, or non-c.,** designates degree of conductivity.

condyloma (kon-dil-ō'-má) [G. *kondylos,* knuckle; *-oma,* tumour]. Papilloma. Condylomata acuminta are acuminate (pointed) dry warts found under prepuce (male), on the vulva and vestibule (female), or on the skin of the perianal region. They are non-venereal. Condylomata lata are the highly infectious, moist, warty excrescences found in moist areas of the body (vulva, anus, axilla, etc.) as a manifestation of late secondary syphilis—condylomatous, adj.; condylomata, pl.

Condy's fluid (kon'-dēz). A proprietary preparation consisting of a solution of sodium permanganate (potassium permanganate is commonly substituted for it); it is antiseptic, disinfectant and deodorant.

confabulation (kon-fab-ū-lā'-shun) [L. *confabulatio,* a talking together]. A symptom common in confusional states when there is impairment of memory for recent events. The gaps in the patient's memory are filled in with fabrications of his own invention. Occurs in senile and toxic confusional

states, cerebral trauma and Korsakoff's syndrome (q.v.).

confection (kon-fek'-shun) [L. *confectio,* a composing]. A preparation in which drugs are mixed with sugar, syrup and honey, e.g. c. of senna.

conflict (kon'-flikt) [L. *confligere,* to strike together]. In psychiatry, presence in the unconscious of two incompatible and contrasting wishes or emotions. When the conflict becomes intolerable, repression (q.v.) of one of the wishes may occur. Mental conflict and repression form the basic causes of many neuroses, especially hysteria.

confluent (kon'-floo-ent) [L. *confluere,* to flow together]. Becoming merged; flowing together; a uniting as of neighbouring pustules—confluence, n.

confusion (kon-fū'-zhun) [L. *confusio,* disorder]. Used to describe the mental state which is out of touch with reality and associated with a clouding of consciousness. Often present following epileptic fits, in cerebral arteriosclerosis, trauma, severe toxaemia.

congenital (kon-jen'-it-al) [L. *congenitus,* born together with]. Existing from birth or before. **c. dislocation of the hip** is due to faulty formation of the acetabulum. **c. heart disease,** developmental abnormalities in the anatomy of the heart, resulting postnatally in imperfect oxygenation of blood, manifested by cyanosis and breathlessness. Later there is clubbing of the fingers. See 'BLUE BABY'. **c. syphilis** is acquired by the fetus from the infected mother just after the 4th month of intrauterine life.

congestion (kon-jest'-yun) [L. *congestio,* from *congerere,* to heap up]. Hyperaemia. Passive congestion results from obstruction or slowing down of venous return, as in the lower limbs or the lungs—congest, v.i., v.t.; congestive, adj.

congestive heart failure. A chronic inability of the heart to maintain an adequate output of blood from one or both ventricles resulting in manifest congestion and overdistension of certain veins and organs with blood, and in an inadequate blood supply to the body tissues.

conization (kōn-īz-ā'-shun) [G. *konos,* cone]. Removal of a cone-shaped part of the cervix by the knife or cautery.

conjugate (kon-joo'-gāt) [L. *conjugare,* to yoke together]. A measurement of the bony pelvis. **diagonal c.,** the clinical measurement taken in pelvic assessment, from the lower border of the symphysis pubis to the sacral promontory= 110.5 to 133.3 mm. It is 18.9 mm greater than obstetrical conjugate. **obstetrical c.**, the available space for the fetal head, i.e. the distance from the sacral promontory to the posterior surface of the top of the symphysis pubis = 107.9 to 114.2 mm. **true c.**, the distance from the sacral promontory to the summit of the symphysis pubis = 110.5 mm.

conjunctiva (kon-jungk-tī′-vá) [L. *conjunctivus*, serving to connect]. The delicate transparent membrane which lines the inner surface of the eyelids (**palpebral c.**) and reflects over the front of the eyeball (**bulbar** or **ocular c.**)—conjuctival, adj.

conjunctivitis (kon-jungk-ti-vī′-tis) [L. *conjunctivus*, serving to connect; *itis*, inflammation]. Inflammation of the conjunctiva. **inclusion c.**, or inclusion blennorrhoea, occurs in countries with low standards of hygiene. The reservoir of infection is the urogenital tract. See TRIC AGENT.

Conn's syndrome. Too much aldosterone. Muscular weakness, hypertension, renal failure but no oedema. [J. Conn, American physician, 20th century.]

Conotrane (kon′-ō-trān). A cream containing a silicone and penotrane (q.v.).

consanguinity (kon-sang-gwin′-i-ti) [L. *con*, with; *sanguis*, blood]. Blood relationship—consanguineous, adj.

consolidation (kon-sol-i-dā′-shun) [L. *consolidare*, to make firm]. Becoming solid, as, for instance, the state of the lung due to exudation and organization in lobar pneumonia.

constipation (kon-sti-pā′-shun) [L. *constipare*, to press closely together]. An implied chronic condition of infrequent and often difficult evacuation of faeces due to insufficient food or fluid intake, or to sluggish or disordered action of the bowel musculature or nerve supply, or to habitual failure to empty the rectum. Acute constipation signifies obstruction or paralysis of the gut of sudden onset.

consumption (kon-sump′-shun) [L. *consumere*, to consume]. 1. Act of consuming or using up. 2. Popular term for pulmonary tuberculosis (which 'consumed' the body)—consumptive, adj.

contact (kon′-takt) [L. *contactum*, from *contingere*, to touch]. 1. Direct or indirect exposure to infection. 2. A person

who has been so exposed. **c. lens**, of glass or plastic, worn under the eyelids in direct contact with conjunctiva (in place of spectacles) for therapeutic or cosmetic purposes.

contagion (kon-tāj′-un) [L. *contagio*, to touch]. Communication of disease from body to body—contagious, adj.; contagiousness, n.

contraceptive (kon-trá-sep′-tiv) [L. *contra*, against; *conceptio*, conception]. An agent used to prevent conception, e.g. condom, spermaticidal vaginal pessary or cream, rubber cervical cap, intrauterine contraceptive device (see IUCD), oral female medication—contraception, n.

contract (kon-trakt′) [L. *contractum*, from *contrahere*, to draw together]. 1. Draw together; shorten; decrease in size. 2. Acquire by contagion or infection.

contractile (kon-trak′-tīl) [L. *contractum*]. Possessing the ability to shorten—usually when stimulated, special property of muscle tissue—contractility, n.

contraction (kon-trak′-shun) [from L. *contrahere*, to draw together]. Shortening, especially applied to muscle fibres.

contracture (kon-trak′-tūr) [L. *contractus*, from *contrahere*, to draw together]. Shortening of muscle or scar tissue, producing deformity. **Dupuytren's c.**, painless, chronic flexion of the digits, especially the third and fourth, towards the palm; aetiology uncertain. Some cases associated with hepatic cirrhosis. See VOLKMANN. [Guillame Dupuytren, French surgeon, 1777–1835.]

contraindication (kon′ trn in-dik-ā′-shun) [L. *contra*, opposite to; *indicare*, to indicate]. A sign or symptom suggesting that a certain line of treatment (usually used for that disease) should be discontinued or avoided.

contralateral (kon-tra-lat′-er-al) [L. *contra*, opposite to; *latus*, side]. On the opposite side—contralaterally, adv.

contre-coup (kong′-tr-koo) [F.]. Injury or damage at a point opposite the impact, resulting from transmitted force. More likely to occur in an organ or part containing fluid, as the skull.

controlled cord traction. Used after the firm contraction of the uterus is felt following delivery and in response to an oxytocic. One hand holds the lower uterus with the index finger and exerts upward pressure on the corpus. Steady pressure downwards on the cord (using other hand) counteracts this upward pressure on the uterus and the placenta is usually delivered easily. Some people call this method a modified Brandt Andrews technique.

contusion (kon-tū'-zhun) [l. *contusus*, crushed]. A bruise; slight bleeding into tissues whilst the skin remains unbroken—contuse, v.t.

convection (kon-vek'-shun) [L. *convectio*, from *convehere*, to carry together]. Transfer of heat from the hotter to the colder part; the heated substance (air or fluid), being less dense tends to rise. The colder portion, flowing in to be heated, rises in its turn, thus c. currents are set in motion.

conversion (kon-vėr'-shun) [L. *conversio*, turn round]. Psychological conflict manifesting as a physical symptom.

convolutions (kon-vō-loo'-shunz) [L. *convolutum*, to roll together]. Folds, twists or coils as found in the intestine, renal tubules and surface of brain—convoluted, adj.

convulsions (kon-vul'-shunz) [L. *convulsus*, from *convellere*, to rend]. Involuntary contractions of muscles resulting from abnormal cerebral stimulation from many causes. Occur with or without loss of consciousness. **clonic c.** show alternating contraction and relaxation of muscle groups. **tonic c.** reveal sustained rigidity—convulsive, adj.

convulsive therapy (kon-vul'-siv ther'-a-pi). Electroplexy; electrotherapy, electroconvulsive therapy (ECT). One of the most useful physical methods of treatment for mental disorders, notably depressive states, mania, stupor. Introduced in 1937 by Cerletti and Bini. Injections of cardiazol or metrazol also produce convulsions, and were introduced by Meduna in 1934 and widely used until the introduction of ECT.

Cooley's anaemia. Mediterranean anaemia or thalassaemia (q.v.). [Thomas Benton Cooley, American physician, 1871–1945.]

co-ordination (kō-awr-din-ā'-shun) [L. *cum*, together; *ordinare*, to regulate]. Moving in harmony. **muscular c.,** the harmonious action of muscles, permitting free, smooth and efficient movements under perfect control.

copper. Present in traces in all animal tissues. Copper salts have little use in medicine except the sulphate. This is used occasionally as an astringent lotion, and in phosphorus poisoning. Copper sulphate is also used in Benedict's and Fehling's solutions for testing urine for glucose.

coprolalia (kop-rō-lā'-li-á) [G. *kopros*, dung; *lalia*, speech]. Filthy or obscene speech. Occurs as a symptom most commonly in cerebral deterioration or trauma affecting frontal lobes of the brain.

Coprolax (kop'-rō-laks). Dioctyl sodium sulphosuccinate (q.v.).

coproporphyrin (kop-rō-por-fī'-rin) [G. *kopros*, dung; *porphyros*, purple]. Naturally occurring porphyrin in the faeces.

copulation (kop-ū-lā'-shun) [L. *copulare*, to bind together]. Sexual intercourse.

Coramine (kor'-a-min). Nikethamide (q.v.).

cord [G. *chorde*, string]. A thread-like structure. **spermatic c.,** that which suspends the testicles in the scrotum. **spinal c.,** a cord-like structure which lies in the spinal column, reaching from the foramen magnum to the first or second lumbar vertebra. It is a direct continuation of the medulla oblongata and is about 45.72 cm long in the adult. **umbilical c.,** the navel-string, attaching the fetus to the placenta. **vocal c.,** the membranous bands in the larynx, vibrations of which are responsible for the voice.

Cordilox (kor'-dil-oks). Verapamil (q.v.).

cordotomy (kor-dot'-om-i) [G. *chorde*, string; *tome*, a cutting]. See CHORDOTOMY.

core (kawr). Central portion, usually applied to the slough in the centre of a boil.

Corlan (kor'-lan). Hydrocortisone (q.v.).

corn (kawrn) [L. *cornu*, horn]. A cone-shaped, overgrowth and hardening of epidermis, with the point of the cone in the deeper layers; produced by friction or pressure. **hard c.** usually occurs over a toe joint. **soft c.** occurs between the toes.

cornea (kor'-ni-á) [L. *corneus*, horny]. The outwardly convex transparent membrane forming part of the anterior outer coat of the eye. It is situated in front of the iris and pupil and merges backwards into the sclera—corneal, adj.

corneal graft (kor'-ni-al) [L. *corneus*, horny; O.F. *greffe*, from G.*graphein*, to write]. Corneal opacity excised and replaced by healthy, transparent, human cornea from a donor. Keratoplasty.

corneoplasty (kor-ni-ō-plas'-ti) [L. *corneus*, horny; G. *plassein*, to form]. Syn. keratoplasty. See CORNEAL GRAFT.

corneoscleral (kor'-ni-ō-sklē'-rál) [L. *corneus*, horny; G. *skleros*, hard]. Pertaining to the cornea and sclera, as the circular junction of these structures.

coronary (kor'-on-a-ri) [L. *corona*, crown]. Crown-like; encircling, as of a vessel or nerve. c. arteries, those supplying the heart, the first pair to be given off by the aorta as it leaves the left ventricle. Spasm or narrowing of these vessels produces angina pectoris. c. sinus, channel receiving most cardiac veins and opening into the right atrium. c. thrombosis, occlusion of a coronary vessel by a clot of blood.

coronaviruses (kor-ō-na-vī'-rus-es). A newly recognized group of viruses that can cause the common cold.

cor pulmonale (kor pul-mon-ā'-lē) [L. *cor*, heart; *pulmo*, lung]. Heart disease following on disease of lung (emphysema, silicosis, etc.) which strains the right ventricle.

corpus (kor'-pus)[L.]. A body. c. luteum, the yellow body formed in the ovary after rupture of a Graafian follicle and subsequent expulsion of the ovum. The false c. l. is formed in the non-pregnant state and persists for approximately one month, when it is reabsorbed. The true c. l. occurs in pregnancy and persists for 12 wks. See FOLLICLE.—corpora, pl.

corpuscle (kor-pus'-l) [L. *corpusculum*, small body]. A microscopic mass of protoplasm. There are many varieties but the term generally refers to the red and white blood cells. See ERYTHROCYTES and LEUCOCYTES—corpuscular, adj.

corrective (kor-ek'-tiv) [L. *correctum*, from *corrigere*, to correct]. Changes, counteracts or modifies something harmful.

Corrigan's pulse. See PULSE.

corrosive sublimate (kor-rō'-ziv sub'-lim-āt). Perchloride of mercury (q.v.).

cortex (kor'-teks) [L. rind or bark]. 1. The outer bark or covering of a plant. 2. The outer layer of an organ beneath its capsule or membrane—cortices, pl.; cortical, adj.

corticoid (kor'-ti-koid). A name for the

several groups of natural hormones produced by the adrenal cortex and for synthetic compounds with similar actions. Examples of the three main groups are hydrocortisone, cortisone, prednisolone and prednisone in the first, deoxycortone acetate (DCA or DOCA) in the second, and the sex hormones in the third.

corticosteroids (kor-ti-kō-stēr'-oids). Hormones which are steroids and produced by the adrenal cortex.

corticotrophin (kor-ti-kō-trōf'-in). The hormone of the anterior pituitary gland which specifically stimulates the adrenal cortex to produce corticoids. Available commercially as a purified extract of animal anterior pituitary glands (ACTH). Only active by injection.

cortisol (kor'-ti-zol). Hydrocortisone, an adrenal cortical steroid essential to life. Increased in malignant phase hypertension but not in other forms of hypertension.

cortisone (kor'-ti-zōn). One of the principal hormones of the adrenal gland. Converted into cortisol before use by the body. It has powerful antiinflammatory properties, and is used in ophthalmic conditions, rheumatoid arthritis, pemphigus and Addison's disease. Side effects, such as salt and water retention, may limit therapy, and newer derivatives are now preferred for some conditions.

Corynebacterium (kor-ī'-nē-bak-tēr'-i-um). A bacterial genus: Gram-positive, rod-shaped bacteria averaging 3 microns in length, showing irregular staining in segments (metachromatic granules). Many strains are parasitic and some are pathogenic, e.g. *Corynebacterium diphtheriae*, producing a powerful exotoxin.

coryza (kor-ī'-zá) [G. *koruza*, running at nose]. An acute upper respiratory infection of short duration; highly contagious; causative viruses include rhinoviruses, coronaviruses and adenoviruses (q.v.).

cosmetic (kos-met'-ik) [G. *kosmesis*, an adorning]. That which is done to improve the appearance or prevent disfigurement.

costive (kos'-tiv) [O.F. *costive*, from L. *constipare*, to press together]. Lay term for constipation—costiveness, n.

costoclavicular (kos-tō-klav-ik'-ūl-är) [L. *costa*, rib; *clavicula*, small key].

Pertaining to the ribs and the clavicle. **c. syndrome**, syn. for cervical rib syndrome. See CERVICAL.

co-trimoxazole (kō-trī-moks'-a-zōl). Active against most urinary pathogens.

cotyledon (kot-il-ē'-don) [G. *kotyledon* any cup-shaped' hollow]. One of the subdivisions of the uterine surface of the placenta.

Coumadin (koo'-mà-din). A proprietary brand of warfarin. Derivative of discoumarol (q.v.).

counterextension (kown'-tèr-eks-ten'-shun) [L. *contra*, against; *extendere*, to extend]. Traction upon the proximal extremity of a fractured limb opposing the pull of the extension apparatus on the distal extremity.

counterirritant (kown-tė-ir'-it-ant) [L. *contra*, against; *irritare*, to irritate]. An agent, which, when applied to the skin, produces an inflammatory reaction (hyperaemia) relieving congestion in underlying organs—counterirritation, n.

Cowper's glands (kow'-pèrz). Bulbourethral glands. Two in number, lying lateral to the membranous urethra, below the prostrate gland, and deep to the perineal membrane. They open via short ducts into the anterior (penile) uretha. [William Cowper, English surgeon, 1666–1709.]

coxa (koks'-à) [L.]. The hip joint. **c. valga**, an increase in the normal angle between neck and shaft of femur. **c. vara**, a decrease in the normal angle plus torsion of the neck, e.g. slipped femoral epiphysis—coxae, pl.

coxalgia (koks-al'-ji-à) [L. *coxa*, hip; G. *algos*, pain]. Literally pain in the hip joint. Often used as syn. for hip disease.

coxitis (koks-ī'-tis) [L. *coxa*, hip; G. *-itis*, inflammation]. Inflammation of the hip joint.

Coxsackie viruses. First isolated at Coxsackie, N.Y. One of the three groups included in the family of enteroviruses. Divided into groups A and B. Many in group A appear to be non-pathogenic. Others cause aseptic meningitis and herpangina. Those in group B also cause aseptic meningitis, Bornholm disease and myocarditis.

crab louse (krab lows). Pediculus pubis (q.v.).

cramp (kramp) [O.F. *crampe*]. Spasmodic contraction of a muscle or group of muscles, involuntary and painful:

may result from fatigue. Occurs in tetany, food poisoning and cholera. **occupational c.** is such as occurs amongst miners and stokers.

craniofacial (krā-ni-ō-fāsh'-al) [G. *kranion*, skull; L. *facies*, face, external form]. Pertaining to the cranium and the face.

craniometry (krā-ni-om'-et-ri) [G. *kranion*, skull; *metron*, a measure]. The science which deals with the measurement of skulls.

craniopharyngioma (krā-ni-ō-far-in'-ji-ō-mà) [G. *kranion*, skull; *pharygx*, pharynx; *-oma*, tumour]. A tumour which develops between the brain and the pituitary gland.

cranioplasty (krā-ni-ō-plas'-ti) [G. *kranion*, skull; *plassein*, to form]. Operative repair of a skull defect—cranioplastic, adj.

craniosacral (krā-ni-ō-sā'-kràl) [G. *kranion*, skull; L. *sacer*, sacred]. Pertaining to the skull and sacrum. Applied to the parasympathetic nervous system.

craniosynostosis (krā'-ni-ō-sin-os-tō'-sis). Premature ossification of skull bones with closure of suture lines, giving rise to facial deformities. See APERT'S SYNDROME.

craniotabes (krā-ni-ō-tā'-bēz) [G. *kranion*, skull; L. *tabes*, a wasting away]. A thinning or wasting of the cranial bones occurring in infancy. Can occur in rickets, syphilis and marasmus—craniotabetic, adj.

craniotomy (krā-ni-ot'-om-i) [G. *kranion*, skull; *tome*, a cutting]. A surgical opening of the skull in order to remove a growth, relieve pressure, evacuate blood clot or arrest haemorrhage. See LEUCOTOMY.

cranium (krā-n'i-um) [G. *kranion*, skull]. The part of the skull enclosing the brain. It is composed of eight bones: the occipital, two parietals, frontal, two temporals, sphenoid and ethmoid—cranial, adj.

Crasnatin (kras'-nat-in). Asparaginase extracted from *E. coli*. Antileukaemic.

creatine (krē'-at-in) [G. *kreas*, flesh]. A protein derivative found in muscle. The serum c. is raised in hyperthyroidism, values above 0.6 mg per 100 ml of blood being suggestive.

creatinine (krē-at'-in-ēn) [G. *kreas*, flesh]. A waste product of protein (endogenous) metabolism found in normal urine. Probably derived from creatinine of muscle.

creatinuria (krē-at-in-ū′-ri-á) [G. *kreas,* flesh; *ouron,* urine]. Discovery of creatinine in the urine. Occurs in conditions in which muscle is rapidly broken down, e.g. acute fevers, starvation—creatinuric, adj.

Credé's method (krě′-dez). A method of delivering the placenta by gently rubbing the fundus uteri until it contracts, and then, by squeezing the fundus, expressing the placenta into the vagina from whence it is expelled. [Karl Seigmund Franz Credé, German obstetrician, 1819-92.]

creosote (krē′-ō-sōt). A phenolic antiseptic obtained from beechwood. Occasionally used as a deodorant antiseptic and expectorant.

crepitation (krep-i-tā′-shun) [L. *crepitare,* to crackle]. 1. Grating of bone ends in fracture. 2. Crackling sound in joints, e.g. in osteoarthritis. 3. Crackling sound heard via stethoscope in lung infections. 4. Crackling sound elicited by pressure on emphysematous tissue.

cresol (krē′-sol). Principal constituent of lysol (q.v.).

cretinism (kret′-in-izm) [F. *crétin*]. Due to congenital thyroid deficiency; results in a dull-looking child, underdeveloped mentally and physically, dwarfed, large head, thick legs, pug nose, dry skin, scanty hair, swollen eyelids, short neck, mute, short thick limbs, clumsy uncoordinated gait—cretin, n.

cribriform (krib′-ri-form) [L. *cribrum,* sieve; *forma,* shape]. Perforated, like a sieve. **c. plate,** that portion of ethmoid bone allowing passage of fibres of olfactory nerve.

cricoid (krī′-koid) [G. *krikos,* ring; *eidos,* form]. Ring-shaped. Applied to the cartilage forming the inferior posterior part of larynx.

'cri du chat' syndrome. Produced by partial loss of one of the number 5 chromosomes leading to mental subnormality. There are certain physical abnormalities and curious flat, toneless cat-like cry in infancy.

crisis (krī′-sis) [G. *krysis,* turning point]. 1. The turning point of a disease—as the point of defervescence in fever, the arrest of an anaemia. 2. Muscular spasm in tabes dorsalis referred to as visceral crisis (gastric, vesical, rectal, etc.). 3. Dietl's crises (q.v.). **oculogyric**

c., see OCULOGYRIC. **thyrotoxic c.,** sudden return of symptoms of thyrotoxicosis, due to shock, injury or thyroidectomy. **myasthenic c.,** sudden deterioration with weakness of respiratory muscles due to an increase in severity of myasthenia. **cholinergic c.,** respiratory failure resulting from overtreatment with anticholinesterase drugs. The latter two crises are distinguished by 10 mg Tensilon i.v. Marked improvement confirms myasthenic c. Cholinergic c. needs 1 mg atropine sulphate i.v. and immediate mechanical respiration.

Crohn's disease. See ILEITIS. [Burrill Bernard Crohn, American gastroenterologist, 1884-   .]

cromoglycate (krō-mō-glī′-kāt). Disodium cromoglycate (q.v.).

Crosby capsule. Used for intestinal biopsy.

crotamiton BP. (krō-tá-mīt′-on). Effective for scabies, especially in infants, as in kills the mite and prevents itching. Is usually recognized as Eurax.

croup (kroop). Laryngeal obstruction. Croupy breathing in a child is often called 'stridulous', meaning noisy or harsh-sounding. Narrowing of the airway which gives rise to the typical attack with crowing inspiration may be the result of oedema or spasm, or both.

cruciate (kroo′-shi-āt) [L. *crux,* cross]. Shaped like a cross.

crus (kroos) [L. leg]. Leg-like; root-like. Applied to various parts of body, e.g. crus of the diaphragm—crural, adj.; crura, pl.

'crush' syndrome. Traumatic uraemia. A condition resulting from damage to the renal tubules because their blood supply has been interfered with. Following an extensive trauma to muscle, there is a period of delay before the effects of renal damage manifest themselves. There is an increase of non-protein nitrogen of the blood, with oliguria, proteinuria and urinary excretion of myohaemoglobin. Loss of blood plasma to damaged area is marked. See TUBULAR NECROSIS.

crutch palsy. Paralysis of extensor muscles of wrist, fingers and thumb from repeated pressure of a crutch upon the radial nerve in the axilla.

cryoanalgesia (krī-ō-an-al-jē-zi-á) [G. *kryos,* cold; *a-,* not; *algos,* pain]. Relief of pain achieved by use of a cryosurgical probe to block peripheral nerve function.

cryogenic (kri-ō-jen'-ik) [G. *kryos*, cold; *genos*, origin]. Anything produced by low temperature. Also used to describe any means or apparatus involved in the production of low temperature.

cryopexy (krī-ō-peks'-i) [G. *kryos*, cold; *pexein*, to clip]. Surgical fixation with freezing as replacement of a detached retina.

cryophake (krī'-ō-fāk) [G. *kryos*, cold; *phagein*, to eat]. Cataract extraction using freezing.

cryoprecipitate therapy (krī-ō-pres-ip'-i-tāt ther'-a-pi). Use of Factor VIII to prevent or treat bleeding in haemophilia. The term refers to the preparation of Factor VIII for injection. Sub-Arctic temperatures make it separate from plasma.

cryoprobe (krī'ō-prōb) [G. *kryos*, cold; L. *probo*, to test]. Freezing probe. Can be used for biopsy. A flexible metal tube attached to liquid nitrogen equipment. The cryoprobe has tips of various sizes which can be cooled to a temperature of –180° C. Causes less tissue trauma and 'seeding' of malignant cells.

cryosurgery (krī-ō-sur'-je-ri) [G. *kryos*, cold; *kheirourgia*, surgery]. The use of intense, controlled cold to remove or destroy diseased tissue. Instead of a knife or guillotine a cryoprobe is used.

cryothalamectomy (krī-ō-thal-am-ek'-to-mi) [G. *kryos*, cold; *thalamos*, chambers; *ektome*, excision]. Freezing applied within the thalamus for Parkinson's disease and other hyperkinetic conditions.

Cryptococcus (krip-to-kok'-us) [G. *kryptos*, hidden; *kokkos*, berry]. A genus of fungi. *Cryptococcus neoformans* is pathogenic to man. It has a marked predilection for the central nervous system causing subacute or chronic disease.

cryptogenic (krip'-tō-jen'-ik) [G. *kryptos*, hidden; *genos*, origin]. Of unknown or obscure cause.

cryptomenorrhoea (krip'-tō-men-o-rē'-a) [G. *kryptos*, hidden; *men*, month; *rheein*, to flow]. Retention of the menses due to a congenital obstruction, such as an imperforate hymen or atresia of the vagina. Syn., haematocolpos.

cryptorchism (kript-or'-kizm) [G. *kryptos*, hidden; *orchis*, testis]. A developmental defect whereby the testes do not descend into the scrotum; they are retained within the abdomen or inguinal canal—cryptorchid, cryptorchis, n.

crystal violet (kris'-tal vī'-ō-let). Antiseptic dye, used as 0.5 per cent solution for ulcers and skin infections.

crystallin (kris'-ta-lin) [G. *krystallos*, ice]. A globulin, principal constituent of lens of eye.

crystalline (kris'-tal-īn) [G. *krystallos*, ice]. Like a crystal; transparent. Applied to various structures. **c. lens**, a biconvex body, oval in shape, which is suspended just behind the iris of the eye, and separates the aqueous from the vitreous humor. It is slightly less convex on its anterior surface and it refracts the light rays so that they focus directly on to the retina.

crystalluria (kris-tal-ū'-ri-a) [G. *krystallos*, ice; *ouron*, urine]. Excretion of crystals in the urine—crystalluric, adj.

CTAB. Cetrimide (q.v.).

CTG. Cardiotocograph.

cubitus (kū'-bi-tus) [L.]. The forearm; elbow—cubital, adj.

cuboid (kū'-boid) [G. *kybos*, cube; *eidos*, form]. Shaped like a cube.

cuirass (kwir-as') [F. *cuirrasse*, a breastplate]. A mechanical apparatus fitted to the chest for artificial respiration.

culdocentesis (kul-dō-sen-tē'-sis) [F. *cul-de-sax; kentesis*, puncture]. Aspiration of the pouch of Douglas via the posterior vaginal wall.

culdoscope (kul'-dō-skōp). An endoscope used via the vaginal route.

culdoscopy (kul-dos'-kō-pi) [F. *cul-de-sax*; G. *skopein*, to examine]. A form of peritoneoscopy, laparoscopy. Passage of a culdoscope through the posterior vaginal fornix, behind the uterus to enter the peritoneal cavity, for viewing same—culdoscopic, adj.; culdoscopically, adv.

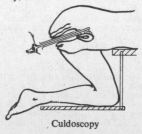

Culdoscopy

culture (kul'-tūr) [L. *cultura, colere,* to till]. The development of micro-organisms on artificial media under ideal conditions for growth.

cumulative action (kū-mū-lā-tiv). If the dose of a slowly excreted drug is repeated too frequently, an increasing action is obtained. This can be dangerous as, if the drug accumulates in the system, toxic symptoms may occur, sometimes quite suddenly. Long acting barbiturates, strychnine, mercurial salts and digitalis are examples of drugs with a cumulative action.

cupping (kup'-ping) [L. *cupa,* tub]. A method of counterirritation. A small bell-shaped glass (in which the air is expanded by heating, or exhausted by compression of an attached rubber bulb) is applied to the skin, resultant suction producing hyperaemia—dry c. When the skin is scarified before application of the cup it is termed 'wet c'.

curare (kū-rár'-i). The crude extract from which tubocurarine is obtained.

curettage (kū-ret'-āzh') [F.]. The scraping of unhealthy or exuberant tissue from a cavity. This may be treatment or may be done to establish a diagnosis.

curette (kū-ret') [F. *curer,* to cleanse]. A spoon-shaped instrument or a metal loop which may have sharp, and/or blunt edges for scraping out (curetting) cavities.

curettings (kū-ret'-ingz). The material obtained by scraping or curetting and usually sent for examination in the pathology department.

Cushingoid. Used to describe the moon face and central obesity common in people with elevated levels of plasma corticosteroid from whatever cause. See CUSHING'S DISEASE and SYNDROME.

Cushing's disease. A rare disorder, mainly of females, characterized principally by virilism, obesity, hyperglycaemia, glycosuria and hypertension. Due to extrinsic and excessive hormone stimulation of the adrenal cortex by tumour, or by hyperplasia, of the anterior pituitary gland.

Cushing's syndrome. A disorder clinically similar to Cushing's disease, but more common. It is due to elevated levels of plasma corticosteroid and is divided into two main groups dependent on exposure or non-exposure to excessive ACTH. 1. ACTH-dependent causes can be iatrogenic due to exces-sive doses; or the secretion of ACTH by non-endocrine tumours such as bronchial carcinoma. 2. Non ACTH-dependent causes can also be iatrogenic due to excessive doses of corticosteroids; or can be due to adenomas or carcinomas of the adrenal cortex.

cusp (kusp) [L. *cuspis,* pointed end]. A projecting point, such as the edge of a tooth or the segment of a heart valve. The tricuspid valve has three, the mitral valve two cusps.

cutaneous (kū-tān'-i-us) [L. *cutis,* skin]. Relating to the skin. c. ureterostomy, the ureters are transplanted so that they open on to the skin of the abdominal wall. This may be done prior to a complete cystectomy.

cuticle (kū'-tik-l) [L. *cutis,* skin]. The epidermis (q.v.); dead epidermis, as that which surrounds a nail—cuticular, adj.

cyanocobalamin (sī-an-ō-kō-bal'a mēn). Vitamin B_{12}. Present in food and absorbed from intestine only when gastric intrinsic factor present. Stored in liver. Deficiency results in megaloblastic erythropoiesis, e.g. pernicious anaemia which responds to intramuscular injection.

cyanosis (sī-an-ō'-sis) [G. *kyanos,* blue; *-osis,* condition]. A bluish tinge manifested by hypoxic tissue, observed most frequently under the nails, lips and skin. It is always due to lack of oxygen, and the causes of this are legion. central c., blueness seen on warm surfaces such as the oral mucosa and tongue. Increases with exertion—cyanosed, cyanotic, adj.

cycle (sī-kl) [G. *kyklos,* circle]. A regular series of movements or events; a sequence which recurs cardiac c., the series of movements through which the heart passes in performing one heart beat which corresponds to one pulse beat and takes about one second. See DIASTOLE and SYSTOLE. menstrual c., the periodically recurring series of changes in breasts, ovaries and uterus culminating in menstruation.

cyclical syndrome (sī'-klik-āl-sin'-drōm). Currently used for premenstrual symptoms complex, to emphasize that these symptoms are due to normal physiological interaction between several endocrine glands under the cyclical control of the hypothalamus and pituitary.

cyclical vomiting (sī'-klik-ál vom'-it-ing). Periodic attacks of vomiting in children, associated with ketosis: no demonstrable pathological cause. Occurs in nervous children.

Cyclimorph 10 (sī'-kli-morf). Ampoules of 1 ml of solution for injection, containing morphine tartrate 10 mg and cyclizine tartrate (histamine, antiemetic) 50 mg. For relief of pain without causing nausea or vomiting.

Cyclimorph 15. In each ampoule of 1 ml there is 15 mg morphine tartrate and 50 mg cyclizine tartrate.

cyclitis (sī-klī'-tis) [G. *kyklos,* circle;*-itis,* inflammation]. Inflammation of the ciliary body of the eye, shown by deposition of small collections of white cells on the posterior cornea called 'keratitic precipitates' (KP). Often co-existent with inflammation of the iris. See IRIDOCYCLITIS.

cyclizine (sī'-kli-zēn). See ANTIHISTAMINES.

cyclobarbitone (sī-klō-bår'-bit-ōn). A short-acting barbiturate, useful when the onset of sleep is delayed. The general properties of these drugs are described under barbiturates (q.v.).

cyclodialysis (sī-klō-dī-al'-i-sis) [G. *kyklos,* circle; G., a separating]. Establishment of communication between anterior chamber and perichoroidal space to relieve intraocular pressure in glaucoma.

cyclodiathermy (sī-klō-dī-a-ther'-mi) [G. *kyklos,* circle; *dia,* through; *therme,* heat]. Destruction by diathermy of the ciliary body.

Cyclogyl (sī'-klō-jil). Cyclopentolate hydrochloride q.v.

cyclopenthiazide (sī-klō-pen-thī'-a-zīd). Diuretic. Decreases reabsorption of sodium and chloride in kidney tubules. Effective orally.

cyclopentolate hydrochloride (sī-klō-pen'-tol-āt hī-drō-klor'-īd). A synthetic, spasmolytic drug. Causes cycloplegia and mydriasis.

cyclophosphamide (sī-klō-fos'-fa-mīd). Cytotoxic agent. A nitrogen mustard. Alkylating agent that interferes with synthesis of nucleic acid in cell chromosomes, particularly in rapidly dividing cells such as those which occur in bone marrow, skin, gastrointestinal tract and fetal tissues. The main side effects therefore occur in these tissues causing anorexia, nausea, vomiting, diarrhoea, depression of bone marrow and alopecia. Main indications are disorders of lymphoid tissue.

cycloplegia (sī-klō-plē'-ji-à) [G. *kyklos,* circle; *plege,* stroke]. Paralysis of the ciliary muscle of the eye—cycloplegic, adj.

cycloplegics (sī-klō-plē'-jiks) [G. *kyklos,* circle;*plege,* stroke]. Drugs which cause paralysis of the ciliary muscle, e.g. atropine, homatropine, scopolamine and lachesine.

cyclopropane (sī'-klō-prō'-pān). A highly inflammable, gaseous anaesthetic, supplied in orange-coloured cylinders. Induction is rapid and recovery prompt. Used with closed circuit apparatus.

cycloserine (sī-klō-sēr'-in). Antitubercular antibiotic. Given orally. Useful in some non-tubercular urinary tract infections. Hepatotoxicity guarded against by SGOT tests twice weekly. Can be epileptogenic. Can give rise to gastrointestinal side effects.

cyclospasmol (sī-klō-spas'-mol). Vasodilator used particularly for cerebral vascular disorders.

cyclothymia (sī-klō-thī'-mi-à) [G. *kyklos,* circle; *thymos,* mind]. A tendency to alternating mood swings between elation and depression such as occur in the manic-depressive psychoses.

cyclotomy (sī-kloṭ'-om-i) [G. *kyklos,* circle; *tome,* a cutting]. A drainage operation for the relief of glaucoma, consisting of an incision through the ciliary body.

cyesis (sī-ē'-sis) [G. *kyesis,* conception]. Pregnancy. **pseudo c.,** signs and symptoms simulating those of early pregnancy occurring in a childless person with an overwhelming desire to have a child.

Cyklokapron (sī-klō-kap'-ron). More powerful than Epsikapron (q.v.).

cylindroma (sil'-in-drō-mà) [G. *kylindros,* cylinder; *-oma,* tumour]. A tumour containing elongated twisted cords of hyaline material, found in malignancy of salivary flands, basal cell carcinomas and endotheliomas.

Cyllin (si'-lin). A disinfectant of the black-fluid type. These products are solutions of coal-tar acids in soap.

Cynomel (sin'-ō-mel). A preparation of liothyronine (q.v.), that has a standardized activity.

cyst (sist) [G. *kystis,* bladder]. A sac with membranous wall, enclosing fluid or semisolid matter. **branchial c.,** in the neck region arising from anomalous development of the embryonal branchial cleft(s). **chocolate c.**, an endometrial cyst containing altered blood. The ovaries are the most usual site. **dermoid c.**, congenital in origin, usually in the ovary, containing elements of hair, nails, skin, teeth, etc. **hydatid c.** is the envelope in which *Taenia echinococcus* (tapeworm) produces its larvae—usually in the human liver. **meibomian c.**, see CHALAZION. **ovarian c.**, ovarian new growth. Most are cystic, but some such as the fibroma are solid. To be differentiated from a cystic ovary (q.v.), o. c. is enucleated from the ovary which is conserved. **papilliferous c.**, an ovarian cyst in which there are nipple-like (papillary) outgrowths from the wall. May be benign or malignant. **retention c.**, caused by blocking of a duct, as a ranula (q.v.). **sebaceous c.**, retention cyst of a sebaceous gland (wen). **thyroglossal c.**, cystic distension of thyroglossal duct near the hyoid bone, in the neck region.

cystadenoma (sist-ad-en-ō'-má) [G. *kystis*, bladder; *aden*, gland; *-oma*, tumour]. An innocent cystic new growth of glandular tissue. Liable to occur in the female breast.

cystathioninuria (sis-tá-thī-on-in-ū'-ri-á). Inherited excessive excretion of thionine, an intermediate product in conversion of methionine to cysteine. Associated with mental subnormality.

cystectomy (sis-tek'-tom-i) [G. *kystis*, bladder; *ektome*, excision]. Usually refers to the removal of part or the whole of the urinary bladder. This may involve the transplantation of one or both ureters—cutaneously or into the bowel.

cystic (sis'-tik) [G. *kystis*, bladder]. Pertaining to or resembling a cyst (q.v.). **c. duct**, the tube connecting the gallbladder to the hepatic and common bile ducts. It conveys bile to and from the gall-bladder. **c. disease of lung**, fibrosis of pancreas, due to a recessive gene mutation. Affects about one child in 2500 live births. The control of pulmonary infection is the key to survival. See MUCOVISCIDOSIS.

cysticerosis (sis-ti-ser-kō'-sis) [G. *kystis*, bladder; *-osis*, condition]. Infection of man with cysticercus.

cysticercus (sis-ti-ser'-kus) [G. *kystis*, bladder; *kerkos*, tail]. The larval form of tapeworms. After ingestion, the ova do not develop beyond this form in man, but form 'cysts' in subcutaneous tissues, skeletal muscles and the brain where they provoke epilepsy.

cystine (sis'-tēn). A sulphur-containing amino acid, produced by the breaking down of proteins during the digestive process.

cystinosis (sis-tin-ō'-sis) [G. *kystis*, bladder; *-osis*, condition]. Metabolic disorder in which crystalline cystine is deposited in the body. Cystine and other aminoacids are excreted in the urine. Fanconi syndrome. See AMINOACIDURIA.

cystinuria (sis-tin-ū'-ri-a) [G. *kystis*, bladder; *ouron*, urine]. Metabolic disorder in which cystine appears in the urine. A cause of renal stones—cystinuric, adj.

cystitis (sis-tī'-tis) [G. *kystis*, bladder; *-itis*, inflammation]. Inflammation of the urinary bladder, exciting cause usually bacterial. The condition may be acute or chronic, primary or secondary to stones, etc. More frequent in females as the urethra is short.

cystitome (sis'-ti-tom). Delicate ophthalmic instrument for incision of the lens capsule.

cystocele (sis'-tō-sēl) [G. *kystis*, bladder; *kele*, hernia]. Prolapse of the posterior wall of the urinary bladder into the anterior vaginal wall. See COLPORRHAPHY.

cystodiathermy (sis'-tō-dī-ath-ér'-mi) [G. *kystis*, bladder; *dia*, through; *therme*, heat]. The application of a cauterizing electrical current to the walls of the urinary bladder through a cystoscope, or by open operation.

cystogram (sis'-tō-gram) [G. *kystis*, bladder; *gramma*, letter]. An X-ray film demonstrating the urinary bladder. **micturating c.**, taken during the act of passing urine.

cystography (sis-tog'-ra-fi) [G. *kystis*, bladder; *graphein*, to write]. Radiographic examination of the urinary bladder, after it has been rendered radio-opaque—cystographic, adj.; cystographically, adv.

cystolithiasis (sis-tō-lith-ī'-as-is) [G. *kystis*, bladder; *lithos*, stone; N.L. *-iasis*, condition]. The presence of a stone or stones in the urinary bladder.

cystometrogram (sis-tō-met'-rō-gram) [G. *kystis*, bladder; *metron*, a measure; *gramma*, letter]. A record of the changes in pressure within the urinary bladder under various conditions; used in the study of certain disorders of paraplegia.

cystometry (sis-tom'-et-ri) [G. *kystis,* bladder; *metron,* a measure]. The study of pressure changes within the urinary bladder—cystometric, adj.

cystopexy (sis-tō-peks'-i) [G. *kystis,* bladder; *pexy,* fixation]. A 'sling' operation for stress incontinence whereby the bladder neck is supported from the back of the symphysis pubis.

cystoplasty (sis'-tō-plas-ti) [G. *kystis,* bladder; *plassein,* to form]. Surgical repair of the bladder—cystoplastic, adj.

cystoscope (sis'-tō-skōp) [G. *kystis,* bladder; *skopein,* to examine]. An endoscope (q.v.) used in diagnosis and treatment of bladder, ureter and kidney conditions—cystoscopy, n.; cystoscopic, adj.; cystoscopically, adv.

cystostomy (sis-tos'-to-mi) [G. *kystis,* bladder; *stoma,* mouth]. The operation whereby a fistulous opening is made into the bladder via the abdominal wall. Usually the fistula can be allowed to heal when its purpose has been achieved.

cystotomy (sis-tot'-o-mi) [G. *kystis,* bladder; *tome,* a cutting]. Incision into the urinary bladder, often done to fulgurate a papilloma or to pass retrograde bougies, etc.

cystourethritis (sis-tō-ū-rē-thrī'-tis) [G. *kystis,* bladder; *ourethron,* urethra; *-itis,* inflammation]. Inflammation of the urinary bladder and urethra.

cystourethrogram (sis-tō-ū-rē'-thrō-gram) [G. *kystis,* bladder; *ourethra,* urethra; *gramma,* letter]. An X-ray film demonstrating the urinary bladder and urethra.

cystourethrography (sis-tō-ū-rē-throg'-ra-fi) [G. *kystis,* bladder; *ourethra,* urethra; *graphein,* to write]. Radiographic examination of the urinary bladder and urethra, after they have been rendered radio-opaque—cystourethrographic, adj.; cystourethrographically, adv.

cystourethropexy (sis-tō-ūr-ēth'-rō-peks-i). Forward fixation of the bladder and upper urethra in an attempt to combat incontinence of urine.

Cytamen (sīt'-a-men). Cyanocobalamin (q.v.).

cytarabine (sī-ta'-ra-bēn). See CYTOSINE ARABINOSIDE.

cytodiagnosis (sī-tō-dī-ag-nō'-sis) [G. *kytos,* cell; *dia,* through; *gnosis,* recognizing]. Diagnosis by microscopic study of cells—cytodiagnostic, adj.

cytogenetics ((sī-tō-jen-et'-iks). Laboratory examination of a person's chromosomes by culture techniques, using either lymphocytes or a piece of tissue such as skin. Some abnormal chromosomes can be linked with physical and mental disorder—cytogenesis, n.

cytology (sī-tol'-oj-i) [G. *kytos,* cell; *logos,* discourse]. Subdivision of biology, consisting of the microscopic study of the body cells. **exfoliative c.,** microscopic study of cells from the surface of an organ or lesion after suitable staining.

cytolysis (sī-tol'-i-sis) [G. *kytos,* cell; *lysis,* a loosening]. The degeneration, destruction, disintegration or dissolution of cells—cytolytic, adj.

cytomegalovirus (sī-tō-meg'-al-ō-vīr'-us) [G. *kytos,* cell; *megas,* large; L.]. Belongs to the same group of viruses as herpes simplex. Can cause latent and symptomless infection. Virus excreted in urine and saliva. Congenital infection is the most severe form of c. infection.

cytomegalovirus infection. Predominantly affects children and infants, but it has been found in adults undergoing open-heart surgery. Evidence of symptomless infection in pregnant women has also been described. It is characterized by the presence of intracellular inclusion bodies in the cells of many organs, so that the cells become grossly enlarged—hence the name a virus causing large cells. The respiratory tract, kidneys, adrenals, liver, gastrointestinal tract, blood, eyes and CNS—especially the brain—may be involved. In premature and neonatal infants the inclusion bodies are best seen in the kidneys. Virus may be present in saliva of patients for 4 weeks after infection and in urine for 2 years. It has also been recovered from normal infants. There is an increased incidence in children with mental or developmental retardation and blood disorders. It has been described in relation to Rh incompatibility and hepatitis in newborn infants and after intrauterine transfusions. Although in the majority of cases the condition is congenital the mode of transmission is uncertain, whether by blood or amnion. As a rule the mothers are not ill. Recovery of the virus from urine and cervix is more frequent in primipara than multipara. Affected infants are premature or below average weight and present with a large spleen and liver, jaundice, anaemia and purpura. Cerebral calcification, hydrocephalus and microcephaly are common. Pneumonitis and enterocolitis occur in older children. Outlook grave and fatality high. Permanent brain damage occurs in many survivors. Management of the infection is at present unsatisfactory due to lack of precise knowledge and virus-killing drugs.

cytopathic (sī-tō-path'-ik) [G. *kytos*, cell; *pathos*, disease]. Pertaining to disease of the living cell.

cytoplasm (sī-tō-plazm) [G. *kytos*, cell; *plasma* from *plassein*, to mould]. The living material of the cell external to the nucleus — cytoplasmic, adj.

cytosar (sī-tō-sâr). See CYTOSINE ARABINOSIDE

cytosine arabinoside (sīt'-o-sēn ar-ab-in'-o-sīd). Antimetabolite; used in acute leukaemia. Interrupts DNA synthesis. Also termed cytarabine, cytosar or Ara-C.

cytostasis (sī-tō-stā'-sis) [G. *kytos*, cell; *stasis*, a standing still]. Arrest or hindrance of cell development — cytostatic, adj.

cytotoxic (sī-tō-toks'-ik) [G. *kytos*, cell; *toxikon*, poison]. Any substance which is toxic to cells. Applied to the drugs used for the treatment of carcinomas and the reticuloses. Two main groups: (1) antimetabolites which block action of an enzyme system, e.g. methotrexate, fluouracil, mercaptopurine; (2) alkylating agents which poison cell directly, e.g. cyclophosphamide, mustine, Thiotepa.

cytotoxins (sī'-tō-toks'-inz) [G. *kytos*, cell; *toxikon*, poison]. See ANTIBODIES.

D

D860. Tolbutamide (q.v.).

Da Costa's syndrome. Cardiac neurosis. An anxiety state (q.v.) in which palpitations are the most prominent symptom. [Jacob Mendes Da Costa, American surgeon, 1883–1900.]

dacry(o)adenitis (dak'-ri-(ō)-ad-en-ī'-tis) [G. *dakryon*, tear; *aden*, gland; *-itis*, inflammation]. Inflammation of a lacrimal gland. It is a rare condition which

may be acute or chronic. May occur in mumps.

dacryocyst (dak'-ri-ō-sist) [G. *dakryon*, tear; *kystis*, bladder]. Old term for the tear sac (lacrimal sac). The word is still used in its compound forms. See below.

dacryocystectomy (dak-ri-ō-sis-tek'-tomi) [G. *dakryon*, tear; *kystis*, bladder; *ektome*, excision]. Excision of any part of the lacrimal sac.

dacryocystitis (dak-ri-ō-sis-tī'-tis) [G. *dakryon*, tear; *kystis*, bladder; *-itis*, inflammation]. Inflammation of the tear sac, which usually results in abscess formation and obliteration of the tear duct, giving rise to epiphora (q.v.).

dacryocystography (dak-ri-ō-sis-tog'-rafi) [G. *dakryon*, tear; *kystis*, bladder; *graphein*, to write]. Radiographic examination of the tear drainage apparatus after it has been rendered radioopaque—dacryocystographic, adj.; dacryocystographically, adv.; dacryocystogram, n.

dacryocystorhinostomy (dak'-ri-ō-sis'-tō-rin-os'-tom-i) [G. *dakryon*, tear; *kystis*, bladder; *rhis*, nose; *stoma*, mouth]. An operation to establish drainage from the lacrimal sac into the nose when there is obstruction of the nasolacrimal duct. Toti's operation. [Addeo Toti, Italian ophthalmologist and laryngologist, 1861–1946.].

dacryolith (dak'-ri-ō-lith) [G. *dakryon*, tear; *lithos*, stone]. A concretion in the lacrimal passages.

dactyl (dak'-til) [G. *daktylos*, finger]. A digit, finger or toe—dactylar, dactylate, adj.

dactylion (dak-til'-i-on). Syndactyly (q.v.).

dactylitis (dak-til-ī'-tis) [G. *daktylos*, finger; *-itis*, inflammation]. Inflammation of finger or toe. The digit becomes swollen due to periostitis. Met with in congenital syphilis, tuberculosis, sarcoid, etc.

dactylology (dak-til-ol'-o-ji) [G. *daktylos*, finger; *logos*, discourse]. The finger sign method of communication with deaf and dumb people.

Daltonism (dawl'-ton-izm). Colour blindness, named after John Dalton, English chemist and physicist [1766–1844], who was afflicted with it.

dandruff (dand'-ruff). The common scaly condition of the scalp. Called 'scurf'. May be the forerunner of skin diseases of the seborrhoeic type, such as flexural dermatitis.

dandy fever (dan'-di fē'-vėr). Dengue (q.v.).

Dangerous Drugs Act. Replaced by the MISUSE OF DRUGS ACT (q.v.).

Dantrium (dan'-tri-um). Dantrolene sodium (q.v.).

dantrolene sodium (dan'-trō-lēn sō'-di-um). Antispasmodic.

Daonil (dā'-on-il). Glibenclamide (q.v.).

dapsone (dap'-sōn). A sulphone derivative used mainly in leprosy, but also valuable in dermatitis herpetiformis. Prolonged treatment may produce haemolytic anaemia with Heinz body formation, clinical signs of which are cyanosis of the lips; the patient is generally off-colour.

Daptazole (dap'-taz-ol). Aminophenazole (q.v.).

Darabdin (dar'-ab-din). Given intramuscularly to encourage appetite.

Daranide (dar'-á-nīd). Dichlorphenamide (q.v.).

Daraprim (da'-ra-prim). Pyrimethamine (q.v.).

Dartalan (dár'-tal-an). Thiopropazate (q.v.).

daunorubicin (daw-nō-roo'-bi-sin). Similar to adriamycin (q.v.). Antibiotic used in acute leukaemia. Believed to act by inhibiting DNA synthesis. Can cause severe bone marrow depression and toxicity of heart muscle.

day hospital. Patients attend daily. Recreational and occupational therapy and physiotherapy often provided. Greatest use is in the geriatric and psychiatric fields.

DBH. Dopamine-β-hydroxylase. An enzyme present in blood, increased in high blood pressure.

DBI. Phenformin (q.v.).

DDS. Diaminodiphenylsulphone (q.v.).

DDT. Dicophane (q.v.).

deamination (dē-am-in-ā'-shun). A process occurring in the liver whereby amino acids are broken down and urea formed.

Debendox (deb'-en-docks). Dicyclomine hydrochloride (q.v.) with doxylamine (q.v.) and pyridoxine hydrochloride (q.v.). Useful for nausea and vomiting in pregnancy.

debridement (dā-brēd'-mong) [F]. In surgery, thorough cleansing of a wound with removal of all foreign matter and injured or infected tissue.

debrisoquine (deb-ris'-ō-kwin). Hypotensive agent. Interferes with transmission in sympathetic adrenergic nerves, especially sympathetically mediated vascular reflexes, thus can lead to postural hypotension.

Deca-Durabolin (dek'-á-dū-rō-bol'-in). Synthetic androgen; anabolic. Given intramuscularly. Neutralizes oestrogen uptake by cancer cells.

decalcification (dē-kal-si-fik-ā'-shun) [L. de- away; calx, lime; facere, to make]. Removal of mineral salts, as from teeth in dental caries, bone in disorders of calcium metabolism.

decannulation (dē-kan-ū-tā'-shun). A term currently in use for the introduction of decreasingly smaller tubes to wean an infant from reliance on the original tracheostomy tube.

decapsulation (dē-kap-sū-lā'-shun) [L. de-, away; capsula, little box]. Surgical removal of a capsule.

Decaspray (dek'-á-sprā). Aerosol containing dexamethasone and neomycin for topical application.

decerebrate (dē-sėr'-ē-brāt) [L. de-, away; cerebrum, brain]. Without cerebral function; a state of deep unconsciousness. **d. posture,** a condition of the unconscious patient in which all four limbs are spastic and which indicates severe damage to the cerebrum.

Decholin (dek'-o-lin). Dehydrocholic acid. Cholagogue (q.v.).

Decicain (des'-i-kān). Amethocaine (q.v.).

decidua (dē-sid'-ū-á) [L. deciduas, from decidere, to fall off]. The endometrial lining of the uterus thickened and altered for the reception of the fertilized ovum. It is shed when pregnancy terminates. **d. basalis,** that part which lies under the embedded ovum and forms the maternal part of the placenta. **d. capsularis,** that part that lies over the developing ovum. **d. vera,** the decidua lining the rest of the uterus—decidual, adj.

deciduoma malignum (dē-sid-ū-ō'-má mal-ig'-num) [L. deciduus, a falling off; G. -oma, tumour]. Chorionepithelioma (q.v.).

Declinax (de-klīn'-aks). Debrisoquine (q.v.).

decompensation (dē-kom-pen-sā'-shun) [L. de-, away; compensare, to compensate]. A failure of compensation in heart disease.

decompression (dē-kom-presh'-un) [L. *de-*, away; *compressus*, from *comprimere*, to compress]. Removal of pressure or a compressing force. **abdominal d.** currently being used in pregnancy and labour. Apparatus applied to anterior abdominal wall. Improves blood supply and results in shorter and less painful labour. Of value in pre-eclamptic toxaemia. **d. of brain** achieved by trephining the skull; **d. of bladder** in cases of chronic urinary retention, by continuous or intermittent drainage via catheter inserted per urethra. **d. chamber** used when returning deep-sea divers to the surface. See CAISSON DISEASE.

decongestion (dē-kon-jest'-yun) [L. *de-*, reversing, separating; *congerere*, to bring together] Relief of congestion—decongestive, adj.

decortication (dē-kort-ik-ā'-shun) [L. *decorticare*, to deprive of bark]. Surgical removal of cortex or outer covering of an organ. **d. of lung** carried out when thickening of the visceral pleura prevents re-expansion of lung as may occur in chronic empyema. The visceral pleura is peeled off the lung, which is then re-expanded by positive pressure through an anaesthetic apparatus.

decubitus (de-kū'-bit-us) [L., from *decumbere*, to lie down]. The recumbent position; lying down. **d. ulcer**, pressure sore (q.v.)—decubital, adj; decubiti, pl.

decussation (dē-kus-ā'-shun) [L. *decussare*, to cross]. Intersection; crossing of nerve fibres at a point beyond their origin as in the optic and pyramidal tracts. Chiasma.

defaecation (dē-fē-kā'-shun) [L. *de-*, away; *faeces*, dregs, excrement]. Voiding of faeces per anus—defaecate, v.t.

defervescence (dē-fèr-ves'-ens) [L. *defervescere*, to cease boiling]. The time during which a fever is declining. If the body temperature falls rapidly it is spoken of as 'crisis'; if it falls slowly the term 'lysis' is used.

defibrillation (dē-fib-ril-ā'-shun) [L. *fibrilla*, dim. of *fibra*, a fibre]. The arrest of fibrillation of the cardiac muscle (atrial or ventricular), and restoration of normal cycle—defibrillate, v.

defibrillator (dē-fib'-ril-ā-tor). Any agent, e.g. an electric shock, which arrests ventricular fibrillation and restores normal rhythm.

defibrinated (dē-fī'-brin-āt-ed) [L. *de-*, away; *fibra*, fibre]. Rendered free from fibrin (q.v.). A necessary process in the preparation of serum (q.v.)—defibrinate, v.

deficiency disease. Disease resulting from dietary deficiency of any substance essential for good health, especially the vitamins.

degeneration (dē-jen-ėr-ā'-shun) [L. *degenerare*, to depart from]. Deterioration in quality or function. Regression from more specialized to less specialized type of tissue. **afferent d.**, degeneration spreading up sensory nerves. **amyloid d.**, a wax-like change in tissues. **caseous d.**, cheese-like tissue resulting from atrophy in a tuberculoma or gumma. **colloid d.**, mucoid degeneration of tumours. **fatty d.**, in which droplets of fat occur in atrophic tissue, as in the myocardium. **hyaline d.**, affecting connective tissue, especially of blood vessels, in which the tissue takes on a homogeneous or formless appearance. **senile d.** is the clinical picture of old age in which the acuity of thought and performance is blunted. **subacute combined d.**, of the spinal cord, heralded by paraesthesis (q.v.)., is a complication of untreated pernicious anaemia—degenerative, adj; degenerate, v.i.

deglutition (dē-gloo-tish'-un) [L. *deglutire*, to swallow down]. The process of swallowing, partly voluntary, partly involuntary.

Degranol (dē-grān'-ol). Mannomustine (q.v.).

dehiscence (de-his'-ens) [L. *dehiscere*, to gape]. The process of splitting or bursting open, as of a wound.

dehydration (de-hīd-rā'-shun) [L. *de-*, away; G. *hydor*, water]. Loss or removal of fluid. In the body this condition arises when the fluid intake fails to replace fluid loss. This is liable to occur when there is bleeding, diarrhoea, excessive exudation from a raw area, excessive sweating, polyuria or vomiting, and usually upsets the body's electrolyte balance. If suitable fluid replacement cannot be achieved orally then parenteral administration must be instituted—dehydrate, v.t.

dehydrocholic acid (dē-hīd-rō-kol'-ik as'-id). Cholagogue (q.v.).

déjà vu phenomenon [F. seen before]. Occurs in epilepsy involving temporal lobes of the brain and in certain epileptic dream states. An intense feeling of familiarity as if everything had happened before.

Deladroxate (del-a-droks'-āt). Contains hormones, similar to those in the once-daily contraceptive pills. Given as monthly injection.

Delhi boil. See ORIENTAL SORE.

deliquescent (del-i-kwes'-ent). Capable of absorption, thus becoming fluid.

delirium (dē-lir'-i-um) [L.]. Abnormal mental condition based on hallucinations or illusion. May occur in high fever, in mental disease, or be toxic in origin. **d. tremens** results from alcoholic intoxication and is represented by a picture of confusion, terror, restlessness and hallucinations—delirious, adj.

Delta-Cortef (del'-tá-kawr'-tef). Prednisolone (q.v.).

Delta-Cortelan (del'-tá-kawr'-tē-lan). Prednisone (q.v.).

Deltacortone (del'-tá-kawr'-tōn). Prednisone (q.v.).

deltoid (del'-toid) [G. *delta*, fourth letter of the G. alphabet *Δ*; *eidos*, form]. Triangular. **d. muscle**, base lies over shoulder region, apex inserted into midshaft of humerus.

delusion (de-lū'-zhun) [L. *delusum*, from *deludere*, to deceive]. A false belief which cannot be altered by argument or reasoning. Found as a psychotic symptom in several types of insanity, notably schizophrenia, paraphrenia, paranoia, senile psychoses, mania and depressive states including involutional melancholia.

demarcation (dē-már-kā-'shun). An outlining of the junction of diseased and healthy tissue, and usually referring to gangrene.

dementia (dē-men'-shi-á) [L. being out of one's mind]. Irreversible organic deterioration of mental faculties. **d. paralytica**, general paralysis of the insane. See GENERAL. **d. praecox**, see SCHIZOPHRENIA. **presenile d.**, Alzheimer's disease. Dementia occurring in the under fifties. Due to hyaline degeneration of medium and smaller cerebral blood vessels. [Alois Alzheimer, German physician, 1864–1915.]

demethylchlortetracycline (dē-mēth'-īl-klawr-tet-rá-sī'-klin). One of the tetracyclines (q.v.).

demography (dem-og'-ra-fi) [G. *demos*, the people; *graphein*, to write]. Social science, including vital statistics.

demulcent (dē-mul'-sent) [L. *demulcere*, to stroke down]. A slippery, mucilaginous fluid which allays irritation and soothes inflammation, especially of mucous membranes.

demyelinization (dē-mī-el-in-īz-ā'-shun). Destruction of the myelin sheaths surrounding nerve fibres; occurs in multiple sclerosis. See SCLEROSIS.

dendrite or **dendron** (den'drīt; den'-dron) [G. *dendron*, tree]. One of the branched filaments which are given off from the body of a nerve cell. That part of a neurone which transmits an impulse to the nerve cell—dendritic, adj.

dendritic ulcer. Linear corneal ulcer that sends out tree-like branches. Caused by herpes simplex. See IDOXURIDINE.

denervation (dē-ner-vā'-shun). The means by which a nerve supply is cut off. Usually refers to incision, excision or blocking of a nerve.

dengue (deng'-gā). Disease of the tropics. Causative agent is an arbovirus conveyed by a mosquito. Characterized by rheumatic pains, fever and a skin eruption. Sometimes called 'break-bone fever.'

Dennis Browne splints. Splints used to correct congenital talipes equinovarus. The splints are of metal, padded with felt, with a joining bar, to which the baby's feet are strapped. [Dennis Browne, British surgeon, 1892–1967.]

dentine (den'-tēn) [L. *dens*, tooth]. The calcified tissue enclosing the pulp cavity of a tooth.

dentition (den-tish'-un) [L. *dentitio*, from *dentire*, to teethe]. Teething. **primary d.**, eruption of the deciduous, 'milk' or temporary teeth. **secondary d.**, eruption of the 'adult' or permanent teeth.

deodorant (dē-ōd'-or-ant) [L. *de-*, away; *odor*, smell]. Any substance which destroys or masks an (unpleasant) odour. Potassium permanganate and hydrogen peroxide are deodorants by their powerful oxidizing action; chlorophyll has some reputation as a deodorant for foul-smelling wounds, but its value in masking other odours is doubtful—deodorize, v.t.

deoxycortone (dē-oks-i-kor'-tōn). An important hormone of the adrenal cortex, controlling the metabolism of sodium and potassium. Used mainly in the management of Addison's disease. DOCA.

deoxygenation (dē-oks-i'-jen-ā-shun) [L.

de-, away; G. *oxys*, sharp; *genesthai*, to be produced]. The removal of oxygen— deoxygenated, adj.

deoxyribonucleic acid (dē-oks-i-rī-bō-nūk´-li-ik). DNA. The natural carbohydrate constituent of cell nuclei. In conjunction with deoxyribonucleoprotein it makes up the autoreproducing component of chromosomes and many viruses. Together they are fundamental components of living tissue.

depersonalization (dē-pér-son-al-ī-zā´-shun). A subjective feeling of having lost one's personality, sometimes that one no longer exists. Occurs in schizophrenia and more rarely in depressive states.

depilate (dep´-il-āt) [L. *de-*, away; *pilus*, hair]. To remove hair from—depilatory, adj., n.; depilation, n.

depilatories (dē-pil´-at-or-iz). Substances usually made in pastes (e.g. barium sulphide) which remove excess hair only temporarily; they do not act on the papillae, consequently the hair grows again. See EPILATION.

Depo-Provera (dep´-ō-prō´-vér-á). Medroxyprogesterone acetate (q.v.).

depression (de-presh´-un) [L. *depressus*, from *deprimere*, to depress]. 1. A hollow place or indentation. 2. Diminution of power or activity. 3. A low condition, either mental or physical. In psychiatry, emotional disorder. Of two distinct types, neurotic and psychotic. The neurotic type, **reactive d.**, occurs as a reaction to stress. The psychotic type, **endogenous d.**, arises spontaneously in the mind. The symptoms are almost the same in both conditions and vary from mild to fatal and are: insomnia, headaches, exhaustion, anorexia, irritability, emotionalism or loss of affect, loss of interest, impaired concentration, feelings that life is not worth living, and suicidal thoughts. **involution d.**, that occurring at the climacteric.

deprivation syndrome. Usually the result of parental rejection of offspring. Includes dwarfism, malnutrition with potbelly, gluttonous appetite, superficial affectionate attachment to any adult, old healed sores on buttocks, chilblain scars on fingers and toes, very thin hair.

deptropin citrate (dep-trō´-pēn sit´-rāt). Tablets and injection for bronchorrhoea, bronchial asthma, vasomotor rhinitis and maintenance therapy in bronchitis.

Derbyshire neck (dár´-bi-shér). Goitre (q.v.).

derealization (dē-rē-al-īz-ā´-shun) [L. *de-*, away from; *res*, thing]. Feelings of unreality, such as occur to normal people during dreams. A symptom often found in schizophrenia and depressive states.

dereistic (dē-rē-is´-tik). Thinking not adapted to reality. Autistic thinking.

dermatitis (dér-ma-tī´-tis) [G. *derma*, skin; *-itis*, inflammation]. Inflammation of the skin (by custom limited to an eczematous reaction). **d. herpetiformis**, an intensely itchy skin eruption of unknown cause, most commonly characterized by vesicles, bullae and pustules on urticarial plaques, which remit and relapse. When occurring in pregnancy it is known as 'hydrogravidarum'. **juvenile d. herpetiformis**, recurrent bullous eruption on genitalia, lower abdomen, buttocks and face, mainly in children under 5, boys being affected more often than girls. In Great Britain the incidence is higher in northern parts of country. Treatment is dapsone possibly until puberty; maintenance dose that prevents new lesions appearing. **industrial d.** is a term used in the National Insurance (Industrial Injuries) Act to cover occupational skin conditions '...due to dust or liquids'.

dermatoglyphics (der-mat-ō-gli´-fiks) [G. *derma*, skin; *glyphos*, carved]. Study of the ridge patterns of the skin of the fingertips, palms and soles to discover developmental anomalies.

dermatographia (dér-mat-ō-graf-i-á). See DERMOGRAPHIA.

dermatologist (dér-mat-ol´-oj-ist) [G. *derma*, skin; *logos*, discourse]. One who studies skin diseases and is skilled in their treatment. A skin specialist.

dermatology (dér-mat-ol´-o-ji) [G. *derma*, skin; *logos*, discourse]. The science which deals with the skin, its structure, functions, diseases and their treatment—dermatological, adj.; dermatologically, adv.

dermatome (dér´-mat-ōm) [G. *derma*, skin; *tome*, a cutting]. An instrument for cutting slices of skin of varying thickness, usually for grafting.

dermatomycosis (dér-mat-ō-mī-kō´-sis) [G. *derma*, skin; *mykes*, fungus; *-osis*, condition]. Fungal infection of the skin—dermatomycotic, adj.

dermatomyositis (dér´-mat-ō-mī-os-īt´-

is) [G. *derma*, skin; *mys*, muscle; *-itis*, inflammation]. An acute inflammation of the skin and muscles which presents with oedema and muscle weakness. May result in the atrophic changes of scleroderma (q.v.). See COLLAGEN.

dermatophytes (dėr-mat-ō-fitz') [G. *derma*, skin; *phyton*, a plant]. A group of fungi which invade the superficial skin.

dermatophytosis (dėr'-mat-ō-fī-tō'-sis) [G. *derma*, skin; *phyton*, a plant; *-osis*, condition]. Syn., athlete's foot. See TINEA PEDIS.

dermatosis (dėr-mat-ōs'-is). [G. *derma*, skin; *-osis*, condition]. Generic term for skin disease—dermatoses, pl.

dermis (dėr'-mis) [G. *derma*, skin]. The true skin; the cutis vera; the layer below the epidermis.

dermographia (dėr-mō-gráf'-i-á) [G. *derma*, skin; *graphein*, to write]. A condition in which weals occur on the skin after a blunt instrument or fingernail has been lightly drawn over it. Seen in vasomotor instability and urticaria.

dermoid (dėr'-moid) [G. *derma*, skin; *eidos*, form]. Pertaining to or resembling skin. See CYST.

Dermo-jet (der'-mō-jet) Apparatus for delivery of fluid under pressure into the dermis. It is a painless method, twice as fast as needle injection and free from the danger of hepatitis transmission.

dermovate (dėr'-mō-vāt). Clobetasol propionate (q.v.).

desensitization (dē-sen-sit-īz-ā'-shun). The neutralization of acquired hypersensitiveness to some agent acting on the skin or internally. Used in asthma and for treatment of people who have become allergic to drugs such as penicillin and streptomycin. **systematic d.**, of phobic patients using i.v. methohexitone sodium to achieve psychological relaxation. In this state the phobic situation is imagined without fear and the patient 'unlearns' his irrational fear—densensitize, v.t.

Deseril (des'-er-il). Methysergide (q.v.).

desferrioxamine (des-fer-ri-oks'-á-mēn). Used in iron poisoning and haemosiderosis (q.v.) (p. 137).

desipramine. See ANTIDEPRESSANT.

deslanoside (des-lan'-ō-sīd). Natural glycoside. Cardiac therapeutic agent.

Desmopressin (des-mō-press'-in). Antidiuretic. See VASOPRESSIN.

desoxycorticosterone. Deoxycortone (q.v.).

desquamation (des-kwá-mā'-shun) [L. *desquamare*, to scale off]. Shedding; flaking off; casting off—desquamate, v.i., v.t.

detergent (dē-tėr'-jent) [L. *detergere*, to wipe off]. A cleansing agent. Is often applied to drugs of the cetrimide type, which have both antiseptic and cleaning properties, and so are valuable in removing grease, dirt, etc., from skin and wounds, and scabs and crusts from skin lesions. **d. application,** useful for removing greasy ointments from the skin; contains arachis oil, emulsifying wax and water.

detoxication (dē-toks-ē-kā'-shun) [L. *de-*, away; G. *toxikon*, poison]. The process of removing the poisonous property of a substance—detoxicant, adj., n.; detoxicate, v.

detritus (det-rī'-tus) [L. *detritum*, from *deterere*, to wear away]. Matter produced by detrition; waste matter from disintegration.

detrusor (dē-troo'-sėr) [L. *detrudere*, to thrust from]. The muscle of the urinary bladder.

Dettol. A non-caustic antiseptic of the chloroxylenol type.

dexamethasone. Thirty times as active as cortisone in suppressing inflammation. Less likely to precipitate diabetes than the other steroids. Sometimes given to unconscious patients to prevent cerebral oedema.

dexamphetamine (deks-am-fet'-a-mēn). Central stimulant similar to amphetamine (q.v.), and used for similar purposes. Sometimes used as an appetite depressant in obesity.

Dexedrine. Dexamphetamine (q.v.).

dextran (deks'-tran). A blood plasma substitute, obtained by the action of a specific bacterium on sugar solutions. Used as a 6 or 10 per cent solution in haemorrhage, shock, etc.

dextranase (deks'-tran-ās). An enzyme that stops sugar from leaving the sticky deposit which sets free the acid that eats into tooth enamel and cannot be brushed away. Made from a mould related to that producing penicillin.

dextrin (deks'-trin). A soluble polysaccharide formed during the hydrolysis of starch.

dextrocardia (deks-trō-kár'-di-á) [L. *dexter*, right; G. *kardia*, heart]. Transposition of the heart to the right side of the thorax—dextrocardial, adj.

dextromoramide (deks-trō-mor'-a-mīd). Substitute for morphine. Can cause drug dependence.

dextropropoxyphene (deks'-trō-prō-poks'-i-fēn). Milder type of analgesic used as morphine substitute.

dextrose (dcks'-trōs). Glucose, a soluble carbohydrate (monosaccharide) widely used by intravenous infusion in dehydration, shock and postoperatively. Also given orally as a readily absorbed sugar in acidosis and other nutritional disturbances.

DFP. Dyflos (q.v.).

DF 118. Dihydrocodeine tartrate (q.v.).

dhobie itch (dō'-bē). Tinea cruris (q.v.). Derived from belief that ringworm of the groin originated from infection of the Indian laundryman (dhobie).

diabetes (dī-a-bē'-tēz) [G. diabainein, to cross through]. A disease characterized by polyuria. Used without qualification it means d. mellitus. d. innocens, renal glycosuria, where there is unusual permeability of the kidneys to glucose, the concentration in the blood remaining within normal limits. d. insipidus, a disease (congenital or following injury or infection) of the posterior pituitary gland or its adnexa. There is dehydration, polydipsia, polyuria, urine being pale and of low specific gravity. nephrogenic d. insipidus, brought to medical attention 25 years ago, is, like haemophilia, inherited through females but appears only in males. Afflicted persons known as 'water drinkers'. Characterized by polydipsia and polyuria but there is normal secretion of antidiuretic hormone. d. mellitus, a condition characterized by hyperglycaemia due to deficiency or diminished effectiveness of insulin. The hyperglycaemia leads to glycosuria, which in turn causes polyuria and polydipsia. Severe dehydration, sometimes sufficient to cause unconsciousness (hyperosmolar non-ketoacidotic diabetic coma), may occur. Impaired utilization of carbohydrate is associated with increased secretion of antistorage hormones such as glucagon and growth hormone in an attempt to provide alternative metabolic substrate. Glycogenolysis, gluconeogenesis and lipolysis are all increased. The latter results in excessive formation of ketone bodies which in turn leads to acidosis. If untreated this will eventually cause coma (ketoacidotic diabetic coma) and death. Two main clinical types are recognized: **Juvenile-onset diabetes** usually develops before the age of 40 and is characterized by complete lack of insulin. Such patients require treatment with insulin. **Maturity-onset diabetes** usually appears in middle-aged or elderly patients who are often obese. They have a variable, although less than normal amount of plasma insulin and can usually be controlled by dietary means alone, or by an oral hypoglycaemic drug. *Potential diabetics* have a normal glucose tolerance test but are at increased risk of developing diabetes for genetic reasons. *Latent diabetics* have a normal glucose tolerance test but are known to have had an abnormal test under conditions imposing a burden on the pancreatic beta cells, e.g. during infection or pregnancy. In the latter instance the term *gestational diabetes* is commonly used.

diabetic (dī-ab-et'-ik). Pertaining to diabetes.

diabetogenic (dī-a-bet-ō-jen'-ik) [G. diabainein, to cross through; gignesthai, to be produced]. 1. Causing diabetes. 2. Applied to an anterior pituitary hormone.

Diabinese (dī'-ab-in-ēz). Chlorpropamide (q.v.).

diacetic acid (dī-a-sē'-tik as'-id). Syn., acetoacetic acid (q.v.).

Diaginol (dī-aj' in-ol). Sodium acetrizoate (q.v.).

diagnosis (dī-ag-nō'-sis) [G. dia, through; gnosis, recognizing]. The art or act of distinguishing one disease from another. differential d., arriving at a correct decision between diseases presenting a similar clinical picture—diagnose, v.t.; diagnosis, pl.; See CYTO-DIAGNOSIS.

diagnostic (dī-ag-nos'-tik) [G. dia, through; gnosis, recognizing]. 1. Pertaining to diagnosis. 2. Serving as evidence in diagnosis—diagnostician, n.

diaguanides (dī'-a-gwan-īds). See BIGUANIDES.

Dial (dī'-al). Allobarbitone (q.v.).

dialysis (di-al'-i-sis) [G. a separating]. Separation of substances in solution by taking advantage of their differing diffusability through a porous membrane as in the artificial kidney. **peritoneal d.**, a method of irrigating the peritoneum; urea and other waste products are exuded into the irrigation fluid and withdrawn from the abdominal cavity—dialyse, v.t.; dialyses, pl. See HAEMODIALYSIS.

diaminodiphenylsulphone. Synthetic drug for use against resistant strains of malaria; and for leprosy.

diamorphine (dī-a-mor′-fēn). Heroin, a derivative of morphine, but liable to cause addiction. Valuable in severe pain, and as a cough depressant in useless cough.

Diamox (dī′-a-moks). Acetazolamide (q.v.).

Dianabol (dī-an′-á-bol). Methandienone (q.v.).

Diandrone (dī′-an-drōn). Dehydroisoandrosterone. Endocrine useful in psychoneurosis, neurasthenia and schizophrenia.

diapedesis (dī-a-pe-dē′-sis) [G. *dia,* through; *pedesis,* springing]. The passage of blood cells through the vessel walls into the tissues—diapedetic, adj.

diaphoresis (dī-af-or-ē′-sis) [G. *dia,* through; *phorein,* to carry]. Perspiration.

diaphoretic (dī-af-or-et′-ik) [G. *dia,* through; *phorein,* to carry]. An agent which induces diaphoresis.

diaphragm (dī′-a-fram) [G. *diaphragma,* partition]. 1. The dome-shaped muscular partition between the thorax above and the abdomen below. 2. Any partitioning membrane or septum—diaphragmatic, adj.

diaphysis (dī-af′-i-sis) [G. a growing through]. The shaft of a long bone—diaphyseal, adj.; diaphyses, pl.

diaplacental (dī-a-pla-sen′-tal) [G. *dia,* through; L. *placenta,* cake]. Through the placenta.

diarrhoea (dī-á-rē′-á) [G. *diarrhoia,* a flowing through]. Deviation from established bowel rhythm characterized by an increase in frequency and fluidity of the stools. Epidemic diarrhoea of the newborn is a highly contagious infection of maternity hospitals. The gastroenteritis is probably the result of virus infection.

diarthrosis (dī-ár-thrō′-sis) [G. articulation]. A synovial, freely movable joint—diarthrodial, adj.; diarthroses, pl.

diasonograph (dī-á-sōn′-o-graf). Ultrasound machine used to show position of organs inside body.

diastase (dī′-as-tās) [G. *diastasis,* a separation]. An amylase produced by animal, plant and bacterial cells. **pancreatic d.** is excreted in the urine (and saliva) and therefore estimation of urinary diastase may be used as a test of pancreatic function.

diastasis (dī-as′-tas-is) [G. separation]. A separation of bones without fracture: dislocation.

diastole (dī-as′-to-li) [G. *diastole,* difference]. The relaxation period of the cardiac cycle, as opposed to systole—diastolic, adj.

diathermy (dī-á-thér′-mi) [G. *dia,* through; *therme,* heat]. The passage of a high frequency electric current through the tissues whereby heat is produced. When both electrodes are large, the heat is diffused over a wide area according to the electrical resistance of the tissues. In this form it is widely used in the treatment of inflammation, especially when deeply seated (e.g. sinusitis, pelvic cellulitis). When one electrode is very small the heat is concentrated in this area and becomes great enough to destroy tissue. In this form (surgical diathermy) it is used to stop bleeding at operation by coagulation of blood, or to cut through tissue in operation for malignant disease.

diazepam (dī-az′-ē-pam). Tranquillosedative with muscle relaxant properties. Useful in i.v. infusion for status epilepticus and tetanus.

diazoxide (dī-az-oks′-īd). Supresses activity of insulin-producing beta cells, therefore useful in hypoglycaemia from pancreatic tumour. Its main use is as a hypotensive agent by rapid i.v. injection in hypertensive emergencies.

Dibenyline (dī-ben′-il-in). Phenoxybenzamine (q.v.).

Dibistin. This is a mixture of antazoline and tripelennamine. Antiallergic.

Dibotin (dib′-o-tin). Phenformin (q.v.).

dibromomannitol (dī-brō-mō-man′-it-ol). Oral drug which has an action similar to busulphan and may be effective when busulphan has been used previously.

dicephalous (dī-kef′-a-lus). Two-headed.

dichloralphenazone (dī-klor-al-fen′-á-zōn). Causes less gastric irritation than chloral hydrate. Hypnotic of the chloral group. Particularly suitable for children.

dichlorophen (dī-klor′-ō-fen). Synthetic

anthelmintic effective against tapeworm. Preliminary fasting and purging as with filix mas, is unnecessary.

dichlorphenamide (dī-klor-fen'-a-mīd). Oral diuretic of short duration. Carbonic anhydrase inhibitor. Used for systemic treatment of glaucoma.

dichuchwa. Term for non-venereal syphilis used in Bechuanaland.

dicloxacillin (dī-cloks-a-sil'-in). See FLUCLOXACILLIN.

Diconal (dī-kōn'-al). Dipipanone hydrochloride (q.v.). and cyclizine (q.v.).

dicophane (dī'-ko-fān). Dichlorodiphenyltrichloroethane (DDT). Well-known insecticide, used against pediculosis capitis and other body parasites as lotion or dusting powder.

dicoumarol (dī-koo'-mar-ol) Early orally effective anticoagulant. Now largely replaced by more controllable drugs.

dicrotic (dī-kro'-ik) [G. dikrotos, double beating]. Pertaining to, or having a double beat, as indicated by a second expansion of the artery during diastole. **d. wave,** the second rise in the tracing of a dicrotic pulse.

dicyclomine (dī-sī'-klō-mēn). An antispasmodic resembling atropine, but less potent. Used in pylorospasm and gastric hypermotility.

Dicynene (dī'-sin-ēn). Ethamsylate (q.v).

dienoestrol (dī-nē'-strol). A synthetic oestrogen similar to stilboestrol, but less active.

dietetics (dī-e-tet'-iks) [G. diata, mode of living, from diatoein, to support life]. The interpretation and application of the scientific principles of nutrition to feeding in health and disease.

diethazine (dī-eth'-a-zen). Synthetic anti-Parkinson drug.

diethylcarbamazine (dī-eth'-il-kar-bam-az-ēn). Oral filaricide especially active against young worms. Can kill roundworms.

diethylpropion hydrochloride (dī-eth'-il-prō'-pi-on hī-drō-klor'-īd). CNS stimulant used as an appetite suppressant.

dietitian (dī-e-tish'-un). One who applies the principles of nutrition to the feeding of an individual or a group of individuals in a heterogeneous setting of economics or health, e.g. in schools, hospitals, institutions, restaurants, hotels, food factories, and in the World Health Organization.

Dietl's crisis (dēt'-lz krī'-siz). A complication of 'floating kidney' (nephroptosis). Kinking of the ureter is thought to be responsible for the severe colic produced in the lumbar region. [Józef Dietl, Polish physician, 1804–78.]

differential blood count. The estimation of the relative proportions of the different leucocyte cells in the blood. The normal differential count is: polymorphs, 65 to 70 per cent; lymphocytes, 20 to 25 per cent; monocytes, 5 per cent; eosinophils, 0 to 3 per cent; basophils, 0 to 0.5 per cent. In childhood the proportion of lymphocytes is higher.

diffusion (dif-fū'-zhun) [L. diffundere, to pour]. 1. The process whereby gases and liquids of different densities intermingle when brought into contact, until the density is equal throughout. 2. Dialysis.

digestion (di-jest'-chun) [L. digestio, distribution]. The process by which food is rendered absorbable—digestible, digestive, adj.; digestibility, n.; digest, v.t., v.i.

digit (dij'-it) [L. digitus, finger]. A finger or toe—digital, adj.

Digitaline (dij-it-al'-ēn). Digitoxin.

digitalis (dij-it-ā'-lis). Leaf of the common foxglove. Powerful cardiac tonic, widely used in congestive heart failure and atrial fibrillation. Large initial doses are sometimes given.

digitalization (dij-it-al-ī-zā'-shun). Physiological saturation with digitalis, to obtain optimum therapeutic effect.

Digitoxin (dij-it-oks'-in). Glycoside of digitalis.

Digoxin (dij-oks'-in). Glycoside of digitalis.

diguanides (dī'-gwan-īds). Oral hypoglycaemic agents, thought to function as such by increasing glucose uptake in muscle and skin.

Diguanil (dī'-qwan-il). Metformin (q.v.).

dihydrocodeine tartrate (dī-hī-drō-kō'-dēn tar'-trāt). Non-habit forming analgesic, useful for suppression of cough, respiratory infections and painful wounds. Can be given orally or by injection.

dihydromorphinone (dī-hī'-drō-mor'-fin-ōn). A morphine-like analgesic of high potency but short action. It has little hypnotic effect. Occasionally used as a depressant in severe cough. Considered less habit-forming than morphine.

dihydrostreptomycin (dī-hī'-drō-strep'-tō-mī-sin). A derivative of streptomycin and used for similar purposes. A mixture of both antibiotics is sometimes employed to reduce any neurotoxic effects.

dihydrotachysterol (dī-hī-drō-tak-is-tē'-rol). Prepared in oil; used to raise the blood calcium, especially in parathyroid tetany.

diiodohydroxyquinoline (dī'-ī-ō'-dō-hī-droks'-i-kwin'-o-lin). Used chiefly in amoebic dysentery in association with emetine.

dilatation (dī-la-tā'-shun) [L. *dilatare,* to spread out]. Stretching or enlargement. May occur physiologically, pathologically or be induced artificially.

Dilaudid (di-law'-did). Dihydromorphinone (q.v.).

dill water. Aqua anethi. Popular preparation of a volatile oil used as a carminative for infants to relax muscular tone in digestive colic or flatulence.

diloxanide furoate (dil-oks'-an-īd-fū'-rō-āt). For amoebic dysentery.

Dimelor (dim-ē'-lor). Acetohexamide (q.v.).

dimenhydrinate (dī-men-hīd'-rin-āt). Powerful antiemetic for travel sickness, vomiting of pregnancy and vertigo.

dimercaprol (dī-mer'-kā-prol). An organic compound used as an antidote for poisoning by arsenic and gold. Also useful in mercury poisoning if treatment is prompt, but it is not suitable for lead poisoning. It forms soluble compounds with the metals, which are then rapidly excreted. Syn., BAL.

Dindevan (din'-dē-van). Pheninidione (q.v.).

Dioctyl-Medo (dī-ok'-til-med-ō). Dioctyl sodium sulphosuccinate (q.v.).

dioctylsodium sulphosuccinate (dī-ok'-til-sō'-di-um sul-fō-suks'-in-āt). Wetting agent helpful in prevention of faecal impaction. Should be taken regularly for this purpose.

diodone (dī'-ō-dōn). Organic iodine compound used as X-ray contrast agent in intravenous pyelography.

Diodoquin (dī-od'-o-kwin). Di-iodohydroxyquinoline (q.v.).

dioptre (dī-op'-tėr) [G. *dioptra,* an optical instrument]. A unit of measurement in refraction. A lens of one dioptre has a focal length of 1 metre.

dioxide (dī-oks'-īd). Oxide formed by combination of two atoms of oxygen with one of metal or non-metal.

Diparcol (dī-par'-kol). Diethazine (q.v.).

diphenhydramine (dī-fen-hīd'-ra-min). One of the first antihistamines (q.v.). Widely used in allergic conditions and travel sickness. Also has sedative action.

diphenoxylate (dī-fen-oks'-i-lāt). Prescribed for acute and chronic diarrhoea, and gastrointestinal upsets. It has some morphine-like actions: 1. It depresses the respiratory centre; 2. It acts as a cortical depressant; 3. It reduces intestinal mobility. Atropine is included to provide dryness of the mouth should patient take an overdose.

diphenylhydantoin (dī-fen-il-hīd'-an-toin). Used in digitalis poisoning. See p. 344.

diphtheria (dif-thē'-ri-á) [G. *diphthera,* leather, membrane]. An acute, specific, infectious, notifiable disease caused by *Corynebacterium diptheriae.* Characterized by a grey, adherent, false membrane growing on a mucous surface, usually that of the upper respiratory tract. Locally there is pain, swelling and may be suffocation. Systemically the toxins attack the heart muscle and nerves—diphtheritic, adj.

diphtheroid (dif'-thėr-oid) [G. *diphthera,* leather; *eidos,* form]. Any bacterium morphologically and culturally resembling *Corynebacterium diphtheriae.*

dipipanone (dī-pi-pan'-ōn). Synthetic morphine substitute with both sedative and pain relieving properties.

diplegia (dī-plē'-ji-á) [G. *dis,* twice; *plege,* a stroke]. Symmetrical paralysis of legs, usually associated with cerebral damage—diplegic, adj. (Cf. paraplegia.)

diplococcus (dip-lō-kok'-us) [G. *diploos,* double; *kokkos,* grain]. A coccal bacterium characteristically occurring in pairs. Diplococcus may be used in a binominal to describe a characteristically paired coccus, e.g. *Diplococcus pneumoniae* = pneumococcus.

diplopia (dip-lō'-pi-á) [G. *diploos,* double; *opsis,* vision]. Double vision.

diprophylline (dī-prof'-i-lin). Diuretic. Xanthine derivative. Can be given orally, intravenously and as a suppository.

dipsomania (dip-sō-mā'-ni-á) [G. *dipsa,* thirst; *mania,* madness]. Alcoholism in which the drinking occurs in bouts, often with long periods of sobriety between—dipsomaniac, adj., n.

dipyridamole (dī-pir-id'-á-mōl). Inhibits platelet thrombus formation on dialyser membranes and reduces the frequency of embolic complications in patients with prosthetic heart valves.

Direma (dir-ē-'má). Hydrochlorothiazide (q.v.).

Disablement Resettlement Officer. Appointed by the Department of Employment to ensure the local operation of the Disabled Persons Employment Acts, 1944 and 1958.

disaccharide (dī-sak'-ár-īd). A sugar (carbohydrate, e.g. lactose, maltose, sucrose) which yields two molecules of monosaccharide on hydrolysis.

Disalcid (dī-sal'-sid). An ester of salicylic acid which is insoluble in gastric juice therefore less likely than aspirin to cause gastric irritation and erosion.

disarticulation (dis-árt-ik-ū-lā'-shun) [L. *dis*, asunder; *articulus*, joint]. Amputation at a joint.

discectomy (dis-sek'-to-mi). Surgical removal of a disc, usually an intervertebral disc.

discission (dis-si'-shun) [L. *discissum*, from *discindere*, to tear]. Rupturing of lens capsule to allow absorption of lens substance in the condition of cataract. Syn., needling.

discogenic (dis-kō-jen'-ik). Arising in or produced by a disc, usually an intervertebral disc.

discogram (dis'-kō-gram). See DISCOGRAPHY.

discography (dis-kog'-ra-fi) [G *diskos*, disc; *graphein*, to write]. X ray of an intervertebral disc after it has been rendered radio-opaque. Normal disc accepts not more than 0.5 ml; damaged disc may accept 2 to 3 ml. Injection frequently reproduces pain -discographic, adj.; discographically, adv.; discograph, n.

disinfectants (dis-in-fēk'-tants) [L. *dis*, the reverse of; *infestare*, to infest]. Germicides which are too corrosive or toxic to be applied to tissues, but which are suitable for application to inanimate objects.

disinfection (dis-in-fek'-shun) [F. *desinfecter*]. The destruction of all microorganisms, except spores, and can refer to the action of antiseptics as well as disinfectants.

disinfestation (dis-in-fes-tā-shun) [L. *dis*, the reverse of; *infestare*, to infest]. Extermination of infesting agents, especially lice. Delousing.

Disipal (di'-si-pal). Orphenadrine (q.v.).

disipidin (dī-sip'-i-din). Posterior pituitary snuff. Useful in enuresis, diabetes insipidus and nocturnal frequency in the aged.

dislocation (dis-lō-kā'-shun) [L. *dis*, separation; *locare*, to place]. A displacement of organs or articular surfaces, so that all apposition between them is lost. It may be congenital, spontaneous, traumatic, or recurrent. Syn., luxation -dislocated, adj.; dislocate, v.t.

disobliteration (dis-ob-lit er-ā'-shun). Rebore. Removal of that which blocks a vessel, most often intimal plaques in an artery, when it is called endarterectomy (q.v.).

disodium cromoglycate (dī-sōd'-i-um krō-mō-glī'-cāt). Useful in allergic airway disease. It is not anti-inflammatory, nor is it a bronchodilator. It inhibits the effects of some specific types of reaginic antibody-antigen reactions. Gives relief of bronchospasm in asthma.

disorientation (dis-or-i-en-tā'-shun) [l *dis*, separation; *oriens*, East]. Loss of orientation (q.v.)

dissection (dis-sek'-shun) [L. *dis-secare*, to cut in pieces]. Separation of tissues by cutting. block d. of glands, the total excision of a group of lymph nodes, usually part of the treatment of carcinoma.

disseminated sclerosis (dis-em'-in-āt'-ed skler-ō'-sis) See SCLEROSIS.

dissociation (dis-sō-shi-ā'-shun) [L. *dissociare*, to separate from fellowship]. In psychiatry an abnormal mental process by which the mind achieves non-recognition and isolation of certain unpalatable facts. This involves the actual splitting off from consciousness of all the unpalatable ideas so that the individual is no longer aware of them. Dissociation is a common symptom in hysteria but is seen in its most exaggerated form in delusional psychoses, e.g. a woman who, being deluded, believes she is the Queen cheerfully scrubbing the ward floor. Her royal status and the fact that she is charring are completely separated or dissociated in her mind and she does not recognize the incongruity.

distal (dis'-tal) [L. *distare*, to be distant]. Farthest from the head or source—distally, adv.

Distalgesic (dis-tal-jēz'-ik) Dextropropoxyphene with paracetamol. Useful analgesic, especially for chronic conditions.

Distaquaine (dis'-ta-qwān). Various preparations of penicillin (q.v.).

distichiasis (dis-tik-ī'-as-is) [G.*dis*, twice; *stichos*, row]. An extra row of eyelashes at the inner lid border, which is turned inward against the eye.

distractibility (dis-trak-tib-il'-i-ti)[L.*distractus*, from *distrahere*, to draw apart]. A psychiatric term applied to a disorder of the power of attention when it can only be applied momentarily.

disulfiram (dī-sulf'-ir-am): A sulphur compound that in the presence of alcohol causes nausea and vomiting. Hence used in alcoholism.

dithranol (dī-thrā'-nol). Similar to chrysarobin (q.v), but more powerful. Sensitivity tests necessary before treatment begins.

diuresis (dī-ū-rē'-sis) [G. *diourein*, to pass urine]. Increased secretion of urine. **forced d.**, term used when diuresis is part of intensive therapy, particularly in poisoning.

diuretic (dī-ū-ret'-ik) [G, *diouretikos*, diuretic]. 1. Increasing the flow of urine. 2. An agent which increases the flow of urine.

divaricator (dī-var'-i-kā-tor) [L. *divaricare*, to spread asunder]. A hinged wooden splint, permitting various degrees of divarication in congenital dislocation of the hip.

diverticulitis (dī-vår-tik-ū-lī'-tis) [L. *diverticulum*, a bypath; *-itis*, inflammation]. Inflammation of a diverticulum.

diverticulosis (dī-vér-tik-ū-lō'-sis) [L. *diverticulum*, a bypath; *-osis*, condition]. A condition in which there are many diverticula, especially in the intestines.

diverticulum (dī-vér-tik'-ū-lum) [L.]. A pouch or sac protruding from the wall of a tube or hollow organ. May be congenital or acquired—diverticula, pl.

Dixarit (diks'-ar-it). Clonidine (q.v.).

DNA. Deoxyribonucleic acid (q.v.).

dobutamine (do-bū-ta-mēn). A directly acting stimulant of heart muscle which augments myocardial contractility in severe cardiac failure and shock syndrome, e.g. after myocardial infarction.

Dobutrex. Dobutamine (q.v.).

DOCA. Deoxycortone (q.v.).

Döderlein's bacillus (*Lactobacillus acidophilus*). Gram-positive rod bacterium which produces acid; occurs in the normal vagina, and the pH of the vaginal secretions is largely due to the growth of the organism. Also found in the intestine and the bacilli are especially numerous if the diet is rich in milk or milk products. Non-pathogenic. [Albert Döderlein, German obstetrician and gynaecologist, 1860–1941.]

Dogger Bank itch. Sensitization dermatitis due to Alcyonidium (seaweed family). Clinical features include a papular and vesicular rash on hands and forearms with facial erythema and oedema.

dolor (dō'-lor) [L.]. Pain.

Doloxene (dol'-oks-ēn). Dextropropoxyphene (q.v.).

dominant (dom'-in-ant) [L. *dominans*, ruling]. A character possessed by one parent, which, in the offspring, masks the corresponding alternative character derived from the other parent. Opp. recessive. See MENDEL'S LAW.

domiphen bromide (dom'-i-fen brō'-mīd). White, uncoated lozenges for mouth and throat infections.

Donovan's bodies. See LEISHMAN-DONOVAN.

dopamine (dōp'-a-min). A catecholamine neurotransmitter, closely related to adrenaline and noradrenaline. Increases cardiac output and renal blood flow but does not produce peripheral vasoconstriction. Most valuable in hypotension and shock of cardiac origin. Normally present in high concentration in those regions of the brain which are selectively damaged in Parkinsonism.

Doppler ultrasound technique. Machine sends out ultrasounds, which pick up the velocity of blood flow through the vein and are transmitted as sound. If the vein is completely occluded, no sound is transmitted as there is no flow.

Doptone (dop'-tōn). Instrument using echo-sounder principles to detect fetal heart at very early stage.

Dorbanex (dor'-ban-eks). Contains faecal-softening agent and laxative for constipation. Available as capsules and in two strengths of highly palatable liquid.

Doriden (do'-ri-den). Glutethemide (q.v.).

dorsal (dor'-sal) [L. *dorsum*, back]. Pertaining to the back, or the posterior part of an organ.

dorsiflexion (dor-si-flek'-shun) [L. *dorsum*, back; *flectere*, to bend]. Bending backwards. In the case of the great toe—upwards. See BABINSKI'S REFLEX.

dorsocentral (dor-sō-sen'-tral) [L. *dorsum*, back; G. *kentron*, centre of a circle]. At the back and in the centre.

dorsolumbar (dor-sō-lum'-bar) [L. *dorsum*, back; *lumbus*, loin]. The lumbar region of the back.

douche (doosh) [F.]. A stream of fluid directed against the body externally or into a body cavity.

Dover's powder. A time-honoured remedy containing 10 per cent of opium and ipecacuanha. Once used extensively as a diaphoretic, but is now prescribed less often. [Thomas Dover, English physician, 1660–1742.]

Down's syndrome. Mongol (q.v.).

doxepin (doks'-e-pin). One of the tricyclic antidepressants. Effective after 3 to 15 days medication.

doxycycline (doks-i-sī'-klin). New, rapidly excreted tetracycline.

D-penicillamine (pen-i-sil'-a-mēn). Drug of first choice in 'rheumatoid factor-positive' rheumatoid arthritis. See PENICILLAMINE

dracontiasis (dra-kon-tī'-a-sis). Infestation with *Dracunculus medinensis* (Guinea worm), a nematode parasite which infests man from contaminated drinking water. From the patient's intestine the adult female migrates to the skin surface to deposit her larvae, producing a cord-like thickening which ulcerates. Common in India and Africa.

Dracunculus medinensis. Nematode parasite responsible for dracontiasis (q.v.).

Dramamine (dram'-a-mēn). Dimenhydrinate (q.v.).

DRO. Disablement Resettlement Officer (q.v.).

Droleptan (drō-lep'-tan). Droperidol (q.v.).

Dromoran (drom'-or-an). Levorphanol (q.v.).

drop attacks. Periodic falling because of sudden loss of postural control of the lower limbs, without vertigo or loss of consciousness. Usually followed by sudden return of normal muscle tone, allowing the person to rise, if uninjured. See VERTEBROBASILAR INSUFFICIENCY.

droperidol (drop-er'-i-dol). A butyrophenone compound. Neuroleptic agent. Can be used as a pre-operative premedication. Induces state of mental detachment without loss of consciousness or effect upon respiratory system.

dropsy (drop'-si) [G. *hydrops*, from *hydor*, water]. See ANASARCA, ASCITES and OEDEMA—dropsical, adj.

drostanolone (dros-tan'-ō-lōn). Anabolic agent. Has less virilizing effect than Durabolin or deca-Durabolin.

drug dependence. A state arising from repeated administration of a drug on a periodic or continuous basis (WHO, 1964). Drug dependence now a preferable term to d. addiction and d. habituation.

'drug fast'. A term used to describe resistance of microbial cells to the action of anti-microbial drugs.

Ducrey's bacillus (*Haemophilus ducreyi*) (dū-crā'-i). Gram-negative rod. The causative organism of soft chancre (chancroid), a venereal disease. [Augosto Ducrey, Italian dermatologist, 1860–1940.]

ductless glands (dukt'-les). See ENDOCRINE GLANDS.

ductus arteriosus (duk'-tus ár-tē-ri-ō'-sus). A blood vessel connecting the left pulmonary artery to the aorta, to bypass the lungs, in the fetal circulation. **patent d. a.** is a form of congenital heart defect wherein this 'shunt' remains open.

Duhamel's operation. For Hirschsprung's disease (q.v.).

Dulcolax (dul'-ko-laks). A synthetic laxative that is effective without griping. Bisacodyl.

'dumping syndrome.' The name given to the symptoms which often follow a partial gastrectomy, bilious vomiting and a feeling of faintness and weakness after meals.

duodenitis (dū-ō-dēn-ī'-tis) [L. *duodeni*, twelve; *-itis*, inflammation]. Inflammation of the duodenum.

duodenojejunal (dū-ō-dē-nō-je-joo'-nal) [L. *duodeni*, twelve; *jejunus*, empty]. Pertaining to the duodenum and jejunum.

duodenopancreatectomy (dū-ō-dē'-nō-pan-krē-at-ek'-to-mi) [L. *duodeni,* twelve; G. *pankreas,* pancreas; *ektome,* excision]. Surgical excision of the duodenum and part of the pancreas, carried out in cases of cancer arising in the region of the head of the pancreas (e.g. lower end of common bile duct).

duodenostomy (dū-ō-dē-nos'-to-mi) [L. *duodeni,* twelve; G. *stoma,* mouth]. A surgically made fistula between the duodenum and another cavity, e.g. cholecystoduodenostomy, a fistula between the gall-bladder and duodenum made to relieve jaundice in inoperable cancer of the head of the pancreas.

duodenum (dū-ō-dē'-num) [L. *duodeni,* twelve]. The fixed, curved, first portion of the small intestine, connecting the stomach above to the jejunum below—duodenal, adj.

Duogastrone (dū-ō-gas'-trōn). Carbenoxolone. Capsules for duodenal ulcer. Swell to twice their size in stomach and 'pop' to release drug.

Dupuytren's contraction (dū'-pwi-trens). Contracture of the palmar fascia, which bends and fixes one or more fingers.

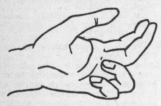

Dupuytren's contraction

Durabolin (dūr'-a-bol-in). An agent with testosterone-like activity. Useful for secondary cancer deposits in bone. Metabolically a protein sparer; used where there is extensive tissue damage, e.g. burns and scalds.

Duvadilan (dū-va-dil'-an). Isoxuprine hydrochloride (q.v.).

D-Vac antigens (an'-ti-jens). Used for desensitization in conditions of allergy.

DVT. Deep vein thrombosis (q.v.). See THROMBOPHLEBITIS.

dwarf (dwawrf) [A.S. *dweorg*]. Person of stunted growth. Condition is found in achondroplasia, hypothyroidism (cretinism), congenital heart disease, etc. Two types due to underactivity of ante-rior pituitary gland. **Lorain d,** delayed skeletal growth; retarded sexual development; alert; intelligent. **Frolich's d,** stunted growth; obesity; arrested sexual development; lethargic; somnolent; mentally subnormal—dwarfism,n.

dyflos (dif'-los). A fluorine derivative with an action similar to that of eserine and neostigmine. Used mostly as a 0.1 per cent solution in oil for glaucoma, when a very long action is required. As an organophosphorous compound, it is used as an insecticide in agriculture. Powerful and irreversible anticholinesterase action. Potentially dangerous to man for this reason.

dynamic psychology (dī-nam'-ik sī-kol'-o-ji) [G. *dynamis,* strength; *psyche,* soul; *logos,* study]. A psychological theory which stresses the element of energy in mental processes.

dynamometer (dī-nam-om'-ē-tėr) [G. *dynamis,* strength; *metron,* measure]. Apparatus to test the strength of grip.

dysaesthesia (dis-ės-thēz'-i-á) [G. *dys-,* difficult; *aisthesis,* sensation]. Impairment of touch sensation.

dysarthria (dis-árth'-ri-á) [G. *dys-,* difficult; *arthron,* joint]. Impairment of articulation. Stammering.

dysarthrosis (dis-ár-thrō'-sis) [G. *dys-,* difficult; *arthron,* joint; *-osis,* condition]. Any joint condition limiting movement.

dyschezia (dis-kē'-zi-á) [G. *dys-,* difficult; *chezein,* to go to stool]. Difficult or painful defaecation.

dyschondroplasia (dis-kon-drō-plá'-zi-á) [G. *dys,* difficult; *chondros,* cartilage; *plassein,* to form]. Normal trunk, short arms and legs.

dyscoria (dis-kor'-ē-á) [G. *dys-,* abnormal *kore,* pupil]. Abnormality of the pupil.

dyscrasia (dis-krā-zi-á) [G. *dys-,* difficult; *krasis,* mixing]. A morbid general state resulting from the presence of toxic materials in the blood. **blood d.,** usually refers to abnormality of the blood cells.

dysentery (dis'-en-tėr-i) [G. *dys-* difficult; *enteron,* intestine]. Inflammation of the bowel with evacuation of blood and mucus, accompanied by tenesmus and colic. **amoebic d.** is caused by the protozoon *Entamoeba histolytica.* **bacillary d.** is caused by the bacillus of Shiga, Flexner or Sonne. Disease results from poor sanitation and the house-fly carries the infection from faeces to food. See AMOEBIASIS—dysenteric, adj.

dysfunction (dis-fungk'-shun) [G. *dys-*, abnormal; L. *functus*, from *fungi*, to perform]. Abnormal functioning of any organ or part.

dysgammaglobulinaemia (dis-gam'-maglob'-ū-lin-ē'-mi-à). Syn., antibody deficiency syndrome. Disturbance of gammaglobulin production. Can be transient, congenital or acquired. Normally there is transfer of IgG from mother to baby, the amount so transferred gradually falls. This can lead to transient hypogammaglobulinaemia with repeated respiratory infections. Injections of gammaglobulin are given until normal levels occur. Congenital agammaglobulinaemia is a sex-linked recessive genetic variety and is the commonest type of total deficiency. The lymph nodes and spleen are abnormal. Males are solely affected, females being carriers of the abnormal gene. As yet there is no means of detecting carriers. The disease usually presents in the second or third years as severe, recurrent bacterial infections with high fever. Virus infections are handled well, because the defence mechanism is different. Acquired agammaglobulinaemia occurs at any age and in either sex. Cause unknown. Secondary agammaglobulinaemia may occur in lymphoma, leukaemia and myeloma, especially after chemotherapy or radiation. It may also be found in bullous skin disorders such as pemphigus and eczema and after burns when it is due to excessive loss of protein in the exuded fluid.

dysgenesis (dis-jen'-es-is) [G *dys-*, abnormal, *genesis*, descent]. Malformation during embryonic development—dysgenetic, adj.; dysgenetically, adv.

dysgerminoma (dis-jér-min-ō'-mà) [G. *dys-*, abnormal; L. *germen*, germ; G. *-oma*, tumour]. A tumour of the ovary of low grade malignancy. It is not hormone secreting, as it is developed from cells which date back to the undifferentiated state of gonadal development, i.e. before the cells have either male or female attributes.

dyshidrosis (dis-hid-rō'-sis) [G. *dys-*, abnormal; *hidrosis*, sweating]. A vesicular skin eruption, thought to be caused by blockage of the sweat ducts at their orifice.

dyskaryosis (dis-kar-i-ō'-sis). Term used for the first stage of abnormality in a cervical smear. Follow-up tests may revert to normal, but some may become positive and demand biopsy.

dyskinesia (dis-ki-nē'-zi-à) [G. *dys-*, difficult; *kinesis*, motion]. Impairment of voluntary movement—dyskinetic, adj.

dyslalia (dis-lã'-li-à) [G. *dys-*, difficult; *lalein*, to talk]. Difficulty in talking due to defect of speech organs. Immature articulation—dyslalic, adj.

dyslexia (dis-leks'-i-à) [G. *dys-*, difficult; *lexis*, word]. Impairment of reading ability. The child usually has difficulty with groups of letters, but intelligence is unimpaired. Often associated with mirror-writing—dyslexic, adj.

dysmaturity (dis-mat-ūr'-it-i) [G. *dys-*, difficult; L. *maturare*, to make ripe]. Signs and symptoms of growth retardation at birth. 'Small for dates'.

dysmelia (dis-mēl'-ı-à) [G. *dys-*, difficult; *melos*, limb]. Limb deficiency.

dysmenorrhoea (dis-men-ô-rē'-à) [G. *dys-*, difficult; *men*, month; *rhein*, to flow]. Painful menstruation. **spasmodic d.**, comes on during the first day of a period, often within an hour or two of the start of bleeding. It comes in spasms of acute colicky pain in the lower part of the abdomen, and sometimes in the back and inner parts of the thighs. The spasms can be bad enough to cause fainting and vomiting. The victims, with some exceptions, are immature shy girls, with small breasts, pale nipples and not much pubic hair. **congestive d.**, caused not by too little oestrogen, but by too little progesterone. Sufferers know several days in advance that their period is coming, because they have a dull aching pain in the lower abdomen, increasing heaviness, perhaps constipation, nausea and lack of appetite. There may also be breast tenderness, headache and backache. The sufferers, again with exceptions, tend to have rounded, feminine hips, large breasts with dark nipples, ample pubic hair, with a marked maternal instinct and the wish for a large family (though each pregnancy seems to make the dysmenorrhoea get worse, not better). Fluid retention at this time leads to typical oedema and weight gain; this can be helped by the use of diuretics but the principal treatment is with progesterone.

dysmorphogenic (dis-mor-fō-jen'-ik) [G. *dys*, difficult; *morphe*, form; *gignesthai*, to be produced]. Now preferred to teratogenic (q.v.) when applied to drugs taken during pregnancy.

dysopia (dis-ō'-pi-ă) [G. *dys-*, difficult; *opsis*, vision]. Painful or defective vision.

dysorexia (dis-o-reks'-i-ă) [G. *dys-*, abnormal *orexis*, appetite]. An abnormal or unnatural appetite.

dyspareunia (dis-par-ū'-ni-ă) [G. *dys-*, difficult; *pareunos*, lying beside]. Painful or difficult coitus.

dyspepsia (dis-pep'-si-ă) [G. *dys-*, difficult; *peptein, pessein*, to cook]. Indigestion—dyspeptic, adj.

dysphagia (dis-fā'-ji-ă) [G. *dys-*, difficult; *phagein*, to eat]. Difficulty in swallowing—dysphagic, adj.

dysphasia (dis-fā'-zi-ă) [G. *dys-*, difficulty; *phasis*, speech]. Incomplete language function. **motor d.**, patient is aware of what is said, knows what he wants to reply, but is unable to assemble the symbols of language (speech) in any coherent order, thus giving the impression that he does not understand. In **receptive d.**, patient unable to put any meaning to the words he hears though he may well be able to understand other forms of communication, such as miming, drawing and writing—dysphasic, adj.

dysplasia (dis-plăz'-i-ă) [G. *dys-*, difficult; *plasis*, a moulding]. Formation of abnormal tissue—dysplastic, adj.

dyspnoea (disp-nē'-ă) [G. *dys-*, difficult; *pnoia*, breath]. Difficulty in, or laboured breathing; can be mainly of an inspiratory or expiratory nature—dyspnoeic, adj.

dysrhythmia (dis-rith'-mi-ă) [G. *dys-*, abnormal; *rhythmos*, rhythm]. Disordered rhythm—dysrhythmic, adj.

dystaxia (dis-taks'-i-ă) [G. *dys-*, difficult; *taxis*, arrangement]. Difficulty in controlling voluntary movements—dystaxic, adj.

dystocia (dis-tōs'-i-ă) [G. *dys-*, difficult; *tokos*, birth]. Difficult or slow labour.

dystonic reaction. Refers to 'mental' drugs. Disorder of tissue tonicity. May be above or below normal.

dystrophy (dis'-trō-fi) [G. *dys-*, faulty; *trophe*, nourishment]. Defective nutrition. **muscular d.**, genetically determined primary degenerative myopathy—dystrophic, adj.

dysuria (dis-ū'-ri-ă) [G. *dys-*, difficult;

ouron, urine]. Difficult or painful micturition—dysuric, adj.

Dytac (dī'tak). Triamterene (q.v.).

Dytide (dī'-tīd). Triamterene (q.v.) 50 mg and benzthiazide (q.v.) 25 mg.

dytransin (di-tran'-sin). Mild anti-inflammatory agent. No gastro-intestinal irritation with continued use. A few cases of hepatic toxicity have been reported. Occasional SGOT estimations advised. Useful for the chronic rheumatic disorders.

E

E_3. Lachesine (q.v.).

EACA. Epsilon aminocaproic acid (q.v.).

Eaton agent. Isolated in 1944 from pleural secretions of patients with non-bacterial pneumonia. In 1962 identified as PPLO (q.v.). already assigned the generic name Mycoplasma. *Mycoplasma pneumoniae*, proposed as alternative to E. a.

EBI. Emetine bismuth iodide.

EB virus (vī-rus). See EPSTEIN BARR VIRUS.

ecbolic (ek-bol'-ik) [G. *ekbole*, a throwing out]. Any agent which stimulates contraction of the gravid uterus and hastens expulsion of its contents.

ecchondroma (ek-kon-drō'-mă) [G. *ek*, out of; *chondros*, cartilage; *-oma*, tumour]. A benign tumour composed of cartilage which protrudes from the surface of the bone in which it arises—ecchondromata, pl.

ecchymosis (ek-i-mō'-sis) [G. *ek*, out of; *chymos*, juice; *-osis*, condition]. An extravasation of blood under the skin. Syn., bruise—ecchymoses, pl.

ECG. Electrocardiogram. See ELECTROCARDIOGRAPH.

Echinococcus (ek-i'-nō-kok'-us) [G. *echinos*, hedgehog]. A genus of tapeworms, the adults infesting a primary host, e.g. a dog. In man (secondary host) the encysted larvae cause 'hydatid disease'.

echoencephalography (ek-ō-en-kef-al-og'-ra-fi) [G. *echo; egkephalos*, brain; *graphein*, to write]. Passage of penetrating sound waves across the head. Can detect abscess, blood clot, injury or tumour within brain.

echolalia (ek-ō-lā'-li-ă) [G. *echo; lalia*, talk]. Repetition, almost automatically of words or phrases heard. Occurs most commonly in schizophrenia and dementia; sometimes in toxic delirious states. A characteristic of all infants' speech—echolalic, adj.

echophony (ek-of'-o-ni) [G. *echo*, echo; *phone*, voice]. The echo of a vocal sound heard during auscultation of the chest.

echopraxia (ek-ō-prak'-si-á) [G. *echo: praxis*, action]. Involuntary mimicking of another's movements.

echoviruses. Enteric Cytopathic Human Orphan. This name was given because these viruses were originally found in the stools of diseaseless children. They have caused meningitis and mild respiratory infection in children. At least 30 types.

eclampsia (ek-lamp'-si-á) [G *eklampsis*, a shining forth]. 1. A severe manifestation of toxaemia of pregnancy, associated with fits and coma. 2, A sudden convulsive attack—eclamptic, adj.

ecmnesia (ek-nē'-zi-á) [G. *ek*, out of; *amnesia*, forgetfulness]. Impaired memory for recent events with normal memory of remote ones. Common in old age and in early cerebral deterioration.

Economycin (ek-on-ō-mī'-sin). Tetracycline (q.v.).

ecraseur (ā-krá-zèr) [F.]. An instrument with a wire loop that can be tightened round the pedicle of a new growth to sever it.

ECT. Electroconvulsive therapy. See ELECTROTHERAPY.

ecthyma (ek-thī'-má) [G. *ekthyma*, pustule]. A crusted eruption of impetigo contagiosa on the legs, producing necrosis of the skin, which heals with scarring. A similar condition occurs in syphilis.

ectoderm (ek'-tō-dèrm) [G. *ektos*, without; *derma*, skin]. The external primitve germ layer of the embryo. From it are developed the skin structures, the nervous system, organs of special sense, pineal gland and part of the pituitary and adrenal glands—ectodermal, adj.

ectodermosis (ek-tō-derm-ō-'sis) [G. *ektos*, outside; *derma*, skin; *osis*, condition]. Disease of any organ or tissue derived from the ectoderm.

ectogenous (ek-toj'-en-us). Originating outside the organism. Opp. to endogenous.

ectoparasite (ek-tō-par'-a-sīt) [G. *ektos*, outside; *parasitos*, parasite]. A parasite that lives on the exterior surface of its host—ectoparasitic, adj.

ectopia (ek-tō'-pi-á) [G. *ektopos*, away from a place]. Malposition of an organ or structure, usually congenital. e. vesicae, an abnormally placed urinary bladder which protrudes through or opens on to the abdominal wall—ectopic, adj.

ectopic pregnancy (ek-top'-ik preg'-nan-si). Extrauterine gestation, the Fallopian tube being the most common site. At about the 6th week the tube ruptures, constituting a 'surgical emergency'.

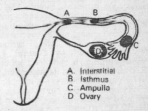

A. Interstitial
B. Isthmus
C. Ampulla
D. Ovary

Sites of ectopic pregnancy

ectozoa (ek-tō-zō'-á) [G. *ektos*, outside; *zoon*, animal]. External parasites.

ectrodactylia (ek-trō-dak-til'-i-á) [G. *ektrosis*, miscarriage; *daktylos*, finger]. Congenital absence of one or more fingers or toes or parts of them.

ectropion (ek-trō'-pi-on) [G. *ek*, out of; *trepein*, to turn]. An eversion or turning outward, especially of the lower eyelid or of an unhealed lesion of the cervix uteri.

eczema (ek'-zē-má) [G. *ek*, out; *zeo*, boil]. Precise meaning has not been agreed upon. Some medical men use the term as synonymous with 'dermatitis' (q.v.). Others regard it as one form of dermatitis, describing it as the 'eczema reaction' to an irritant on an already susceptible skin. The reaction begins with erythema, then vesicles appear. These rupture, forming crusts or leaving pits which ooze serum. This is the exudative or weeping stage. In the process of healing, the area becomes scaly. Some authorities limit term 'eczema' to the cases with internal causes while those caused by external contact factors are called dermatitis.

A. Internal causes:
1. Atopic
2. Seborrhoeic
3. Discoid
4. Gravitational.
B. External causes:
5. Contact
   (a) by primary irritation
   (b) by allergic sensitization.

atopic e. is an inflammatory skin condition in which the skin becomes red and small vesicles, crusts and scales may develop on the skin surface. The skin is very itchy causing scratching, usually at night. It is found mostly on the face and in the flexor areas of the arms and legs. usually does not occur under 6 months of age. **infantile e.,** an allergic eczema of infants aged between 2 months and 2 years, often limited to the cheeks and forehead and which is very irritating. Such infants should not be vaccinated or inoculated with a foreign serum. May be followed by **flexural e.,** (Besnier's prurigo) in childhood. **seborrhoeic e.,** is confined to the napkin area and the face. This form is not itchy but the skin looks very dry. The prognosis is very good as the condition clears in a relatively short time. **e.-asthma syndrome,** affected infants begin with infantile eczema and in childhood develop asthma as the eczema remits; frequently the asthma remits at puberty—eczematous, adj.

EDD. Expected date of delivery (q.v.).

Edecrin (ed'-ē-krin). Ethacrynic acid (q.v.).

edentulous (ed-ent'-ū-lus). Without teeth.

Edosol (ed'-os-ol). Salt-free dried milk.

Edward's syndrome. Autosomal trisomy associated with mental subnormality. The cells have 47 chromosomes. Sometimes called trisomy E.

EEG Electroencephalogram. See ELECTROENCEPHALOGRAPH.

Efcortesol (ef-kor'-ti-sol). Hydrocortisone phosphate in stabilized solution for intravenous use.

effector (ē-fek'-tor) [L. *efficere,* to carry out]. A motor or secretory nerve ending in a muscle, gland or organ.

efferent (ef'-ėr'-ent) [L. *effere,* to carry away]. Carrying, conveying, conducting away from a centre. Opposite to afferent (q.v.).

effort syndrome (ef'-fort sin'-drŏm). A form of anxiety neurosis, manifesting itself in a variety of cardiac symptoms including precordial pain, for which no pathological explanation can be discovered.

effusion (ef-fū'-zhun) [L. *effundere,* to pour out]. Extravasation of fluid into body tissues or cavities.

ego (eg'-ō) [L. I]. Refers to the unconscious self, the 'I', that part of personality that deals with reality and is influenced by social forces. It modifies behaviour by unconscious compromise between the primitive instinctual urges (the id) and the conscience.

Ehrlich's theory of immunity. Postulated that tissue cells received molecules of antigen by means of receptors. Under certain conditions these receptors were overproduced and released into the body-fluids. The free receptor groups became the antibodies and were capable of combining specifically with antigen molecules. **E's diazo reagent,** used for the detection of urobilinogen in urine **E's '606'** Salvarsan, discovered in 1909 as a result of the 606th experiment. See NEOARSPHENAMINE. [Paul Ehrlich, German bacteriologist and pathologist, 1854–1915.]

ejaculation (ē-jak-ū-lā'-shun) [L. *ex,* from; *jaculatus,* thrown out]. A sudden emission of semen.

ejaculatory ducts (ē-jak'-ū-lāt-or-i dukts). Two fine tubes, one on either side, commencing at the union of the seminal vesicle with the vas deferens, and terminating at their union with the prostatic urethra.

Elase ointment. A cleansing agent used in the debridement of necrotic debris and purulent exudates from wounds.

Elastoplast (ē-lás'-tō-plást). Elastic cotton cloth without rubber threads, with porous adhesive and non-fray edges. **E. bandages** are applied firmly in the ambulatory treatment of varicose ulcers and after injection treatment of veins; the compression reduces oedema and pain and promotes healing. Removal of the bandages should be carefully carried out by cutting with special flat-bladed scissors. **E. dressings** are elastic, porous, adhesive dressings for surgical purposes, with a central pad impregnated with Domiphen Bromide BPC (0.15 per cent) on an elastic cotton cloth, and spread with porous adhesive. **E. extension plaster,** 2.743 m length of elastic cotton cloth spread with porous adhesive in which the stretch is *across* the width: rigid lengthwise for skin traction in orthopaedic conditions.

Electra complex. Excessive emotional attachment of daughter to father. The name is derived from Greek mythology.

electrocardiograph (ē-lek-trō-kár'-di-ō-gráf) [G. *electron,* amber; *cardia,* heart; *graphein,* to write].An instrument containing a string galvanometer through which passes the electrical current produced by the heart's contraction. A permanent record (electrocardiogram, ECG) of these oscillations is made on a moving drum of graph paper -electrocardiographic, adj.; electrocardiographically, adv.

electrocoagulation (ē-lek-trō-kō-ag-ū-lā'-shun). Technique of surgical diathermy. Coagulation, especially of bleeding points, by means of electrodes.

electrocochleography (ē-lek-trō-kok-lē-oq'-ra-fi). ECoG. Direct recording of movement in the fluid in the internal ear.

electrocorticography (ē-lek-trō-kor-ti-kog'-ra-fi). Direct recording from the cerebral cortex during operation -electrocorticographic, adj.; electrocorticographically, adv.

electrode (ē-lek'-trōd) [G. *electron,* amber; *hodos,* path]. A conductor in the form of a pad or plate, whereby electricity enters or leaves the body in electrotherapy.

electrodessication (ē-lek-trō-des-i-kā'-shun). Technique of surgical diathermy. There is drying and subsequent removal of tissue, e.g. papillomata.

electrodiagnosis (ē-lek'-trō-dī-ag-nō'-sis). The use of graphic recording of electrical irritability of tissues in diagnosis—electrodiagnostic, adj.

electroencephalograph (ē-lek'-trō-en-kef'-al-ō-gráf) [G. *electron,* amber; *egkephalos,* brain; *graphein,* to write]. An instrument by which electrical impulses derived from the brain can be amplified and recorded on paper, in a fashion similar to that of the electrocardiograph. The record is an electroencephalogram (EEG)—electroencephalographic, adj.; electroencephalographically, adv.

electrolysis (ē-lek-trol'-is-is) [G. *electron,* amber; *luein,* to loose]. 1. Chemical decomposition by electricity. 2. Destruction of individual hairs (epilation); eradication of moles, spider naevi, etc., using electricity.

electrolyte (ē-lek'-trō-līt). A liquid or solution of a substance which is capable of conducting electricity. On passing an electric current through the substance a chemical change always takes place. The change is 'electrolysis' (q.v.). **e. balance,** a normal state in which the action and reaction of two or more electrolytes is of normally balanced proportions—electrolytic, adj.

electromyography (el-ek-trō-mī-og'-ra-fi) [G. *electron,* amber; *myos,* muscle; *graphein,* to write]. Graphic recording of electrical currents generated in active muscle EMG electromyogram, n.; electromyographical, adj.; electromyographically, adv.

electro-oculogram (ē-lek-trō-ok'-ū-lō-gram). Graphic record of eye position and movement, and potential difference between front and back of eyeball using electrodes placed on skin near socket. Can be used as an electrodiagnostic test.

electroplexy ((ē-lek-trō-pleks'-i) [G. *electron,* amber; *plassein,* to form]. See ELECTROTHERAPY.

electropyrexia (ē-lek'-trō-pī-rek'-si-á) [G. *electron,* amber; *pur,* fire]. A high body temperature produced by an electrical apparatus. (Keltering cabinet or inductotherm.)

electroretinogram (ē-lek-trō-ret'-in-ō-gram) [G. *electron,* amber; L. *rete,* net; G. *gramma,* letter]. ERG. Graphic record of electrical currents generated in active retina.

electrosection (ē-lek-trō-sek'-shun). Technique of surgical diathermy for cutting the skin or parting soft tissues.

electrotherapy (ē-lek-trō-ther'-a-pi) [G. *elektron,* amber; *therapeia,* treatment]. Electrical treatment. Syn., ECT, electroplexy, electroshock. A form of physical treatment widely used by psychiatrists in the treatment of depression, acute mania and toxic confusional states. Also used in cases of stupor and certain types of schizophrenia. An apparatus is used which delivers a definite voltage for a precise fraction of a second to electrodes placed on the head, producing a convulsion. **modified e.,** the convulsion is modified with an intravenous anaesthetic and a muscle relaxant, e.g. scoline. **unilateral ECT** is being tried to avoid the sequela of amnesia for recent events. The mechanism for memory of recent events is probably in the dominant cerebral hemisphere which is the left in practically all people. ECT is therefore applied to the right hemisphere to minimize memory disturbance. See CONVULSIVE THERAPY.

element (el'-ē-ment). One of the constituents of a compound. The elements are the primary substances which in pure form, or combined into compounds, constitute all matter.

elephantiasis (el-ef-an-tī'-a-sis) [G. *elephas,* elephant; *-iasis,* condition]. The swelling of a limb, usually a leg, as a result of lymphatic obstruction (lymphoedema), followed by thickening of the skin (pachydermia) and subcutaneous tissues. A complication of filariasis in tropical countries, but by no means rare in Britain as a result of syphilis or recurring streptococcal infection (e.nostras). See BARBADOS LEG.

elixir (e-liks'-ėr). A sweetened, aromatic solution of a drug, often containing an appreciable amount of alcohol. Elixirs differ from syrups in containing very little sugar, and in requiring dilution before use.

elliptocytosis (el-ip-tō-tō-sī-tō'-sis). Anaemia in which the red blood cells are oval.

Eltroxin (el-troks'-in). A preparation of thryoxine (q.v.) that has a standardized activity.

emaciation (ē-mā-shi-ā'-shun) [L. *macies,* thinness]. Excessive leanness, or wasting of body tissue—emaciate, v.t.

emasculation (ē-mas-kū-lā'-shun) [L. *emasculare,* to make impotent]. Castration.

Embequin (em'-bē-quin). Di-iodo-hydroxyquinoline (q.v.).

embolectomy (em-bol-ek'-to-mi) [G. *embolos,* plug; *ektome,* excision]. Surgical removal of an embolus.

embolic (em-bol'-ik) [G. *embolos,* plug]. Pertaining to an embolism or an embolus.

embolism (em'-bol-ism) [G. *embolos,* plug]. Obstruction of a blood vessel by the impaction of a solid body (e.g. thrombi, fat globules, tumour cells) or an air bubble.

embologenic (em-bol-ō-jen'-ik) [G. *embolos,* plug; *genesis,* descent]. Capable of producing an embolism.

embolus (em'-bol-us)[G.*embolos,* plug]. Solid body or air bubble transported in the circulation. See EMBOLISM—emboli, pl.

embryo (em'-bri-ō) [G. *embruon,* embryo]. The term applied to the developing ovum during the early months of gestation—embryonic, adj.

embryology (em-bri-ol'-oj-i) [G. *embruon,* embryo; *logos,* discourse]. Study of the development of an organism from fertilization to extrauterine life—embryological, adj.; embryologically, adv.

embryoma (em-bri-ō'-má) [G. *enbruon,* embryo; *-oma,* tumour]. Teratoma (q.v.).

embryopathy (em-bri-op'-ath-i) [G. *embruon,* embryo; *pathos,* disease]. Disease or abnormality in the embryo. More serious if it occurs in the first three months. Includes the 'rubella syndrome'—embryopathic, adj.; embryopathically, adv.

embryotomy (em-bri-ot'-o-mi) [G. *embruon,* embryo; *tome,* a cutting]. Mutilation of the fetus to facilitate removal from womb, when natural birth is impossible.

emepronium bromide (em-ē-prō'-ni-um brō'-mīd). Atropine-like drug with inhibitory influence on bladder contraction. Reduces nocturnal frequency of micturition.

emesis (em'-i-sis) [G.]. Vomiting.

emetic (ē-met'-ik) [G. *emetikos,* provoking sickness]. Any agent used to produce vomiting.

emetine (em'-e-tēn). Principal alkaloid of ipecacuanha. Used in amoebic dysentery, often in association with other amoebicides.

EMI scan. Non-invasive technique which produces a pictorial print-out revealing the density of tissues, thereby demonstrating the presence or absence of a tumour.

emission (ē-mish'-un) [L.]. An ejaculation or sending forth. An involuntary ejaculation of semen.

emmetropia (em-met-rōp'-i-á) [G. *emmetros,* in measure; *ops,* eye]. Normal or perfect vision—emmetropic, adj.

emollient (ē-mol'-i-ent) [L. *emollire,* to soften]. An agent which softens and soothes skin or mucous membrane.

emotion (ē-mō'-shun) [L. *emovere* to stir up]. The tone of feeling recognized in ourselves by certain bodily changes, and in others by tendencies to certain characteristic behaviour. Aroused usually by ideas or concepts.

emotional (ē-mō'-shun-al). Characteristic of or caused by emotion. **e. bias,** tendency of e. attitude to affect logical judgement. **e. state,** effect of emotions on normal mood, e.g. agitation.

empathy (em'-pa-thi) [G. *empatheia*, passion]. Identifying oneself with another person or the actions of another person.

emphysema (em-fi-sē'-má) [G. inflation]. Gaseous distension of the tissues. **pulmonary e.,** alveolar distension: (1) generalized—often accompanying chronic bronchitis; (2) localized—either distal to partial obstruction of a bronchus or bronchiole (obstructive e.) or in alveoli adjacent to a segment of collapsed lung (compensatory e.). **surgical e.,** air in the subcutaneous tissue planes following trauma of surgery or injury -emphysematous, adj.

empirical (em-pir'-ik-al) [G. *empeirikos*, experience]. Based on observation and experience and not on scientific reasoning.

empyema (em-pi-e'-má). [G. *empuos*, discharging matter]. A collection of pus in a cavity, hollow organ or space.

emulsion (ē-mul'-shun) [L. *emulgere*, to milk out]. A uniform suspension of fat or oil particles in an aqueous continuous phase (O/W emulsion) or aqueous droplets in an oily continuous phase (W/O emulsion).

emylcamate. Striatran. Tranquillizer.

enamel (ē-nam'-el). The hard external covering of the crown of a tooth.

encapsulation (en-kap-sū-lā'-shun) [G. *en,* in; *capsula,* small box]. Enclosure within a capsule.

encephalitis (en-kef-a-lī'-tis) [G. *egkephalos,* brain; *-itis,* inflammation]. Inflammation of the brain.

encephalocele (en-kef'-al-ō-sēl) [G. *egkephalos,* brain; *kele,* hernia]. Protrusion of brain substance through the skull. Often associated with hydrocephalus when the protrusion occurs at a suture line.

encephalogram (en-kef'-al-ō-gram) [G. *egkephalos,* brain; *gramma,* letter]. See PNEUMOENCEPHALOGRAPHY.

encephalography (en-kef-al-og'-ra-fi) [G. *egkephalos,* brain; *graphein,* to write]. See PNEUMOENCEPHALOGRAPHY.

encephaloma (en-kef-al-ō'-má) [G. *egkephalos,* brain; *-oma,* tumour]. A tumour of the brain—encephalomata, pl.

encephalomalacia (en-kef'-al-ō-mal-ās-i-á) [G. *egkephalos,* brain; *malakia,* softness]. Softening of the brain.

encephalomyelitis (en-kef'-al-ō-mī-e-lī'-tis) [G. *egkephalos,* brain; *myelos,* marrow; *-itis,* inflammation]. Inflammation of the brain and spinal cord.

encephalomyelopathy (en-kef-al-ō-mī-el-op'-ath-i) [G. *egkephalos,* brain; *myelos,* marrow; *pathos,* disease]. Disease affecting both brain and spinal cord—encephalomyelopathic, adj.

encephalon (en-kef'-a-lon) [G. *egkephalos*]. The brain.

encephalopathy (en-kef-al-op'-a-thi) [G. *egkephalos,* brain; *pathos,* disease]. Any disease of the brain—encephalopathic, adj.

enchondroma (en-kon-drō'-má) [G. *en,* in; *chondros,* cartilage; *-oma,* tumour]. A cartilaginous tumour—enchondromata, pl.

encopresis (en-kō-prē'-sis) [G. *en,* in; *kopros,* dung]. Involuntary passage of faeces—encopretic, adj., n.

Endamoeba (en-da-mē'-bá) [G.*endon,* within; *amoibe,* change]. Syn., Entamoeba.

endarterectomy (end-árt-e-rek'-to-mi) [G. *endon,* within; *arteria,* artery; *ektome,* excision]. Surgical removal of an atheromatous core from an artery. Disobliteration or 'rebore.' **gas e.,** or carbo-dissection, the use of carbon dioxide gas to separate the occlusive core.

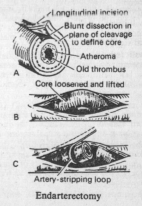

Endarterectomy

endarteritis (end-árt-e-rī'-tis) [G. *endon*, within; *arteria*, artery; *-itis*, inflammation]. Inflammation of the intima or lining coat of an artery. **e. obliterans,** the new intimal connective tissue obliterates the lumen.

endaural (end-awr'-al) [G. *endon*, within; L. *auris*, ear]. Pertaining to the inner portion of the external auditory canal.

endemic (en-dem'-ik) [G. *endemos*, dwelling in a place]. Recurring in a locality. (Cf. epidemic.)

endemiology (en-dem-i-ol'-o-ji) [G. *endemos*, dwelling in a place; *logos*, discourse]. The special study of endemic diseases.

endocarditis (en-dō-kár-dī'-tis) [G. *endon*, within; *kardia*, heart; *-itis*, inflammation]. Inflammation of the inner lining of the heart (endocardium) most commonly due to rheumatic fever. **valvular e.,** when one or more heart valves are affected. See SUBACUTE.

endocardium (en-dō-kár'-di-um) [G. *endon*, within; *kardia*, heart]. The lining membrane of the heart, which covers the valves.

endocervical (en-dō-sér-vī'-kal) [G. *endon*, within; L. *cervix*, neck]. Pertaining to the inside of the cervix uteri.

endocervicitis (en-dō-sér-vi-sī'-tis) [G. *endon*, within; L. *cervix*, neck; G. *-itis*, inflammation]. Inflammation of the mucous membrane lining the cervix uteri.

endocrine (en'-do-krīn) [G. *endon*, within; *krinein*, to separate]. Secreting internally. **e. glands,** the ductless glands of the body; those which make an internal secretion or hormone which passes into the blood stream and has an important influence on general metabolic processes: e.g. the pineal, pituitary, thyroid, parathyroids, thymus, adrenals, ovaries, testes and pancreas. The last-mentioned has both an internal and external secretion. Opp. to exocrine—endocrinal, adj.

endocrinology (en-dō-krin-ol'-o-ji) [G. *endon*, within; *krinein*, to separate; *logos*, discourse]. The study of the ductless glands and their internal secretions.

endocrinopathy (en-dō-krin-op'-ath-i) [G. *endon*, within; *krinein*, to separate; *pathos*, disease]. Abnormality of one or more of the endocrine glands or their secretions.

endogenous (en-doj'-en-us) [G. *endon*, within; *genesthai*, to be produced]. Originating within the organism. Opp. to ectogenous.

endolymph (en'-dō-limf) [G. *endon*, within; L. *lympha*, water]. The fluid contained in the membranous labyrinth of the internal ear.

endolymphatic shunt (en-dō-lim-fat'-ik). Drainage of excess endolymph from the semicircular canals to the subarachnoid space where it flows to join the cerebrospinal fluid. Performed for patients with Ménière's disease.

endolysin (en-dō-lī'-sin) [G. *endon*, within; *lysis*, a loosening]. An intracellular, leucocytic substance which destroys engulfed bacteria.

endometrioma (en-dō-mē-tri-ō'-má) [G. *endon*, within; *metra*, womb; *-oma*, tumour]. A tumour of misplaced endometrium. Adenomyoma (q.v.). See CYST (chocolate)—endometriomata, pl.

endometriosis (en-dō-mēt-ri-ōs'-is) [G. *endon*, within; *metra*, womb; *-osis*, condition]. The presence of endometrium in abnormal sites. See CYST (chocolate).

endometritis (en-dō-mē-trī'-tis) [G. *endon*, within; *metra*, womb; *-itis*, inflammation]. Inflammation of the endometrium.

endometrium (en-do-mēt'-ri-um) [G. *endon*, within; *metra*, womb]. The lining mucosa of the uterus—endometrial, adj.

endomyocardium (en-dō-mī-ō-kar'-di-um) [G. *endon*, within; *mys*, muscle; *kardia*, heart]. Relating to the endocardium and myocardium—endomyocardial, adj.

endoneurium (en-do-nū'-ri-um) [G. *endon* within; *neuron*, nerve]. The delicate, inner connective tissue surrounding the nerve fibres.

endoparasite (en'-dō-par'-a-sīt) [G. *endon*, within; *parasitos*, parasite]. Any parasite living within its host—endoparasitic, adj.

endophlebitis (en-dō-flē-bī'-tis) [G. *endon*, within; *phleps*, vein; *-itis*, inflammation]. Inflammation of internal lining of vein. Can occur after prolonged intravenous infusion.

endophthalmitis (en-dof-thal-mī'-tis) [G. *endon*, within; *ophthalmos*, eye; *-itis*, inflammation]. Internal infection of eye globe, usually as a result of a perforating injury.

endoscope (en'-do-skōp) [G. *endon*, within; *skopein*, to examine]. An instrument for visualization of body cavities or organs. If of the fibre-optic variety, light is transmitted by means of very fine glass fibres along a flexible tube. It can permit examination, photography and biopsy of the cavities or organs of a relaxed conscious person. See PHOTO-ENDOSCOPE—endoscopic adj.; endoscopy, n.

endospore (en'-do-spōr) [G. *endon*, within; *sporos*, seed]. A bacterial spore which has a purely vegetative function. It is formed by the loss of water and probable rearrangement of the protein of the cell, so that metabolism is minimal and resistance to environmental conditions, especially high temperature, desiccation and antibacterial drugs, high. The only genera which includes pathogenic species that form spores are Bacillus and Clostridium

endothelioid (en-do-thē'-li-oid) [G. *endon*, within; *thele*, nipple; *eidos*, form]. Resembling endothelium.

endothelioma (en-dō-thē-li-ō'-ma) [G. *endon*, within; *thele*, nipple; *-oma*, tumour]. A malignant tumour derived from endothelial cells.

endothelium (en-dō-thē'-li-um) [G. *endon*, within; *thele*, nipple]. The lining membrane of serous cavities, heart, blood and lymph vessels—endothelial, adj.

endotoxin (en-dō-toks'-in) [G. *endon*, within; *toxikon*, poison]. A toxic product of bacteria which is associated with the structure of the cell, and can only be obtained by destruction of the cell—endotoxic, adj. Opp. to exotoxin.

endotracheal (en-dō-trak-ē'-al) [G. *endon*, within; *trachus*, rough]. Within the trachea.

Enduxana (en-doks-àn'-à). Cyclophosphamide (q.v.).

Enduron (en'-dūr-on). Methyclothiazide. See CHLOROTHIAZIDE.

Enduronyl (en-dūr'-on-il). Methyclothiazide. See CHLOROTHIAZIDE.

enema (en'-e-má) [G. injection]. The injection of a liquid into the rectum, to be returned or retained. It can be further designated according to the function of the fluid—A small bowel enema can be given after duodenal intubation (q.v.). Followed by radiography of the small and, if necessary, the large bowel—enemas, enemata, pl.

Englate (eng'-lāt). Theophylline sodium glycinate. See THEOPHYLLINE.

enophthalmos (en-of-thal'-mos) [G. *en*, in; *ophthalmos*, eye]. Abnormal retraction of an eyeball within its orbit.

enostosis (en-os-tō'-sis) [G. *en*, in; *osteon*, bone; *-osis*, condition]. A bony growth within the medulary canal of a bone. See EXOSTOSIS.

Enpac (en'-pak). Antidiarrhoeal.

ensiform (en'-si-form) [L. *ensis*, sword; *forma*, shape]. Sword shaped; xiphoid.

Entamoeba (en-ta-mē'-bà). A genus of protozoon parasites, three species infesting man: *Entamoeba coli*, non-pathogenic, infesting intestinal tract; *E. gingivalis* non-pathogenic, infesting mouth; *E. hystolytica*, pathogenic causing amoebic dysentery (q.v.). Syn., Endamoeba (q.v.).

enteral (en'-tèr-àl) [G. *enteron*, intestine]. Within gastrointestinal tract.

enteric (en-ter'-ik) [G. *enteron*, intestine]. Pertaining to the intestine. **e. fever** includes typhoid and paratyphoid fever (q.v.).

enteritis (en-te-rī'-tis) [G. *enteron*, intestine; *-itis*, inflammation]. Inflammation of the intestines. **regional e.**, currently preferred term to Crohn's disease (q.v.).

entero-anastomosis (en'-te-ro-an-as-tom-ō'-sis) [G. *enteron*, intestine; *anastomosis*, opening]. Intestinal anastomosis.

enterobiasis (en-ter-ō-bī'-as-is). Infestation with threadworms.

Enterobius vermicularis (en-ter-ō'-bi-us ver-mik-ū-lar'-is) [G. *enteron*, intestine; *bios*, life; L. *vermiculus*, little worm]. A nematode which infests the small and large intestine. Threadworm. Because of autoinfective life-cycle, treatment aims at complete elimination. Each member of household given three single dose treatments at weekly intervals of either piperazine citrate, 75 mg per kg, or viprymium embonate (Vanquin) 5 mg per kg. Latter gives red stools. Hygiene measures necessary to prevent. re-infestation during treatment.

enterocele (en'-ter-ō-sēl) [G. *enteron*, intestine; *kele*, tumour]. Prolapse of intestine. Can be into the upper third of vagina.

enteroclysis (en-te-rō-klī'-sis) [G. *enteron*, intestine; *klysis*, a drenching]. The introduction of fluid into the rectum. Syn., proctoclysis.

enterococcus (en-te-rō-kok'-us) [G. *enteron,* intestine; *kokkos,* seed]. A Gram-positive coccus which occurs in short chains and is relatively resistant to heat. Enterococci belong to Lancefield's group D, and occur as commensals in human and warm-blooded animal intestines, and sometimes as pathogens in infections of the urinary tract, ear and wounds and, more rarely, in endocarditis.

enterocolitis (en-ter-ō-kol-ī'-tis) [G. *enteron,* intestine; *kolon,* colon; *-itis,* inflammation]. Inflammation of the small intestine and colon.

enterokinase (en-te-rō-kī'-nās) [G. *enteron,* intestine; *kinein,* to move]. An enzyme in intestinal juice. It converts inactive trypsinogen into active trypsin.

enterolith (en'-te-rō-lith) [G. *enteron,* intestine; *lithos,* stone]. An intestinal concretion.

enterolithiasis (en-te-rō-lith-ī'-a-sis) [G. *enteron,* intestine; *lithos,* stone; N.L. *-iasis,* condition]. The presence of intestinal concretions.

enteron (en'-te-ron) [G. intestine]. The gut.

enterostomy (en-te-ros'-to-mi) [G.*enteron,* intestine; *stoma,* mouth]. A surgically established fistula between the small intestine and some other surface. gastro-e., a fistula between stomach and jejunum, sometimes made in the treatment of duodenal ulcer. See DUODENOSTOMY, ILEOSTOMY, JEJUNOSTOMY —enterostomal, adj.

enterotomy (en-te-rot'-o-mi) [G. *enteron,* intestine; *tome,* a cutting]. An incision into the small intestine.

enterotribe (en'-te-rō-trīb) [G. *enteron,* intestine; *tribein,* to crush]. A metal clamp which causes necrosis of the spur of a double-barrelled colostomy, as a preliminary to its closure.

Entero-Vioform (en-te-rō-vī'-ō-form). An antidiarrhoeal which was promoted for traveller diarrhoea but is now restricted due to its association with SMON, a disease which occurs particularly in Japan.

enteroviruses ((en'-te-rō-vī'-rus-es) [G. *enteron,* intestine; L. *virus,* poison]. Enter the body by the alimentary tract. Comprise the poliomyelitis, Coxsackie and ECHO groups of viruses. They tend to invade the central nervous system. Enteroviruses, together with rhinoviruses, are now to be called picornaviruses.

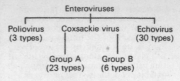

Enteroviruses

enterozoa (en-te-rō-zō'-á) [G. *enteron,* intestine; *zoion,* living being]. Any animal parasites infesting the intestines— enterozoon, sing.

Entonox (en'-to-noks). Inhalant analgesic. Mixture of 50 per cent nitrous oxide and 50 per cent oxygen.

entropion (en-trō'-pi-on) [G. *en,* in; *trepein,* to turn]. Inversion of an eyelid so that the lashes are in contact with the globe of the eye.

enucleation (ē-nū-klē-ā'-shun) [L. *e,* out of; *nucleus,* kernel]. The removal of an organ or tumour in its entirety, as of an eyeball from its socket.

enuresis (en-ū-rē'-sis) [G. *enourein,* to make water in]. Incontinence of urine, especially bed-wetting.

Envacar (en'-va-kar). Guanoxan sulphate (q.v.).

environment (en-vī'-ron-ment) [F. *environ,* about]. External surroundings. Environmental factors are conditions influencing an individual from without.

enzyme (en'-zīm) [G. *en,* in; *zyme,* leaven]. Soluble colloidal protein produced by living cells. See CATALYST.

enzymology (en'-zīm-ol'-oj-i) [G. *en,* in; *zyme,* leaven; *logos,* discourse]. The science dealing with the structure and function of enzymes—enzymological, adj.; enzymologically, adv.

eosin (ē'-ō-sin) [G. *eos,* dawn]. A red staining agent used in histology and laboratory diagnostic procedures.

eosinophil (ē-ō-sin'-ō-fil) [G. *eos,* dawn; *philein,* to love]. 1. Cells having an affinity for eosin. 2. A type of polymorphonuclear leucocyte containing eosin-staining granules—eosinophilic, adj.

eosinophilia (ē-ō-sin-ō-fil'-i-á) [G. *eos,* dawn; *philein,* to love]. Increased eosinophils in the blood.

Epanutin (ep-a-nū'-tin). Phenytoin (q.v.).

ependymoma (ep-end-im-ō'-má) [G. *ependyma,* an upper garment; *-oma,* tumour]. Neoplasm arising in the lining of the cerebral ventricles or central canal of spinal cord. Occurs in all age groups.

ephedrine (ef'-ed-rin). Widely used in asthma and bronchial spasm for its relaxant action on bronchioles; raises blood pressure by peripheral vasoconstriction. Useful in hay fever.

ephelides (e-fe'-lids) [G. *ephelis*]. Freckles—ephelis, sing.

epicanthus (ep-i-kan'-thus) [G. *epi*, on; *kanthos*, corner of the eye]. The congenital occurrence of a fold of skin obscuring the inner canthus of the eye—epicanthal, adj.

epicardium (ep-i-kär'-di-um) [G. *epi*, on; *kardia*, heart]. The visceral layer of the pericardium—epicardial, adj.

epicritic (ep-i-krit'-ik) [G. *epi*, on; *krinein*, to separate]. The term applied to the finer sensations of heat, touch, etc. As opposed to protopathic (q.v.).

epidemic (ep-i-dem'-ik) [G. *epi*, on; *demos*, people]. Simultaneously affecting many people in an area. (Cf. endemic.)

epidemiology (ep-i-dem-i-ol'-o-ji) [G. *epi*, on; *demos*, people; *logos*, discourse]. The scientific study of the distribution of diseases—epidemiological, adj.; epidemiologically, adv.

epidermis (ep-i-děr'-mis) [G. *epi*, on; *derma*, skin]. The external non-vascular layer of the skin; the cuticle. Also known as the 'scarf-skin'—epidermal, adj.

Epidermophyton (ep-i-der-mŏ'-fī-ton) [G. *epi*, on; *derma*, skin; *phyton*, plant]. A genus of fungi which affects the skin and nails.

epidermophytosis (ep-i-der-mŏ-fī-tŏ'-sis) [G. *epi*, on; *derma*, skin; *phyton*, plant; *-osis*, condition]. Infection with fungi of the genus Epidermophyton.

epididymectomy (ep-i-did-i-mek'-to-mi) [G. *epi*, on; *didumoi*, twins, *ektome*, excision]. Surgical removal of the epididymis.

epididymis (ep-i-did'-i-mis) [G. *epi*, on; *didumoi*, twins]. A small oblong body attached to the posterior surface of the testes. It consists of the tubules which convey the spermatozoa from the testes to the vas deferens.

epididymitis (ep-i-did-i-mī'-tis) [G. *epididymis; -itis*, inflammation]. Inflammation of the epididymis (q.v.).

epididymo-orchitis (ep-i-did'-i-mŏ-or-kī'-tis) [G. *epididymis; orchis*, testis; -*itis*, inflammation]. Inflammation of the epididymis and the testis.

epidural (ep-i-dūr'-al) [G. *epi*, on; L. *durus*, hard]. Upon or external to the dura. **e. block**, injection of local anaesthetic, usually in the lumbar or caudal region prior to rectal examination and surgery, a forceps delivery or Caesarean section. Currently used for crush injuries to chest; the analgesia can be maintained for a week or more.

epidurography (ep-i-dūr-og'-ra-fi) [G. *epi*, on; L. *durus*, hard; G. *graphein*, to write]. Radiographs taken after epidural injection of contrast medium.

epigastrium (ep-i-gas'-tri-um) [G. *epi*, on; *gaster*, stomach]. The abdominal region lying directly over the stomach—epigastric, adj.

epiglottis (ep-i-glot'-is) [G. *epi*, on; *glottis*]. The thin leaf-shaped flap of cartilage behind the tongue which, during the act of swallowing, covers the opening leading into the larynx.

epiglottitis (ep-i-glot-ī'-tis) [G. *epi*, on; *glottis; -itis*, inflammation]. Inflammation of the epiglottis.

epilation (ep-il-ā'-shun) [L. *e*, out; *pilus*, hair]. Extraction or destruction of hair roots, e.g. by coagulation necrosis, electrolysis or forceps—epilate, v.t.

epilatory (ep-il'-a-tor-i) [L. *e*, out; *pilus*, hair]. An agent which produces epilation.

epilepsy (ep-i-lep'-si) [G. *epilepsis*, seizure]. Correctly called the epilepsies. Result from disordered electrical activity of brain. The 'fit' is caused by an abnormal electrical discharge that disturbs cerebration and usually results in loss of consciousness. **major e.** (grand mal), loss of consciousness with generalized convulsions. When patient does not regain consciousness between attacks the term status epilepticus is used. **focal e. (Jacksonian)**, motor seizure begins in one part of body, can spread to other muscle groups so that the fit is similar to clonic stage of major epilepsy. Fits can be sensory, i.e. abnormal *feeling* in one part, which spread to other parts. **psychomotor e., temporal lobe e., limbic disorder,** 'psychic' warning of fit consists of feelings of unreality, déjà-vu, auditory, visual, gustatory or olfactory hallucinations. Jerking not as severe as in major epilepsy. **minor e.** (petit mal), characterized by transitory interruption of consciousness without convulsions. Characteristic spike and wave pattern on EEG. Any seizure not conforming to this definition is not petit mal. The term is widely misused. All except petit mal can be symptomatic or idiopathic, but focal and temporal lobe epilepsy carry a higher incidence of symptomatic causes. Petit mal is always idiopathic. See AKINETIC—epileptic, adj.

epileptic (ep-i-lep'-tik). Pertaining to epilepsy. **e. aura,** premonitory subjective phenomena (tingling in the hand or visual or auditory sensations) which precede an attack of grand mal. **e. cry,** the croak or shout heard from the epileptic person as he falls unconscious.

epileptogenic (ep-il-ep-tō-jen'-ik) [G. *epilepsis,* seizure; *genesis,* production]. Agent capable of causing epilepsy.

epileptiform (ep-i-lep'-ti-form). Resembling epilepsy.

epiloia (ep'-il-oi-á). An inherited abnormality of brain tissue, resulting in mental defect. May be associated with epilepsy. Also known as 'tuberose sclerosis.'

epimenorrhoea (ep-i-men-or-rē'-á) [G. *epi,* on; *men,* month; *rheein,* to flow]. Reduction of the length of the menstrual cycle.

epinephrine (ep-i-nef'-rin). Adrenaline (q.v.).

epiphora (ē-pif'-o-rá) [G. *epi,* on; *pherein,* to carry]. Pathological overflow of tears on to the cheek.

epiphysis (ē-pif'-i-sis) [G. *epi,* on; *phyein,* to grow]. The growing part of a bone, especially long bones. Separated from the main shaft (diaphysis) by a plate of cartilage (epiphyseal plate) which disappears due to ossification when growth ceases. **slipped e.,** displacement of an epiphysis, especially the upper femoral—epiphyses, pl.; epiphyseal, adj.

epiphysitis (ē-pif-i-sī'-tis) [G. *epi,* on; *phyein,* to grow; *-itis,* inflammation]. Inflammation of an epiphysis.

epiploon (ep-i-plō'-on) [G.]. The great omentum (q.v.)—epiploic, adj.

episclera (ep-i-sklē'-rá) [G. *epi,* on; *skleros,* hard]. Loose connective tissue between the sclera and conjunctiva—episcleral, adj.

episcleritis (ep-i-sklē-rī'-tis). Inflammation of the episclera.

episiorrhaphy (e-pēs-i-or'-raf-i) [G.

epision, pubic region; *raphe,* a suture]. Surgical repair of a lacerated perineum.

episiotomy (e-pēs-i-ot'-o-mi) [G. *epision,* pubic region; *tome,* a cutting]. A perineal incision made during the birth of a child when the vaginal orifice does not stretch sufficiently.

epispadias (ep-i-spā'di'as) [G. *epi,* on; *spaein,* to draw]. A congenital opening of the urethra on the anterior (upper side) of the penis. (Cf. hypospadias.)

epispastic (ep-i-spas'-tik) [G. *epi,* on; *spaein,* to draw]. A blistering agent.

epistaxis (ep-i-staks'-is) [G. *epi,* on; *stazein,* to drip]. Bleeding from the nose—epistaxes, pl.

epithelioma (ep-i-thēl-i-ō'-má) [G. *epi,* on; *thele,* nipple; *-oma,* tumour]. A malignant growth arising in epithelial tissue, usually the skin; a squamous cell carcinoma.

epithelialization (ep-i-thē-li-ál-ī-zā'-shun). The growth of epithelium over a raw area; the final stage of healing.

epithelium (ep-i-thēl'-i-um) [G. *epi,* on; *thele,* nipple]. The surface layer of cells covering cutaneous, mucous and serous surfaces. It is classified according to the arrangement and shape of the cells it contains—epithelial, adj.

Epodyl (ep'-ō-dil). Ethoglucid (q.v.).

Epontol (ep'-on-tol). Intravenous anaesthetic agent; in about 5s causes unconsciousness which is maintained for 3 to 5 min. Patient awakens quickly without nausea and vomiting.

Eppy (ep'-i). Neutral adrenaline eye drops for use in open angle glaucoma.

Epsikapron (ep-si-kap'-ron). Epsilon aminocaproic acid (q.v.).

epsilon aminocaproic acid (ep'-sil-on am-īn'-ō-kap-rō-ik as'-id). EACA. Prevents formation of fibrinolysin (q.v.), hence used in attempts to arrest bleeding.

Epsom salts. Magnesium sulphate (q.v.).

Epstein Barr virus (ep'-stīn bar vī'rus). Causative agent of infectious mononucleosis (q.v.). A versatile herpes virus which infects many people throughout the world; does not always produce symptoms. Cancer research workers have discovered EBV genome in the malignant cells of Burkitt's lymphoma and nasopharyngeal carcinoma.

epulis (ep'-ū-lis) [G. *epi,* on; *oulon,* gum]. A tumour growing on or from the gums.

Equagesic (e-kwa-jēz'-ik). Ethoheptazine (q.v.); meprobamate (q.v.); aspirin (q.v.); and calcium carbonate. Analgesic and relaxant; useful for musculoskeletal disorders.

Equanil (e-kwan'-il). Meprobamate (q.v.).

Eraldin (èr'-al-din). Practolol (q.v.). Now restricted to emergency i.v. use only, due to the occurrence of a serious adverse reaction syndrome following long-term oral use.

Erb's palsy. See PALSY.

erectile (ē-rek'-tīl) [L. *erigere*, to raise up]. Upright; capable of being elevated. **e. tissue**, highly vascular tissue, which, under stimulus, becomes rigid and erect from hyperaemia.

erection (ē-rek'-shun). The state achieved when erectile tissue is hyperaemic.

erector (ē-rek'-tor). A muscle which achieves erection of a part.

erepsin (ē-rep'-sin). A proteolytic enzyme in succus entericus.

Ergodryl. Antimigraine.

ERG. Electroretinogram (q.v.).

ergography (er-gog'-ra-fi) [G. *ergon*, work; *graphein*, to write]. A method of measuring and recording the state of muscle by its output of effort to an electrical stimulus.

ergometrine (èr-gō-met'-rin). Main alkaloid of ergot (q.v.). Widely used in obstetrics to reduce haemorrhage and improve contraction of uterus.

ergometry (er-gom'-et-ri) [G. *ergon*, work; *metron*, measure]. Measurement of work done by muscles—ergometric, adj.

ergonomics (er gō nom' iks). The application of various biological disciplines in relation to man and his working environment.

ergosterol (èr-gos'-tèr-ol). A provitamin present in the subcutaneous fat of man and animals. On irradiation it is converted into vitamin D_2 which has antirachitic properties.

ergot (èr'-got). A fungus found on rye. Widely used as ergometrine for postpartum haemorrhage.

ergotamine (èr-got'-a-min). An alkaloid of ergot used in the treatment of migraine. Early **e**. treatment of an attack is more effective, especially when combined with antiemetics.

ergotism (èr'-got-izm). Poisoning by ergot.

Ergotrate (èr'-go-trāt). Ergometrine (q.v.).

eructation (e-ruk-tā'-shun) [L. *eructare*, to belch forth]. Noisy, oral expulsion of gas from the stomach.

erysipelas (e-ri-sip'-e-las) [Etym. dub. G. *erythros*, red; L. *pellis*, skin]. An acute, specific, infectious disease, in which there is a spreading, streptococcal inflammation of the skin and subcutaneous tissues, accompanied by fever and constitutional disturbances.

erysipeloid (e-ri-sip'-e-loid). A skin condition resembling erysipelas. It occurs in butchers, fishmongers or cooks. The infecting organism is the Erysipelothrix of swine erysipelas.

erythema (e-ri-thē'-má) [G.]. Reddening of the skin—erythematous, adj. **e. induratum** is Bazin's disease (q.v.). **e. multiforme** is a form of toxic or allergic skin eruption which breaks out suddenly and lasts for days. the lesions are in the form of violet-pink papules or plaques and suggest urticarial weals. Severe form called Stevens-Johnson syndrome (q.v.). **e. nodosum** is an eruption of painful red nodules on the front of the legs. It occurs in young women, and is generally accompanied by rheumaticky pains. It may be a symptom of many diseases including tuberculosis, acute rheumatism, gonococcal septicaemia, etc. **e. pernio**, chilblain (q.v.).

erythraemia (e-rith-rē'-mi-á) [G. *erythros*, red; *haima*, blood]. See ERYTHROCYTHAEMIA.

erythroblast (e-rith'-rō-blast) [G. *erythros*, red; *blastos*, germ]. A nucleated red blood cell found in the red bone marrow and from which the erythrocytes are derived—erythroblastic, adj.

erythroblastosis fetalis (e-rith-rō-blas-tō'-sis fē-tā'lis) [G. *erythros*, red; *blastos*, germ; L. *fetus*, offspring]. A pathological condition in the newborn child due to rhesus incompatibility between the child's blood and that of its mother. Red blood cell destruction occurs with anaemia, often jaundice and an excess of erythroblasts or primitive red blood cells in the circulating blood. Immunization of women at risk, using gammaglobulin containing a high titre of anti-D, prevents EF.

Erythrocin (e-rith'-rō-sin). Erythromycin (q.v.).

erythrocyanosis frigida (e-rith-rō-sī-an-ō'-sis frig'-id-á) [G. *erythros*, red; *kyanos*, blue; *-osis*, condition; L. *frigus*, cold]. Vasospastic disease with hypertrophy of arteriolar muscular coat—erythrocyanotic, adj.

erythrocytes (e-rith'-rō-sitz) [G. *erythros,* red; *kytos,* cell]. The normal nonnucleated red cells of the circulating blood; the red blood corpuscles—erythrocytic, adj.

Eurax (ū'-raks). Crotamiton (q.v.).

erythrocythaemia (ē-rith-rō-si-thē'-mi-á) [G. *erythros,* red; *kytos,* cell; *haima,* blood]. Overproduction of red cells. 1. This may be a physiological response to a low atmospheric oxygen tension (high altitudes), or to the need for greater oxygenation of the tissues (congenital heart disease) and is then referred to as erythrocytosis. 2. The idiopathic condition is polycythaemia vera (erythraemia)—erythrocythaemic, adj.

erythrocytopenia (ē-rith-rō-sī-tō-pē'-ni-á) [G. *erythros,* red; *kytos,* cell; *penia,* want]. Deficiency in the number of red blood cells—erythrocytopenic, adj.

erythrocytosis (ē-rith-rō-sī-tō'-sis) [G. *erythros,* red; *kytos,* cell; *-osis,* condition]. See ERYTHROCYTHAEMIA.

erythroedema polyneuritis (ē-rith-rē-dē'-má pol-i-nū-rī'-tis) [G. *erythros,* red; *oidema,* swelling; *polys,* many; *neuron,* tendon; *-itis,* inflammation]. A disease of infancy characterized by red, swollen extremities. Nervous irritability is extreme, leading to anorexia and wasting. Syn., pink disease. Swift's disease.

erythroderma (ē-rith'-rō-dermá) [G. *erythros,* red; *derma,* skin]. Excessive redness of the skin.

erythrogenic (ē-rith-rō-jen'-ik) [G. *erythros,* red; *genesis,* production]. 1. Producing or causing a rash. 2. Producing red blood cells.

erythromycin (ē-rith-rō-mī'-sin). An orally active antibiotic, similar to penicillin in its range of action. Best reserved for use against organisms resistant to other antibiotics. Risk of jaundice, particularly with e. estolate.

erythropoiesis (ē-rith'-rō-poi-ē-sis) [G. *erythros,* red; *poiesis,* production]. The production of red blood cells. See HAEMOPOIESIS.

Esbach's albuminometer (es'-báks al-bū-min-om'-et-ér). A graduated glass tube in which albumin in urine is precipitated in 24 hours by the addition of E.'s reagent. See APPENDIX ON URINE TESTING. [George H. Esbach, Paris physician, 1843–90.]

Esbatal (es'-bat-al). Bethanidine (q.v.).

eschar (es'-kár) [G. *eschara,* scab]. A slough, as results from a burn, application of caustics, diathermy, etc.

escharotic (es-kár-ot'-ik) [G. *eschara,* scab]. Any agent capable of producing an eschar.

Escherichia (esh-er-ik'-i-á). A genus of bacteria. Motile, Gram-negative rod bacteria which are widely distributed in nature, especially in the intestinal tract of vertebrates. Some strains are pathogenic to man, causing enteritis, peritonitis, pyelitis, cystitis and wound infections. The type species is *E. coli.*

eserine (es'-e-rēn). Physostigmine (q.v.).

Esidrex. Hydrochlorothiazide (q.v.).

Esmarch's bandage. A rubber roller bandage used to procure a bloodless operative field in the limbs. [Johann Friedrich August von Esmarch, German military surgeon, 1823–1908.]

esmodil (es'-mō-dil). Antispasmodic drug similar to carbachol.

ESN. Educationally subnormal. May attend a special school, or a special class in an ordinary school.

espundia (es-pun'-dē-á). South American mucocutaneous leishmaniasis (q.v.). Causes ulceration of the legs with later involvement of nose and throat.

ESR. Erythrocyte sedimentation rate. Citrated blood is placed in a narrow tube. The red cells fall, leaving a column of clear supernatant serum, which is measured at the end of an hour and reported in millimetres. Tissue destruction and inflammatory conditions cause an increase in the ESR.

essence (es'-ens). A solution of a volatile oil in rectified spirit.

Estigyn (es'-ti-jin). Ethinyloestradiol (q.v.).

Estopen (es-to-pen'). A penicillin and iodine compound, with a selective affinity for lung tissue.

Estrovis (es-trō-vis'). Quinestrol (q.v.).

ethacrynic acid (eth-a-krin'-ik). Diuretic with a wider range of effectiveness than the thiazide group. Called a 'loop' diuretic because it prevents the concentration of urine by an action on the loop of Henle.

ethamsylate (eth-am'-sil-āt). Systemic haemostatic agent.

ethambutol (eth-am-būt'-ol). Synthetic antituberculosis drug. Oral. Highly effective when used with isoniazid for tuberculosis. Almost non-toxic, but occasionally its toxic effect is retrobulbar neuritis.

ethanolamine oleate (eth'-ăn-ōl-â-min ol'-e-āt). A sclerosing agent used in varicose vein therapy.

ether (ē'-ther) [G. *aither,* pure air]. Inflammable liquid; one of the oldest volatile anaesthetics and less toxic than chloroform. Occasionally used orally for its carminative action.

ethlazide (eth'-i-a-zīd). See CHLOROTHIAZIDE.

ethics (eth'-iks) [G. *ethos,* custom]. A code of moral principles derived from a system of values and beliefs. nursing e., the code governing a nurse's behaviour, especially to her patients, visitors and colleagues. Ethics apply to national groups and to smaller ones, e.g. professional and business.

Ethinamate (eth-in'-am-āt). Tranquillizer. One of the carbamates. For poisoning see p. 337.

ethinyloestradiol (eth-in-il'-es-trā-di-ol). Powerful orally effective oestrogen, usually well tolerated.

ethionamide (eth-i-on'-a-mīd). Expensive synthetic antitubercular compound. Oral. Hepatotoxicity guarded against by twice weekly SGOT tests. Like isoniazid, e. can be neurotoxic. It can produce gastrointestinal side effects.

ethisterone (eth-i-stē'-rōn). An orally active compound with progesterone-like properties. The average dose is six times that of progesterone by injection.

ethmoid (eth'-moid) [G. *ethmos,* sieve; *eidos,* form]. A spongy bone forming the lateral walls of the nose and the upper portion of the bony nasal septum.

ethmoidectomy (eth'-moid-ek'-to-mi) [G. *ethmos,* sieve; *eidos,* form; *ektome,* a cutting]. Surgical removal of a part of the ethmoid bone, usually that forming the lateral nasal walls.

ethoglucid (eth-ō-gloo'-sid). Intraarterial, anticancer, neurotoxic agent.

ethoheptazine (ē-thō-hep'-ta-zēn). Analgesic that relieves muscle spasm. Related to pethidine. Zactirin.

ethopropazine (ē-thō-prō'-pa-zēn). An antispasmodic used chiefly in rigidity of Parkinsonism. May have more side effects than other drugs.

ethosuximide (eth-ō-suks'ī-mīd). Anti-

convulsant useful in petit mal.

ethotoin (eth'-ō-toin). For major, focal and psychomotor epilepsy.

ethyl biscoumacetate (eth'-il bis-koom-as'-ē-tāt). A blood anticoagulant of the dicoumarol type, but with a more rapid and controllable action.

ethyl carbamate (eth'-il-kâr'-bâm-āt). Urethane (q.v.).

ethyl chloride (eth'-il klōr'-id). A volatile general anaesthetic for short operations, and a local anaesthetic by reason of the intense cold produced when applied to the skin; useful in sprains.

ethyloestrenol (eth-il-ēs'-tren-ol). An anabolic steroid; useful for treating severe weight loss, debility and osteoporosis.

ethyloleamine oleate (eth-il-ōl'-a-mēn ol'-ē-āt). Sclerosing agent.

ethyl pyrophosphate (eth'-il pī-rō-fos'-fāt). Organo-phosphorous compound used as insecticide in agriculture. Powerful and irreversible anticholinesterase action. Potentially dangerous to man for this reason.

ethynodiol diacetate (eth-in-ō'-di-ol dī-as'-âs'-e-tat). Controls uterine bleeding.

etiology (ē-ti-ol'-o-ji). See AETIOLOGY.

Etophylate (et-ō-fil'-āt). Theophylline (q.v.).

EUA. Examination (of the uterus) under anaesthetic.

eucalyptus oil (ū-ka-lip'-tus). Has mild antiseptic properties, and is sometimes used in nasal drops for catarrh.

Eucortone (ū-kor'-tōn). Adrenal cortex extract.

Eudemine (ū'-de-mēn). Diazoxide (q.v.).

euflavine (ū-flā'-vēn). See ACRIFLAVINE.

eugenics (ū-jen'-iks) [G. *eu,* well; *genos,* birth]. The science dealing with those factors which improve successive generations of the human race—eugenic, adj.

Euglucon (ū-glū'-kon). Glibenclamide (q.v.).

Eugynon (ū-gī'-non). Low oestrogen oral contraceptive.

Eumydrin (ū'-mid-rin). Atropine methonitrate (q.v.). Specially useful in pylorospasm.

eunuch (ū'-nuk) [G. *eunouchos,* guarding the couch]. A human male from whom the testes have been removed; a castrated male.

eupepsia (ū-pep'-si-á) [G. *eu*, well; *peptein*, to digest]. Normal digestion.

euphoria (ū-for'-ē-á) [G. *eu*, well; *pheresthai*, to turn out]. In psychology, an exaggerated sense of well-being—euphoric, adj.

eurhythmics (ū-rith'-miks) [G. *euruthmia*, good rhythm]. Harmonious bodily movements performed to music.

eusol (ū'-sol). Antiseptic solution prepared from chloride of lime and boric acid. Effective when freshly prepared, but solutions lose strength rapidly.

Eustachian (ū-stā'-ki-an). A canal, partly bony, partly cartilaginous, measuring 38.0 to 50.8 mm in length, connecting the pharynx with the tympanic cavity. It allows air to pass into the middle ear, so that the air pressure is kept even on both sides of the eardrum. **E. catheter**, an instrument used for dilating the Eustachian tube when it becomes blocked. [Bartolommeo Eustachius, Italian anatomist, 1520–74.]

euthanasia (ū-than-ā'-zi-á) [G. *eu*, well; *thanatos*, death]. 1. A good, inferring a painless death. 2. Frequently interpreted as the painless killing of a patient suffering from an incurable disease.

euthyroid state (ū-thī'-roid stāt). Denoting normal thyroid function.

eutocia (ū-tō'-si-á) [G. *eu*, well; *tokos*, childbirth]. A natural and normal labour without any complications.

Eutonyl. MAOI (q.v.).

EVA. Evacuation (of the uterus) under anaesthetic.

evacuant (e-vak'-ū-ant) [L. *evacuare*, to empty out]. An agent which causes an evacuation, particularly of the bowel. **e. enema** fluid injected into the rectum, to be returned, as distinct from retained.

evacuation (e-vak-ū-ā'-shun) [L. *evacuare*, to empty out]. The act of emptying a cavity; generally referred to the discharge of faecal matter from the rectum.

evacuator (e-vak'-ū-ā-tor) [L. *evacuare*, to empty out]. An instrument for procuring evacuation, e.g. the removal from the bladder of a stone, crushed by a lithotrite.

evaporate (e-vap'-o-rāt) [L. *e*, out; *vaporare*, to fill with steam]. To convert from the liquid to the gaseous state by means of heat.

evaporating lotion (e-vap'-o-rāt-ing lō'-shun). One which, applied as a compress, absorbs heat in order to evaporate, and so cools the skin.

eversion (ē-ver'-shun) [L. *evertere*, to turn out]. A turning outwards, as of the upper eyelid to expose the conjunctival sac.

evisceration (ē-vis-e-rā'-shun) [L. *eviscerare*, to disembowel]. Removal of internal organs.

evulsion (ē-vul'-shun) [L. *evulsus* from *evellere*, to tear out]. Forcible tearing away of a structure.

Ewing's tumour. Sarcoma involving shaft of long bone before twentieth year. Current view holds that it is a secondary bone deposit from a malignant neuroblastoma of the adrenal gland. [James Ewing, American pathologist, 1866–1943.]

exacerbation (eks-as-ér-bā'-shun) [L. *exacerbare*, to irritate]. Increased severity, as of symptoms.

exanthema (eks-an-thēm'-á) [G. eruption]. A skin eruption—exanthemata, pl.; exanthematous, adj.

excision (ek-sizh'-un) [L. *excidere*, to cut out]. Removal of a part by cutting—excise, v.t.

excitability (ek-sīt-a-bil'-i-ti) [L. *excitare*, to arouse]. Rapid response to stimuli; a state of being easily irritated—excitable, adj.

excitation (ek-sī-tā'-shun) [L. *excitare*, to arouse]. The act of stimulating an organ or tissue.

excoriation (eks-kōr-i-ā'-shun) [L. *ex*, from; *corium*, hide; so *excoriare*, to fray]. See ABRASION.

excrement (eks'-krē-ment). Faeces (q.v.).

excrescence (eks-kres'-ens) [L. *excrescere*, to grow out]. An abnormal protuberance or growth of the tissues.

excreta (eks-krē'-tá). The waste matter which is normally discharged from the body, particularly urine and faeces.

excretion (eks-krē'-shun). The elimination of waste material from the body, and also the matter so discharged—excretory, adj., n.; excrete, v.t.

exenteration (eks-en-te-rā'-shun) [L. *exenterare*, from G. *ex*; out of; *enteron*, intestine]. Removal of the viscera. **pelvic e.**, a radical operation for advanced cancer of the pelvic organs.

exfoliation (eks-fō-li-ā'-shun) [L. *exfoliare*, to strip off leaves]. The scaling off of tissues in layers—exfoliative, adj. See CYTOLOGY.

exhibitionism (eks-i-bish'-un-izm) [L. *exhibere*, to hold forth]. Any kind of 'showing off'; extravagant behaviour to attract attention including such perverted behaviour . as indecent exposure—exhibitionist, n.

exocrine (eks'-ō-krīn) [G. *exo*, outside; *krinein*, to separate]. Glands from which the secretion passes via a duct. Secreting externally. Opp. to endocrine—exocrinal, adj.

exogenous (eks-oj'-en-us) [G. *exo*, outside; *genes*, producing]. Of external origin.

Exolan (eks' ō lan). Non-staining, non-burning form of dithranol.

exomphalos (cks-om'-fal-os) [G. *ex*, out; *omphalos*, navel]. A condition present at birth and due to failure of development of the abdominal wall. The intestines protrude through a gap in the umbilical region, covered only by a thin membrane.

exophthalmos (eks-of-thal'-mos) [G. *ex*, out; *ophthalmos*, eye]. Protrusion of the eyeball. See GOITRE—exophthalmic, adj.

exostosis (cks-os-tō'sis) [G. *ex*, out; *osteon*, bone; *-osis*, condition]. An overgrowth of bone tissue forming a tumour.

exotoxin (eks-ō-toks'-in) [G. *exo*, outside; *toxikon*, poison]. A toxic product of bacteria which is passed into the environment of the cell during growth. Opp. to endotoxin—exotoxic, adj.

expected date of delivery. Usually dated from the first day of the last normal menstrual period, even though for the next 14 days there is really no pregnancy.

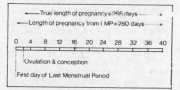

Expected date of delivery chart

expectorant (eks-pek'-to-rant) [L. *expectorare*, to drive from the breast]. A drug which promotes or increases expectoration.

expectoration (eks-pek-tor-ā'-shun) [L. *expectorare*, to drive from the breast].

1. The elimination of secretion from the respiratory tract by coughing. 2. Sputum (q.v.)—expectorate, v.t.

expiration (eks-pi-rā'-shun) [L. *expirare*, to breathe out]. The act of breathing out air from the lungs—expire, v.t., v.i.; expiratory, adj.

exploration (eks-plor-ā'-shun) [L. *explorare*, to spy out]. The act of exploring for diagnostic purposes, particularly in the surgical field—exploratory, adj.

Expranolol (eks-pran'-o-lol). Propranolol (q.v.).

expression (eks-presh'-un) [L. *ex*, out; *premere*, press]. 1. Expulsion by force as of the placenta from the uterus; milk from the breast, etc. 2. Facial disclosure of feelings, mood, etc.

exsanguination (eks-sang-gwin-a'-shun [L. *exsanguis*, deprived of blood]. The process of rendering bloodless—exsanguinate, v.t.

extension (eks-ten'-shun) [L. *extendere*, to stretch out]. 1. Traction upon a fractured or dislocated limb. 2. The straightening of a flexed limb or part.

extensor (eks-ten'-sor) [L. from *extendere*, to stretch out]. A muscle which on contraction extends or straightens a part. Opp. to flexor.

extirpation (eks-tėr-pā'-shun) [L. *exstirpare*, to pluck out]. Complete removal or destruction of a part.

extra-articular (eks-tra-ăr-tīk'-ū-lar) [L. *extra*, outside of; *articulus*, dim. of *aitus*, joint]. Outside a joint.

extracapsular (eks-tra-kap'-sū-lar) [L. *extra*, outside of; *capsula*, small box]. Outside the capsule.

extracardiac (eks-tra-kăr'-di-ak) [L. *extra*, outside of; G. *kardia*, heart]. Outside the heart.

extracellular (eks-tra-sel'-ū-lár) [L. *extra*, outside of; *cellula*, little cell]. Occurring outside the cell.

extracorporeal (eks-tra-kor-por'-ri-al) [L. *extra*, outside; *corporeus*, bodily, material]. Outside the body. See CIRCULATION.

extracorpuscular (eks-tra-kor-pus'-kū-lár) [L. *extra*, outside; *corpusculum*, small body]. Outside corpuscles (q.v.).

extract (eks'-trakt) [L. *extrahere*, to draw out]. A preparation obtained by evaporating a solution of a drug.

extraction (eks-trak'-shun) [L. *extrahere*, to draw out]. The act of drawing out. **e. of lens,** surgical removal of the lens. **extracapsular e.,** the capsule is ruptured prior to delivery of the lens. **intracapsular e.,** the lens is removed within its capsule.

extradural (eks-tra-dūr'-al) [L. *extra,* outside of; *durus,* hard]. External to the dura mater.

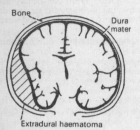

Bone

Dura mater

Extradural haematoma

extragenital (eks-tra-jen'-it-al) [L. *extra,* outside of; *genitalis,* genital]. On areas of the body apart from genital organs. **e. chancre** is the primary ulcer of syphilis occurring on the finger, the lip, the breast, etc.

extrahepatic (eks-tra-hep-at'-ik) [L. *extra,* outside of; G. *hepar,* liver]. Outside the liver.

extramural (eks-tra-mūr'-al) [L. *extra,* outside of; *murus,* wall]. Outside the wall of a vessel or organ—extramurally, adv.

extraperitoneal (eks-tra-per-it-on-ē'-ál) [L. *extra,* outside of; G. *peri,* round; *teinein,* to stretch]. Outside the peritoneum—extraperitoneally, adv.

extrapleural (eks-tra-ploo'-ral) [L. *extra,* outside of; G. *pleura,* side]. Outside the pleura, i.e. between the parietal pleura and the chest wall. See PLOMBAGE.

extrarenal (eks-tra-rē'-nal) [L. *extra,* outside of; *renalis,* of the kidney]. Outside the kidney.

extrasystole (eks-tra-sis'-to-li) [L. *extra,* outside of; G. *systole,* a drawing together]. Premature beats in the pulse rhythm: the cardiac impulse is initiated in some focus apart from the sinoatrial node.

extrathoracic (eks-tra-thor-as'-ik) [L. *extra* outside of; G. *thorax*]. Outside the thoracic cavity.

extrauterine (eks-tra-ū'-ter-īn) [L. *extra,* outside of; *uterus,* womb]. Outside the uterus. See ECTOPIC PREGNANCY.

extravasation (eks-trav-a-sā'-shun) [L. *extra,* outside of; *vas,* vessel]. An escape of fluid from its normal enclosure into the surrounding tissues.

extravenous (eks'-tra-vēn'-us) [L. *extra,* outside; *vena,* vein]. Outside a vein.

extrinsic (eks-trin'-sik) [L. *extrinsecus,* on the outside]. Developing or having its origin from without; not internal. **e. factor,** vitamin B_{12} (cyanocobalamin), which is normally present in the diet and absorbed from the gut; it is essential for normal haemopoiesis.

extroversion (eks-tro-vėr'-shun) [L. *extra,* outside of; *vertere,* to turn]. Turning inside out. **e. of the bladder,** ectopia vesicae (q.v.). In psychology, the direction of thoughts to the external world.

extrovert (eks'-tro-vėrt) [L. *extra,* outside; *vertere,* to turn]. Sometimes **extra-vert.** Used by Jung to describe one extreme of personality dimension. The person described as e. regulates his behaviour in response to other people's attitude to him.

exudate (eks'-ū-dāt) [L. *exudare,* to sweat out]. The product of exudation.

exudation (eks-ū-dā'-shun) [L. *exudare,* to sweat out]. The oozing out of fluid through the capillary walls, or of sweat through the pores of the skin—exudate, n.; exude, v.t., v.i.

eye-teeth. The canine teeth in the upper jaw.

F

facet (fas'-et) [F. *facette,* little face]. A small, smooth, flat surface of a bone or a calculus. **f. syndrome,** dislocation of some of the gliding joints between vertebrae causing pain and muscle spasm.

facial (fāsh'-al) [L. *facies,* face, external form]. Pertaining to the face. **f. nerve,** seventh pair of cranial nerves. **f. paralysis,** paralysis of muscles supplied by f. nerve. See PALSY (BELL'S).

facies (fā'-sēz) [L. *facies,* face, external form]. The appearance of the face, used especially of the subject of congenital syphilis with saddle nose, prominent brow and chin. **adenoid f.,** open mouthed, vacant expression due to deafness from enlarged adenoids. **f. hippocratica,** the drawn, pale, pinched appearance, indicative of approaching death. **Parkinson f.,** a mask-like appearance; saliva may trickle from the corners of the mouth.

facultative (fak'-ul-tā-tiv) [L. *facultas*, faculty]. Conditional; having the power of living under different conditions.

faecalith (fē'-ka-lith) [L. *faeces*, dregs; G. *lithos*, stone]. A concretion formed in the bowel from faecal matter.

faeces (fē'-sēz) [L. *faeces*, dregs]. The waste matter excreted from the bowel, consisting mainly of indigestible cellulose, unabsorbed food, intestinal secretions, water and bacteria—faecal, adj.

Fahrenheit (fár'-en-hīt). A thermometric scale; the freezing point of water is 32° and its boiling point 212°. [Gabriel Fahrenheit, German physicist, 1686–1736.]

failure to thrive. Blanket term replacing marasmus. Afflicted children do not progress because of difficulty in absorbing the basic nutritional requirements.

faint (fānt). A swoon; a state of temporary unconsciousness. Syn., syncope.

Fairbank's splint. Used for treatment of Erb's palsy, where baby's arm is immobilized in abduction and external rotation of the shoulder, flexion of the elbow to 90°, supination of the forearm and extension of the wrist.

falciform (fal'-si-form) [L. *falx*, sickle; *forma*, shape]. Sickle-shaped.

Fallopian tubes (fal-lō'-pi-an). Two tubes opening out of the upper part of the uterus. Each measures 10.16 cm and the distal end is fimbriated and lies near the ovary. Their function is to convey in the ova into the uterus. [Gabriel Fallopius, Italian anatomist, 1523–63.]

Fallot's tetralogy (fal'-ōs tet-ral'-o-ji). Congenital heart defect comprising interventricular septal defect, pulmonary stenosis, right ventricular hypertrophy and malposition of the aorta. [Etienne L. A. Fallot, French physician, 1850–1911.]

falx (fal-ks) [L. sickle]. A sickle-shaped structure. **f. cerebri,** that portion of the dura mater separating the two cerebral hemispheres.

familial (fam-il'-i-al) [L. *familia*, household]. Pertaining to the family, as of a disease affecting several members of the same family.

Fanconi syndrome. See AMINOACIDURIA. [Guido Fanconi, Swiss paediatrician, 1892–   .]

fang. The root of a tooth.

fantasy (fan'-ta-si) [G. *phantasia*]. Imagination, where images or chains of images are directed by the desire or pleasure of the thinker, normally accompanied by a feeling of unreality. Occurs pathologically in schizophrenia.

farinaceous (far-in-ā'-shus) [L. *farina*, flour]. Pertaining to cereal substances, i.e. made of flour or grain. Starchy.

farmer's lung. A form of pneumoconiosis arising from the dust of mouldy hay or other mouldy vegetable produce. Recognized as an industrial disease.

fascia (fash'-i-à) [L. band]. A connective tissue sheath consisting of fibrous tissue and fat which unites the skin to the underlying tissues. It also surrounds and separates many of the muscles, and, in some cases, holds them together—fascial, adj.

fasciculation (fas-ik-ū-lā-shun). Visible flickering of muscle; can occur in the upper and lower eyelids.

fasciculus (fas-sik'-ū-lus) [L. small bundle]. A little bundle, as of muscle or nerve—fascicular, adj.; fasciculi, pl.

fasciotomy (fash-i-ot'-om-i) [L. *fascia*, band; G. *tome*, a cutting]. Incision of a fascia.

fastigium (fas-tij'-i-um) [L. summit]. The highest point of a fever; the period of full development of a disease.

fat. An oil which may be of animal or vegetable origin, and may be either solid or liquid f. soluble vitamins A, D, E and K. See CALORIFIC—fatty, adj.

fatigue (fa-tēg') [L. *fatigare*, to tire]. Weariness. Term used in physiological experiments on muscle to denote diminishing reaction to stimulus applied—fatigability, n.

fatty degeneration. Degeneration (q.v.) of tissues which results in appearance of fatty droplets in the cytoplasm: found especially in disease of liver, kidney and heart.

fauces (faw'-sēz) [L. throat]. The opening from the mouth into the pharynx, bounded above by the soft palate, below by the tongue. Pillars of the f., anterior and posterior, lie laterally and enclose the tonsil—faucial, adj.

favism (fā'-vizm) [from It *fava*, bean]. Reduced amount of enzyme G6PD (glucose-6-phosphate dehydrogenase) in red blood cells. Afflicted people develop a severe haemolytic anaemia when they eat fava beans.

favus (fā'-vus) [L. honeycomb]. A type of ringworm not common in Britain; caused by *Trichophyton schoenleini*.

Yellow cup-shaped crusts (scutula) develop especially on the scalp.

febrile (feb'-rīl) [L. *febris*, fever]. Feverish; accompanied by fever.

fecundation (fe-kun-dā'-shun) [L. *fecundus*, fertile]. Impregnation. Fertilization.

fecundity (fe-kun'-di-ti) [L. *fecundus*, fertile]. The power of reproduction; fertility.

Fehling's solution (fā'-lings). An alkaline, copper solution used for the detection and estimation of amount of sugars. [Herman von Fehling, German chemist, 1812–85.]

Felty's syndrome. Enlargement of liver, spleen and lymph nodes as a complication of rheumatoid arthritis. [Augustus Roi Felty, American physician, 1895–   .]

Felypressin (fel-i-pres'-in). Vasoconstrictor. Related to posterior pituitary hormone vasopressin. Sometimes combined with local anaesthetic.

Femergin (fem'-er-gin). Ergotamine tartrate (q.v.).

femoropopliteal (fem-or-ō-pop-lit-ē'-al) [L. *femur*, thigh bone; *poples*, ham]. Usually referring to the femoral and popliteal vessels.

femur (fē'-mur) [L.]. The thighbone; the longest and strongest bone in the body—femoral, adj., femora, pl.

fenestra (fen-es'-trà) [L. window]. A window-like opening. **f. ovalis**, an oval opening between the middle and internal ear. Below it lies the **f. rotunda**, a round opening.

fenestration (fen-es-trā'-shun) [L. *fenestra*, window]. 1. The surgical creation of an opening (or fenestra) in the inner ear for the relief of deafness in otosclerosis. 2. A type of walking seen in such nervous diseases as paralysis agitans, when patient trots along in little bursts, getting faster and faster until he has to stop and then start off again, otherwise he would fall over.

fenfluramine hydrochloride (fen-flū'-ra-mēn). Appetite depressant. Free from the disadvantages of the amphetamines.

Fentazin. Perphenazine (q.v.). Closely allied to chlorpromazine (q.v.).

ferment (fer'-ment). See CATALYST.

fermentation (fer-men-tā'-shun) [L. *fermentum*, ferment]. The chemical changes brought about by the action of ferments, usually accompanied by liberation of heat and gas. Excellent examples are the making of bread, cheese and wine.

ferric (fer'-ik) [L. *ferrum*, iron]. Pertaining to trivalent iron, as of its salts and compounds.

Ferrivenin (fer-ri-ven'-in). A solution of saccharated iron oxide, used by intravenous injection for severe iron deficiency anaemia.

ferrous (fer'-rus) [L. *ferrum*, iron]. Pertaining to divalent iron, as of its salts and compounds. Ferrous carbonate, f. fumarate, f. gluconate, f. succinate and f. sulphate are oral preparations for iron-deficiency anaemias.

fertilization (fer-til-ī-zā'-shun) [L. *fertilis*, fertile]. The impregnation of an ovum by a spermatozoon.

fester (fes'-ter). To become inflamed; to suppurate.

festination (fes-tin-ā'-shun) [L. *festinare*, to hasten]. An involuntary hastening in gait as seen in paralysis agitans.

fetishism (fet'-ish-izm). A condition in which a particular object is regarded with an irrational fear or a strong emotional attachment.

fetor (fē'-tor) [L. offensive smell]. Offensive odour, stench, **f. oris**, bad breath. Also foetor.

fetus (fē'-tus) [T.]. An unborn child. **f. papyraceous**, a dead fetus, one of a twin which has become flattened and mummified—fetal, adj.

fever (fē'-ver) [L. *febris*, fever]. An elevation of body temperature above normal. Syn., pyrexia. Designates some infectious conditions, e.g. **paratyphoid f.**, **scarlet f.**, **typhoid f.**, etc.

Fibogel (fī'-bō-jel). A hydrophyllic gel which is a mucilaginous polysaccharide.

fibre (fī'-ber) [L. *fibra*, fibre]. A threadlike structure—fibrous, adj.

fibril (fī'-bril) [L. *fibra*, fibre]. A component filament of a fibre. A small fibre.

fibrillation (fī-bril-ā'-shun). Uncoordinated quivering contraction of muscle; referring usually to atrial (auricular) f. in the myocardium wherein the atria (auricles) beat very rapidly and are not synchronized with the ventricular beat. The result is a total irregularity of the pulse.

fibrin (fī'-brin). The matrix on which a blood clot is formed. The substance is formed from soluble fibrinogen of the blood by the catalytic (enzymatic) action of thrombin—fibrinous, adj.

fibrin foam. A white, dry, spongy material made from fibrinogen. It is used in conjunction with thrombin as a haemostatic in brain and lung surgery.

fibrinogen (fī-brin'-ō-jen). A soluble protein of the blood from which is produced the insoluble protein called fibrin (q.v.), essential to blood coagulation.

fibrinogenopenia (fī-brin-ō-jen-ō-pē'-ni-à) [L. *fibra*, fibre; G. *genesthai*, to be produced; *penia*, poverty]. Lack of blood plasma fibrinogen. Can be congenital or due to liver disease. Fibrinopenia. Hypofibrinogenaemia.

fibrinolysin (fī-brin-ō-līs'-in) [L. *fibra*, fibre; G. *lysis*, a loosening]. Blood stream enzyme thought to dissolve fibrin occurring after minor injuries. Has been administered intravenously in thrombosis.

fibrinolysis (fī-brin-ol'-i-sis) [L. *fibra*, fibre; G. *lysis*, a loosening]. The dissolution of fibrin—fibrinolytic, adj.

fibroadenoma (fī-brō-ad-e-nō'-má) [L. *fibra*, fibre; G. *aden*, gland; *-oma*, tumour]. A benign tumour containing fibrous and glandular tissue.

fibroblast (fī'-brō-blast) [L. *fibra*, fibre; G. *blastos*, germ]. A cell which gives rise to connective tissue. Syn., fibrocyte—fibroblastic, adj.

fibrocartilage (fī-brō-kár'-til-āj) [L. *fibra*, fibre; *cartilago*, cartilage]. Cartilage containing fibrous tissue—fibrocartilaginous, adj.

fibrocaseous (fī-brō-kā'-sē-us) [L. *fibra*, fibre; *caseus*, cheese]. A soft, cheesy mass infiltrated by fibrous tissue, formed by fibroblasts.

fibrochondritis (fī-brō-kon-drī'-tis) [L. *fibra*, fibre; G. *chondros*, cartilage; *-itis*, inflammation]. Inflammation of fibrocartilage.

fibrocyst (fī'-brō-sist) [L. *fibra*, fibre; G. *kystis*, bladder]. A fibroma which has undergone cystic degeneration—fibrocystic, adj.

fibrocystic (fī-brō-sis'-tik). Pertaining to a fibrocyst. **f. disease of bone,** cysts may be solitary or generalized. The latter condition, when accompanied by decalcification of bone, is due to hyperparathyroidism. **f. disease of breast,** see MASTITIS. **f. disease of pancreas,** see MUCOVISCIDOSIS.

fibrocyte (fī'-brō-sīt) [L. *fibra*, fibre; G.

kytos, cell]. See FIBROBLAST—fibrocytic, adj.

fibroid (fī'-broid) [L. *fibra*, fibre; G. *eidos*, form]. A fibromuscular benign tumour usually found in the uterus. An interstitial uterine f. is embedded in the wall of the uterus (intramural)—if extended to the outer surface it becomes subperitoneal (subserous), if to the inner or endometrial surface it becomes submucous or even a f. polypus.

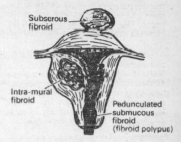

Uterine fibroids

fibroma (fī-brō'-má) [L. *fibra*, fibre; G. *-oma*, tumour]. A benign tumour composed of fibrous tissue—fibromatous, adj.; fibromata, pl.

fibromuscular (fī-brō-mus'-kū-lár) [L. *fibra*, fibre; *musculus*, muscle]. Pertaining to fibrous and muscle tissue.

fibromyoma (fī-brō-mī-ō'-má) [L. *fibra*, fibre; G. *mys*, muscle; *-oma*, tumour]. A benign tumour consisting of fibrous and muscle tissue—fibromyomata, pl.; fibromyomatous, adj.

fibrosarcoma (fī-brō-sár-kō'-má) [L. *fibra*, fibre; G. *sarx*, flesh; *-oma*, tumour]. A form of sarcoma. A malignant tumour derived from fibroblastic (fibrocytic) cells—fibrosarcomata, pl.; fibrosarcomatous, adj.

fibrosis (fī-brō'-sis) [L. *fibra*, fibre; G. *-osis*, condition]. The formation of excessive fibrous tissue in a structure—fibrotic, adj.

fibrositis (fī-brō-sī'-tis) [L. *fibra*, fibre; G. *-itis*, inflammation]. Pain of uncertain origin which affects the soft tissues of the limbs and trunk. It is generally associated with muscular stiffness and local tender points—fibrositic nodules. Cause unknown; some disturbance in immunity may be a factor, as may be gout. Non-specific factors include chill, postural trauma, muscular strain and psychological stress especially in tense, anxious people. Syn., muscular rheumatism. See BORNHOLM DISEASE, LUMBAGO, PLEURODYNIA.

fibrovascular (fī-brō-vas'-kū-lár) [L. *fibra,* fibre; *vasculum,* small vessel]. Pertaining to fibrous tissue, which is well supplied with blood vessels.

fibula (fib'-ū-lá) [L. clasp]. One of the longest and thinnest bones of the body; situated on the outer side of the leg and articulating at the upper end with the lateral condyle of the tibia and at the lower end with the lateral surface of the talus (astragalus) and tibia—fibular, adj.

field of vision. The area in which objects can be seen by the fixed eye.

Filaria (fil-ā'-ri-á). Parasitic, thread-like worms, found mainly in the tropics and subtropics. The adults of *Filaria bancrofti* and *Brugia malayi* live in the lymphatics, connective tissues or mesentery, where they may cause obstruction, but the embryos migrate to the blood stream. Completion of the lifecycle is dependent upon passage through a mosquito—filarial, adj.

filariasis (fil-ér-ī'-á-sis) infestation with Filaria. See ELEPHANTIASIS.

filaricide (fil-ér'-i-sīd) [L. *filum,* thread; *coedere,* to kill]. An agent which destroys Filaria.

filiform (fi'-li-form) [L. *filum,* thread; *forma,* shape]. Threadlike. **f. papillae,** small projections ending in several minute processes; found on the tongue.

filipuncture (fi-li-pungk'-tūr) [L. *filum,* thread; *punctura,* puncture]. Insertion of wire thread, etc. into an aneurysm to produce coagulation of contained blood.

filix mas (fi'-liks mas). Male fern extract, used to expel tapeworm.

filtrate (fil'-trāt). That part of the substance which passes through the filter.

filtration (fil-trā'-shun). The process of straining through a filter. The act of passing fluid through a porous medium. **f. under pressure** occurs in the kidneys, due to the pressure of blood in the glomeruli.

filum (fi'-lum) [L. thread]. Any filamentous or thread-like structure. **f. terminale,** a strong, fine cord blending with the spinal cord above, and the periosteum of the sacral canal below.

fimbria (fim'-bri-á) [L. fringe]. A fringe or frond; resembling the fronds of a fern; e.g. the fimbriae of the Fallopian tubes—fimbrial, fimbriated, adj.; fimbriae, pl.

finger (fing'-gér). A digit. **clubbed f.,** swelling of terminal phalanx which occurs in many lung and heart diseases.

fission (fish'-un) [L. *fissus,* from *findere,* to split]. A method of reproduction common among the bacteria and protozoa.

fissure (fish'-ur) [L. *fissura,* cleft]. A split or cleft. **anal f.,** a linear ulcer on the margin of the anus. **palpebral f.,** the opening between the eyelids.

fistula (fis'-tū-lá) [L. tube]. An abnormal communication between two body surfaces or cavities, e.g. gastrocolic f., between the stomach and colon; colostomy, between the colon and the abdominal surface—fistular, fistulous, adj.; fistulae, pl.

fits. Convulsions. See EPILEPSY.

fixation (fiks-ā'-shun) [L. *fixus,* from *figere,* to fix]. In optics, the direct focusing of one or both eyes on an object so that the image falls on the retinal disc. As a psychoanalytical term, an emotional attachment, generally sexual, to a parent, causing difficulty in forming new attachments later in life. **complement f.,** when antigen and homologous antibody unite to form a complex, complement may unite with such a complex, and this is referred to as fixation.

flaccid (flak'-sid) [L. *flaccus,* flabby]. Soft, flabby, not firm. See PARALYSIS—flaccidity, n.

flagellum (fla-jel'-um) [L.]. A fine, hairlike appendage capable of lashing movement. Characteristic of spermatozoa, certain bacteria and protozoa—flagella, pl.

Flagyl. Metronidazole (q.v.).

flail chest. Unstable thoracic cage due to fracture. See RESPIRATION.

flat-foot. A congenital or acquired deformity marked by depression of the arches of the feet. See TALIPES.

flat pelvis. A pelvis in which the anteroposterior diameter of the brim is reduced, causing pelvic contraction.

flatulence (flat'-ū-lens) [L. *flatus,* a blowing]. Gastric and intestinal distension with gas—flatulent, adj.

flatus (flā'-tus) [L.]. Gas in the stomach or intestines.

flavine (flā'-vēn). See ACRIFLAVINE.

flavoxate (flav-oks'-āt). Oral urinary antiseptic.

Flaxedil (flaks'-ē-dil). Gallamine (q.v.).

flea (flē). A blood-sucking wingless insect of the order Siphonaptera; it acts as a host and transmits disease. Its bite leaves a portal of entry for infection. **human f.**, *Pulex irritans.* **rat f.**, *Xenopsylla cheopis,* transmitter of plague (q.v.).

flex. Bend.

flexibilitas cerea (fleks-ib-il'-it-as sā'-rē-ä). Literally waxy flexibility. A condition of generalized hypertonia of muscles found in catatonic schizophrenia. When fully developed, the patient's limbs retain positions in which they are placed, remaining immobile for hours at a time. Occasionally occurs in hysteria as hysterical rigidity.

flexion (flek'-shun) [L. *flexus,* bent]. The act of bending.

Flexner's bacillus (*Shigella flexneri*). A pathogenic, Gram-negative rod bacterium, which is the most common cause of bacillary dysentery epidemics, and sometimes infantile gastroenteritis. It is found in the faeces of cases of dysentery and carriers, from whence it may pollute food and water supplies, or be transferred by contact. [Simon Flexner, American pathologist, 1863–1946.]

flexor (fleks'-or) [L. *flexus,* bent]. A muscle which on contraction flexes or bends a part. Opp. to extensor.

flexure (fleks'-ūr) [L. *flexura,* a bending]. A bend. **left colic** or **splenic f.** is situated at the junction of the transverse and descending parts of the colon. It lies at a higher level than the **right colic** or **hepatic f.**, the bend between the ascending and transverse colon, beneath the liver. **sigmoid f.**, the S-shaped bend at the lower end of the descending colon. It is continuous with the rectum below—flexural, adj.

floaters (flō'-ters). Floating bodies in the vitreous humor (of the eye) which are visible to the person.

floating kidney. Abnormally mobile kidney. See NEPHROPEXY.

flocculation (flok-ul-ā'-shun). The coalescence of colloidal particles in suspension resulting in their aggregation into larger discrete masses which are often visible to the naked eye.

flooding. A popular term to describe excessive bleeding from the uterus.

floppy infant (benign congenital hypoto-

nia). Usually no demonstrable muscular neural pathology is present.

florid (flor'-id) [L. *floridus,* flowery]. Flushed, high coloured.

flowmeter. A measuring instrument for flowing gas or liquid.

Floxapen (flok'-sa-pen). Flucloxacillin (q.v.).

flucloxacillin (floo-cloks-a-sil'-lin). An isoxazole penicillin, active against penicillinase-producing strains of *Staphylococcus aureus.* Well absorbed in man after oral and intramuscular administration. The chlorine of cloxacillin has been replaced with fluorine.

fluctuation (fluk-tū ā'-shun) [L. *fluctuare,* to move as a wave]. A wave-like motion felt on digital examination of a fluid-containing tumour, e.g. abscess—fluctuant, adj.

fludrocortisone (floo-drō-kor'-ti-zōn). Sodium-retaining tablets. Useful in some cases of Addison's disease.

flufenamic acid (floo-fen'-a-mik). Nonsteroidal, anti-inflammatory, antipyretic analgesic, especially useful for disorders of the musculoskeletal system. Does not interfere with uricosuric action of sulphinpyrazone, therefore useful in gout.

fluke (flook). A trematode worm of the order Digenea. The European or sheep f. (*Fasciola hepatica*) usually ingested from water-cress. There is fever, malaise, a large tender liver and eosinophilia. No satisfactory treatment though chloroquine helps. The Chinese f. (*Clonorchis sinensis*) is usually ingested with raw fish. The adult fluke lives in the bile ducts and while it may produce cholangitis, hepatitis and jaundice, it may be asymptomatic, or be blamed for vague digestive symptoms. **lung f.** (Paragonimus) usually ingested with raw crab in China and Far East.

fluocinolone (floo-ō-sin'-ō-lōn). Cortisone derivative for topical application.

fluocortolone (floo-o-kor'-to-lōn). Topical corticosteroid.

fluorescein (floo-or-es'-in). Red substance that forms green fluorescent solution. Used as eye drops to detect corneal lesions, which stain green.

fluoridation (floo-or-īd-ā'-shun). The addition of fluorine. When added to water to prevent dental caries, it is used in a 1:1 000 000 dilution.

fluoride (floo-or-īd). A salt sometimes present in water. It prevents caries but in gross excess causes mottling of the teeth.

5-fluorocystosine (floo-or-ō-sī'-to-sēn). Antifungal agent.

fluorohydrocortisone (floo-or-ō-hī-drō-kor'-ti-zōn). 125 times as active as cortisol in causing sodium retention, therefore useful in Addison's disease.

fluoroscopy (floo-or-os'-ko-pi) [L. *fluere,* to flow; G. *skopein,* to examine]. X-ray examination by means of fluorescent screen commonly called 'screening.'

fluorouracil, 5-FU (floo-o-rō-ū'-ra-sil). Antimetabolite cytotoxic agent.

Fluothane (floo'-o-thān). Halothane (q.v.).

fluphenazine enanthate (floo-fen'-á-zēn en'-an-thāt). Used in psychiatry. Can be given as a depot injection. A newer preparation is **f. deconoate.**

flupenthixol deconoate/enanthate (floo-pen-thiks'-ol dek-on-ō-āt/en'-an-thāt). Less likely than fluphenazine d. and e. to produce extrapyramidal side effects and has a mild antidepressant action.

flurbiprofen (flurb-i-prō'-fen). A nonsteroidal anti-inflammatory agent.

flux (fluks) [L. *fluxum,* from *fluere,* to flow]. Any excessive flow of any of the body excretions.

foetor (fē'-tor). See FETOR.

foetus (fē'-tus) [L.]. See FETUS.

Föelling's disease. Phenylpyruvic oligophrenia. [Asbjorn Föelling, Contemporary Norwegian Professor.]

folic acid (fō'-lik as'-id) [L. *folium,* leaf]. A member of the vitamin B complex abundant in green vegetables, yeast and liver. Absorbed from small intestine and an essential factor for normal haemopoiesis and cell division generally. Used in treatment of megaloblastic anaemias (q.v.) other than those due to vitamin B_{12} deficiency.

Folicin (fō'-lis-in). Folic acid and antianaemia compounds especially for prevention of anaemia in pregnancy.

folie à deux. A rare psychiatric syndrome, in which one member of a close pair has a psychosis and imposes his delusions on the other.

follicle (fol'-ikl) [L. *folliculus,* small sac]. 1. A small secreting sac. 2. A simple tubular gland. **follicle stimulating hormone** (FSH), secreted in the anterior pituitary gland; it is trophic to the ovaries in the female, where it develops the ovum-containing (Graafian) follicles; and to the testes in the male, where it is responsible for sperm production. **Graafian f.**, minute vesicles contained in the stroma of an ovary, each containing a single ovum. When an ovum is extruded from a G.f. each month, the corpus luteum is formed under the influence of luteotrophin from the anterior pituitary gland. If fertilization occurs, the corpus luteum persists for 12 weeks, if not it only persists for 12 to 14 days. **hair f.**, the sheath in which a hair grows—follicular, adj.

folliculitis (fol-ik-ūl-ī'-tis) [L. *folliculus,* small sac; G. *-itis,* inflammation]. Inflammation of follicles, such as the hair follicles.

folliculosis (fol-ik-ūl-ō-sis) [L. *folliculus,* small sac; G. *-osis,* condition]. Hypertrophy of follicles. **conjunctival f.**, overgrowth of conjunctival follicles.

fomentation (fō-men-tā'-shun) [L. *fomentum,* poultice]. A hot, wet application to produce hyperaemia. When the skin is intact, strict cleanliness is observed (medical f); when the skin is broken, aseptic technique is used (surgical f.).**fomite** (fō'-mit) [L. *fomes,* touchwood]. Any article which has been in contact with infection and is capable of transmitting same.

fomite (fō-mīt) [L. *fomes,* touchwood]. Any article which has been in contact with infection and is capable of transmitting same.

fontanelle (fon-ta-nel') [F. a little fountain]. A membranous space between the cranial bones. The diamond-shaped anterior f. (bregma) is at the junction of the frontal and two parietal bones. It ossifies during the second year of life. The triangular posterior f. (lambda) is at the junction of the occipital and two parietal bones. It ossifies within a few weeks of birth.

food poisoning. Vomiting, with or without diarrhoea, resulting from eating food contaminated with chemical poison, preformed bacterial toxin, or live bacteria; or poisonous natural vegetation, e.g. berries, toad stools (fungi).

foot. That portion of the lower limb below the ankle. **athlete's foot,** tinea pedis (q.v.). **foot drop,** inability to dorsiflex foot, as in severe sciatica and nervous disease affecting lower lumbar regions of the cord. **madura f.,** mycetoma (q.v.). **trench f.,** immersion f., occurs in frost-bite or other conditions of exposure where there is local deprivation of blood supply.

foramen (for-ā′-men) [L.]. A hole or opening. Generally used with reference to bones. **foramen magnum,** the opening in the occipital bone through which the spinal cord passes. **obturator f.,** found in the anterior portion of the innominate bone. **foramen ovale,** a fetal cardiac, interatrial communication. Closes at birth—foramina, pl.

forceps (for′-seps) [L. pincers]. Surgical instruments with two opposing blades which are used to grasp or compress tissues, swabs, needles and many other surgical appliances. The two blades are controlled by direct pressure on them (tong-like), or by handles (scissor-like).

forensic medicine. Also called 'legal m.' The application of medical knowledge to questions of law.

foreskin (fōr′-skin). The prepuce or skin covering the glans penis.

formaldehyde (for-mal′-de-hīd). Powerful germicide. Formalin is a 40 per cent solution; used mainly for room disinfection and the preservation of pathological specimens.

formication (for-mi-kā′-shun) [L. *formica,* ant]. A sensation as of ants running over the skin. Occurs in nerve lesions, particularly in the regenerative phase.

formula (form′-ū-lá) [L. small pattern]. A prescription. A series of symbols denoting the chemical composition of a substance—formulae, formulas, pl.

formulary (form′-ū-la-ri). A collection of formulas. The **British National F.** is produced by the Joint Formulary Committee.

fornix (for′-niks) [L. arch]. An arch; particularly referred to the vagina, i.e. the space between the vaginal wall and the cervix of the uterus. **conjunctival f.,** the line of reflection of the conjunctiva from the eyelids on to the eyeball—fornices, pl.

Fortral (for′-tral). Pentazocine (q.v.).

fossa (fos′-sa) [L. ditch]. A depression or furrow—fossae, pl.

Fothergill's operation. Anterior colporrhaphy, amputation of part of the cervix and posterior colpoperineorrhaphy performed for genital prolapse. [William Edward Fothergill, English gynaecologist, 1865–1926.]

Fouadin (fū′-a-din). Stibophen (q.v.).

fourchette (foor′-shet) [F.]. A membranous fold connecting the posterior ends of the labia minora.

fovea (fō′-vi-á) [L. a small pit]. A small depression or fossa; particularly the fovea centralis retinae, the site of most distinct vision.

FPL 670. Disodium cromoglycate (q.v.).

fracture (frak′-tūr) [L. *fractura*]. Breach in continuity of a bone. **Bennett's f.,** of proximal end of first metacarpal involving the articular surface. Simulates a dislocated thumb. **closed (simple) f.,** there is no communication with external air. **Colles' f.,** of the lower end of radius giving typical 'dinner fork' deformity. **comminuted f.,** the bone is broken into several pieces. **complicated f.,** there is injury to surrounding organs and structures. **compression f.,** usually of lumbar or dorsal region due to hyper-

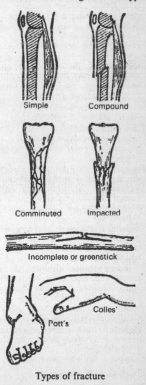

Simple   Compound

Comminuted   Impacted

Incomplete or greenstick

Pott's   Colles'

Types of fracture

flexion of spine; the anterior vertebral bodies are crushed together. **depressed f.**, the broken bone presses on an underlying structure, such as brain or lung. **impacted f.**, one end of the broken bone is driven into the other. **incomplete f.**, the bone is only cracked or fissured—called 'greenstick f,' when it occurs in children. **open (compound) f.**, there is a wound permitting communication of broken bone end with air. **pathological f.**, one caused by local disease of bone. **Pott's f.**, occurs at the lower end of the fibula; often accompanied by dislocation of the tarsal bones and injury to the ligaments. **spontaneous f.**, one occurring without appreciable violence; may be synonymous with pathological f.

fraenotomy (frēn-ot'-om-i) [L. *frenum,* bridle; G. *tome,* a cutting]. Surgical severance of a fraenum, particularly for tongue-tie. Also FRENOTOMY.

fraenum (frē'-num) [L. a bridle]. A fold of membrane which checks or limits the movement of an organ, e.g. **f. linguae**, from the undersurface of the tongue to the floor of the mouth. Also **frenum**.

fragilitas (fraj-il'-i-tas) [L.]. Brittleness. **fragilitas ossium**, congenital disease characterized by abnormal fragility of bone, multiple fractures and a chinablue colouring of the sclera.

framboesia (fram-bē'-zi-à). [F. *framboise,* raspberry]. Yaws (q.v.).

framycetin (frà-mī-sēt'-in). Closely related to neomycin. Used as a local application or orally for its effect on the bowel flora.

Franol (frā'-nol). Ephedrine hydrochloride, theophylline and phenobarbitone. For chronic bronchitis and asthma. **Franol plus**, F. plus an antihistamine. **Franol expect.**, F. plus a mucolytic expectorant.

Freamine (frē'-à-mēn). Mainly synthetic preparation of those amino acids normally ingested as protein in egg, meat and fish.

Freiberg's disease. Osteochondritis of the second metatarsal head. [Albert Henry Freiberg, American orthopaedic surgeon, 1868–1940.]

French chalk. Talc (q.v.).

Frenkel's exercises. Exercises for tabes dorsalis to teach muscle and joint sense. [Heinrich Frenkel, Swiss neurologist, 1860–1931.]

frenotomy. See FRAENOTOMY.

Frenquel. Azacyclonal (q.v.).

frenulum (fren'-ū-lum) [L. *frenum,* a bridle]. A small fraenum (q.v.).

frenum. See FRAENUM.

Freud (froid). The originator of psychoanalysis and the psychoanalytical theory of the causation of neuroses. He first described the existence of the unconscious mind, censor, repression, the theory of infantile sexuality, and worked out in detail many mental mechanisms of the unconscious which modify normal, and account for abnormal human behavour. [Sigmund Freud, Austrian psychiatrist, 1856–1939.]

Freyer's operation. Suprapubic transvesical type of prostatectomy (q.v.). [Peter Johnston Freyer, English surgeon, 1851–1921.]

friable (frī'-abl) [L. *friare,* to break into small pieces]. Easily crumbled; readily pulverized.

Friar's balsam (frī'-ars bawl'-sam). Ancient remedy for bronchitis. Contains benzoin, storax, aloes and balsam of Tolu, dissolved in alcohol. It is added to hot water and the vapour is inhaled. Of dubious value.

friction (frik'-shun) [L. *fricere,* to rub]. Rubbing. **friction murmur**, heard through the stethoscope when two rough or dry surfaces rub together, as in pleurisy and pericarditis.

Friedländer's bacillus (*Klebsiella pneumoniae*). A large Gram-negative rod bacterium occasionally found in the upper respiratory tract, of which it can cause inflammation. Pneumonia so caused (less than 1 per cent of all cases) is severe, with tissue necrosis and abscess formation. [Carl Friedländer, German pathologist, 1847–87.]

Friedreich's ataxia. A progressive familial disease of childhood, in which there develops a sclerosis of the sensory and motor columns in the spinal cord, with consequent muscular weakness and staggering (ataxia). [Nikolaus Friedreich, German neurologist, 1825–82.]

frigidity (frij-id'-it-i) [L. *frigus,* cold]. Lack of normal sexual desire. Used mainly in relation to the female.

frog plaster. Conservative treatment of a congenital dislocation of the hip, whereby the dislocation is reduced by gentle manipulation and both hips are immobilized in plaster of Paris, both limbs abducted to 80 degrees.

Fröhlich's syndrome or **dystrophia adiposogenitalis.** Uncommon but recognized syndrome resulting from anterior pituitary insufficiency secondary to hypothalamic neoplasm. Characterized by obesity, stunted growth, arrested sexual development and knock-knees. [Alfred Fröhlich, Vienna neurologist, 1871–1953.]

frontal (fron'-tal) [L. *frons,* forehead]. Pertaining to the front of a structure; the bone of the forehead. **frontal sinus,** a cavity at the inner aspect of each orbital ridge on the frontal bone.

frost-bite (frost'-bīt). Freezing of the skin and superficial tissues resulting from exposure to extreme cold. The lesion is similar to a burn and may become gangrenous.

frozen shoulder. Cause unknown. Initial pain followed by stiffness, lasting several months. As pain subsides, exercises are intensified until full recovery is gained.

fructose (fruk'-tōs) [L. *fructus,* fruit]. A monosaccharide found with glucose in plants. It is the sugar in honey and is a constituent of cane sugar. Syn., laevulose.

frusemide (frū'-sē-mīd). Produces prompt and effective diuresis. Lasts approximately 4 h after oral administration, and 2 h after parenteral administration. Valuable in pulmonary and cerebral oedema, and in congestive heart failure when the response to other diuretics is inadequate. Acts by inhibition of active chloride transport in the thick limb of the loop of Henle. It has been reported to cause a fall in glomerular filtration rate during diuresis. In consequence, handling of drugs which are removed from the body predominantly by glomerular filtration may be altered by coincidental frusemide therapy. Potassium supplements are given routinely in prolonged f. therapy.

FSH. Follicle stimulating hormone. See FOLLICLE

Fucidin (fūs'-i-din). Sodium salt of fusidic acid. A steroid antibiotic with high activity against Staphylococcus. Can be given intravenously, orally or locally.

fugue (fūg) [L. *fuga,* a fleeing from]. An attempt to escape from reality. A period of loss of memory.

fulguration (ful-gūr-ā'-shun) [L. *fulgur,* lightning]. Destruction of tissue by diathermy.

full term. Mature—when pregnancy has lasted 40 weeks.

fulminant (ful'-min-ant); **fulminating** (ful'-min-ā-ting) [L. *fulminare,* to thunder and lighten]. Developing quickly and with an equally rapid termination.

fumigation (fū-mi-gā'-shun) [L. *fumigare,* to smoke]. Disinfection by exposure to the fumes of a vaporized disinfectant.

function (fungk'-shun) [L. *functio,* performance]. The special work performed by an organ or structure in its normal state.

functional (fungk'-shun-al). In general sense, pertaining to function. Disorder of the function but not the structure of an organ. As psychiatric term, of neurotic origin, i.e. psychogenic, without primary organic disease.

fundus (fun'-dus) [L. *bottom*]. The basal portion of a hollow structure; the part which is distal to the opening—fundi, pl.; fundal, adj.

fungicide (fun'-ji-sīd) [L. *fungus,* mushroom; *coedere,* to kill]. An agent which is lethal to fungi—fungicidal, adj.

fungiform (fun'-ji-form) [L. *fungus,* mushroom; *forma,* form]. Resembling a mushroom.

Fungilin (fun'-ji-lin). Amphotericin B (q.v.)

fungistatic (fun-ji-stat'-ik) [L. *fungus,* mushroom; G. *statikos,* causing to stand]. An agent which inhibits the growth of fungi.

Fungizone (fung'-i-zōn). Amphotericin B (q.v.).

fungus (fung'-gus) [L. *mushroom*]. A low form of vegetable life including many microscopic organisms capable of producing superficial and systemic disease in man. **ray f.,** the original term for the Actinomyces genus, descriptive of the radial arrangement of the filaments which make up the 'sulphur granules' or colonies of the organism in pus. See ACTINOMYCOSIS, RINGWORM—fungi, pl.; fungal, adj.

funiculitis (fū-nik-ū-lī'-tis). [L. *funis,* a cord; G. *-itis,* inflammation]. Inflammation of the spermatic cord.

funiculus (fū-nik'-ū-lus) [L.]. A cord-like structure.

funnel chest. A congenital deformity in which the breast-bone is depressed towards the spine. (Pectus excavatum.)

Furacin (fū'-ra-sin). Nitrofurazone (q.v.). Available as dressings or ointment.

Furadantin (fū-ra-dan'-tin). Nitrofurantoin (q.v.).

Furamide (fū'-ra-mīd). Diloxanide furoate (q.v.).

furazolidone (fū-ra-zol'-i-dōn). Used for non-specific diarrhoeas, bacillary dysentery and bacterial food poisoning.

furor (fūr-or') [L.]. Fury, madness, rage.

Furoxone (fū-roks'-ōn). Furazolidone (q.v.).

furuncle (fūr'-ung-kl) [L. *furunculus*, boil]. See BOIL.

furunculosis (fūr-ung-kū-lō'-sis) [L. *furunculus*, boil; G. *-osis*, condition]. A condition of affliction due to boils.

furunculus orientalis (fūr-un'-kū-lus o-ri-en-ta'-lis). Oriental sore (q.v.).

fusiform (fū'-zi-form) [L. *fusus*, a spindle; *forma*, shape]. Resembling a spindle.

G

gag. An instrument placed between the teeth to keep the mouth open.

gait (gāt). A manner or style of walking. **ataxic g.**, an incoordinate or abnormal gait. **cerebellar g.**, reeling, staggering, lurching. **scissors g.**, one in which the legs cross each other in progression. **spastic g.**, stiff, shuffling, the legs being held together. **tabetic g.**, the foot is raised high then brought down suddenly, the whole foot striking the ground. See FESTINATION.

galactagogue (ga-lak'-ta-gog) [G. *gala*, milk; *agrogos*, leading]. An agent inducing or increasing the flow of milk.

galactin (ga-lak'-tin) [G. *gala*, milk]. Syn., prolactin (q.v.).

galactocele (ga-lak'-tō-sēl) [G. *gala*, milk; *kele*, tumour]. A cyst containing milk, or fluid resembling milk.

galactorrhoea (gal-ak-tor-rē'-á)[G. *gala*, milk; *rheein*, to flow.] Excessive flow of milk. Usually reserved for abnormal or inappropriate secretion of milk.

galactosaemia (gal-ak-tos-ēm'-i-á) [G. *gala*, milk; *haima*, blood]. Excess of galactose in the blood. Normally lactase in the small intestine converts lactose into glucose and galactose. In the liver another enzyme system converts galactose into glucose. Galactosaemia is the result of congenital deficiency of this system and is one cause of mental subnormality—galactosaemic, adj.

galactose (gal-ak'-tōs) [G. *gala*, milk]. A monosaccharide found with glucose in lactose or milk sugar.

gall. See BILE. **gall-bladder** a pear-shaped bag on the undersurface of the liver. It concentrates and stores the bile. **gall-stones**, concretions formed within the g.-bladder; they are often multiple and faceted.

gallamine (gal'-a-min). A muscle relaxant resembling tubocurarine, but with a shorter action. Widely used in surgery, as it is well tolerated and side effects are few. The action can be neutralized if required by neostigmine.

Gallie's operation (gal'-ēs). The use of fascial strips from the thigh for radical cure after reduction of a hernia. [William Edward Gallie, surgeon of Toronto, Canada, 1882–1959.]

gallipot (gal'-i-pot). A small vessel for lotions.

galls (gawls'). The excrescences which form on certain oak trees, and from which tannic acid (q.v.) is obtained. Ung. Gallae c Opio is an astringent ointment used mainly for haemorrhoids.

galvanocauterization (gal-van'-ō-kaw-tér-ī-zā'-shun). The use of a wire heated by galvanic current to destroy tissue.

galvanometer (gal-van-om'-et-ér). An instrument for measuring an electrical current.

gamete (ga'-mēt) [G. *gamein*, to marry]. A male or female reproductive cell. See OVA, SPERMATAZOON.

gamgee (gam'-jē). A brand of absorbent, white cotton wool enclosed in a fine gauze mesh.

gamma-benzene hexachloride (gam'-ma-ben'-zēn heks-a-klor'-īd). Used as shampoo for treatment of head lice. Less irritant than benzyl benzoate for scabies; requires only one application.

gamma-encephalography (gam-ma-en-kef-al-og'-ra-fi) [*gamma*, G. third letter of alphabet; *egkephalos*, brain]. A small dose of isotope is given. It is concentrated in many cerebral tumours. The pattern of radioactivity is then measured.

gammaglobulin (gam-ma-glob'-ū-lin). One of the several protein globulins (A, D, E, G and M). Often referred to as immunoglobulins, abbreviated to IgA, etc. They take part in various immune responses of the body to antigens, which can be bacteria, when we speak of immunity; a foreign substance, when we speak of allergy; a substance produced by the body, when we speak of autoimmunity. When the substance produced by the body is in response to transposed tissue, e.g. organ transplant, we speak of rejection. **anti-D g.** (anti-Rh₀) clears injected Rh-positive cells from the recipient's circulation. Used to prevent formation of antibodies in an Rh-negative mother delivered of an Rh-positive baby.

Gammexane (gam'-eks-ān). A powerful insecticide similar to DDT but not so toxic.

ganglion (gang'-li-on) [G. a swelling]. 1. A mass of nerve tissue forming a subsidiary nerve centre which receives and sends out nerve fibres, e.g. the ganglionic masses forming the sympathetic nervous system. 2. Localized cyst-like swelling near a tendon, sheath or joint. Contains a clear, transparent, gelatinous or colloid substance, sometimes occurs on the back of the wrist due to strain such as excessive practice on the piano. 3. An enlargement on the course of a nerve such as is found on the receptor nerves before they enter the spinal cord. 4. An enlarged lymphatic gland. **Gasserian g.**, deeply situated within the skull, on the sensory root of the fifth cranial nerve. It is involved in trigeminal neuralgia—ganglia, pl.; ganglionic, adj. [Johann Leurentius Gasser, Professor of Anatomy in Vienna, 1723–63.]

ganglionectomy (gang-li-on-ek'-tom-i) [G. *ganglion*, swelling; *ektome*, a cutting]. Surgical excision of a ganglion.

gangliosidosis (gang-li-ō-sid-ō'-sis). See TAY-SACHS' DISEASE.

gangrene (gang-grēn) [G. *gag-graina*]. Death of part of the tissues of the body. Usually the result of inadequate blood supply, but occasionally due to direct injury (traumatic g.) or infection (e.g. gas g.). Deficient blood supply may result from pressure on blood vessels (e.g. tourniquets, tight bandages and swelling of a limb), from obstruction within healthy vessels (e.g. arterial embolism; frost-bite, where the capillaries become blocked), from spasm of the vessel wall (e.g. ergot poisoning), or from thrombosis due to disease of the vessel wall (e.g. arteriosclerosis in arteries; phlebitis in veins). **dry g.** occurs when the drainage of blood from the affected part is adequate; the tissues become shrunken and black. **moist g.** occurs when venous drainage is inadequate so that the tissues are swollen with fluid—gangrenous, adj.

Ganser state (gan'-ser). A hysterical condition—simulating dementia, approximate answers to questions are given which show that the correct answers are known.

Gantrisin (gan'-tri-sin). Sulphafurazole (q.v.).

Gardenal (gar'-den-ăl). Phenobarbitone (q.v.).

gargle (gár'-gl). The act of washing the throat. A solution used for washing the throat.

gargoylism (gar'-goul-izm) [L. *gurgulio*, gullet]. Congenital mucopolysaccharide disorder of metabolism with recessive or sex-linked inheritance. The polysaccharides chondroitin sulphate 'B' and heparitin sulphate are excreted in the urine. Characterized by skeletal abnormalities, coarse features, enlarged liver and spleen, mental subnormality. ACTH useful. Hunter-Hurler syndrome.

Garoin. Phenytoin sodium and phenobarbitone sodium. For grand-mal epilepsy, psychomotor seizures.

Gärtner's bacillus (*Salmonella enteritidis*). A motile Gram-negative rod bacterium, widely distributed in domestic and wild animals, particularly rodents, and sporadic in man as a cause of food poisoning. [August Gärtner, German bacteriologist, 1848–1934.]

gas. One of the three states of matter. It retains neither shape nor volume when released. **gas and air analgesia,** an authorized inhalation to lessen the pain of uterine contraction in labour. **laughing g.,** nitrous oxide (q.v.). **marsh g.,** methane, liberated in the activated sludge method of sewage disposal and converted into electricity—gaseous, adj.

gas gangrene. A wound is infected by anaerobic organisms, especially *Clostridium welchii,* normally found in the intestine of man and animals, consequently there are many sources from which infection can arise, including operation on the intestine. See GANGRENE.

gasserectomy (gas-er-ek'-to-mi). Surgical excision of the Gasserian ganglion (q.v.).

gastralgia (gas-tral'-ji-ă) [G. *gaster*, belly; *algos*, pain]. Pain in the stomach.

gastrectomy (gas-trek'-to-mi) [G. *gaster*,

belly; *ektome,* excision]. Removal of a part or the whole of the stomach. **billroth I** is a partial g., least commonly performed and usually reserved for ulcer on the lesser curvature. **polya partial g.** (known in America as **billroth II**) is the most commonly performed g. Used for duodenal ulcer and as a palliative procedure for gastric cancer. Transverse colon and its mesentery intervene between stomach and jejunum. A hole can be made in the mesentery so that the anastomosis lies behind the transverse colon, **retrocolic g.**; or the loop of jejunum can be lifted up anterior to the transverse colon, **antecolic g. total g.** is carried out only for cancer of the stomach. See ROUX-EN-Y OPERATION.

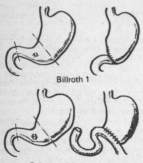

Billroth 1

Polya partial gastrectomy

Types of gastrectomy

gastric (gas'-trik) [G. *gaster,* belly]. Pertaining to the stomach. **gastric crisis,** see CRISIS. **gastric juice** is acid in reaction and contains two proteolytic enzymes. **gastric influenza,** a term used when gastrointestinal symptoms predominate. **gastric suction,** may be intermittent or continuous to keep the stomach empty after some abdominal operations. **gastric ulcer,** see ULCER.

gastrin (gas'-trin) [G. *gaster,* belly]. A hormone secreted by the gastric mucosa on entry of food, which causes a further flow of gastric juice.

gastritis (gas-trī'-tis) [G. *gaster,* belly; *-itis,* inflammation]. Inflammation of the stomach, especially the mucous membrane lining.

gastrocnemius (gas-trok-nē'-mi-us) [G. *gaster,* belly; *kneme,* tibia]. The large two-headed muscle of the calf.

gastrocolic (gas-trō-kol'-ik) [G. *gaster,* belly; *kolon,* colon]. Pertaining to the stomach and the colon. **gastrocolic reflex,** sensory stimulus arising on entry of food into stomach, resulting in strong peristaltic waves in the colon.

gastroduodenal (gas-trō-dū-ō-dēn'-ál) [G. *gaster,* belly; L. *duodeni,* twelve at once]. Pertaining to the stomach and duodenum.

gastroduodenostomy (gas-trō-dū-ō-dēn-os'-to-mi) [G. *gaster,* belly; L. *duodeni,* twelve at once; G. *stoma,* mouth]. A surgical anastomosis between the stomach and the duodenum.

gastrodynia (gas-trō-din'-i-á) [G. *gaster,* belly; *odyne,* pain]. Pain in the stomach.

gastroenteritis (gas-trō-en-tėr-ī'-tis) [G. *gaster,* belly; *enteron,* intestine; *-itis,* inflammation]. Inflammation of mucous membranes of stomach and small intestine: although sometimes the result of dietetic error, the cause is usually a bacterial infection.

gastroenterology (gas-trō-en-ter-ol'-o-ji) [G. *gaster,* belly; *enteron,* intestine; *logos,* discourse]. Study of the stomach and intestines and their diseases—gastroenterological, adj.; gastroenterologically, adv.

gastroenteropathy (gas-trō-en-te-rop'-a-thi) [G. *gaster,* belly; *enteron,* intestine; *pathos,* disease]. Disease of the stomach and intestine—gastroenteropathic, adj.

gastroenteroscope (gas-trō-en'-ter-ō-skōp) [G. *gaster,* belly; *enteron,* intestine; *skopein,* to examine]. An endoscope (q.v.) for visualization of stomach and intestine—gastroenteroscopic, adj.; gastroenteroscopically, adv.

gastroenterostomy (gas-trō-en-tėr-os'-to-mi) [G. *gaster,* belly; *enteron,* intestine; *stoma,* mouth]. A surgical anastomosis between the stomach and small intestine.

gastrografin (gas-trō-grā'-fin). Sodium and meglumine diatrizoates Can be used early in patients with haematemesis. Its detergent and purgative effects are used in meconium ileus, when it is given as an enema.

gastrointestinal (gas-trō-in-tes-tin'-al) [G. *gaster,* belly; L. *intestinum,* intestine]. Pertaining to the stomach and intestine.

gastrojejunostomy (gas-trō-je-joon-os'-to-mi) [G. *gaster,* belly; L. *jejunus,* empty; *stoma,* mouth]. A surgical anastomosis between the stomach and the jejunum.

gastro-oesophageal (gas-trō-ē-sof'-a-jēl) [G. *gaster*, belly; *oisophagos*, gullet]. Pertaining to the stomach and oesophagus as g. reflux in heartburn.

gastropathy (gas-trop'-ath-i) [G. *gaster*, belly; *pathos*, disease]. Any disease of the stomach.

gastropexy (gas-trō-peks'-i) [G. *gaster*, belly; *pexein*, to clip, fix]. Surgical fixation of a displaced stomach.

gastrophrenic (gas-trō-fren'-ik) [G. *gaster*, belly; *phren*, midriff]. Pertaining to the stomach and diaphragm.

gastroplasty (gas'-trō-plas-ti) [G. *gaster*, belly; *plassein*, to form]. Any plastic operation on the stomach. Currently used for reconstruction of the cardiac orifice of the stomach, where fibrosis prevents replacement below the diaphragm in cases of hiatus hernia.

gastroplication (gas-trō-plik-ā'-shun) [G. *gaster*, belly; L. *plicare*, to fold]. An operation for the cure of dilated stomach by pleating the wall.

gastroptosis (gas-trop-tō'-sis) [G. *gaster*, belly; *ptosis*, a falling]. Downward displacement of the stomach.

gastropylorectomy (gas-trō-pī-lor-ek'-tō-mi) [G. *gaster*, belly; *pylouros*, gatekeeper; *ektome*, excision]. Excision of the pyloric end of the stomach.

gastroscope (gas'-trō-skōp) [G. *gaster*, belly; *skopein*, to examine]. See ENDOSCOPE—gastroscopic, adj.; gastroscopy, n.

gastrostomy (gas-tros'-to-mi) [G. *gaster*, belly; *stoma*, mouth]. A surgically established fistula between the stomach and the exterior abdominal wall; usually for artificial feeding.

gastrotomy (gas-trot'-o-mi) [G. *gaster*, belly; *tome*, a cutting]. Incision into the stomach.

gastrula (gas'-troo-lá). Next stage after blastula in embryonic development.

Gaucher's disease (gō'-shā). A rare familial disorder mainly in Jewish children, characterized by a disordered lipoid metabolism (lipid reticulosis) and usually accompanied by very marked enlargement of the spleen. Diagnosis follows sternal marrow puncture and the finding of typical Gaucher cells (distended with lipoid). [Phillippe Charles Ernest Gaucher, French physician, 1854–1918.]

gauze (gawz). A thin open-meshed material used in all surgical procedures.

Gee's linctus (jēz ling'-tus) [L. *linctus*, a licking]. A cough suppressant containing camphorated tincture of opium, squill and syrup of Tolu balsam. [Samuel Gee, British physician, 1839–1911.]

gefarnate (gef'-ar-nāt). Heals gastric ulcer.

Gefarnil (gef'-ar-nil). Gefarnate (q.v.).

Geiger–Müller counter (gī'-gér, mil'-ér kown'-ter). A device for detecting and registering radioactivity.

gelatin(e) (jel'-a-tēn) [L. *gelare*, to freeze]. The protein-containing, glue-like substance obtained by boiling bones, skins and other animal tissues. Used as a base for pessaries; as the adhesive constituent of Unna's paste, and in jellies and pastilles—gelatinous, adj.

gene (jēn) [G. *genesis*, descent]. A factor in the chromosome responsible for transmission of hereditary characteristics. **dominant g.**, capable of transmitting its characteristics, irrespective of the genes from the other parent. **recessive g.**, can transmit characteristics only if they are present in a similar recessive g. from the other parent.

general paralysis of the insane (GPI). Involvement of the brain by syphilitic infection with consequent dementia. The onset may be slow or rapid; loss of memory is an early sign and there is disintegration of the personality. See BACTERIOTHERAPY, MALARIAL THERAPY.

generative (jen'-ér-at-iv) [L. *generare*, to beget]. Pertaining to reproduction.

genetic code (jen-et'-ik kōd). Name given to arrangement of genetic material stored in the DNA molecule of the chromosome.

genetics (jen-et'-iks) [G. *genesis*, descent]. Study of the part played by nuclear and extranuclear cellular structures in human heredity.

genital (jen'-it-al) [G. *genesis*, descent]. Pertaining to the organs of generation.

genitalia (jen-it-ā'-li-á) [G.]. The organs of generation.

genitocrural (jen-it-ō-kroo'-ral) [L. *genitalis*, from *gignere*, to beget; *crus*, leg]. Pertaining to the genital area and the leg.

genitourinary (jen-it-ō-ū'-rin-a-ri) [L. *genitalis*, from *gignere*, to beget; *urina*, urine]. Pertaining to the reproductive and urinary organs.

genome (jen'-ōm) [G. *genos,* birth]. A complete set of chromosomes derived from one parent.

Genophyllin (jen-of'-il-in). Aminophylline (q.v.).

genotype (jen'-o-tīp). The inherent endowment of the individual.

gentamicin (jen-ta-mī'-sin) Antibiotic produced by *Micromonospora purpurea.* Antibacterial, especially against Pseudomonas and staphylococci resistant to other antibiotics. Given intramuscularly and as eye and ear drops. Ototoxic and dangerous in renal failure.

gentian violet (jen'-shun). A brilliant violet-coloured, antiseptic, aniline dye. Syn., crystal violet (q.v.).

Genticin (jen'-tis-in). Gentamicin (q.v.).

genu (jen'-ū) [L.]. The knee. **genu valgum,** knock-knee. **genu varum,** bowleg.

genus (je'-nus) [L. race]. A classification ranking between the family (higher) and the species (lower).

geriatrician (jer-i-at-rish'-n) [G. *geras,* old age]. One who specializes in geriatrics.

geriatrics (jer-i-at'-riks) [G. *geras,* old age; *iatrikos,* healing]. The branch of medical science dealing with old age and its diseases.

germ (jėrm) [L. *germen,* bud]. A unicellular micro-organism, especially used for a pathogen.

German measles. See RUBELLA.

germicide (jėr'-mi-sīd) [L. *germen,* bud; *coedere,* to kill]. An agent which kills germs—germicidal, adj.

gerontology (jer-on-tol'-oj-i) [G. *geron,* old man; *logos,* discourse]. The scientific study of ageing—gerontological, adj.

gestation (jes-tā'-shun) [L. *gestare,* to carry]. Pregnancy—gestational, adj. **ectopic g.,** extrauterine pregnancy, usually in the Fallopian tube.

Gestyl (jes'-til). Serum gonadotrophin.

Ghon focus. Primary lesion of tuberculosis in lung. [Anton Ghon, Austrian pathologist, 1866–1936.].

GH-RIH. Growth-hormone-release-inhibiting hormone. See SOMATOSTATIN.

giant cell arteritis. See ARTERITIS.

giardiasis (ji-ar-di'-a-sis). Infection with the flagellate *Giardia intestinalis.* Often symptomless, especially in adults. Can cause diarrhoea with steatorrhoea, Treatment is mepacrine hydrochloride or metronidazole orally. Syn. lambliasis.

gigantism (jī-gan'-tizm) [G. *gigas,* giant]. An abnormal overgrowth, especially in height. May be associated with anterior pituitary tumour if the tumour develops before fusion of the epiphyses.

Gilliam's operation. A method of correcting retroversion by shortening the round ligaments of the uterus. [David Tod Gilliam, American gynaecologist, 1844–1923]

ginger (jin'-jėr). An aromatic root with carminative properties. Used as syrup or tincture for flavouring purposes.

gingiva (jin-jī'-va) [L.]. The gum; the vascular tissue surrounding the necks of the teeth.

gingivectomy (jin-jiv-ek'-to-mi) [L. *gingiva,* gum; G. *ektome,* excision]. Excision of a portion of the gum, usually for pyorrhoea.

gingivitis (jin-ji-vī'-tis) [L. *gingiva,* gum; G. *-itis,* inflammation]. Inflammation of the gums. **pregnancy g.** occurs due to hormonal changes.

Giovannetti diet. Used for patients with chronic renal failure; protein intake lowered to 20g per day which although less than the recommended intake, can achieve normal balance. This is because the 20g is chosen from proteins containing the essential amino acids, and uraemic patients can synthesize more non-essential amino acids (utilizing ammonia split from urea in the gut) than normal people. Urea production from exogenous protein can be kept at a minimum and a little of the excess urea is used up synthesizing the non-essential amino acids.

girdle (gėr'-dl). A belt. **g. pain,** a constricting pain round the waist region, occurring in tabetic persons. **pelvic g.,** comprises the two innominate bones, sacrum and coccyx. **shoulder g.,** comprises the two clavicles and scapulae.

Girdlestone's operation. Pseudoarthrosis of hip for osteoarthritis. Part of the acetabulum and the femoral head and neck are removed. A muscle mass is stitched between the bone ends. [Gathorne Robert Girdlestone, English surgeon, 1881–1950.]

gland [L. *glans,* an acorn]. An organ or structure capable of making an internal or external secretion. **lymphatic g.** (node) does not secrete, but is concerned with filtration of the lymph. See ENDOCRINE—glandular, adj.

glanders (glan'-derz). A contagious, febrile, ulcerative disease communicable from horses, mules and asses to man.

glandular fever syndrome (gland'-ū-lår fē'-vėr sin'-drōm). A contagious self limiting disease almost certainly due to infection with the Epstein-Barr virus. Most common in children and adolescents. Characterized by fever, sore throat, enlargement of superficial lymph nodes and appearance of atypical lymphocytes in the blood. Agglutination tests, Paul-Bunnell and monospot slide test are useful in diagnosis. Syn., infectious mononucleosis.

glans (glanz) [L.]. The bulbous termination of the clitoris and penis.

Glauber's salts (glaw'-bėrs). Sodium sulphate (q.v.).

glaucoma (glaw-kō'-må) [G. *glaukos*, blue-green]. A condition where the intraocular pressure is raised. In the acute stage the pain is severe—glaucomatous, adj.

glenohumeral (glē-nō-hū'-mėr-ål) [G. *glene*, socket; L. *humerus*]. Pertaining to the glenoid cavity of scapula and the humerus.

glenoid (glē'-noid) [G. *glene*, socket; *eidos*, form]. A cavity on the scapula into which the head of the humerus fits to form the shoulder joint.

glia (glī'-á) [G., glue]. Neuroglia (q.v.)—glial, adj.

glibenclamide (glī-ben'-klá-mīd). Potent oral hypoglycaemic agent.

glioblastoma multiforme (glī-ō-blas-tō'-ma mul-ti-form) [G. *glia*, glue; *blastos*, germ; *-oma*, tumour; L. *multus*, many; *forma*, form]. A highly malignant brain tumour.

glioma (glī-ō'-má) [G. *glia*, glue; *-oma*, tumour]. A malignant growth which does not give rise to secondary deposits. It arises from neuroglia. One form occurring in the retina is hereditary—gliomata, pl.

gliomyoma (glī-ō-mī-ō'-má) [G. *glia*, glue; *mys*, muscle; *-oma*, tumour]. A tumour of nerve and muscle tissue—gliomyomata, pl.

globin (glō'-bin) [L. *globus*, ball]. A protein which combines with haematin to form haemoglobin.

globulin (glob'-ū-lin) [L. *globulus*, little ball]. A fraction of serum or plasma protein from which antibody is formed. There are several varieties designated by the letters A, D, E, G and M. See GAMMAGLOBULIN.

globulinuria (glob-ūl-in-ū'-ri-á) [L. *globulus*, little ball; G. *ouron*, urine]. The presence of globulin in the urine.

globus hystericus (glō'-bus his-ter'-ik-us). Subjective feeling of neurotic origin of a lump in the throat. Can also include difficulty in swallowing and is due to tension of muscles of deglutition. Occurs in hysteria, anxiety states and depression. Sometimes follows slight trauma to throat, e.g. scratch by foreign body.

glomerulitis (glom-ėr-ū-lī'-tis) [L. *glomus*, ball; G. *-itis*, inflammation]. Acute suppurative inflammation of the glomeruli of the kidney.

glomerulonephritis (glom-ėr-ū-lō-nef-rī'-tis) [L. *glomus*, ball; G. *nephros*, kidney; *-itis*, inflammation]. A term used in bilateral, non-suppurative inflammation of the glomeruli of the kidneys. Preceded by streptococcal infection of the skin and throat in the majority of cases.

glomerulosclerosis (glom-ėr-ū-lō-skler-ō'-sis). Fibrosis of the glomeruli of the kidney, the result of inflammation. **intercapillary g.** is a common pathological finding in diabetics. See NEPHROTIC SYNDROME—glomerulosclerotic, adj.

glomerulus (glom-ėr'-ū-lus). A coil of minute arterial capillaries held together by scanty connective tissue. It invaginates the entrance of the uriniferous tubules in the kidney cortex—glomerular, adj., glomeruli, pl.

glossa (glos'-a) [G.]. The tongue—glossal, adj.

glossectomy (glos-ek'-to-mi) [G. *glossa*, tongue; *ektome*, excision]. Excision of the tongue.

glossitis (glos'-ī-tis) [G. *glossa*, tongue; *-itis*, inflammation]. Inflammation of the tongue.

glossodynia (glos-ō-din'-i-á) [G. *glossa*, tongue; *odyne*, pain]. Name used for painful tongue when there is no visible change.

glossopharyngeal (glos-ō-far-in'-ji-al) [G. *glossa*, tongue; *pharynx*, throat]. Pertaining to the tongue and pharynx. The ninth pair of cranial nerves.

glossoplegia (glos-ō-plē'-ji-ă) [G. *glossa,* tongue; *plege,* stroke]. Paralysis of the tongue.

glottis (glot'-is) [G.]. That part of the larynx associated with voice production. **rimaglottidis,** the opening between the free margins of the vocal cords—glottic, adj.

glucagon (gloo'-ka-gon). Hormone produced in alpha cells of pancreatic islets of Langerhans. Causes breakdown of glycogen into glucose thus preventing blood sugar from falling too low during fasting. Can now be obtained commercially from the pancreas of animals. Given to accelerate breakdown of glycogen in the liver and raise blood sugar rapidly. As it is a polypeptide hormone, it must be given by injection.

glucocorticoid (gloo-kō-kor'-ti-koid). Any steroid hormone which promotes gluconeogenesis (i.e. the formation of glucose and glycogen from protein) and which antagonizes the action of insulin. Occurring naturally in the adrenal cortex as cortisone and hydrocortisone, and produced synthetically as, for example, prednisone and prednisolone.

glucogenesis (gloo-kō-jen'-e-sis). Production of glucose.

gluconeogenesis (gloo-kō-nē-ō-jen'-e-sis). The formation of sugar from protein or fat when there is lack of available carbohydrate.

Glucophage (gloo'-kō-fāg). Metformin (q.v.).

glucose (gloo'-kōs). Dextrose or grape sugar. A monosaccharide. The form in which carbohydrates are absorbed through the intestinal tract and circulated in the blood. It is stored as glycogen in the liver.

glucoronic acid (gloo-kūr-on'-k). An acid which acts on bilirubin to form conjugated bilirubin.

glutaminase (gloo-tam'-in-āz). An amino acid-degrading enzyme, being used in the treatment of cancer.

gluteal (gloo'-tē-al) [G. *gloutos,* buttock]. Pertaining to the buttocks.

gluten (gloo'-ten) [L.]. A protein constituent of wheat flour. Insoluble in water but an essential component of the elastic 'dough.' It is not tolerated in coeliac disease (q.v.).

glutethimide (gloo-teth'-i-mīd). Hypnotic of medium action. Useful when an alternative to the barbiturates is required.

glycerin(e) (glis'-e-rin). A clear, syrupy liquid prepared synthetically or obtained as a by-product in soap manufacture. It has a hygroscopic action. **glycerine and borax,** useful for softening sordes (q.v.). **glycerine and honey,** useful as a softening agent for oral toilet. **glycerine and ichthyol,** used to relieve inflammation. **glycerine and magnesium sulphate,** useful for boils, etc.

glycerophosphates (glis-er-ō-fos'-fātz). Appetite stimulant.

glyceryl trinitrate (glis'-er-il trī-nīt'-rāt). Vasodilator used in angina pectoris. Given mainly as tablets which should be chewed, or dissolved under the tongue.

glycine (glī'-sēn). A non-essential amino acid (q.v.).

glycinuria (glī-sin-ū'-ri-ă). Excretion of glycine in the urine. Associated with mental subnormality.

glycogen (glī'-kō-jen) [G. *glykys,* sweet]. Animal starch, the form to which glucose is linked in branched chains for storage in the body. **glycogen storage disease,** inborn error of carbohydrate metabolism. Associated with mental subnormality.

glycogenase (glī-kō-jen-āz) [G. *glykys,* sweet; *genesis,* descent]. An enzyme necessary for the conversion of glycogen into glucose.

glycogenesis (glī-kō-jen'-e-sis). Glycogen formation from blood glucose.

glycogenosis (glī-kō-jen-ō'sis) [G. *glykys,* sweet; *genesis,* descent; *-osis,* condition]. Metabolic disorder leading to increased storage of glycogen. Leads to glycogen myopathy.

glycolysis (glī-kol'-i-sis) [G. *glykys,* sweet; *lysis,* a loosening]. The hydrolysis of sugar in the body—glycolytic, adj.

glyconeogenesis (glī-kō-nē-ō-jen'-e-sis) [G. *glykys,* sweet; *neos,* new; *genesis,* descent]. Gluconeogenesis (q.v.).

glycosides (glī'-kō-sīdz). Natural substances composed of a sugar with another compound. The non-sugar fragment is termed an 'aglycone,' and is sometimes of therapeutic value. Digoxin is a familiar example of a glycoside.

glycosuria (glī-kō-sū'-ri-ă) [G. *glykys,* sweet; *ouron,* urine]. The presence of sugar in the urine.

glycyrrhiza (glis-i-rī'-za) [G. *glykys,* sweet; *rhiza,* root]. Liquorice root, demulcent, slightly laxative, expectorant and used as a flavouring agent. Results in an increase in extracellular fluid, retention of sodium and increased excretion of potassium.

glymidine (glī'-mi-dēn). Oral antidiabetic agent.

gnathalgia (nath-al'-ji-á) [G. *gnathos,* jaw; *algos,* pain]. Pain in the jaw.

gnathoplasty (nath'-ō-plas-ti) [G. *gnathos,* jaw; *plassein,* to form]. Plastic surgery of the jaw.

goblet cells. Special secreting cells, shaped like a goblet, found in the mucous membranes.

Goeckerman régime (gā'-kėr-man). A method of treatment for psoriasis; exposure to ultraviolet light alternating with the application of a tar paste.

goitre (goi'-ter) [L. *guttur,* throat]. An enlargement of the thyroid gland. **simple g.,** in which the patient does not show any signs of excessive thyroid activity. **toxic g.,** in which the enlarged gland secretes an excess of thyroid hormone. The patient is nervous, loses weight and often has palpitations and exophthalmos. See COLLOID.

goitrogens (goi'-tro-jens) [L. *guttur,* throat; G. *genesis,* descent]. Agents causing goitre. Some occur in plants, e.g. turnip, cabbage, brussels sprouts and peanuts. Drugs, e.g. propylthiouracil, carbimazole, potasium perchlorate and thiocyanate, iodide.

golden eye ointment. Ung. hyd. ox. flav. Yellow oxide of mercury ointment.

gold injections. See AUROTHIOMALATE.

Goldthwait belt. Wide belt with steel support for back injuries.

Goldthwait strap. Strap to support foot injuries. [Joel Goldthwait, American orthopaedic surgeon, 1866–1961.].

gonad (gon'-ad) [G. *gone,* generation]. A male or female sex gland. See OVARY, TESTIS—gonadal, adj.

gonadotrophic (gon-ad-ō-trō'-fik) [G. *gone,* generation; *atrophe,* nourishment]. Having an affinity for, or influence on the gonads.

gonadotrophin (gon-a-dō-trō'-fin) [G. *gone,* generation; *trophe,* nourishment]. Any gonad-stimulating hormone. See FOLLICLE STIMULATING HORMONE.

Gonadyl seric. Serum gonadotrophin for oral administration for acne. An

extended course of treatment is essential.

Gonan. Serum gonadotrophin.

Gondafon (gon'-da-fon). Glymidine (q.v.).

gonioscopy (gon-i-os'-kop-i) [G. *gonia,* angle; *skopein,* to examine]. Measuring angle of anterior chamber of eye with a gonioscope.

goniotomy (gon-i-ot'-o-mi) [G. *gonia,* angle; *tome,* a cutting]. Operation for glaucoma. Incision through the anterior chamber angle to the canal of Schlemm.

Gonococcus (gon-ō-kok'us) (*Neisseria gonorrhoeae*). A Gram-negative diplococcus, the causative organism of gonorrhoea. It is a strict parasite. Occurs characteristically inside polymorph leucocytes in the tissues—gonococci, pl.; gonococcal, adj.

gonorrhoea (gon-or-rē'-á)[G. *gone,* generation; *rheein,* to flow]. An infectious disease of venereal origin in adults. In children infection is accidental, e.g. gonococcal ophthalmia of the newborn, gonococcal vulvovaginitis of girls before puberty. Chief manifestations of the disease in the male are a purulent urethritis with dysuria. In the female, urethritis and endocervicitis which may be symptomless. Incubation period is usually 2 to 5 days—gonorrhoeal, adj.

gonorrhoeal (gon-or-rē'-ál). Resulting from gonorrhoea. **gonorrhoeal arthritis** is a metastatic manifestation of gonorrhoea. **gonorrhoeal ophthalmia** is one form of ophthalmia neonatorum.

Goodpasture's syndrome. Association of haemorrhagic lung disorder with glomerulonephritis. [Ernest W. Goodpasture. American pathologist, 1886–1960.]

Gordh needle (gort'). An intravenous needle with a rubber diaphragm. Through it repeated injections can be given.

gouge (gowj). A chisel with a grooved blade for removing bone.

gout (gowt) [L. *gutta,* drop). A form of metabolic disorder in which sodium biurate is deposited in the cartilages of the joints, the ears, and elsewhere. The big toe is characteristically involved and becomes acutely painful and swollen. See TOPHUS, PURINS, URIC ACID.

GPI. General paralysis of the insane (q.v.).

Graafian follicle. See FOLLICLE.

Graefe's knife (grā'-fes). Finely pointed knife with narrow blade, used for making incisions across anterior chamber of eye prior to removal of cataract. [Albrecht von Graefe, German ophthalmologist, 1828–70.]

graft [G. *graphein*, to write]. A tissue or organ which is transplanted to another part of the same animal (autograft), to another animal of the same species (homograft), or to another animal of a different species (heterograft). Only autografts and homografts are used in man.

gramicidin (gram-is-ī'-din). A mixture of antibiotic substances obtained from tyrothricin. Too toxic for systemic use, but valuable for topical application when local antibiotic therapy is required.

Gram's stain. A bacteriological stain for differentiation of germs. Those retaining the stain are Gram-positive (+), those unaffected by it are Gram negative (−). [Hans Christian Joachim Gram, Danish physician, 1853–1938.]

grand mal (grong mal). Major epilepsy. See EPILEPSY.

granulation (gran-ū-lā'-shun) [L. *granulum*, small grain]. The outgrowth of new capillaries and connective tissue cells from the surface of an open wound. **g. tissue,** the young, soft tissue so formed—granulate, v.t., v.i.

granulocyte (gran'-ū-lō-sīt) [L. *granulum*, small grain; G. *kytos*, cell]. A cell containing granules in its cytoplasm. Used as syn. for polymorphonuclear leucocytes which have neutrophil, eosinophil or basophil granules.

granulocytopenia (gran-ū-lō-sīt-ō-pē'-ni-à). [L. *granulum*, small grain; G. *kytos*, cell; *penia*, want]. Decrease of granulocytes (polymorphs) not sufficient to warrant the term agranulocytosis (q.v.).

granuloma (gran-ū-lō'-má) [L. *granulum*, small grain; G. *-oma*, tumour]. A tumour formed of granulation tissue. **g. venereum,** see LYMPHOGRANULOMA—granulomata, pl.; granulomatous, adj.

gravel (grav'l). A sandy deposit which, if present in the bladder, may be passed with the urine.

Graves' disease. Thyrotoxicosis (q.v.). [Robert James Graves, Irish physician, 1797–1853.]

gravid (grav'-id) [L. *gravis*, heavy or pregnant]. Pregnant.

gravitational (gra-vi-tā'-shun-ál). Being attracted by force of gravity. **g. ulcer,** varicose ulcer (q.v.).

gravity (gra'-vi-ti) [L. *gravis*, heavy]. Weight. **specific g.,** the weight of a substance compared with that of an equal volume of water.

Grawitz tumour. Hypernephroma (q.v.). [Paul Albert Grawitz, German pathologist, 1850–1932.]

green monkey disease. See MARBURG DISEASE.

gregarious (gre-gār'-i-us) [L. *grex*, a herd]. Showing a preference for living in a group, liking to mix. The g. or herd instinct is an inborn tendency on the part of various species including man.

Griffith's types. Antigenic subdivisions of Lancefield group A streptococci by virtue of their characteristic M protein antigens.

grinders (grīn'-dérz). The molars or double teeth.

grinder's asthma. One of the many popular names for silicosis arising from inhalation of metallic dust.

gripe (grīp). Colic.

Griseofulvin (grī-sē-ō-ful'-vin). An oral fungicide, useful in ringworm.

grocer's itch. Contact dermatitis, especially from flour or sugar.

groin. The junction of the thigh with the abdomen.

group psychotherapy. See PSYCHOTHERAPY.

growing pains. Pain in the limbs during youth; differential diagnosis rheumatic fever.

guanethidine (gwan-eth'-i-dēn). A hypotensive, sympathetic blocking agent. Gives sustained reduction of intraocular pressure in glaucoma. Applied locally to block the sympathetic fibres to the eye in exophthalmos. Absorbed more regularly and permits a smoother control of hypertension than mecamylamine.

Guanimycin (gwan-i-mī'-sin). Streptomycin, sulphaguanidine and kaolin. Antidiarrhoeal.

guanoclor (gwan'-ō-klor). Antihypertensive.

guanoxan sulphate (gwan-oks'-an-sul'-fāt). Antihypertensive.

guillotine (gil'-o-tēn). A surgical instrument for excision of the tonsils.

guinea worm (gin'-i). *Dracunculus medinensis* (q.v.).

gullet (gul'-et). The oesophagus.

gumma (gum'-á). A localized area of vascular granulation tissue which develops in the later stages (tertiary) of syphilis. Obstruction to the blood supply results in necrosis, and gummata near a surface of the body tend to break down, forming chronic ulcers, e.g. on the nose, the lower leg, the palate, etc. Probably these ulcers are not infectious.

gut. The intestines.

gynaecography (gī-ne-kog'-ra-fī) [G. *gyne*, woman; *graphein*, to write]. Radiological visualization of internal female genitalia after pneumoperitoneum—gynaecographical, adj.; gynaecographically, adv.

gynaecologist (gī-ne-kol'-oj-ist). A surgeon who specializes in gynaecology.

gynaecology (gī-ne-kol'-o-ji) [G. *syne*, woman; *logos*, discourse]. The science dealing with the diseases which are peculiar to women.

gynaecomastia (gī-ne-ko-mas'-ti-á) [G. *gyne*, woman; *mastos*, breast]. Enlargement of the male mammary gland.

Gypsona (jip-sō'-ná). Ready-made quick setting plaster of Paris bandage made by impregnating fine plaster of Paris into specially woven (interlock) cotton cloth. For immobilization in fracture treatment and orthopaedic conditions generally.

gypsum (jip'-sum). Plaster of Paris (calcium sulphate).

gyrectomy (jī-rek'-to-mi) [G. *gyros*, circle; *ektome*, excision]. Surgical removal of a gyrus, a convoluted portion of cerebral cortex.

H

habit (ha'-bit) [L. *habitus*, state]. A constant automatic response in a given situation acquired by frequent repetition. When applied to thoughts, thinking habits become attitudes. **habit training**, used in mental hospitals for deteriorated patients who relearn personal hygiene by constant repetition with encouragement.

habituation (ha-bit-ū-ā'-shun). See DRUG DEPENDENCE.

haem (hēm). The pigment-carrying portion of haemoglobin.

haemangioma (hēm-an-ji-ō'-má) [G. *haima*, blood; *aggeion*, vessel; *-oma*, tumour]. A malformation of blood vessels which may occur in any part of the body. When in the skin it is one form of birthmark, appearing as a red spot or a 'port wine stain'—haemangiomata, pl.

haemarthrosis (hē-már-thrō'-sis) [G. *haima*, blood; *arthron*, joint; *-osis*, condition]. The presence of blood in a joint cavity. The irritant effect of haemoglobin and the chondrolytic effect of plasmin destroy the joint—haemarthroses, pl.

haematemesis (hē-ma-tem'-e-sis) [G. *haima*, blood; *emesis*, vomiting]. The vomiting of blood.

haematin (hē'-ma-tin) [G. *haima*, blood]. An iron-containing constituent of haemoglobin It may crystallize in the kidney tubules when there is excessive haemolysis.

haematinic (hē-ma-tin'-ik) [G. *haima*, blood]. Any substance which is required for the production of the red blood cell and its constituents.

haematite—miner's lung (hē'-ma-tīt, mī'-nêrs). A form of silicosis (q.v.) occurring in the haematite (iron ore) industry.

haematocele (hē-mat'-ō-sēl) [G. *haima*, blood; *kele*, tumour]. A swelling filled with blood.

haematocolpos (hē-mat-o-kol'-pos) [G. *haima*, blood; *kolpos*, vagina]. See CRYPTOMENORRHOEA.

haematogenous (hē-mat-oj'-en-us) [G. *haima*, blood; *genesis*, descent]. 1. Concerned with the formation of blood. 2, Carried by the blood stream.

haematology (hē-mat-ol'-o-ji) [G. *haima*, blood; *logos*, discourse]. The science dealing with the formation, composition, functions and diseases of the blood—haematological, adj.; haematologically, adv.

haematoma (hē-ma-tō'-má) [G. *haima*, blood; *-oma*, tumour]. A swelling filled with blood—haematomata, pl.

haematometra (hē-ma-tō-mē'-trá) [G. *haima*, blood; *metra*, womb]. An accumulation of blood (or menstrual fluid) in the uterus.

haematopoiesis (hē-ma-tō-poi-ē'-sis). See HAEMOPOIESIS.

haematosalpinx (hē-ma-tō-sal'-pinks) [G. *haima*, blood; *salpigx*, trumpet]. Blood in the Fallopian tube.

haematozoa (hē-ma-tō-zō'-á) [G. *haima*, blood; *zoion*, living thing] Parasites, living in the blood—haematozoon, sing.

haematuria (hē-ma-tū'-ri-á) [G. *haima*,

blood; *ouron,* urine]. Blood in the urine—haematuric, adj.

haemochromatosis (hē-mō-krō-ma-tō'-sis) [G. *haima,* blood; *chroma,* colour; *-osis,* condition]. A congenital error in iron metabolism with increased iron deposition in tissues, resulting in brown pigmentation of the skin and cirrhosis of the liver. Syn., 'bronzed diabetes.'—haemochromatotic, adj.

haemoconcentration (hē-mō-kon-sen-trā'-shun) [G. *haima,* blood; L. *con,* together; *centrum,* centre]. Relative increase of volume of red blood cells to volume of plasma, usually due to loss of the latter.

haemocytometer (hēm-ō-sī-tom'-et-ẻr) [G. *haima,* blood; *kytos,* cell; *metron,* a measure]. An instrument for measuring the number of blood corpuscles.

haemodialysis (hē-mō-dī-al'-is-is) [G. *haima,* blood; *dialysis,* a separating]. A process of removing waste products from, and replacing essential constituents in blood by a process of dialysis (q.v.). Such a technique is used in the artificial kidney.

haemoglobin (hē-mō-glō'-bin) [G. *haima,* blood; L. *globus,* ball]. The respiratory pigment in the red blood corpuscles. It is composed of an iron-containing substance called 'haem', combined with globin. It has the reversible function of combining with, and releasing oxygen. See OXYHAEMOGLOBIN.

haemoglobinaemia (hē-mō-glō-bin-ē'-mi-à). Haemoglobin in the blood plasma—haemoglobinaemic, adj.

haemoglobinometer (hē-mō-glō-bin-om'-et-ẻr) [G. *haima,* blood; *globus,* ball; *metron,* a measure]. An instrument for estimating the percentage of haemoglobin in the blood.

haemoglobinopathy (hē-mō-glōb-in-op'-ath-i) [G. *haima,* blood; *globus,* ball; *pathos,* disease]. Abnormality of the haemoglobin—haemoglobinopathic, adj.

haemoglobinuria (hē-mō-glob-in-ū'-ri-à) [G. *haima,* blood; *globus,* ball; *ouron,* urine]. Haemoglobin in the urine—haemoglobinuric, adj.

haemolysin (hē-mō-lī'-sin) [G. *haima,* blood; *lysis,* a loosening]. An agent which causes disintegration of erythrocytes. See ANTIBODIES.

haemolysis (hē-mol'-is-is) [G. *haima,* blood; *lysis,* a loosening]. Disintegra-tion of red blood cells, with liberation of contained haemoglobin. Laking. See ANAEMIA, HAEMOGLOBINAEMIA—haemolytic, adj.

haemolytic disease of the newborn. A pathological condition in the newborn child due to rhesus incompatibility between the child's blood and that of the mother. Red blood cell destruction occurs with anaemia, often jaundice and an excess of erythroblasts or primitive red blood cells in the circulating blood. Immunization of women at risk, using gammaglobulin containing a high titre of anti-D can prevent haemolytic disease of the newborn. Exchange transfusion of the infant may be essential.

haemopericardium (hē-mō-per-ri-kàr'-di-um) [G. *haima,* blood; *peri,* around; *kardia,* heart]. Blood in the pericardial sac.

haemoperitoneum (hē-mō-per-it-on-ē'-um) [G. *haima,* blood; *peri,* around; *teinein,* to stretch]. Blood in the peritoneal cavity.

haemophilia (hē-mō-fil'-i-à) [G. *haima,* blood; *philein,* to love.] Deficiency of antihaemophilic globulin (AHG Factor VIII). An inherited bleeding disease found only in males and transmitted through carrier females, who are daughters of affected males. Under special genetic circumstances, females with haemophilia may be produced. Patient is subject to prolonged bleeding following even minor injuries—haemophiliac, adj.

Haemophilus (hē-mof'-il-us) [G. *haima,* blood; *philein,* to love]. A genus of bacteria. Small Gram-negative rods which show much variation in shape (pleomorphism). They are strict parasites, and accessory substances present in blood, are usually necessary for growth. They are found in the respiratory tracts of vertebrates and are often associated with acute and chronic disease, e.g. *Haemophilus influenzae.* See DUCREY'S BACILLUS.

haemophthalmia (hē-mof-thal'-mi-à) [G. *haima,* blood; *ophthalmos,* eye]. Bleeding into the eyeball.

haemopneumothorax (hē-mō-nū-mō-thor'-aks) [G. *haima,* blood; *pneumon,* lung; *thorax,* thorax]. The presence of blood and air in the pleural cavity causing compression of lung tissue.

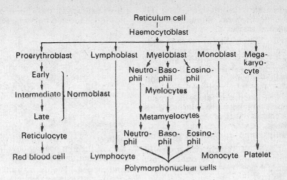

Formation of blood

haemopoiesis (hē-mō-poi-ē'-sis) [G. *haima*, blood; *poiesis*, production]. The formation of blood—haemopoietic, adj.

haemoptysis (he-mop'-tis-is) [G. *haima*, blood; *ptysis*, spitting]. The coughing up of blood—haemoptyses, pl.

haemorrhage (hem'-or-rāj) [G. *haima*, blood; *rhegnynai*, to burst]. The escape of blood from a vessel. Arterial, capillary, venous designates the type of vessel from which it escapes. **primary h.,** that which occurs at the time of injury or operation. **reactionary h.,** that which occurs within 24 hours of injury or operation. **secondary h.,** that which occurs within 7 to 10 days of injury or operation. **accidental antepartum h.,** bleeding from separation of a normally situated placenta, after the 28th week of pregnancy. The term placental abruption now preferred. **antepartum h.,** vaginal bleeding after the 28th week and before labour. **intrapartum h.,** that occurring during labour. **postpartum h.,** excessive bleeding after delivery of child. In Great Britain it must be at least 500 ml to qualify as haemorrhage. **secondary postpartum h.,** excessive uterine bleeding more than 24 hours after delivery—haemorrhagic, adj.

haemorrhagic disease of the newborn. Characterized by gastrointestinal, pulmonary or intracranial haemorrhage occurring from the second to the fifth day of life. Due to a physiological variation in clotting power due to change in prothrombin content which falls on second day, and returns to normal at end of first week when colonization of gut with bacteria results in synthesis of vitamin K, thus permitting formation of prothrombin by the liver. Responds to administration of vitamin K.

haemorrhoidal (hem-or-roid'-ăl) [G. *haima*, blood; *rheein*, to flow]. 1. Pertaining to haemorrhoids. 2. Applied to blood vessels and nerves in the anal region.

haemorrhoidectomy (hem-or-roid-ek'-to-mi) [G. *haima*, blood; *rheein*, to flow; *ektome*, excision]. Surgical removal of haemorrhoids.

haemorrhoids (hem'-or-roidz) [G. *haima*, blood; *rheein*, to flow]. Varicosity of the veins around the anus; piles. **external h.,** those outside the anal sphincter covered with skin. **internal h.,** those inside the anal sphincter covered with mucous membrane.

haemosalpinx (hē-mō-sal'-pinks). See HAEMATOSALPINX.

haemosiderosis (hē-mō-sid-er-ōs'-is) [G. *haima*, blood; *sideros*, iron]. Iron deposits in the tissues.

haemospermia (hē-mō-sper'-mi-a) [G. *haima*, blood; *sperma*, seed]. The discharge of blood-stained semen.

haemostasis (hē-mō-stā'-sis) [G. *haima*, blood; *stasis*, a standing]. 1. Arrest of bleeding. 2. Stagnation of blood within its vessel.

haemostatic (hē-mō-stat'-ik) [G. *haima*, blood; *statikos*, causing to stand]. Any agent which arrests bleeding. **haemostic forceps,** artery forceps.

haemothorax (hē-mō-thor'-aks) [G. *haima*, blood; *thorax*, thorax]. Blood in the pleural cavity.

hair (hār). Thread-like appendage present on all parts of human skin except palms, soles, lips, glans penis and that surrounding the terminal phalanges. **exclamation-mark h.**, the broken-off stump found at the periphery of spreading bald patches in alopecia areata. Atrophic thinning of the hair shaft gives this characteristic shape—hence its name.

Haldol (hal'-dol). Haloperidol (q.v.).

halibut liver oil. A very rich source of vitamins A and D. The smaller dose required makes it more acceptable than cod liver oil.

halitosis (hal-i-tō'-sis) [L. *halitus*, breath; G. *-osis*, condition]. Bad breath.

hallucination (hal-ū-sin-ā'-shun) [L. *alucinari*, to wander in the mind]. A false perception occurring without any true sensory stimulus. A common symptom in severe psychoses (q.v.) including schizophrenia, paraphrenia, confusional states. Also common in delirium, during toxic states and following head injuries.

hallucinogens (hal-ūs-in'-ō-jens). Chemicals, e.g. mescaline, LSD, capable of producing hallucination. Psychotomimetics.

hallucinosis (hal-ū-sin-ō'-sis) [L. *alucinari*, to wander in the mind; G. *-osis*, condition]. A psychosis in which the patient is grossly hallucinated. Usually a subacute delirious state; the predominant symptoms are auditory illusions (q.v.) and hallucinations.

hallux (hal'-uks) [L. *allex*, big toe]. The great toe. **hallux valgus**, bunion (q.v.). **hallux rigidus**, ankylosis of the metatarsophalangeal articulation caused by osteoarthritis.

halogen (hal'-ō-jen) [G. *hals*, salt, sea]. Any one of the non-metallic elements—bromine, chlorine, fluorine, iodine.

haloperidol (hal-ō-per'-i-dol). Tranquillizer. Useful in acute mania. Useful for premedication.

halothane. A clear colourless liquid used as an inhalation anaesthetic. Advantages: non-explosive and non-inflammable in all circumstances. Odour is not unpleasant. It is non-irritant.

hamamelids (ham-am-el'-ids). Witch hazel. **aqua h.**, 'extract of witch hazel', made from the bark. Astringent lotion.

hamamelids leaf, incorporated in suppositories for non-inflammatory piles.

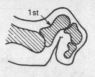

Hammer toe

hammer toe. A permanent hyperextension of the first phalanx and flexion of second and third phalanges.

handicapped. The term applied to a person with a defect that interferes with normal activity and achievement.

Hand-Schuller-Christian disease. A rare condition usually manifesting in early childhood with histiocytic granulomatous lesions affecting many tissues. Regarded as a form of histiocytosis X. Cause unknown and course relatively benign. [Alfred Hand, American paediatrician, 1868–1949. Artur Schuller, Austrian neurologist, 1876–1958. Henry Asbury Christian, Boston internist, 1876–1951.]

hangnail (hang'-nāl). A narrow strip of skin, partly detached from the nail fold.

Hansen's disease and bacillus. See LEPROSY.

hare-lip. A congenital defect in the lip; a fissure extending from the margin of the lip to the nostril; may be single or double, and is often associated with cleft palate.

Harris's operation. A transvesical, suprapubic type of prostatectomy (q.v.). [S. Harvy Harris, Australian surgeon, 1880–1936.]

Hartmann's solution. An electrolyte replacement solution. Contains sodium lactate and chloride, potassium chloride and calcium chloride. [Alexis Hartmann, American physician, 1898–   .]

Hartnup disease. Inborn error of protein metabolism. Associated with mental subnormality. Can be treated with nicotinamide and neomycin.

Hashimoto's disease. Affliction of an enlarged thyroid gland occurring in middle-aged females, and producing mild hypothyroidism. Result of sensitization of patient to her own thyroid protein, thyroglobulin. See AUTO-

IMMUNIZATION. [H. Hashimoto, Japanese surgeon, 1881-1934.]

hashish (hash'-ish). Cannabis indica (q.v.).

haustration (haws-trā'-shun). Sacculation, as of the colon—haustrum, sing.; haustra, pl.

hay fever. A form of allergic rhinitis in which attacks of catarrh of conjunctiva, nose and throat are precipitated by exposure to pollen.

Haygarth's nodes. Swelling of joints sometimes seen in the finger joints of patients suffering from arthritis. [John Haygarth, English physician, 1740-1827.]

HCG. Human chorionic gonadotrophin; obtained from the placenta. Used for cryptorchism.

healing (hē'-ling) [A.S.]. The natural process of cure or repair of the tissues, healing by first intention, when the edges of a clean wound are accurately held together, healing occurs with the minimum of scarring and deformity. healing by second intention, when the edges of a wound are not held together, the gap is filled by granulation tissue before epithelium can grow over the wound—heal, v.t., v.i.

health (helth). World Health Organization states, 'Health is a state of complete physical, mental and social well-being and not merely the absence of disease or infirmity.' Office of Health Economics states, 'A person should be regarded as healthy provided he can remain socially and economically active, even though he may have to suffer some health disability or discomfort.'

heart (hárt) [A.S. heorte]. The hollow muscular organ which pumps the blood through the body; situated behind the sternum, lying obliquely between the two lungs. It weighs 2.24 to 3.36 hg in the female and 2.80 to 3.36 hg in the male. heart-lung, apparatus for extracorporeal oxygenation of the blood. Used with heparin to prevent blood clotting.

heartblock. Partial or complete inhibition of the speed of conduction of the electrical impulse from the atrium to the ventricle of the heart. The cause may be an organic lesion or a functional disturbance. In its mildest form, it can only be detected electrocardiographically, whilst in its complete form the ventricles beat at their own slow intrinsic rate uninfluenced by the atria.

heartburn. See PYROIS and HOT-FAT HEARTBURN SYNDROME.

heat exhaustion. Heat syncope. Collapse, with or without loss of consciousness, suffered in conditions of heat and high humidity; largely resulting from loss of fluid and salt by sweating. If the surrounding air becomes saturated, heat-stroke will ensue.

heat-stroke. Final stage in heat exhaustion. When the body is unable to lose heat, hyperpyrexia occurs and death may ensue. A complication of electropyrexia (q.v.). See STROKE.

hebephrenia (hē-bē-frē'-ni-à) [G. hebe, puberty; phren, mind]. A type of schizophrenia (q.v.)—hebephrenic, adj.

Heberden's disease. Angina pectoris. Heberden's nodes, small osseous swellings at terminal phalangeal joints occurring in many types of arthritis. [William Heberden, English physician, 1710-1801.]

hedonism (hēd'-on-izm) [G. hedone, pleasure]. Excessive devotion to pleasure, so that a person's conduct is determined by an unconscious drive to seek pleasure and avoid unpleasant things.

Hegar's sign. Marked softening of the cervix in early pregnancy. [Alfred Hegar, German gynaecologist, 1830-1914.]

Heinz body. Refractile, irregularly shaped body present in red blood cells in some haemoglobinopathies.

helium (hē'-li-um) [G. helios, the sun]. An inert gas of low density. Sometimes mixed with oxygen for treatment of asthma, as it aids inspiration.

Heller's operation. Division of the muscle coat at the junction between the oesophagus and the stomach; used to relieve the difficulty in swallowing in cases of cardiospasm. [Ernst Heller, Professor of Surgery and Surgeon to St. Georg Hospital, Leipzig, 1877-1964.[

helminthagogue (hel-minth'-a-gog) [G. helmins, worm; agogos, leading]. See ANTHELMINTIC.

helminthiasis (hel-min-thī'-a-sis) [G. helmins, worm; N.L. -iasis, condition]. The condition resulting from infestation with worms.

helminthology (hel-min-thol'-o-ji). [G. helmins, worm; logos, discourse.]. The study of parasitic worms.

heloma (hel-ō'-má) [G. helos, a nail]. Corn, callosity—helomata, pl.

hemeralopia (hem-er-al-ō'-pi-á) [G. *hemera,* day; *alaos,* blind; *ops,* eye]. Defective vision in a bright light. Term has been incorrectly used for nyctalopia, night blindness (q.v.).

hemianopia (hem-i-an-ō'-pi-á) [G. *hemi,* half; *a-,* not; *opsis,* vision]. Blindness in one half of the visual field of one or both eyes.

hemiatrophy (hem-i-at'-ro-fi) [G. *hemi,* half; *atrophia,* lack of food]. Atrophy of one half or one side. **hemiatrophy facialis,** a congenital condition, or a manifestation of scleroderma (q.v.)., in which the structures on one side of the face are shrunken.

hemichorea (hem-i-kor-ē'-á) [G. *hemi,* half; *choreia,* dance]. Choreiform movements limited to one side of the body. See CHOREA.

hemicolectomy (hem-i-kō-lek'-to-mi) [G. *hemi,* half; *kolon,* colon; *ektome,* excision]. Removal of approximately half the colon.

hemicrania (hem-i-krān'-i-á) [G. *hemi,* half; *kranion,* skull]. Unilateral headache as in migraine.

hemidiaphoresis (hem-i-dī-a-for-ē'-sis) [G. *hemi,* half; *diapkerein,* carry through]. Unilateral sweating of the body.

hemiglossectomy (hem-i-glos-ek'-to-mi) [G. *hemi,* half; *glossa,* tongue; *ektome,* excision]. Removal of approximately half the tongue.

Heminevrin (hem-in-ev'-rin). Chlormethiazole (q.v.).

hemiparesis (hem-i-pa-rē'-sis) [G. *hemi,* half; *paresis,* paralysis]. A slight paralysis or weakness of one half of face or body.

hemiplegia (hem-i-plē'-ji-á) [G. *hemi,* half; *plege,* stroke]. Paralysis of one side of the body, usually resulting from a cerebrovascular accident on the opposite side—hemiplegic, adj.

Henoch's purpura (hen'-oks). See PURPURA. [Edvard H. Henoch, German paediatrician, 1820–1910.]

hepar (hē'-pár) [G.]. The liver—hepatic, adj.

heparin (hep'-ar-in). An acid present in liver and lung tissue. When injected intravenously it inhibits coagulation of the blood, and it is widely used in the treatment of thrombosis, often in associated with orally active anticoagulants such as phenindione.

hepatectomy (hep-at-ek'-to-mi) [G. *hepar,* liver; *ektome,* excision]. Excision of part of the liver.

hepatic (hep-at'-ik) [G. *hepar,* liver]. Pertaining to the liver.

hepaticocholedochostomy (hep-at'-ik-ō-kō-lē-dok-os'-tō-mi) [G. *hepar,* liver; *chole,* bile; *docke,* reception; *stoma,* mouth]. End-to-end union of the severed hepatic and common bile ducts.

hepaticoenteric (hep-at'-ik-ō-en-ter'-rik) [G. *hepar,* liver; *enteron,* intestine]. Pertaining to the liver and intestine.

hepaticojejunostomy (hep-at'-ik-ō-je-joon-os'-tō-mi) [G. *hepar,* liver; L. *jejunus,* empty; G. *stoma,* mouth]. Anastomosis of the hepatic duct to a loop of proximal jejunum.

hepatitis (hep-a-tī'-tis) [G. *hepar,* liver; *-itis,* inflammation]. Inflammation of the liver. **infective h.,** syn. 'catarrhal jaundice,' hepatitis-A virus infection of liver with an incubation period of two to six weeks, causing jaundice after a brief influenzalike illness. Notifiable in Britain since 1968. Spread by faecal-oral route. Virus B or SH is spread only by contact or inoculation with human blood products and causes **serum h.** Incubation period six weeks to six months, but infection can be severe, even fatal. It is estimated that 2 to 3 per cent of world adult population are carriers of hepatitis-B virus. **Australia antigen** (an'-ti-jen), associated with hepatitis virus B. Discovered by Dr Blumberg in 1965 in the blood of an Aborigine. In the United Kingdom it is found in about 1/800 to 1/1000 of the population, mostly without manifestations of disease. Rates are higher in tropical areas. The majority of patients with serum hepatitis give a positive reaction to the Australia antigen during the acute phase of illness, but because of technical limitations a negative reaction does not exclude serum hepatitis. Persons whose serum contains the antigen are, through their blood, infective to others. Their blood must never be used for transfusion because of this risk. See JAUNDICE.

hepatization (hep-a-tī-zā'-shun) [G. *hepar,* liver]. Pathological changes in the tissues, which cause them to resemble liver. Occurs in the lungs in pneumonia.

hepatocellular (hep-at-ō-sel'-ū-lar) [G. *hepar,* liver; L. *cellula,* small cell]. Pertaining to, or affecting liver cells.

hepatocirrhosis (hep-at-ō-si-rō'-sis) [G. *hepar,* liver; *kirrhos,* tawny; *-osis,* condition]. Cirrhosis (q.v.) of the liver.

hepatoma (hep-at-ō'-mǎ) [G. *hepar,* liver; *-oma,* condition]. Primary carcinoma of the liver —hepatomata, pl.

hepatomegaly (hep-at-ō-meg'-al-i) [G. *hepar,* liver; *megas,* large]. Enlargement of the liver. It is palpable below the costal margin.

hepatosplenic (hep'-at-ō-splen'-ik) [G. *hepar,* liver; *splen,* spleen]. Pertaining to the liver and spleen.

hepatotoxic (hep-at-ō-toks'-ik) [G. *hepar,* liver; *toxikon,* poison] Having an injurious effect on liver cells—hepatotoxicity, n.

Heptalgin (hep-tal' jin). Phenadoxone (q.v.).

hereditary (he-red'-it-ā-ri) [L. *hereditas,* heirship]. Inherited; capable of being inherited.

heredity (he-red'-i-ti). That factor responsible for the persistence of characteristics in successive generations.

hermaphrodite (hėr-maf'-rō-dīt) [L. *hermaphroditus,* from G. Hermes and Aphrodite]. Individual possessing both ovarian and testicular tissue. Although they may approximate either to male or female type, they are usually sterile from imperfect development of their gonads.

hernia (hėr'-ni-ǎ) [L.]. The abnormal protrusion of an organ, or part of an organ, through an aperture in the surrounding structures; commonly the protrusion of an abdominal organ through a gap in the abdominal wall. **diaphragmatic h.,** protrusion through

the diaphragm, the commonest one involving the stomach at the oesophageal opening (**hiatus h.**). **femoral h.,** protrusion through the femoral canal, alongside the femoral blood vessels as they pass into the thigh. **inguinal h.,** protrusion through the inguinal canal in the male. **strangulated h.,** hernia in which the blood supply to the organ involved is impaired, usually due to constriction by surrounding structures. **umbilical h.,** protrusion through the area of the umbilical scar. See IRREDUCIBLE.

hernioplasty (hėr-ni-ō-plas'-ti) [L. *hernia,* rupture; G. *plassein,* to form]. An operation for hernia, in which an attempt is made to prevent recurrence, by refashioning the structures to give greater strength—hernioplastic, adj.

herniorrhaphy (hėr-nē-or'-raf-i) [L. *hernia,* rupture; G. *rhaphe,* a suture]. An operation for hernia, in which the weak area is reinforced by some of the patient's own tissues, or by some other material.

herniotome (hėr'-nē-o-tōm) [L. *hernia,* rupture; G. *tomos,* a cutting]. A special knife with a blunt tip, used for hernia operations.

herniotomy (hėr-nē-ot'-o-mi) [L. *hernia,* rupture; G. *tome,* a cutting]. An operation to cure hernia, by the return of its contents to their normal position, and the removal of the hernial sac.

heroin (her'-ō-in). Diamorphine (q.v.).

herpangina (her-pan-jīn'-ǎ) [G. *herpein,* to creep; L. *angere,* to strangle]. Minute vesicles and ulcers at the back of the mouth. Short, febrile illness in children caused by Coxsackie viruses

herpes (hėr'-pēz) [G. *herpein,* to creep]. Vesicular eruption due to a virus infection. **herpes facialis, febrilis** and **labialis** are names used when blisters appear around the mouth (cold sores). Caused by the virus of herpes simplex type 1. Can also cause dendritic corneal ulcer. Genital herpes caused by herpes simplex virus type 2. **herpes zoster** (shingles) is caused by varicella-zoster virus; the virus attacks sensory nerves, with severe pain and appearance of vesicles along the distribution of the nerves involved (usually unilateral). herpes simplex virus and varicella-zoster virus often cause recurrent infection as they remain latent in nerve ganglia after the initial infection—herpetic, adj.

herpetiform (hėr-pet'-i-form) [G. *her-*

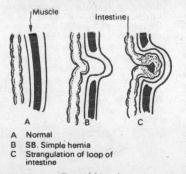

A Normal
B SB. Simple hernia
C Strangulation of loop of
   intestine

Types of hernia

pein, to creep; L.*forma,* form]. Resembling herpes.

hesperidin (hes-per′-i-din). Functions as vitamin P (q.v.). See CITRIN.

hetacillin (het-á-sil′-in). Synthetic antibiotic of the penicinate group. Destroyed by penicillinase, thus not active against Staphylococcus resistant to penicillin G.

heterogenous (het-er-oj′-en-us) [G. *heteros,* other; *genesis,* descent]. Of unlike origin; not originating within the body; derived from a different species, e.g. the use of beef bone pegs in orthopaedic surgery. See AUTOGENOUS, HOMOGENOUS.

heterologous (het-er-ol′-o-gus) [G. *heteros,* other; *logos,* relation]. Of different origin; from a different species.

heterophile (het′-er-ō-fīl) [G. *heteros,* other; *philos,* fond]. Activity of a product of one species against that of another, for example human antigen against sheep's red blood cells.

heteroplasty (het-e-rō-plas′-ti) [G. *heteros,* other; *plassein,* to form]. Plastic operation using a graft from another individual—heteroplastic, adj.

heterosexual (he-te-rō-seks′-ū-al) [G. *heteros,* other; L. *sexus,* sex]. Attracted towards the opposite sex. Opp. homosexual.

Hetrazan (het′-rá-zan). Diethyl carbamazine (q.v.).

hexachlorophane (heks-a-klor′-ō-fān). An antiseptic used in skin sterilization, and in some bactericidal soaps. Any medicinal product containing, hexachlorophane (irrespective of the amount) must bear a warning on the container 'not to be used for babies', or 'not to be administered to a child under 2'. Under suspicion as being a possible cause of brain damage in babies.

hexamethonium bromide (heks-a-meth-ō′-ni-um brō′-mīd). One of the earlier ganglionic blocking agents, used in the treatment of hypertension, given by subcutaneous or intramuscular injection. It is now being replaced by orally active drugs such as pentolinium or mecamylamine (q.v.).

hexamine (heks′-a-mēn). A urinary antiseptic of low toxicity. Action is due to liberation of formaldehyde in the urine, and is increased by acidification. Often prescribed with sodium acid phosphate. **hexamine hippurate,** especially useful before urinary tract surgery.

hexobarbitone (heks-ō-bár′-bit-ōn). A short-acting barbiturate, useful when a prompt but relatively brief action is required.

hexoestrol (heks-ēs′-trol). A synthetic compound related to stilboestrol, and used for similar purposes.

Hexopal (heks′-ō-pal). Nicotinyl alcohol. Vasodilator in peripheral vascular disease.

hexose (heks′-ōs). A class of simple sugars, monosaccharides, $C_9H_{12}O_6$. Examples are glucose, mannose, galactose.

hexylresorcinol (heks-il-rē-sor′-sin-ol). An anthelmintic with a wide range of activity, being effective against threadworm, roundworm, hookworm and intestinal fluke. It is followed by a saline purge. Treatment may have to be repeated at 3 day intervals. Also used in cystitis and other infections of the urinary tract.

HGH. Human growth hormone secreted by pituitary gland. Has now been synthesized.

hiatus (hī-ā′-tus) [L.]. A space or opening. See HERNIA—hiatal, adj.

Hibb's operation. Operation for spinal fixation, following spinal tuberculosis. No bone graft is used (as in Albee's operation), but the split vertebral spines are pressed outwards, and laid in contact with the laminae. Bony union occurs, and the spine is rigid. [Russell Aubra Hibbs, American orthopaedic surgeon, 1869–1932].

Hibitane (hi′-bi-tān). Chlorhexidine (q.v.).

hiccough (hi′-kuf). An involuntary inspiratory spasm of the respiratory organs, ending in a sudden closure of the glottis, with the production of a characteristic sound. Hiccup.

hiccup (hi′-kup). Hiccough (q.v.).

hidrosis (hid-rō′-sis) [G. *hidros,* sweat; *-osis,* condition]. Sweat secretion.

Higginson's syringe. Compression of the rubber bulb forces fluid forward through the nozzle for irrigation of a

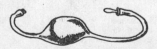

Higginson's syringe

body cavity. [Alfred Higginson, Liverpool surgeon of the 19th century.]

hilum (hī'-lum) [L. a trifle]. A depression on the surface of an organ where vessels, ducts, etc. enter and leave—hilar, adj.; hili, pl.

Hippocrates (hi-pok'-ra-tēz). Famous Greek physician and philosopher (460 to 367 BC) who established a school of medicine at Cos, his birthplace. He is often termed the 'Father of Medicine'.

Hippuran (hip'-ū-ran). One of the iodine-containing media used in X-ray Depts. **radioactive H.,** see RENOGRAM.

Hiprex (hip-reks). Hexamine hippurate (q.v.).

Hirschsprung's disease. Megacolon. Congenital intestinal aganglionosis. There is marked hypertrophy and dilation of the colon. Treated by Swenson's operation (q v.), Duhamel's operation (q.v.). [Harold Hirschsprung, Danish physician, 1830–1916.]

hirsute (hėr'-sūt) [L. *hirsutus*]. Hairy or shaggy.

hirudin (hi-roo'-din). A substance secreted by the leech, which prevents the clotting of blood.

hirudo (hi-roo'-dō) [L.]. The leech.

Hirudoid cream (hī-rū'-doid). Nongreasy cream containing heparin 1g in an absorbable base. Useful for acute and chronic inflammatory skin lesions, haemotoma, haemorrhoids and phlebothrombosis.

Histalog (his'-ta-log). Betazole hydrochloride (q.v.).

histamine (his'-ta-mēn). A naturally occurring chemical substance in body tissues which, in small doses, has profound and diverse actions on muscle, blood capilliaries, and gastric secretion. Sudden excessive release from the tissues, into the blood, is believed to be the cause of the main symptoms and signs in anaphylaxis (q.v.)—histaminic, adj. Used in circulatory and gastric function tests. There are two types of **h. receptor** cells in the body, H_1 in the cells of bronchial muscle, and H_2 in the cells that secrete gastric juice.

histidinaemia (his-ti-din-ēm'-i-á). Genetically determined increase in histidine in blood. Gives rise to speech defects without mental retardation.

histidine (his'-ti-dēn). An essential amino acid which is widely distributed and is present in haemoglobin. It is a precursor of histamine.

histiocytes (his'-ti-ō-sīts). Derived from reticuloendothelial cells; act as scavengers.

histiocytoma (his-ti-ō-sī-tō-má). Benign tumour of histiocytes.

histiocytosis X (his-ti-ō-sīt-ō'-sis). See HAND-SCHULLER-CHRISTIAN DISEASE.

histocompatibility (his-tō-kom-pat-ib-il'-it-i). Cells' ability to be accepted and to function in a new situation; important in organ transplantation.

histology (his-tol'-o-ji) [G. *histos,* web; *logos,* a discourse]. Microscopic study of tissues—histological, adj.; histologically, adv.

histolysis (his-tol'-is-is) [G. *histos,* web; *lysis,* a loosening]. Disintegration of organic tissue—histolytic, adj.

histones (his'-tōns). Recent research shows that h. are a system of proteins that may control genes.

histoplasmosis (his-tō-plas-mō'-sis) [G. *histos,* web; *plasma,* anything formed; *-osis,* condition]. One of the infective reticuloses. Disease involving the reticuloendothelial system, resulting from infection by the fungus *Histoplasma capsulatum.*

hives (hīvs). Nettle-rash; urticaria (q.v.).

hobnail liver. Firm nodular liver, may be found in cirrhosis.

Hodgkin's disease. Lymphadenoma. A malignant lymphoma causing progressive enlargement of lymph nodes and involvement of reticuloendothelial tissues including bone marrow. Some cases show **Pel Ebstein fever** (q.v.). [Thomas Hodgkin, English physician, 1798–1866.]

Homans' sign. Passive dorsiflexion of foot causes pain in calf muscles. Indicative of incipient or established venous thrombosis of leg. [John Homans, American surgeon, 1877–1954.]

homatropine (hōm-at'-rō-pēn). A mydriatic similar to atropine, but with a more rapid and less prolonged effect. Often used as a 2 per cent solution with a similar amount of cocaine, which addition increases the mydriatic action and deadens pain.

homeopathy (hōm-i-op'-ath-i) [G. *homoios,* like; *pathos,* disease]. A method of treating disease by prescribing minute doses of drugs which, in maximum dose, would produce symptoms of the disease. First adopted by Hahnemann—homeopathic, adj.

homicide (hom'-i-sīd) [L. *homo*, man; *coedere*, to kill]. Killing of another person: manslaughter if accidental, murder if intentional.

homocystinuria (hō-mō-sis-tin-ū'-ri-á) [G. *homos*, same; *kystis*, bladder; *ouron*, urine]. Excretion of homocystine (a sulphur containing amino acid, homologue of cystine) in the urine. Gives rise to slow development of mental retardation of varying degree, lens and growth abnormalities and thrombotic episodes which are often fatal in childhood—homocystinuric, adj.

homogeneous (hom-ō-jēn'-ē-us) [G. *homos*, same; *genos*, race]. Of the same kind; of the same quality or consistency throughout.

homogenize (ho-moj'-en-īz). To make into the same consistency throughout.

homogenous (hom-oj'-en-us) [G. *homos*, same; *genos*, race]. Having a like nature, e.g. a bone graft from another human being.

homograft (hō'-mō-graft) [G. *homos*, same]. A tissue or organ which is transplanted from one individual to another of the same species. Syn. allograft.

homolateral (hō-mō-lat'-er-al) [G. *homos*, same; L. *lateralis*, side]. On the same side—homolaterally, adv.

homologous (hom-ol'-ō-gus) [G. *homos*, same; *logos*, word]. Corresponding in origin and structure. **homologous chromosomes**, those that pair during reduction cell division and contain identical arrangement of genes in their DNA pattern.

homonymous (hŏm-on'-im-us) [G. *homos*, same; *enyma*, name]. Corresponding halves.

homosexual (hō-mō-seks'-ū-al) [G. *homos*, same; L. *sexus*, sex]. Of the same sex. Often used to describe a person who indulges in homosexuality.

homosexuality (hō-mō-seks-ū-al'-it-i). Attraction for, and desire to establish an emotional and sexual relationship with a member of the same sex.

homotransplant (hō-mō-trans'-plant) [G. *homos*, same; L. *transplantare*, to transplant]. Tissues or organ transplanted from non-identical members of the same species. Syn. allotransplant; homograft.

homozygous (hom-o-zī'-gus). Having

identical genes in the same locus on one of the chromosome pairs.

Honvan (hon'-van). Stilboestrol diphosphate, broken down by prostatic tissue to release stilboestrol *in situ*, thus reducing systemic side effects.

hookworm. See ANCYLOSTOMA.

hordeolum (hor-dē'-ō-lum) [L. *hordeum*, grain of barley]. A stye; a furuncle on the eyelid.

hormone (hor'-mōn) [G. *hormaein*, to excite]. Specific chemical substance secreted by an endocrine gland and conveyed in the blood to regulate the functions of tissues and organs elsewhere in the body.

hormonotherapy (hor-mō-nō-ther'-a-pi). Treatment by hormones.

Horner's syndrome. Clinical picture following paralysis of cervical sympathetic nerves, on one side. There is myosis, slight ptosis with enophthalmos, and anhidrosis. [Johann Friedrich Horner, Swiss ophthalmologist, 1831–86.]

Horton's syndrome. Severe headache due to the release of histamine in the body. To be differentiated from migraine. [Bayard Taylor Horton, American physician, 1895–   .]

host (hōst) [L. *hospes*]. The organic structure upon which parasites thrive. **intermediate h.**, one in which the parasite passes its larval or cystic stage.

hot-dog headache. Post-prandial; induced by sodium nitrite content of frankfurters.

hot-fat heartburn syndrome. Due to excessive leak from stomach to oesophagus producing hypersensitivity in the oesophageal mucosa: tends to be worse after fatty or fried food or drinking coffee. May be associated with hiatus hernia.

hour-glass contraction. A circular constriction in the middle of a hollow organ (usually the stomach or uterus), dividing it into two portions.

housemaid's knee. See BURSITIS.

HPFSH. Human pituitary follicle (q.v.) stimulating hormone.

HPV-77. High passage virus of the 77th passage level. Attenuated rubella virus used to produce active immunity.

Humatin (hū'-mat-in). Paromomycin (q.v.).

humerus (hū'-mėr-us) [L.]. The bone of the upper arm, between the elbow and shoulder joint—humeral, adj.; humeri, pl.

humidity (hū-mid'-it-i) [L. *humidus,* moist]. The amount of moisture in the atmosphere as measured by a hygrometer. **relative h.,** the ratio of the amount of moisture present in the air to the amount which would saturate it (at the same temperature).

humor (hū'-mor) [L. a liquid]. Any fluid of the body. **aqueous h.,** the fluid filling the anterior and posterior chambers in front of the optical lens. **vitreous h.,** the gelatinous mass filling the interior of the eyeball from the lens to the retina.

hunger (hung'-ger). A longing, usually for food. **air h.,** see air. **hunger pain,** epigastric pain which is relieved by taking food; associated with duodenal ulcer.

Hunter-Hurler syndrome. Gargoylism (q.v.).

Hunterian chancre. The hard sore of primary syphilis. [John Hunter, Scottish surgeon, 1728–93]

Huntington's chorea. Genetically determined heredofamilial disease with slow progressive degeneration of the nerve cells of the basal ganglia and cerebral cortex. Affects both sexes, and is due to a dominant gene of large effect. Develops in middle age, or later, and is associated with progressive dementia. See CHOREA. [George Huntington, American physician, 1862–1927.]

Hutchinson's teeth. Defect of the upper central incisors (second dentition) which is part of the facies of the congenital syphilitic person. The teeth are broader at the gum than at the cutting edge, and each shows an elliptical notch. [Jonathan Hutchinson, English surgeon, 1828–1913.]

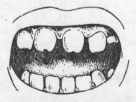

Hutchinson's teeth

Hyalase (hī'-a-lāz). Hyaluronidase (q.v.).

hyaline (hī'-a-lēn) [G.*hyalos,* glass]. Like glass; transparent. **h. membrane dis-**

ease. See RESPIRATORY DISTRESS SYNDROME.

hyalitis (hī-al-ī'-tis) [G. *hyalos,* glass; -*itis,* inflammation]. Inflammation of the optical vitreous humor or its enclosing membrane.

hyaloid (hī'-a-loid) [G. *hyalos,* glass]. Resembling hyaline. **hyaloid membrane,** the transparent capsule enclosing the optical vitreous humor.

hyaluronidase (hī-al-ū-ron'-i-dāz). An enzyme obtained from testes, which when injected subcutaneously, promotes the absorption of fluid. Given with or immediately before a subcutaneous infusion; 1000 units will facilitate the absorption of 500 to 1000 ml of fluid.

Hycal (hī-cal'). Flavoured liquid; protein-free; low-electrolyte; carbohydrate preparation based on demineralized liquid glucose, providing 240 kcal per 100 ml.

hydatid (hī'-dat-id) [G. *hydatis,* watery vesicle]. The cyst formed by larvae of a tapeworm, Echinococcus, found in dogs. The encysted stage normally occurs in sheep but can occur in man after he eats with soiled hands from petting a dog. The cysts are commonest in the liver and lungs. Cysts grow slowly and only do damage by the space they occupy. If they leak, or become infected, urticaria and fever supervene and 'daughter' cysts can result. Treatment surgical. See TEST (CASONI)

hydatidiform (hī-da-tid'-i-form) [G. *hydatis,* watery vesicle; L. *forma,* shape]. Pertaining to or resembling a hydatid. **hydatidiform mole,** see MOLE.

hydraemia (hī-drē'-mi-à) [G. *hydor,* water; *haima,* blood]. A relative excess of plasma volume compared with cell volume of the blood; it is normally present in late pregnancy—hydraemic, adj.

hydramnios (hī-dram'-ni-os) [G. *hydor,* water; *amnion,* membrane around fetus]. An excess of amniotic fluid.

hydrargyrum (hīd-rar'-ji-rum) [L.]. Mercury or quicksilver.

hydrarthrosis (hī-drár-thrō'-sis) [G. *hydor,* water; *arthron,* joint; -*osis,* condition]. A collection of fluid in a joint cavity. **intermittent h.,** afflicts young women; probably due to allergy. Synovitis develops spontaneously, lasts a few days, and disappears as mysteriously.

hydrate (hī'-drāt). Combine with water— hydration, n.

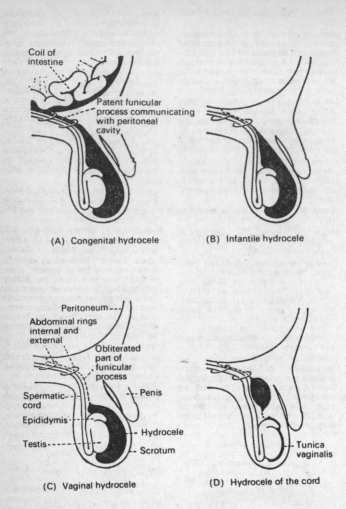

(A) Congenital hydrocele

(B) Infantile hydrocele

(C) Vaginal hydrocele

(D) Hydrocele of the cord

Types of hydrocele

Hydrenox (hī'-dren-oks). Hydroflume-thiazide (q.v.).

hydroa (hī-drō'-á) [G. *hydor*, water; *oion*, egg]. Syn., dermatitis herpetiformis (q.v.). **hydroa aestivale**, or Hutchinson's summer prurigo, is a vesicular or bullous disease occurring in children. It affects exposed parts and probably results from photosensitivity. **hydroa vacciniforme** is a more severe form of this in which scarring ensues.

hydrocele (hī'-drō-sēl) [G. *hydor*, water; *kele*, tumour]. A swelling due to accumulation of serous fluid in the tunica vaginalis of the testis, or in the spermatic cord.

hydrocephalus (hī-drō'-kef'-a-lus) [G. *hydor*, water; *kephale*, head]. 'Water on the brain.' An excess of cerebrospinal fluid inside the skull due to an obstruction to normal CSF circulation. **external h.**, the excess of fluid is mainly in the subarachnoid space. **internal h.**, excess of fluid is mainly in the ventricles of the brain. Spitz-Holter valve (q.v.) used in drainage operations for this condition.—hydrocephalic, adj.

hydrochloric acid (hī-drō-klor'-ik as'-id). Secreted by the gastric oxyntic cells and present in gastric juice (0.2 per cent). The strong acid is caustic, but a 10 per cent dilution is used orally in the treatment of achlorhydria.

hydrochlorothiazide (hī-drō-klor-ō-thī'-a-zīd). More powerful diuretic than chlorothiazide (q.v.).

hydrocortisone (hī-drō-kor'-ti-zōn). Cortisol, an adrenal cortical steroid essential to life. It is more effective locally than cortisone, and is used extensively in inflamed conditions of the skin, eyes and ears, frequently in association with locally effective antibiotics. Also used by intrarticular injection for arthritis and bursitis; intravenously in Addisonian crisis, by retention enema in ulcerative colitis, and as spray or snuff in hay fever.

hydrocyanic acid (hī-drō-sī-an'-ik as'-id). Prussic acid. The dilute acid (2 per cent) has a sedative action on the stomach, and has been given with bismuth carbonate and other antacids in the treatment of vomiting. In large doses, prussic acid is rapidly fatal by causing respiratory and cardiac paralysis.

hydroflumethiazide (hī-dro-flū-meth'-i-azīd). Diuretic. Decreases reabsorption of sodium and chloride in kidney tubules.

hydrogen (hī'-drō-jen). A colourless, odourless, combustible gas. **hydrogen ion concentration**, a measure of the acidity or alkalinity of a solution, ranging from pH 1 to 14, 7 being approximately neutral; the lower numbers denoting acidity; the higher ones denoting alkalinity. **hydrogen peroxide**, H_2O_2, a powerful oxidizing and deodorizing agent, used for cleaning wounds; diluted with 4 to 8 parts of water as a mouthwash, and with 50 per cent alcohol as ear drops.

hydrolysis (hī-drol'-is-is) [G. *hydor*, water, *lysis*, a loosening]. The splitting into more simple substances by the addition of water— hydrolytic, adj.; hydrolyse, v.

hydrometer (hī-drom'-et-ér) [G. *hydor*, water; *metron*, a measure]. An instrument for determining the specific gravity of fluids—hydrometry, n.

hydrometria (hī-drō-mēt'-ri-á) [G. *hydor*, water; *metra*, uterus]. A collection of watery fluid within the uterus.

hydronephrosis (hī-drō-nef-rō'-sis) [G. *hydor*, water; *nephros*, kidney; -*osis*, condition]. Distension of the kidney pelvis with urine, from obstructed outflow. If unrelieved, pressure eventually causes atrophy of kidney tissue. Operations are pyeloplasty (q.v.) and Hamilton Stewart nephroplasty. See NEPHROPLASTY.

hydropericarditis (hī-drō-pe-ri-kárd-ī'lis) [G. *hydor*, water; *peri*, around; *kardia*, the heart, -*itis*, inflammation]. Pericarditis with effusion.

hydropericardium (hī-drō-pe-ri-kárd'-ium) [G. *hydor*, water; *peri*, around; *kardia*, the heart]. Fluid in the pericardial sac in the absence of inflammation. Can occur in heart and kidney failure.

hydroperitoneum (hī-drō-pe-ri-to-nē'-um) [G. *hydor*, water; *peritonaion*, peritoneum]. See ASCITES.

hydrophobia (hī-drō-fō'-bi-á) [G. *hydor*, water; *phobos*, fear]. Rabies in man.

hydropneumothorax (hī-drō-nū-mō-thor'-aks) [G. *hydor*, water; *pneuma*, breath; *thorax*, chest]. Pneumothorax further complicated by effusion of fluid in the pleural cavity. Usually tubercular.

hydrops (hī'-drops) [G.]. Dropsy—hydropic, adj. **hydrops fetalis**, severe form of erythroblastosis fetalis (q.v.).

hydrosalpinx (hī-drō-sal'-pinks) [G. *hydor*, water; *salpigx*, trumpet]. Distension of the Fallopian tube with watery fluid.

Hydrosaluric. Hydrochlorothiazide (q.v.).

hydrotherapy (hī-drō-the′-ra-pi) [G. *hydor,* water; *therapeia,* treatment]. The science of therapeutic bathing for diagnosed conditions.

hydrothorax (hī-drō-thor′-aks) [G. *hydor,* water; *thorax,* chest]. The presence of fluid in the pleural cavity.

hydroureter (hī-drō-ū-rē′-tėr) [G. *hydor,* water; *oureter,* ureter]. Abnormal distension of the ureter with urine.

hydroxocobalamin (hī-droks-ō-kō-bal′-a-mēn). A longer-acting form of vitamin B_{12}. See CYANOCOBALAMIN.

hydroxychloroquine (hī-droks-i-klor′-ō-kwin). Antimalarial. Can cause retinopathy.

hydroxyl (hī-droks′-il). The monovalent group OH, consisting of a hydrogen atom linked to an oxygen atom.

hydroxyprogesterone caproate (hī-droks-i-prō-jes′-ter-ōn kap-rō′-āt). Given intramuscularly for recurrent and threatened abortion.

hydroxystilbamidine (hī-droks-i-stil-bam′-i-dēn). Useful in aspergillosis.

hydroxyurea (hī-droks′-i-ū-rē′-á). Simple compound given orally. Mode of action uncertain, may be of value in patients with chronic myeloid leukaemia who no longer show a response to busulphan.

hydroxyzine (hīd-roks′-i-zēn). Atarax. Tranquillizer. See ATARACTIC.

hygiene (hī′-jēn) [G. *hygieinos,* healthy]. The science dealing with the maintenance of health. **communal h.,** embraces all measures taken to supply the community with pure food and water, good sanitation, housing, etc. **industrial h.** (occupational health) includes all measures taken to preserve the individual's health whilst he is at work. **mental h.** deals with the establishment of healthy mental attitudes and emotional reactions. **personal h.,** includes all those measures taken by the individual to preserve his own health—hygienic, adj.

Hygraphen (hī′-gr-fen). Organic mercurial used when trichomonal infections do not respond to metronidazole.

hygroma (hī-grō′-má) [G. *hygros,* moist; *-oma,* tumour]. A cystic swelling containing watery fluid, usually situated in

the neck and present at birth—hygromata, pl.; hygromatous, adj.

hygrometer (hī-grom′-et-ėr) [G. *hygros,* moist; *metron,* a measure]. An instrument for measuring the amount of moisture in the air. See HUMIDITY.

hygroscopic (hī-grō-skop′-ik) [G. *hygros,* moist; *skopein,* to examine]. Readily absorbing water, e.g. glycerine.

Hygroton (hī-grō′-ton). Chlorthalidone (q.v.).

hymen (hī′-men) [G. membrane]. A membranous perforated structure stretching across the vaginal entrance. **imperforate h.,** a congenital condition leading to haematocolpos. See CRYPT-OMENORRHOEA.

hymenectomy (hī-men-ek′-to-mi) [G., membrane; *ektome,* excision]. Surgical excision of the hymen.

hymenotomy (hī-men-ot′-o-mi) [G., membrane; *tome,* a cutting]. Surgical incision of the hymen.

hyoid (hī′-oid) [G. *y-eidos;* shaped like letter 'Y']. A U-shaped bone at the root of the tongue.

hyoscine (hī′-ō-sēn). A hypnotic alkaloid obtained from belladonna and hyoscyamus. Often used for pre-operative sedation in association with morphine, papaveretum or pethidine. Also **mydriatic** and **cycloplegic.** Syn., scopolamine.

hyoscyamus (hī-ō-sī′-a-mus). Henbane leaves and flowers. Resembles belladonna in its properties. Sometimes given with potassium citrate for urinary tract spasm.

hyperacidity (hī′-pėr-as-id′-it-i) [G. *hyper,* above; L. *acidus,* acid]. Excessive acidity. See HYPERCHLORHYD-RIA.

hyperactivity (hī′-pėr-ak-ti′-vi-ti) [G. *hyper,* above; L. *activus,* active]. Excessive activity.

hyperaemia (hī′-pėr-ē′-mi-á) [G. *hyper,* above; *haima,* blood]. Excess of blood in an area. **active h.** caused by an increased flow of blood to a part. **passive h.** occurs when there is restricted flow of blood from a part—hyperaemic, adj.

hyperaesthesia (hī′-pėr-es-thē′-zi-á) [G. *hyper,* above; *aisthesis,* sensation]. Excessive sensitiveness of a part—hyperaesthetic, adj. (Cf. anaesthesia.)

hyperaldosteronism (hī-pėr-al-dos-tēr′-ōn-izm). Production of excessive aldosterone **primary h.,** see ALDOSTERONE.

secondary h., the adrenal responds to an increased stimulus of extra adrenal origin.

hyperalgesia (hī-pĕr-al-jēz'-i-á) [G. hyper, above; algesis, sense of pain]. Excessive sensibility to pain. Also HYPERALGIA—hyperalgesic, adj.

hyperbaric (hī-pĕr-bar'-ik) [G. hyper, above; baros, weight]. At greater pressure, specific gravity or weight, than normal. hyperbaric oxygen chamber, sealed cylinder containing oxygen under pressure. Accommodates patient, attendant and equipment. In some units surgery can be performed. Anaerobic organisms and their ability to produce toxins are adversely affected by oxygen. O_2 saturated tissues respond better to radiotherapy.

hyperbilirubinaemia (hī'-pĕr-bī-li roo'-bin-ē'-mi-á) [G. hyper, above; L. bilis, bile; ruber, red; G. haima, blood]. Excessive bilirubin in the blood. Present in physiological jaundice of the newborn. See PHOTOTHERAPY—hyperbilirubinaemic, adj.

hypercalcaemia (hī'-pĕr-kal-sē'-mi-á)[G. hyper, above; L. calx, lime; G. haima, blood]. Excessive calcium in the blood. idiopathic h., disorder of calcium storage. Cause unknown. Hypersensitivity to vitamin D has been suggested. Some infants recover. Those who are severely affected show osteosclerosis, developmental retardation and hypertension. Fatal cases show nephrocalcinosis at autopsy. Survivors later present with a typical facies, mental subnormality and aortic stenosis. Treatment includes one of the calcium-free milks. In acute stages, steroids may be useful. Clinical picture may closely resemble renal acidosis (q.v.). Nephrocalcinosis may occur in both. Diagnosis rests on raised blood calcium and urea without a consistently alkaline urine—hypercalcaemic, adj.

hypercalciuria (hī-pĕr-kal-si-ū'-ri-á) [G. hyper, above; L. calx, lime; G. ouron, urine]. Greatly increased calcium excretion in urine, as seen in hyperparathyroidism. idiopathic h., used when there is no known metabolic cause. hypercalciuria of importance in pathogenesis of nephrolithiasis.

hypercapnia (hī'-pĕr-kap'-ni-á) [G. hyper, above; kapnos, smoke]. Excessive CO_2 in the blood—hypercapnic, adj.

hypercarbia (hī-per-kar'-bi-á). Hypercapnia (q.v.).

hypercatabolic (hī-pĕr-kat-ab-ol'-ik) [G. hyper, above; kata, down; ballein, to throw]. Excessive breakdown of complex substances into simpler ones within the body. Can occur in acute renal failure.

hyperchloraemia (hī'-pĕr-klor-ē'-mi-á) [G. hyper, above; chloros, pale green; haima, blood]. Excessive chloride in the blood. One form of acidosis (q.v.)—hyperchloraemic, adj.

hyperchlorhydria (hī'-pĕr-klor-hī'-dri-á) [G. hyper, above; chloros, pale green; hydor, water] Excessive hydrochloric acid in the gastric juice—hyperchlorhydric, adj.

hypercholesterolaemia (hī-pĕr-kol-es-te-rol-ē'-mi-á) [G. hyper, above; chole, bile; stereos, stiff; haima, blood]. Excessive cholesterol in the blood. Predisposes to atheroma and gall-stones. Also found in myxoedema—hypercholesterolaemic, adj.

hyperelectrolytaemia (hī-pĕr-e-lek-trō-līt-ē'-mi-á). Dehydration (not manifested clinically) associated with high serum sodium and chloride levels.

hyperemesis (hī-pĕr-em'-es is) [G. hyper, above; emesis, vomiting]. Excessive vomiting. hyperemesis gravidarum, a complication of pregnancy which may become serious.

hyperextension (hī-pĕr-eks-ten'-shun) [G. hyper, above; L. extendere, to stretch]. Over-extension.

hyperflexion (hī'-pĕr-flek'-shun) [G. hyper, above; L. flexio, a bending]. Excessive flexion.

hyperglycaemia (hī'-pĕr-glī-sē'-mi-á) [G. hyper, above; glykys, sweet; haima, blood]. Excessive sugar in the blood—hyperglycaemic, adj.

hyperglycinaemia (hī-per-glī-sin-ē'-mi-á). Excess glycine in the serum. Can cause acidosis and mental retardation—hyperglycinaemic, adj.

hyperhidrosis (hī'-pĕr-hi-drō'-sis) [G. hyper, above; hidros, sweat; -osis, condition]. Excessive sweating—hyperhidrotic, adj.

hyperinsulinism (hī-pĕr-in'-sul-in-izm) [G. hyper, above; L. insula, island]. Intermittent or continuous loss of consciousness, with or without convulsions. Due to excessive insulin from the pancreatic islets lowering the blood sugar.

hyperinvolution (hī'-pĕr-in-vo-loo'-shun) [G. *hyper*, above; L. *involutus*, infolded]. Reduction to below normal size, as of the uterus after parturition.

hyperkalaemia (hī-pĕr-kal-ē'-mi-á) [G. *hyper*, above; N.L. *kalium*, potassium; G. *haima*, blood]. Excessive potassium in the blood—hyperkalaemic, adj.

hyperkeratosis (hī'-pĕr-ke-ra-tō-sis) [G. *hyper*, above; *keras*, horn; *-osis*, condition]. Hypertrophy of the cornea or the horny layer of the skin—hyperkeratotic, adj.

hyperkinesis (hī-pĕr-kīn-ē'-sis) [G. *hyper*, above; *kinesis*, motion]. Excessive movement—hyperkinetic, adj.

hyperkinetic syndrome. First described in 1962; usually appears between the ages of 2 and 4 years. The child is slow to develop intellectually. There is a marked degree of distractability and a tireless unrelenting exploration of the environment, together with agressivness, especially towards siblings, even if unprovoked. He is fearless and undeterred by threats of punishment. The parents complain of his cold unaffectionate character and destructive behaviour. Condition often responds to chlorpromazine, primidone or amphetamine and can tolerate large doses of these. Many also improve spontaneously between 7 and 10 years old. Some consider that genetic and environmental factors are important, because studies have shown that the child often reacts to changes in his social circumstances.

hyperlipaemia (hī-pĕr-lī-pēm'-i-á) [G. *hyper*, above; *lipos*, fat; *haima*, blood]. Excessive fat in the blood—hyperlipaemic, adj.

hypermagnesaemia (hī-pĕr-mag-nes-ē'-mi-á) [G. *hyper*, above; *Magnesie lithos*, Magnesian stone; *haima*, blood]. Excessive magnesium in the blood—hypermagnesaemic, adj.

hypermetabolism (hī-pĕr-met-ab'-ol-izm) [G. *hyper*, above; *metabole*, change]. Production of excessive body heat. Characteristic of thyrotoxicosis—hypermetabolic, adj.

hypermetropia (hī'-pĕr-me-trō'-pi-á) [G. *hyper*, above; *metron*, a measure; *ops*, eye]. Longsightedness caused by faulty accommodation of the eye, with the result that the light rays are focused beyond, instead of on, the retina—hypermetropic, adj.

hypermobility (hī-pĕr-mō-bil'-i-ti) [G.

hyper, above; L. *mobilitas*, mobility]. Excessive mobility.

hypermotility (hī'-pĕr-mō-til'-i-ti) [G. *hyper*, above; L. *movere*, to move]. Increased movement, as peristalsis.

hypernatraemia (hī'-pĕr-nat-rē'-mi-á) [G. *hyper*, above; *natros*, sodium; *haima*, blood]. Excessive sodium in the blood—hypernatraemic, adj.

hypernephroma (hī'-pĕr-nef-rō'-má) [G. *hyper*, above; *nephros*, kidney; *-oma*, tumour]. Grawitz tumour. A malignant neoplasm of the kidney—hypernephromata, pl.; hypernephromatous, adj.

hyperonychia (hī'-pĕr-on-ik'-i-á) [G. *hyper*, above; *onyx*, nail]. Excessive growth of the nails.

hyperosmolar diabetic coma (hī-pĕr-os-mō'-lar). Coma characterized by a very high blood sugar without accompanying ketosis.

hyperosmolarity (hī'-pĕr-os-mō-lar'-i-ti) [G. *hyper*, above; *osmos*, impulse]. Syn., hypertonicity. A solution exerting a higher osmotic pressure than another, is said to have a hyperosmolarity, with reference to it. In medicine, the comparison is usually made with normal plasma.

hyperostosis (hī'-pĕr-os-tō'-sis) [G. *hyper*, above; *osteon*, bone; *-osis*, condition]. See EXOSTOSIS.

hyperoxaluria (hī-pĕr-oks-al-ū'-ri-á) [G. *hyper*, above; *oxalis*, garden sorrel; *ouron*, urine]. Excessive oxaluria (q.v.)—hyperoxaluric, adj.

hyperparathyroidism (hī'-pĕr-pa-ra-thī'-roid-izm) [G. *hyper*, above; *para*, near; *thureoeides*, shield-shaped]. Overaction of the parathyroid glands with increase in serum calcium levels: may result in osteitis fibrosa cystica with decalcification and spontaneous fracture of bones. See TEST, INTRAVENOUS CALCIUM. **tertiary h.**, development of parathyroid adenomata causing hypercalcaemia on top of reactive or secondary parathyroid hyperplasia due to malabsorption of chronic glomerular failure.

hyperperistalsis (hī'-pĕr-pe-ri-stal'-sis) [G. *hyper*, above; *peri*, around; *stellein*, to draw in]. Excessive peristalsis—hyperperistaltic, adj.

hyperphenylalaninaemia (hī-pĕr-fē-nīl-āl-a-nin-ē'-mi-á). Excess of phenylalanine in the blood.

· hyperphagia (hī'-pĕr-fa'-ji-á) [G. *hyper*, above; *phagein*, to eat]. Overeating.

hyperphosphataemia (hī-pėr-fos-fat-ē'-mia-ā) [G. *hyper*, above; *phosphoros*, light-bringer; *haima*, blood]. Excessive phosphates in the blood—hyperphosphataemic, adj.

hyperpiesis (hī-pėr-pī-ēs'-is) [G. *hyper*, above; *piesis*, pressure]. Hypertension (q.v.).

hyperpigmentation (hī-pėr-pig-men-tā'-shun) [G. *hyper*, above; L. *pigmentum*, pigment]. Increased or excessive pigmentation.

hyperpituitarism (hī'-pėr-pit-ū'-it-ar-izm). Overactivity of the anterior lobe of the pituitary producing gigantism or acromegaly (q.v.).

hyperplasia (hī' pėr-plā'-zi-ā) [G. *hyper*, above; *plasis*, a moulding]. Excessive formation of cells—hyperplastic, adj.

hyperpnoea (hī'-pėrp-nē'-ā) [G. *hyper*, above; *pnoe*, breath]. Rapid, deep breathing; panting; gasping—hyperpnoeic, adj.

hyperpotassaemia (hī'-pėr-pot-as-ē'-mi-ā). Increased potassium in the blood. Hyperkalaemia. Theoretically can cause heart block, cardiac arrest and muscle paralysis—hyperpotassaemic, adj.

hyperpyrexia (hī'-pėr-pī-reks'-i-ā) [G. *hyper*, above; *pyressein*, to be feverish]. Body temperature above 40–41°C (105° F)—hyperpyrexial, adj.

hypersecretion (hī'-pėr-se-krē'-shun) [G. *hyper*, above; L. *secretus*, separated]. Excessive secretion.

hypersensitivity (hī'-pėr-sen-si-ti'-vi-ti) [G. *hyper*, above; L. *sentire*, to feel]. A state of being unduly sensitive to a stimulus or an allergen (q.v.)—hypersensitive, adj.

hypersplenism (hī-pėr-splen'-izm) [G. *hyper*, above; *splen*, spleen]. Term used to describe depression of erythrocyte, granulocyte and platelet counts by enlarged spleen in presence of active bone marrow.

hypertelorism (hī-per-tel'-or-izm) [G. *hyper*, above; *tele*, far off; *horos*, a boundary]. Genetically determined cranial anomaly (low forehead and pronounced vertex) associated with mental subnormality.

Hypertensin (hī-pėr-ten'-sin). Angiotensin (q.v.).

hypertension (hī-pėr-ten'-shun) [G. *hyper*, above; *tendere*, to stretch]. Abnormally high tension, by custom alluding to blood pressure and involving systolic and/or diastolic levels. There is no universal agreement of their upper limits of normal, especially in increasing age. Many cardiologists consider a resting systolic pressure of 160 mm of mercury (mmHg), and/or a resting diastolic pressure of 100 mmHg, to be pathological. The cause may be renal, endocrine, mechanical or toxic (as in toxaemia of pregnancy) but in many cases it is unknown and this is then called 'essential h.' **primary pulmonary h.**, constriction of blood vessels in the lungs with consequent resistance to blood flow which increases pressure in the right cardiac ventricle and atrium. Cause unknown. Usually leads to death from congestive heart failure in two to 10 years—hypertensive, adj.

hyperthermia (hī'-pėr-thėr'-mi-ā) [G. *hyper*, above; *therme*, heat]. Very high body temperature—hyperthermic, adj.

hyperthyroidism (hī'-pėr-thī'-roid-izm) [G. *hyper*, above; *thureoeides*, shield-shaped]. Thyrotoxicosis (q.v.).

hypertonia (hī'-ėr-tō'-ni-ā) [G. *hyper*, above; *tonos*, tension]. Increased tone in a muscular structure—hypertonic, adj.; hypertonicity, n.

hypertonic (hī'-pėr-ton'ik) [G. *hyper*, above; *tonos*, tension]. 1. Pertaining to hypertonia. 2. Pertaining to saline. h. saline has a greater osmotic pressure than normal physiological (body) fluid.

hypertoxic (hī-pėr-toks'-ik) [G. *hyper*, above; *toxikon*, poison]. Very poisonous.

hypertrichiasis (hī'-pėr-trik-ī'-a-sis) [G. *hyper*, above; *thrix*, hair; *-osis*, condition]. Excessive hairiness. Also HYPERTRICHOSIS.

hypertrophy (hī'-pėr-trof-i) [G. *hyper*, above; *trophe*, nourishment]. Increase in the size of tissues or structures, independent of natural growth. It may be congenital (see PYLORIC STENOSIS), compensatory, complementary or functional—hypertrophic, adj.

hyperuricaemia (hī-pėr-ū-ris-ē'-mi-ā). Excessive uric acid in the blood Characteristic of gout. Occurs in untreated reticulosis, but is increased by radiotherapy, cytotoxins and corticosteroids—hyperuricaemic, adj.

hyperventilation (hī'-pėr-ven-til-ā'-shun) [G. *hyper*, above; L. *ventilare*, below]. Syn., hyperpnoea (q.v.).

hypervitaminosis (hī'-pėr-vī-ta-min-ō'-sis) [G. *hyper*, above; L. *vita*, life; G. *-osis*, condition]. Any condition arising from an excess of vitamins, especially vitamin D.

hypervolaemia (hī-per-vol-ē'-mi-à) [G. *hyper,* above; L. *volume,* volume; G. *haima,* blood]. Plethora (q.v.).

hyphaema (hī-fē'-mà) [G. *hypo,* under; *haima,* blood]. Blood in the anterior chamber of the eye.

hypnosis (hip-nō'-sis) [G. *hypnos,* sleep; *-osis,* condition]. A state resembling sleep, brought about by the hypnotist utilizing the mental mechanism of suggestion. Can be used to produce painless labour, dental extractions, and is occasionally utilized in minor surgery and in psychiatric practice—hypnotic, adj.

hypnotherapy (hip-nō-ther'-à-pi) [G. *hypnos,* sleep; *therapeia,* treatment]. Treatment by prolonged sleep or hypnosis.

hypnotic (hip-not'-ik) [G.*hypnos,* sleep]. 1. Pertaining to hypnotism. 2. A drug which produces a sleep resembling natural sleep.

hypoaesthesia (hī-pō-es-thē'-zi-à) [G. *hypo,* below; *aisthesis,* sensation]. Diminished sensitiveness of a part—hypoaesthetic, adj.

hypocalcaemia (hī-pō-kal-sē'-mi-à) [G. *hypo,* under; L. *calx,* lime; G. *haima,* blood]. Decreased calcium in the blood. See TETANY—hypocalcaemic, adj.

hypocapnia (hī-pō-kap'-ni-à) [G. *hypo,* under; *kapnos,* smoke]. Diminished CO_2 content of the blood; can be produced by hyperventilation—hypocapnial, adj.

hypochloraemia (hī-pō-klor-ē'-mi-à) [G. *hypo,* under; *chloros* pale; *haima,* blood]. Reduced chlorides in the circulating blood. A form of alkalosis—hypochloraemic, adj.

hypochlorhydria (hī-pō-klor-hi'-dri-à) [G. *hypo,* under; *chloros,* pale green; *hydor,* water]. Decreased hydrochloric acid in the gastric juice—hypochlorhydric, adj.

hypochlorite (hī-pō-klor'-īt). Salts of hypochlorous acid. They are easily decomposed to yield active chlorine, and have been widely used on that account in the treatment of wounds—Dakin's solution and eusol being examples. Milton is a proprietary product that contains a stabilizer and therefore retains its activity over a longer period.

hypochondria (hī-pō-kon'-dri-à). Excessive anxiety about one's health. Com-

mon in depressive and anxiety states—hypochondriac, adj.; hypochondriasis, n.; hypochondriacal, adj.

hypochondrium (hī-pō-kon'-dri-um). The upper lateral region (left and right) of the abdomen, below the lower ribs—hypochondriac, adj.

hypochromic (hī-pō-krō'-mik) [G. *hypo,* under; *chroma,* colour]. Deficiency in colouring or pigmentation. Decreased haemoglobin in a red blood cell.

hypodermic (hi-pō-dèr'-mik) [G. *hypo,* below, *derma,* skin]. Below the skin. Subcutaneous—hypodermically, adv.

hypofibrinogenaemia (hī-pō-fi-brin'-ō-jen-ē'-mi-à). See AFIBRINOGENAEMIA and ACUTE DEFIBRINATION SYNDROME—hypofibrinogenaemic, adj.

hypofunction (hī-pō-fungk'-shun) [G. *hypo,* below; L. *functio,* performance]. Diminished performance.

hypogammaglobulinaemia (hī-pō-gam-ma-glob'-ū-lin-ē'-mi-à). Decreased gammaglobulin in the blood. Lessens resistance to infection. See DYSGAMMAGLOBULINAEMIA—hypogammaglobulinaemic, adj.

hypogastrium (hī-pō-gas'-tri-um) [G. *hypo,* below; *gaster,* belly]. That area of the anterior abdomen which lies immediately below the umbilical region. It is flanked on either side by the iliac fossae—hypogastric, adj.

hypoglossal (hī-pō-glos'-àl) [G. *hypo,* below; *glossa,* tongue]. Under the tongue. **hypoglossal nerve,** the twelfth pair of cranial nerves.

hypoglycaemia (hī-pō-gli-sē'-mi-à) [G. *hypo,* below; *glykys,* sweet; *haima,* blood]. Decreased blood sugar, attended by anxiety, excitement, perspiration, delirium or coma. **insulin h.** can be produced intentionally (insulin treatment) in schizophrenia. **idiopathic h.,** associated with mental subnormality. ACTH useful. **leucine-induced h.,** a genetic metabolic disorder due to sensitivity to the amino acid leucine—hypoglycaemic, adj.

hypokalaemia (hī-pō-ka-lē'-mi-à) [G. *hypo,* below; L. *kalium,* potassium]. Abnormally low potassium level of the blood—hypokalaemic, adj. See POTASSIUM DEFICIENCY.

hypomagnesaemia (hī-pō-mag-nes-ē'-mi-à) [G. *hypo,* below; *Magnesie lithos,* Magnesian stone; *haima,* blood]. Decreased magnesium in the blood—hypomagnesaemic, adj.

hypomania (hī-pō-mā′-ni-á) [G. *hypo,* below; *mania,* madness]. A less intense form of mania (q.v.), in which the patient is easily distracted—hypomanic, adj.

hypometabolism (hī-pō-met-ab′-ol-izm) [G. *hypo,* below; *metabole,* change]. Decreased production of body heat. Characteristic of myxoedema.

hypomotility (hī-pō-mō-ti′-li-ti) [G. *hypo,* under; L. *movere,* to move]. Decreased movement as of the stomach or intestines.

hyponatraemia (hī-pō-nat-rē′-mi-á) [G. *hypo,* below; *natros,* sodium; *haima,* blood]. Decreased sodium in the blood—hyponatraemic, adj.

hypo-osmolarity (hī-pō-os-mō-lar′-it-i) [G. *hypo,* below; *osmos,* impulse]. Syn., hypotonicity. A solution exerting a lower osmotic pressure than another, is said to have a h.-o. with reference to it. In medicine the comparison is usually made with normal plasma.

hypoparathyroidism (hī-pō-pa-ra-thī′-roid-izm) [G. *hypo,* under; *para,* near; *thureoeides,* shield shaped]. Underaction of the parathyroid glands with decrease in serum calcium levels, producing tetany (q.v.).

hypopharynx (hī-pō-far′-ingks). That portion of the pharynx lying below and behind the larynx, correctly called the laryngopharynx.

hypophoria (hī-pō-fo′-ri-á) [G. *hypo,* below; *phoros,* bearing]. A state in which the visual axis in one eye is lower than the other.

hypophosphataemia (hī-pō-fos-fat-ē′-mi-á) [G. *hypo,* below; *phosphoros,* light-bringer; *haima,* blood]. Decreased phosphates in the blood—hypophosphataemic, adj.

hypophysectomy (hī-pof-i-sek′-to-mi) [G. *hypo,* below; *physis,* growth; *ektome,* excision]. Surgical removal of the pituitary gland.

hypophysis cerebri (hi-pof′-i-sis). The small oval-shaped gland lying in the pituitary fossa of the sphenoid bone and connected to the under surface of the brain by a stalk; the pituitary gland—hypophyseal, adj.

hypopiesis (hī-pō-pī-ēs′-is) [G. *hypo,* below; *piesis,* pressure]. Hypotension (q.v.).

hypopigmentation (hī-pō-pig-men-tā′-shun) [G. *hypo,* below; L. *pigmentum,* pigment]. Decreased or poor pigmentation.

hypopituitarism (hī-pō-pit-ū′-it-ar-izm) [G. *hypo,* under; L. *pituita,* slime]. Pituitary gland insufficiency, especially of the anterior lobe. Absence of gonadotrophins leads to failure of ovulation, uterine atrophy and amenorrhoea. Loss of trophic hormones to other endocrines produces mental inertia, laziness, weakness, lack of sweating, sensitivity to cold (may be hypothermia), oliguria, loss of pubic and axillary hair, hypoglycaemia, pale skin, depigmentation of mammary alveolae and perineum. Can result from post-partum infarction of the pituitary gland.

hypoplasia (hī-pō-plā′-zi-á) [G. *hypo,* under; *plassein,* to form]. Defective development of any tissue—hypoplastic, adj.

hypopotassaemia (hī-pō-pot-as-sē′-mi-á). See HYPOKALAEMIA.

hypoproteinaemia (hī-pō-prō-tēn-ēm′-i-á) [G. *hypo,* below; *proteios,* primary; *haima,* blood]. Deficient protein in blood plasma, from dietary deficiency or excessive excretion (albuminuria)—hypoproteinaemic, adj.

hypoprothrombinaemia (hī-pō-prō-throm-bin-ē′-mi-á) [G. *hypo,* below; *pro,* before; *thrombos,* clot; *haima,* blood]. Deficiency of prothrombin in the blood which retards its clotting ability. See VITAMIN K and JAUNDICE—hypoprothrombinaemic, adj.

hypopyon (hī-pō′-pī-on) [G. *hypo,* below; *pyon,* pus]. A collection of pus in the anterior chamber of the eye.

hyposecretion (hī-pō-sē-krē′-shun) [G. *hypo,* below; L. *secretio,* secretion]. Deficient secretion.

hyposmia (hī-pos′-mi-á) [G. *hypo,* below; *osme,* smell]. Decrease in the normal sensitivity to smell. Has been observed in patients following laryngectomy.

hypospadias (hī-pō-spā′-di-as) [G. *hypo,* below; *spein,* to draw out]. A congenital malformation of the male urethra. Subdivided into two types: (1) penile, when the terminal urethral orifice opens at any point along the posterior shaft of the penis; (2) perineal, when the orifice opens on the perineum and may give rise to problems of sexual differentiation. Cf. epispadias.

hypostasis (hī-pō-stā′-sis) [G. a standing under]. 1. A sediment 2. Congestion of blood in a part due to impaired circulation—hypostatic, adj.

hypotension (hī-pō-ten'-shun) [G. *hypo*, below; L. *tensio*, a stretching]. Low blood pressure (systolic below 110 mmHg, diastolic below 70 mmHg), may be primary, secondary (e.g. shock, Addison's disease) or postural. It can be produced by the administration of drugs to reduce bleeding in surgery—hypotensive, adj.

hypothalamus (hī-pō-thal'-a-mus) [G. *hypo*, below; *thalamos*, chamber]. Below the thalamus. Part of the mid-brain closest to the pituitary. Under control of the emotions and even of the conscious brain.

hypothenar eminence (hī-pō-thē'-nár) [G. *hypo*, below; *thenar*, palm]. The eminence on the ulnar side of the palm below the little finger.

hypothermia (hī-pō-thêr'-mi-à) [G. *hypo*, below; *therme*, heat]. Below normal body temperature, ascertained by a low-reading thermometer. Occurs in the very young and in old people. An artificially induced hypothermia (30° C or 86° F) can be used in the treatment of head injuries and in cardiac surgery. It reduces the oxygen consumption of the tissues and thereby allows greater and more prolonged interference of normal blood circulation. hypothermia of the newborn, failure of the newborn child to adjust to external cold; may be associated with infection. local h. has been tried in the treatment of peptic ulcer. See REFRIGERATION.

hypothyroidism (hī-pō-thī'-roid-izm) [G. *hypo*, below; *thureoeides*, shield-shaped]. Defines those clinical conditions which result from suboptimal circulating levels of one or both thyroid hormones. See THYROXINE, TRIIODO-THYRONINE. Hypothyroidism currently classified as: (1) overt (see MYXOEDEMA); (2) mild; (3) preclinical; (4) autoimmune thyroid disease without thyroid failure. See CRETINISM and MYXOEDEMA.

hypotonic (hī-pō-ton'-ik) [G. *hypo*, below; *tonos*, tension]. Having a low osmotic pressure; less than isotonic; lacking in tone, tension, strength—hypotonia, hypotonicity, n.

Hypovase (hī'-pō-vās). Prazosin (q.v.).

hypoventilation (hī-pō-ven-til-ā'-shun) [G. *hypo*, below; L. *ventilare*, below]. Diminished breathing or underventilation.

hypovitaminaemia (hī-pō-vī-ta-min-ē'-mi-à) [G. *hypo*, below; L. *vita*, life; -amine; *haima*, blood]. Deficiency of vitamins in the blood—hypovitaminaemic. adi.

hypovitaminosis (hī-pō-vī-ta-min-ō'-sis) [G. *hypo*, below; L. *vita*, life; G. *-osis*, condition]. Any condition due to lack of vitamins.

hypovolaemia (hī-pō-vol-ē'-mi-à). See OLIGAEMIA—hypovolaemic, adj.

hypoxaemia (hī-poks-ē'-mi-à) [G. *hypo*, under; *oxys*, sharp; *haima*, blood]. Diminished amount (reduced saturation) of oxygen in the arterial blood—hypoxaemic, adj.

hypoxia (hī-pok'-si-à) [G. *hypo*, under; *oxys*, sharp]. Diminished amount of oxygen in the tissues—hypoxic, adj. anaemic h., resulting from a deficiency of haemoglobin. histotoxic h., interference with the cells in their utilization of O_2, e.g. in cyanide poisoning. hypoxic h., interference with pulmonary oxygenation. stagnant h., a reduction in blood flow, as seen in the finger nails in surgical shock or in cold weather.

hysterectomy (his-ter-ek'-to-mi) [G. *hystera*, womb; *ektome*, excision]. Surgical removal of the uterus. abdominal h., effected via a lower abdominal incision. subtotal h., removal of the uterine body, leaving the cervix in the vaginal vault. Rarely performed because of the risk of a carcinoma developing in the cervical stump. total h., complete removal of the uterine body and cervix. vaginal h., effected per vaginam. Wertheim's h., total removal of the uterus, the adjacent lymphatic vessels and glands, with a cuff of the vagina.

hysteria (his-tē'-ri-à) [G. *hystera*, womb]. A neurosis usually arising from mental conflict and repression (q.v.), and characterized by the production of a diversity of symptoms, e.g. tics, paralysis, anaesthesia, etc. The disorder is characterized by dissociation (q.v.)—hysterical, adj.

hysterography (his-te-rog'-ra-fi) [G. *hystera*, womb; *graphein*, to write]. X-ray examination of the uterus—hysterograph, hysterogram, n.; hysterographical, adj. hysterographically, adv.

hysterosalpingectomy (his-te-rō-sal-pin-jek'-to-mi) [G. *hystera*, womb; *salpigx*, trumpet; *ektome*, excision]. Excision of the womb and usually both uterine tubes (oviducts).

hysterosalpingography   (his-te-rō-sal-ping-og'-ra-fi) [G. *hystera*, womb; *salpigx*, trumpet; *graphein*, to write]. X-ray examination of the uterus and tubes after injection of a contrast medium—hysterosalpingograph, hysterosalpingogram, n.; hysterosalpingographical, adj.; hysterosalpingographically, adv.

hysterosalpingostomy (his-te-rō-sal-ping-os'-to-mi) [G. *hystera*, womb; *salpigx*, trumpet; *stoma*, mouth]. Anastomosis between an oviduct and the uterus.

hysterotomy (his-te-rot'-o-mi) [G. *hystera*, womb; *tome*, a cutting]. Incision of the uterus to remove a pregnancy before the 28th week of gestation.

hysterotrachelorraphy (his-te-rō-trak-el-or'-a-fi) [G. *hystera*, womb; *trachelos*, neck; *rhaphe*, suture]. Repair of lacerated cervix uteri.

hystiocytosis X (his-ti-ō-sī-tō'-sis). See HISTIOCYTOSIS and HAND-SCHULLER-CHRISTIAN DISEASE.

I

iatrogenic (i-at-rō-jen'-ik) [G. *iatros*, physician; a combining form signifying a relation to medicine or physicians]. A secondary condition arising from treatment of a primary condition.

Ibufenac (i-bū-fen'-ac). Dytransin (q.v.).

ibuprofen (ib-ū-prō'-fen). Specific for rheumatoid arthritis. Can be used for osteoarthritis. Can be irritant to the gastrointestinal tract.

ichthammol (ik'-tham-mol). Thick black liquid derived from the destructive distillation of shale. Used as a mild antiseptic ointment for skin disorders and as a solution in glycerin to reduce inflammation.

Ichthyol (ik'-thi-ol). Ichthammol (q.v.).

ichthyosis (ik-thi-ō'-sis) [G. *ichthys*, fish; *-osis*, condition]. A congenital condition of the skin which is dry and scaly. Fish skin. Xeroderma. **ichthyosis hystrix** is a form of congenital naevi with patches of warty excrescences.

icterus (ik'-te-rus) [G. *ikteros*, jaundice]. Jaundice. **icterus gravis**, see ACUTE. **icterus gravis neonatorum** is one of the clinical forms of haemolytic disease of the newborn (erythroblastosis fetalis (q.v.)). **icterus neonatorum** is the normal, or physiological, jaundice occurring in the first week of life as a result of destruction of haemoglobin in excess of the infant's needs. Human albumin is

given as the albumin-bilirubin complex is thought to be too large a molecule to cross the blood-brain barrier, thus reducing the risk of kernicterus.

icterus index. Measurement of concentration of bilirubin in the plasma. Used in diagnosis of jaundice.

id. That part of the unconscious mind which consists of a system of primitive urges (instincts) and according to Freud (q.v.) persists unrecognized into adult life. The suffix -id (or -ide) commonly used to denote allergic skin reaction in existing infection, e.g. syphilide, trichophytid.

idea (ī-dē'-à) [G. form]. The memory of past perceptions. An i. depends upon an image in the same way as a perception (q.v.) depends upon a sensation.

ideation (ī-dē-ā'-shun) [G. *idea*, form]. The process concerned with the highest function of awareness, the formation of ideas. It includes thought, intellect and memory.

identical twins (ī-den'-tik-al). Two offspring of the same sex, derived from a single fertilized ovum. See BINOVULAR and UNIOVULAR.

identification (ī-den-ti-fi-kā'-shun) [L. *idem*, same]. Recognition. In psychology, the way in which we form our personality by modelling it on a chosen person, e.g. identification with the parent of same sex—helping to form one's sex role; identification with a person of own sex in the hero-worship of adolescence.

ideomotor (ī-dē-o-mō'-tor) [G. *idea*, form; L. *movere*, to move]. Mental energy, in the form of ideas, producing automatic movement of muscles, e.g. mental agitation producing agitated movements of limbs.

idioventricular (id-i-ō-ven-trik'-ū-lar) [G. *idios*, one's own; L. *ventriculum*, ventricle]. Pertaining to the cardiac ventricles and not affecting the atria.

idiopathy (id-iō-pa'-thi) [G. *idios*, one's own; *pathos*, disease]. A pathologic state of unknown or spontaneous origin—idiopathic, adj.

idiosyncrasy (id-i-ō-sing'-kra-si) [G. *idios*, own; *synkrasis*, mingling together]. A peculiar variation of constitution or temperament. Unusual individual response to certain drugs, proteins, etc. whether by injection, ingestion, inhalation or contact.

Idoxuridine (ī-doks-ū'-ri-din). 5-Iodo-2-

deoxyuridine. Antiviral chemotherapeutic agent for corneal herpetic ulcers. It interferes with synthesis of DNA in herpes simplex virus and prevents it from multiplying. Active against vaccinia infection.

ileal bladder (īl'-ē-al blad'-ėr). See BLADDER.

ileitis (īl-ē-ī'-tis) [L. *ilia*, flanks; G. *itis*, inflammation]. Inflammation of the ileum. **regional i.**, non-specific chronic recurrent granulomatous disease affecting mainly young adults and characterized by a necrotizing, ulcerating inflammatory process, there usually being an abrupt demarcation between it and healthy bowel. There can be healthy bowel ('skip' area) intervening between two diseased segments.

ileocaecal (ī-lē-ō-sē'-kal) [L. *ilia*, flanks; *caecus*, blind]. Pertaining to the ileum and the caecum.

ileocolic (ī-lē-ō-kol'-ik) [L. *ilia*, flanks; G. *kolon*, colon]. Pertaining to the ileum and the colon.

ileocolitis (ī-lē-ō-kol-ī'-tis) [L. *ilia*, flanks; G. *kolon*, colon; *-itis*, inflammation]. Inflammation of the ileum and the colon.

ileocolostomy (ī-lē-ō-kol-os'-to-mi) [L. *ilia*, flanks; G. *kolon*, colon; *stoma*, mouth]. A surgically made fistula between the ileum and the colon, usually the transverse colon. Most often used to bypass an obstruction or inflammation in the caecum or ascending colon.

ileocutaneous ureterostomy. See BLADDER and URETEROSTOMY.

ileocystoplasty (ī-lē-ō-sis'-to-plas-ti) [L. *ilia*, flanks; G. *kystis*, bladder; *plassein*, to form]. Operation to increase the urinary bladder. See COLOCYSTOPLASTY for diagram—ileocystoplastic, adj.

ileoproctostomy (ī-lē-ō-prok-tos'-to-mi) [L. *ilia*, flanks; G. *proktos*, anus; *stoma*, mouth]. An anastomosis between the ileum and rectum; used when disease extends to the sigmoid colon.

ileorectal (ī-lē-ō-rek'-tal) [L. *ilia*, flanks; *rectus*, straight]. Pertaining to the ileum and the rectum.

ileosigmoidostomy (ī-lē-ō-sig-moid-os'-to-mi) [L. *ilia*, flanks; G. *sigmoides*, E shaped; *stoma*, mouth]. An anastomosis between the ileum and sigmoid colon; used where most of the colon has to be removed.

ileostomy (ī-lē-os'-to-mi) [L. *ilia*, flanks; G. *stoma*, mouth]. A surgically made fistula between the ileum and the anterior abdominal wall; usually a permanent form of artificial anus when the whole of the large bowel has to be removed, e.g. in severe ulcerative colitis. **ileostomy bags**, rubber or plastic bags used to collect the liquid discharge from an ileostomy.

ileo-ureterostomy (ī-lē-ō-ūr-ēt-er-os'-to-mi) [L. *ilia*, flanks; G. *oureter*, ureter; *stoma*, mouth]. Transplantation of the lower ends of the ureters from the bladder to an isolated loop of small bowel which, in turn, is made to open on the abdominal wall. See BLADDER.

ileum (īl'-ē-um) [L. *ilia*, flanks]. The lower three fifths of the small intestine, lying between the jejunum and the caecum—ileal, adj.

ileus (īl'-ē-us) [G. *eileos*, intestinal obstruction]. Intestinal obstruction. Usually restricted to paralytic as opposed to mechanical obstruction and characterized by abdominal distension, vomiting and the absence of pain. See MECONIUM.

iliococcygeal (i-li-ō-koks-ij'-ē-al) [L. *ilium*, flank; G. *kokkyx*, cuckoo]. Pertaining to the ilium and coccyx.

iliofemoral (ī-li-ō-fem'-or-al) [L. *ilium*, flank; *femur*, thigh]. Pertaining to the ilium and the femur.

iliopectineal (i-li-ō-pek-tin'-ē-al) [L. *ilium*, flank; *pecton*, crest]. Pertaining to the ilium and the pubis.

iliopsoas (i-li-ō-sō'-as) [L. *ilium*, flank; G. *psoai*, loins]. Pertaining to the ilium and the loin.

ilium (il'-i-um) [L. flank]. The upper part of the innominate bone, a separate bone in the fetus. The flank—iliac, adj.

illusion (i-lū'-zhun) [L. *illusio-illudere*, to deceive]. A misidentification of a sensation, e.g. of sight, a white sheet being mistaken for a ghost, the sheet being misrepresented in consciousness as a figure.

Ilotycin (i-lō-tī'-sin). Erythromycin (q.v.).

image (im'-āj) [L. imago]. A revived experience of a percept recalled from memory. (Smell and taste.)

imagery (im'-aj-ėr-i) [L. *imago*, image]. Imagination. The recall of mental images of various types depending upon the special sense organs involved when the images were formed, e.g. **auditory i.**,

motor i., visual i. (sight), **tactile i.** (touch), **olfactory i.**

imbalance (im-bal'-ans). Want of balance. Term refers commonly to the upset of acid-base relationship and the electrolytes in body fluids.

Imferon (im'-fer-on).An iron-dextran complexfor parental iron therapy. Used as a total dose infusion to obtain a rapid response in marked iron deficiency anaemia.

imipramine (im-ip'-ra-mēn). Antidepressant, anticholinergic, antihistaminic, anti-Parkinson and antiserotonin properties. Chemically related to chlor promazine. Raises levels of serotonin and catecholamines in brain.

immune (i-mūn') [L. *immunis,* exempt from public burden]. Not susceptible to an infection. **immune body,** antibody. **immune reaction response,** that which causes a body to reject a transplanted organ, to respond to bacterial disease which develops slowly, and to act against malignant cells; cellular immunity is the term used for these various reactions. This does not occur in thymectomized mice.

immunity (im-mūn'-i-ti) [L. *immunis,* exempt from public burden]. A state of relative resistance to an infection. **cellular i.,** produced by the T-lymphocytes (see IMMUNE). **humoral i.,** from antibodies produced by B-lymphocytes. Immunity can be **innate** (from inherited qualities), or it can be **acquired,** actively or passively, naturally or artificially. **active i.** is acquired, naturally during an infectious disease or artificially by vaccination with dead or living organisms. **passive i.** is acquired, naturally when maternal antibody passes to the child via the placenta or in the milk, or artificially by administering immune sera containing antibody—obtained from animals or human beings.

immunization (im-mū-nī-zā'-shun) [L. *immunis,* exempt from public burden]. The process of increasing specific antibody in the tissues.

immunogenesis (im-mūn-ō-jen'-e-sis) [L. *immunis,* exempt from public burden; G. *genesis,* descent]. The process of production of immunity—**immunogenetic,** adj.

immunogenicity (im-mūn-ō-jen-is-i-ti). The ability to produce immunity.

immunoglobulins (im-mūn-ō-glob'-ū-lins). Syn., gammaglobulins (q.v.).

immunology (im-mūn-ol'-oj-i). The special study of immunity— **immunological,** adj.; **immunologically,** adv.

immunopathology (im-mūn-ō-path-ol'-oj-i). Abnormal immune reaction as when a person becomes sensitized.

immunosensitivity (im-mūn-ō-sen-sit-iv'-i-ti). The state produced by immunopathology.

immunosuppressive (im-mūn-ō-sup-res'-iv) [L. *immunis,* exempt from public burden; *supprimere,* to press down]. That which prevents the occurrence of an immune reaction (q.v.).

immunotherapy (im-mūn-ō-ther'-á-pi) Any treatment used to produce immunity.

immunotransfusion (im-mūn-ō-trans-fū'-zhun) [L. *immunis,* exempt from public burden; *transfundere,* to transfuse]. Transfusion of blood from a donor previously rendered immune by repeated inoculations with a given agent from the recipient.

impacted (im-pak'-ted) [L. *impactum,* from *impingere,* to strike against]. Firmly wedged, abnormal immobility, as of faeces in the rectum; fracture; a fetus in the pelvis; a tooth in its socket or a calculus in a duct.

impalpable (im-pal'-pa-bl) [L. *in,* not; *palpare,* to feel] Not palpable. Incapable of being felt by touch (palpation).

imperforate (im-pèr'-for-āt) [L. *in,* not; *perforare,* to bore through]. Lacking a normal opening. **imperforate anus,** absence of an opening into the rectum. **imperforate hymen,** a fold of mucous membrane at the vaginal entrance which has no natural outlet for the menstrual fluid.

impetigo (im-pet-ī'-gō) [L.]. An inflammatory, pustular, skin disease usually caused by Staphylococcus, occasionally by Streptococcus.**impetigo contagiosa,** a highly contagious form of impetigo, commonest on the face and scalp, characterized by bullae which become pustules and then honey-coloured crusts. See ECTHYMA—**impetiginous,** adj.

implantation (im-plan: tā'-shun) [L. *in,* into; *plantare,* to plant]. The insertion of living cells or solid materials into the tissues, e.g. accidental implantation of tumour cells in a wound; implantation of radium or solid drugs.

implants (im'-plantz) [L. *in,* in; *planta,* sprout]. Tissues or drugs inserted surgically into the human body, e.g. implantation of pellets of testosterone under the skin in treatment of carcinoma of the breast, implantation of deoxycortone acetate (DOCA) in Addison's disease.

impotent (im'-pō-tent) [L. *impotentia*, inability]. By custom referring to the male. Absence of sexual power.

impregnate (im'-preg-nāt) [L. *in*, in; *praegnans*, pregnant]. Fill. Saturate, Render pregnant.

impulse (im'puls) [L. *impulsus*, striking against]. 1. The tendency to act without deliberation. 2. A sudden push or communicated force.

Imuran. Azathioprine (q.v.).

inaccessibility (in-ak-ses-ib-il'-i-ti). In psychiatry denotes absence of patient response.

inassimilable (in-as-sim'-a-bl) [L. *in*, in; *assimilare*, to make like]. Not capable of absorption.

incarcerated (in-kár'-se-rā-ted) [L. *in*, in; *carcer*, prison]. The abnormal imprisonment of a part, as in a hernia which is irreducible, and a pregnant uterus held beneath the sacral promontory.

incest (in'-sest) [L. *incestus*, unchaste]. Sexual intercourse between near kindred, whose marriage is prohibited by law.

incipient (in-sip'-i-ent) [L. *incipere*, to begin]. Initial, beginning, in early stages.

incision (in-sizh'-un) [L. *incisio*, cut]. Cutting into body tissue, using a sharp instrument—incise, v.t.; incisional, adj.

incisors (in-sī'-sorz) [L. *incisus*, cut into]. The eight front cutting teeth, four in each jaw.

inclusion bodies (in-klū'-zhun bod'-iz). Minute particles found in the cells of affected tissues.

incompatibility (in-kom-pat-ib-il'-it-i) [L. *in*, not; *compatibilis*, compatible]. Usually refers to the bloods of donor and recipient in transfusion, when antigenic differences in the red cells result in reactions such as haemolysis or agglutination. When two or more medicaments are given concurrently or consecutively they can attenuate, counteract or even potentiate the desired result of one another.

incompetence (in-kom'-pe-tens) [L. *incompetens*, insufficient]. Inadequacy to perform a natural function, e.g. mitral incompetence—incompetent, adj.

incontinence (in-kon'-tin-ens) [L. *incon-*tinentia, inability to retain]. Inability to control the evacuation of urine or faeces. **overflow i.**, dribbling of urine from an overfull bladder. **stress i.**, occurs when the intra-abdominal pressure is raised as in coughing and sneezing; there is usually some weakness of the urethral sphincter muscle coupled with anatomical stretching and displacement of the bladder neck.

incoordination (in-kō-or-din-ā'-shun) [L. *in*, not; *cum*, together; *ordinare*, to regulate.]. Inability to produce smooth, harmonious muscular movements.

incubation (in-kū-bā'-shun) [L. *incubare*, to hatch]. The period from entry of infection to the appearance of the first symptom.

incubator (in'-kū-bā-tor) [L. *incubare*, to hatch]. A temperature-regulated apparatus in which premature or delicate babies can be reared, or bacteria cultured.

Indema (in'-dē-má). Phenindione (q.v.).

Inderal (in'der-al). Propranolol (q.v.).

Indian hemp. Cannabis indica (q.v.). Hashish.

indicanuria (in-di-kan-ū'-ri-á). Excessive potassium salt (indican) in the urine. Traces in normal urine. See INDOLE.

indicator (in'-dik-ā-tor). A substance used to make visible the completion of a chemical reaction.

indigenous (in-dij'-e-nus) [L. *indigena*, a native]. Native to a certain locality or country, e.g. Derbyshire neck (simple colloidal goitre).

indigestion (in-di-jes'-chun). Dyspepsia.

indigocarmine (in-dig-ō-kár'-min). A dye used as an 0.4 per cent solution for testing renal function. Given by intravenous or intramuscular injection. The urine is coloured blue in about 10 min if kidney function is normal.

Indocid (in'-dō-sid). Indomethacin (q.v.).

indol(e) (in'-dol). A product of intestinal putrefaction: it is oxidized to indoxyl in the liver and excreted in urine as indican. See INDICANURIA.

indolent (in'-dō-lent) [L. *in*, not; *dolere*, to feel pain]. A term applied to a sluggish ulcer which is generally painless and slow to heal.

indomethacin (in-dō-meth'-a-sin). An analgesic with anti-inflammatory properties. Useful in the rheumatic disorders. Can be given orally and by suppository.

induction (in-duk'-shun) [L. *inducere*, to lead into]. The act of bringing on or causing to occur, as applied to anaesthesia and labour.

induration (in-dū-rā'-shun) [L. *indurare*, to harden]. The hardening of tissue as in hyperaemia, infiltration by neoplasm, etc.—indurated, adj.

industrial disease. A disease contracted by reason of occupational exposure to an industrial agent known to be hazardous, e.g. dust, fumes, chemicals, irradiation, etc., the notification of, safety precautions against and compensation for which are controlled by law. Syn., occupational disease. See DERMATITIS.

industrial therapy. Current organization of outside industrial working conditions within a unit in a psychiatric hospital. The main purpose is preparation of patients for their return to the working community.

inertia (in-ér'-shi-à) [L. inactivity]. Inactivity. uterine i., lack of contraction of parturient uterus. It may be primary due to constitutional weakness; secondary due to exhaustion from frequent and forcible contractions.

in extremis (in eks-trē'-mis) [L.]. At the point of death.

infant (in'-fant) [L. *infans*, without speech]. A baby or a child of less than 1 year old.

infantile paralysis. See POLIOMYELITIS.

infantilism (in-fant'il-izm) [L. *infantilis*, of infants]. General retardation of development with persistence of childish characteristics into adolescence and adult life.

infarct (in'-fàr-kt) [L. *infarcire*, to stuff into]. Area of tissue affected, when end artery supplying it is occluded, e.g. in kidney or heart. Common complication of subacute endocarditis.

infarction (in-fàrk'-shun) [L. *infarcire*, to stuff into]. Death of a section of tissue because the blood supply has been cut off.

infection (in-fek'-shun) [L. *infectio*, infection]. The successful invasion, establishment and growth of micro-organisms in the tissues of the host.

infectious disease (in-fek'-shus diz-ēz'). A disease caused by a specific, pathogenic organism and capable of being transmitted to another individual by direct or indirect contact. 'Fevers.'

infectious mononucleosis (in-fek'-shus mon-ō-nū-klē-ō'-sis) [L. *infectio*, infection; G *monos*, one; L. *nucleus*, kernel; G-*osis*, condition]. Most common cause of the glandular fever syndrome (q.v.). Infecting agent is the Epstein-Barr virus. Most primary infections occur in childhood and in early adolescence and may be symptomless, but 60 per cent manifest the glandular fever syndrome. As well as production of specific antibodies to EBV in infectious mononucleosis there is an abnormal antibody which has 'heterophile' activity directed against sheeps' red blood cells—the basis of the Paul-Bunnell test (q.v.) which is positive in IM. One attack confers complete immunity and also lifelong harbouring of the virus in the body—as *viral* particles in saliva (hence the synonym 'kissing disease') and in the lymphocytes.

infective (in-fek'-tiv). Infectious. Disease transmissible from one host to another. infective hepatitis, see HEPATITIS

inferior (in-fēr'-i-or) [L.]. Lower; beneath.

inferiority complex. Term first used by Adler to describe a complex (q.v.) arising from conflict between fear and wish for recognition which results often in compensatory or aggressive behaviour.

infertility (in-fer-til'-i-ti) [L. *infertilis*, unfruitful]. Lack of ability to reproduce. Psychological and physical causes play their part. The abnormality can be in the husband and/or wife. Special clinics exist to investigate this condition.

infestation (in-fes-tā'-shun) [L. *infestare*, to infest]. The presence of animal parasites in or on the human body—infest, v.t.

infiltration (in-fil-trā'-shun). Penetration of the surrounding tissues; the oozing or leaking of fluid into the tissues. infiltration anaesthesia, analgesia produced by infiltrating the tissues with a local anaesthetic.

inflammation (in-flam-mā'-shun) [L. *inflammare*, to set on fire]. The reaction of living tissues to injury, infection, or irritation; characterized by pain, swelling, redness and heat—inflammatory, adj.

influenza (in-floo-en'-za) [It. influence]. An acute viral infection of the naso-pharynx and respiratory tract which occurs in epidemic or pandemic form—influenzal, adj.

infrared rays. Long, invisible rays of the spectrum. Used therapeutically for the production of heat in the tissues.

infundibulum (in-fun-dib´-ū-lum) [L.]. Any funnel-shaped passage—infundibular, adj.; infundibula, pl.

infusion (in-fū´-zhun) [L. *infundere*, to pour into]. 1. Fluid flowing by gravity into the body. 2. An aqueous solution containing the active principle of a drug, made by pouring boiling water on the crude drug. 3. **Amniotic fluid i.** (q.v.).

ingestion (in-jest´-chun) [L. *ingestio*, from *ingerere*, to put into]. The act of taking food or medicine into the stomach.

ingrowing toenail. Spreading of the nail into the lateral tissue, causing inflammation.

inguinal (ing´-gwin-al)[L. *inguen*, groin]. Pertaining to the groin. **inguinal canal,** a tubular opening through the lower part of the anterior abdominal wall, parallel to and a little above the i. (Poupart's) ligament. It measures 38.0 mm. In the male it contains the spermatic cord; in the female the uterine round ligaments. **inguinal hernia,** one occuring through the internal abdominal ring of the i. canal.

inhalation (in-hal-ā´-shun) [L. *in*, in; *halare*, breathe]. 1. The breathing in of air, or other vapour, etc. 2. A medicinal substance which is inhaled.

inherent (in-hē´-rent) [L. *inhoerere*, to adhere to]. Innate; inborn.

inhibition (in-hib-i´-shun) [L. *inhibere*, to restrain]. Loss or partial loss of function either mental or physical as a result of mental (psychic) influences.

injected (in-jek´-ted). Congested, with full vessels.

injection (in-jek´-shun) [L. *injectio*]. 1. The act of introducing a fluid (under pressure) into a vessel, cavity or hollow organ. (Air can be injected into a cavity. See PNEUMOTHORAX.) 2. The substance injected. See HYPODERMIC, INTRA-ARTERIAL, INTRACUTANEOUS, INTRADERMAL, INTRAMUSCULAR, INTRATHECAL, INTRAVASCULAR, INTRAVENOUS, SUBCUTANEOUS.

innate (in-āt-) [L. *innatus*, born]. Inborn, dependent on genetic constitution.

innervation (in-nér-vā´-shun) [L. *in*, in; *nervus*, sinew]. The nerve supply to a part.

innocent (in´-nō-sent) [L. *in*, not; *nocere*, to harm]. Benign; not malignant.

innocuous (in-ok´-ū-us) [L. *innocuus*, harmless]. Harmless.

innominate (in-nom´-in-āt) [L. *innominatus*]. Unnamed.

inoculation (in-ok-ū-lā´-shun) [L. *inoculare*, engraft]. Introduction of material (usually vaccine) into the tissues. Introduction of micro-organisms into culture medium for propagation. Mode of entry of bacteria into body.

inorganic (in-or-gan´-ik). Neither animal nor vegetable in origin.

inosital (in-os´-it-ol). A member of the vitamin B_2 complex.

inotropic (ī-nō-trō´-pik). Having an effect on the contractility of muscles.

inotropic agents. Currently being used in a three-year study of left ventricular function during and after open-heart surgery.

inquest (in´qwest). A legal enquiry, held by a coroner, into the cause of sudden or unexpected death.

insecticide (in-sek´-ti-sīd) [L. *insectum*, cut into; *coedere*, to kill]. An agent which kills insects—insecticidal, adj.

insemination (in-sem-in-ā´-shun) [L. *inseminare*, to implant]. Introduction of semen into the vagina, normally by sexual intercourse. **artificial i.,** instrumental injection of semen into the vagina. See AID and AIH.

insensible (in-sens´-i-bl) [L. *insensibilis*]. Without sensation or consciousness. Too small or gradual to be perceived, as i. perspiration (q.v.).

insertion (in-sèr´-shun) [L. *inserere*, to graft into]. The act of setting or placing in. The attachment of a muscle to the bone it moves.

insidious (in-sid´-i-us) [L. *insidiosus*, cunning]. Having an imperceptible commencement, as of a disease with a late manifestation of definite symptoms.

insight (in´-sit). Ability to accept one's limitations but at the same time to develop one's potentialities. In psychiatry means: (1) knowing that one is ill; (2) a developing knowledge of one's present attitudes and past experiences and the connection between them.

in situ (in-sīt´-ū) [L.]. In the correct position; undisturbed.

insomnia (in-som′-ni-à) [L.]. Sleeplessness.

inspiration (in-spi-rā′-shun). The drawing of air into the lungs; inhalation—inspire, v.t.; inspiratory, adj.

inspissated (in′-spis-ā′-ted) [L. *in*, in; *spissare*, to thicken]. Thickened, as by evaporation or withdrawal of water, applied to sputum and culture media used in the laboratory.

instep (in′-step). The arch of the foot on the dorsal surface.

instillation (in-stil-ā′-shun) [L. *instillare*, to pour in drop by drop]. Insertion of drops into a cavity, e.g. conjunctival sac, external auditory meatus.

instinct (in′-stingkt) [L. *instinctus*, incite]. An inborn tendency to act in a certain way in a given situation, e.g. **paternal i.**, to protect children—instinctive, adj.; instinctively, adv.

insufflation (in-suf-flā′-shun) [L. *insufflare*, to breathe out]. The blowing of air along a tube (Eustachian, Fallopian) to establish patency. The blowing of powder into a body cavity.

insulin (in′-sū-lin). A pancreatic hormone, made in the islet cells of Langerhans, secreted into the blood, and having a profound influence on carbohydrate metabolism by stimulating the transport of glucose into cells. The hormone is prepared commercially in various forms and strengths which vary in their speed, length and potency of action and which are used in the treatment of diabetes mellitus (q.v.).

insulinase (in′-sū-lin-āz). An enzyme that inactivates insulin. **insulinase antagonists** and **inhibitors**, growth hormone, cortisol, glucagon, thyroxine and adrenaline.

insulinoma (in-sū-lin-ō′-ma). Adenoma of the islets of Langerhans in the pancreas. Also insuloma.

Intal (in′-tal). Disodium cromoglycate (q.v.).

integrin (in-teg′-rin). Oxypertine (q.v.).

integument (in-teg′-ū-ment) [L.]. A covering, especially the skin.

intellect (in′-tē-lekt) [L. *intellectus*, understanding]. Reasoning power, thinking faculty.

intelligence (in-tel′-i-jens) [L. *intelligentia*]. Inborn mental ability. **intelligence tests**, designed to determine the level of intelligence. **intelligence quotient**, or **IQ**, the ratio of mental age to chronological (actual) age.

interarticular (in-tèr-âr-tik′-ū-lar) [L. *inter*, between; *articulus*, joint]. Between the articulating surfaces of a joint.

interatrial (in-tèr-ā′-tri-al) [L. *inter*, between; *atrium*, hall]. Between the two atria of the heart. Previously interauricular.

interauricular (in-tèr-awr-ik′-ū-lar). See INTERATRIAL.

intercellular (in-tèr-sel′-ū-lar) [L. *inter*, between; *cellula*, little cell]. Between the cells of a structure.

intercostal (in-tèr-kos′-tal) [L. *inter*, between; *costa*, rib]. Between the ribs.

intercourse (in′-tèr-kōrs) [L. *intercurrere*, to run between]. Communication; coitus.

intercurrent (in-tèr-kur′-ent) [L. *inter*, between; *currere*, to run]. A second disease arising in a person already suffering from one disease.

interferon (in-tèr-fē′-ron) [L. *inter*, between; *ferire*, to strike]. A protein effective against most viruses. When a virus infects a cell, it triggers off the cell's production of i. This then interacts with surrounding cells and renders them resistant to virus attack. Available only in very limited amounts for clinical use as bulk production in the laboratory is difficult and expensive.

interlobar (in-tèr-lō′-bar) [L. *inter*, between; *lobos*, lobe]. Between the lobes, e.g. interlobar pleurisy.

interlobular (in-tèr-lob′-ū-lar) [L. *inter*, between; *lobulus*, small lobe]. Between the lobules.

intermenstrual (in-tèr-men′-strū-al) [L. *inter*, between; *menstrualis*, monthly]. Between the menstrual periods.

intermittent (in-ter-mit′-ent) [L. *intermittere*, to leave off]. Occurring at intervals.

internal (in-tèr′-nal) [L. *internus*]. Inside. **internal ear**, that part of the ear which comprises the vestibule, semicircular canals and the cochlea. **internal secretions**, those produced by the ductless or endocrine glands and passed directly into the blood stream; hormones.

interosseous (in-tèr-os′-ē-us) [L. *inter*, between; *os*, bone]. Between bones.

interphalangeal (in-tèr-fal-an′-jē-al). Between the phalanges.

interposition operation. Vein graft to eardrum.

interserosal (in-ter-sē-rōs′-al) [L. *inter*,

between; *serum*, whey]. Between serous membrane as in the pleural, peritoneal and pericardial cavities—interserosally, adv.

intersexuality (in-ter-seks-ū-al'-i-ti) [L. *inter*, between; *sexus*, sex]. The possession of both male and female characteristics. See TURNER'S and KLINEFELTER'S SYNDROME.

interspinous (in-tẽr-spī'-nus) [L. *inter*, between; *spina*, thorn]. Between spinous processes, especially those of the vertebrae.

interstices (in-tẽr'-sti-sēz) [L. *interstitium*, a place between]. Spaces.

interstitial (in-tẽr-stish'-al). Situated in the interstices of a part; distributed through the connective structures.

intertrigo (in-ter-trī'-gō) [L. *inter*, between; *terere*, to rub]. Superficial inflammation occurring in moist skin folds—intertrigenous, adj.

intertrochanteric (in-tẽr-trō-kan'-ter-ik) [L. *inter*, between; G. *trochanter*]. Between trochanters.

interventricular (in-tẽr-ven-trik'-ū-lar) [L. *inter*, between; *ventricula*, small cavity]. Between ventricles, as those of the brain or heart.

intervertebral (in-tẽr-vẽr'-ti-bral) [L. *inter*, between; *vertebra*]. Between the vertebrae, as discs and foramina. See NUCLEUS, PROLAPSE.

intima (in'-tim-a) [L. *intimus*, innermost]. The internal coat of a blood vessel—intimal, adj.

Intocostrin. A curare muscle relaxant. See MUSCLE.

intolerance (in-tol'-e-rans) [L. *intolerans*]. Inability to bear pain or discomfort. Idiosyncrasy (q.v.) to certain drugs, etc.

intra-abdominal (in-tra-ab-dom'-in-al) [L. *intra*, within; *abdomen*, belly]. Inside the abdomen.

intra-amniotic (in-tra-am-ni-ot'-ik) [L. *intra*, within; G. *amnio*, fetal membrane]. Within, or into the amniotic fluid.

intra-arterial (in-tra-ȧrt-ēr'-i-al) [L. *intra*, within; G. *arteria*, artery]. Within an artery—intra-arterially, adv.

intra-articular (in-tra-ȧrt-ik'-ū-lar) [L. *intra*, within; *articulus*, joint]. Within a joint.

intrabronchial (in-tra-brong'-ki-al) [L. *intra*, within; G. *brogchos*, windpipe]. Within a bronchus.

intracanalicular (in-tra-kan-ȧl'-ik'-ū-lȧr) [L. *intra*, within; *canaliculus*, a small channel]. Within a canaliculus.

intracapillary (in-tra-kap-il'-a-ri) [L. *intra*, within; *capillus*, hair]. Within a capillary.

intracapsular (in-tra-kap'-sū-lar) [L. *intra*, within; *capsula*, small box]. Within a capsule, e.g. that of the lens or a joint. Opp. extracapsular.

intracardiac (in-tra-kȧr'-di-ak) [L. *intra*, within; *kardia*, heart]. Within the heart.

intracaval (in-tra-kā'-val). Within the vena cava, by custom referring to the inferior one—intracavally, adv.

intracellular (intra-sel'-ū-lar) [L. *intra*, within; *cellula*, small cell]. Within a cell. Opp. extracellular.

intracerebral (in-tra-ser'-i-bral) [L. *intra*, within; *cerebrum*, brain]. Within the cerebrum.

intracorpuscular (in-tra-kor-pus'-kū-lar) [L. *intra*, within; *corpusculum*, small body]. Within a corpuscle.

intracranial (in-tra-krā-ni-al) [L. *intra*, within; G. *kranion*, skull]. Within the skull.

intracutaneous (in-tra-kū-tā'-nē-us) [L. *intra*, within; *cutis*, skin]. Within the skin tissues—intracutaneously, adv.

intradermal (in-tra-dẽr'-mal) [L. *intra*, within; G. *derma*, skin]. Within the skin—intradermally, adv.

intradural (in-tra-dū'-ral) [L. *intra*, within; *dura mater*, hard mother]. Inside the dura mater.

Intraflodex (in-tra-flō'-deks). Low molecular weight dextran 10 per cent in normal saline or in 5 per cent dextrose solution. Given as i.v. infusion for prevention and treatment of intravascular sludging and to improve capillary circulation.

intragastric (in-tra-gas'-trik) [L. *intra*, within; G. *gaster*, belly]. Within the stomach.

intragluteal (in-tra-glū-tē'-al) [L. *intra*, within; G. *gloutos*, buttock]. Within the gluteal muscle compressing the buttock—intragluteally, adv.

intrahepatic (in-tra-hep-at'-ik) [L. *intra*, within; G. *hepar*, liver]. Within the liver.

Intralipid (in-tra-lī'-pid). Intravenous fluid. ½ litre, 20 per cent contains 1000 kcal. Prepared from soya bean oil and egg yolk phosphatides.

intralobular (in-tra-lob'-ū-lar) [L. *intra*, within; *lobulus*, small lobe.]. Within the lobule, as the vein draining a hepatic lobule.

intraluminal (in-tra-lū'-min-al) [L. *intra*, within; *lumen*, light]. Within the hollow of a tube-like structure—intraluminally, adv.

intralymphatic (in-tra-lim-fat'-ik) [L. *intra*, within; *lympha*, water]. Within a lymphatic gland or vessel.

intramedullary (in-tra-med-ul'-a-ri) [L. *intra*, within; *medulla*, marrow]. Within the bone marrow.

intramural (in-tra mūr' al) [L. *intra*, within; *murus*, wall]. Within the layers of the wall of a hollow tube or organ— intramurally, adv.

intramuscular (in-tra-mus'-kū-lar) [L. *intra*, within; *musculus*, muscle]. Within a muscle—intramuscularly, adv.

intranasal (in-tra-nā'-zal) [L. *intra*, within; *nasus*, nose]. Within the nasal cavity intranasally, adv.

intranatal (in-tra-nā'-tal) [L. *intra*, within; *natus*, birth]. At the time of birth. Syn., intrapartum (q.v.)—intranatally, adv.

intraocular (in-tra-ok'-ū-lar) [L. *intra*, within; *oculus*, eye]. Within the globe of the eye.

intraoral (in-tra-ō'-ral) [L. *intra* within; *os*, mouth]. Within the mouth as an i. appliance—intraorally, adv.

intraorbital (in-tra-orb'-it-al) [L. *intra*, within; *orbita*, orbit]. Within the orbit.

intraosseous (in-tra-os'-ē-us) [L. *intra*, within; *osseus*, of bone]. Inside a bone.

intrapartum (in-tra-pár'-tum) [L. *intra*, within; *partus*, a birth]. During labour, as asphyxia, haemorrhage or infection.

intraperitoneal (in-tra-per-i-ton-ē'-al) [L. *intra*, within; G. *peri*, around; *tein-ein*, to stretch]. Within the peritoneal cavity—intraperitoneally, adv.

intrapharyngeal (in-tra-far-in-jē'-al) [L. *intra*, within; G. *pharygx*, pharynx]. Within the pharynx—intrapharyngeally, adv.

intraplacental (in-tra-pla-sen'-tal) [L. *intra*, within; *placenta*, cake]. Within the placenta—intraplacentally, adv.

intrapleural (in-tra-ploo'-ral) [L. *intra*, within; G. *pleural*, side]. Within the pleural cavity—intrapleurally, adv.

intrapulmonary (in-tra-pul'-mon-a-ri) [L. *intra*, within; *pulmo*, lung]. Within the lungs, as i. pressure.

intrapunitive (in-tra-pūn'-it-iv). Tending to blame oneself.

intraretinal (in-tra-ret'-i-nal) [L. *intra*, within; *rete*, net]. Within the retina.

intraserosal (in-tra-sē-rōs'-al) [L. *intra*, within; *serum*, whey]. Within a serous membrane. See INTERSEROSAL— intraserosally, adv.

intraspinal (in-tra-spī'-nal) [L. *intra*, within; *spina*, thorn]. Within the spinal canal, as i. anaesthesia—intraspinally, adv.

intrasplenic (in-tra-splen'-ik) [L. *intra*, within; G. *splen*, spleen]. Within the spleen.

intrasynovial (in-tra-sī-nō'-vi-al) [L. *intra*, within; N.L. *synovia*]. Within a synovial membrane or cavity—intra-synovially, adv.

intrathecal (in-tra-thē'-kal) [L. *intra*, within; G. *theke*, a case]. Within the meninges; into the subarachnoid space—intrathecally, adv.

intrathoracic (in-tra-thor-as'-ik) [L. *intra*, within; G. *thorax*, chest]. Within the cavity of the thorax.

intratracheal (in-tra-trak-ē'-al) [L. *intra*, within; L.L. *trachia*, windpipe]. Within or through the trachea. **intratracheal anaesthesia**, the administration of an anaesthetic through a special tube passed down the trachea—intratrach-eally, adv.

intratumour (in-tra-tū'-mor) [L. *intra*, within; L. *tumor*, swelling]. Within a tumour.

intrauterine (in-tra-ū'-te-rīn) [L. *intra*, within; *uterus*, womb]. Within the uterus. See IUCD.

intravaginal (in-tra-va-jī'-nal) [L. *intra*, within; *vagina*, sheath]. Within the vagina—intravaginally, adv.

Intraval (in'-tra-val). Thiopentone (q.v.).

intravascular (in-tra-vas'-kū-lar) [L. *intra*, within; *vasculum*, small vessel]. Within the blood vessels—intravascularly, adv.

intravenous (in-tra-vē'-nus) [L. *intra*, within; *vena*, vein]. Within or into a vein—intravenously, adv.

intraventricular (in-tra-ven-trik'-ū-lar) [L. *intra*, within; *ventriculus*, cavity]. Within a ventricle, especially a cerebral ventricle.

intrinsic (in-trin'-sik) [L. *intrinsecus*, inward]. Inherent or inside; from within; real; natural. **intrinsic factor,** a protein released by gastric glands, essential for the satisfactory absorption of the extrinsic factor vitamin B_{12}.

introitus (in-trō'-it-us) [L.]. Any opening in the body; an entrance to a cavity, particularly the vagina.

introjection (in-trō-jek'-shun) [L. *intro*, inward; *jacere*, to throw]. A mental process whereby a person identifies himself with another person or object.

introspection (in-trō-spek'-shun) [L. *intro*, within; *spicere*, look]. Study by a person of his own mental processes. Seen in an exaggerated form in schizophrenia.

introversion (in-trō-vėr'-shun) [L. *introversus*, inward]. The direction of thoughts and interest inwards to the world of ideas, instead of outwards to the external world—introvert, n.

intubation (in-tū-bā'-shun) [L. *in*, in; *tubus*, tube]. Insertion of a tube into a hollow organ, especially into (or via) the larynx. Used, prior to anaesthesia, to promote suction of the respiratory tract, to maintain an airway—See INTRATRACHEAL. **duodenal i.,** a double tube is passed as far as the pyloric antrum under fluoroscopy. The inner tube is then passed along to the duodenojejunal flexure. Barium can then be passed to outline the bowel.

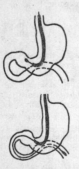

Intubation

intussusception (in-tus-sus-sep'-shun) [L. *intus*, within; *suscipere*, to receive]. A condition in which one part of the bowel slips into (invaginates) the lower part, causing intestinal obstruction. It occurs most commonly in infants.

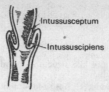

Intussusception

intussusceptum (in-tus-sus-sep'-tum). The invaginated portion of an intussusception.

intussuscipiens (in-tus-sus-sip'-i-ens). The receiving portion of an intussusception.

inunction (in-ungk'-shun) [L. *inunctio*, anointing]. The act of rubbing an oily or fatty substance into the skin.

invagination (in-vaj-in-ā'-shun) [L. *in*, in; *vagina*, sheath]. The act or condition of being ensheathed; a pushing inward, forming a pouch—invaginate, v.t.

invasion (in-vā'-zhun) [L. *invasio*, attack]. The entry of bacteria into the body.

Inversine (in'-ver-sēn). Mecamylamine (q.v.).

inversion (in-vėr'-shun) [L. *inversio*, upside down]. Turning inside out, as i. of the uterus. See PROCIDENTIA.

invertase (in'-ver-tās) [L. *invertere*, to turn into]. A sugar-splitting enzyme in intestinal juice.

in vitro (vi'-trō) [L.]. In glass, as in a test-tube.

in vivo (vī'-vō) [L.]. In living tissue.

involucrum (in-vol-ūk'-rum) [L. covering]. A sheath of new bone, which forms around necrosed bone, in such conditions as osteomyelitis. See CLOACA.

involuntary (in-vol'-un-ta-ri) [L. *involuntarius*]. Independent of the will, as muscle of the chest and abdominal organs.

involution (in-vol-ū'-shun) [L. *involutus*, rolled up]. The normal shrinkage of an organ after fulfilling its functional purpose, e.g. uterus after labour. In psychiatry, the period of decline after middle life—involutional, adj.

Iodatol (ī-ōd'-at-ol). Iodized oil (q.v.).

Iodex (ī'-ō-deks). A non-staining iodine ointment. Used as a counterirritant in sprains, chilblains, etc.

iodides (ī'-ō-dīdz). Compounds of iodine and a base. Potassium and sodium iodide are the most common medicinal iodides.

iodine (ī'-ō-dēn). Powerful antiseptic used as a tincture for skin preparation and emergency treatment of small wounds. Orally it is antithyroid, i.e. it decreases release of the hormones from the thyroid gland. **povidone i.**, antibacterial. See BETADINE. **protein-bound i.** (PBI), estimated in thyroid investigations. **radioactive i.** ([181]I) is used in investigation and treatment of thyrotoxicosis.

iodism (ī'-ō-dizm). Poisoning with iodides; the symptoms are those of a common cold and the appearance of a rash.

iodized oil (ī'-od-izd). Poppy-seed oil containing 40 per cent of organically combined iodine. Should be colourless or pale yellow; darker solutions have decomposed. Used as contrast agent in X-ray examination of bronchial tract, sinuses and other cavities.

iodoform (ī-ō'-dō-form). Antiseptic iodine compound of yellow colour and characteristic odour. Now used chiefly as BIPP (q.v.).

iodopsin (ī-ō-dop'-sin). A protein substance which, with vitamin A, is a constituent of visual purple present in the rods in the retina of the eye.

iodoxyl (ī-ō-doks'-il). A contrast agent containing 50 per cent of combined iodine. Given by slow intravenous injection in pyelography. The solution is irritant, and extravenous injection must be avoided. For this reason diodone (q.v.) is often preferred.

ion (ī'-on). A charged atom which, in electrolysis, passes to one or the other pole, or electrode—ionic, adj.

ionization (ī-on-ī-zā'-shun). Treatment whereby ions of various substances, e.g. zinc, chlorine, iodine, histamine, are introduced into the skin by means of a constant electrical current.

iopanoic acid (ī-ō-pan-ō'-ik-as'-id). A complex iodine derivative of butyric acid; used as a contrast agent in cholecystography. Side reactions are few, and it gives denser shadows than the earlier pheniodol.

ipecacuanha (ip-i-kak-ū-an'-á). Dried root from Brazil and other South American countries. Principal alkaloid is emetine (q.v.). Has expectorant pro-perties, and is widely used in acute bronchitis and relief of dry cough. A safe emetic in larger doses.

IPP. Intermittent positive pressure. Used to inflate the lungs (inspiration). Expiration is by recoil of elastic lung tissue.

iprindol (ip-rin'-dol). Tricyclic antidepressant. Has few side effects; tolerated well by most people; slight risk of jaundice in allergic people.

iproniazid (ip-rō-nī'-az-id). Antidepressant. MAOI. (q.v.). Antituberculosis.

ipsilateral (ip-si-lat'-er-al) [L. *ipse*, self; *latus*, side]. On the same side—ipsilaterally, adv.

IQ. Intelligence (q.v.) quotient.

iridectomy (ir-i-dek'-to-mi) [L. *iris*, rainbow; G. *ektome*, excision]. Excision of a part of the iris, thus forming an artificial pupil.

iridencleisis (ir-id-en-klī'-sis). A filtering operation. Scleral incision made at angle of anterior chamber; meridian cut in iris; either one or both pillars are left in scleral wound to contract as scar tissue. Decreases intraocular tension in glaucoma.

iridocele (ir-id-ō-sēl') [L. *iris*, rainbow; G. *kele*, hernia]. Protrusion of part of the iris through a corneal wound (prolapsed iris). Iridoptosis.

iridocyclitis (ir-id-ō-sī-klī'-tis) [L. *iris*, rainbow; G. *kyklos*, circle;-*itis*, inflammation]. Inflammation of the iris and ciliary body.

iridodialysis (ir-id-ō-dī-al'-i-sis) [L. *iris*, rainbow; G. *dialysis*, a separating]. A separation of the iris from its ciliary attachment.

iridoplegia (ir-id-ō-plē'-ji-a) [L. *iris*, rainbow; G. *plege*, stroke]. Paralysis of the iris.

iridoptosis (ir-id-op-tō'-sis) [L. *iris*, rainbow; G. *ptosis*, a failing]. Prolapse of the iris.

iridotomy (ir-id-ot'-om-i) [L. *iris*, rainbow; G. *tome*, a cutting]. An incision into the iris.

iris (ī'-ris) [L. rainbow]. The circular coloured membrane forming the anterior one-sixth of the middle coat of the eyeball. It is perforated in the centre by an opening named 'the pupil.' Contraction of its muscle fibres regulates the amount of light entering the eye. **iris bombé,** bulging forward of iris due to pressure of aqueous behind, when posterior synechiae are present.

iritis (ī-rī'-tis) [L. *iris*, rainbow; G. *-itis*, inflammation]. Inflammation of the iris.

iron and ammonium citrate. A soluble non-irritant iron complex, now rarely used in the oral treatment of iron deficiency anaemia.

iron gluconate (gloo'-kon-āt). An organic salt of iron, less irritant and better tolerated than ferrous sulphate.

irreducible (ir-rē-dū'-si-bl) [L. *irredux*, does not bring back]. Cannot be brought to desired condition. **irreducible hernia**, when the contents of the sac cannot be returned to the appropriate cavity, without surgical intervention.

irritable (ir'-it-abl) [L. *irritare*, to irritate]. Capable of being excited to activity; responding easily to stimuli—irritability, n.

irritant (Ir'-it-ant) [L. *irritare*, to irritate]. Any agent which causes irritation.

ischaemia (is-kē'-mi-à) [G. *ischein*, to check; *haima*, blood]. Deficient blood supply. See ANGINA, VOLKMANN—ischaemic, adj.

ischiorectal (is-ki-ō-rek'-tal) [G. *ischion*, hip; *rectus*, straight]. Pertaining to the ischium and the rectum, as an i. abscess which occurs between these two structures.

ischium (is'-ki-um) [G. *ischion*, hip]. The lower part of the innominate bone of the pelvis; the bone on which the body rests when sitting—ischial, adj.

islets of Langerhans (ī'-letz lan'-ger-hans). Collections of special cells scattered throughout the pancreas. They secrete insulin which is poured directly into the blood stream. [Paul Langerhans, German pathologist, 1847-88.]

Ismelin (is'-me-lin). Guanethidine (q.v.).

isocarboxazid (ī-zō-kar-boks'-a-zid). Antidepressant. MAOI.

I-so-gel (ī'-sō-jel). Granules prepared from the husks of mucilaginous seeds, and used as a bulk-forming laxative in chronic constipation.

isoimmunization (ī-sō-im-mū-nī-zā'-shun) [G. *isos*, equal; L. *immunis*, exempt from public burden]. Development of anti-Rh agglutins in the blood of an Rh-negative person who has been given an Rh-positive transfusion, or who is carrying an Rh-positive fetus.

isolator (ī'-sō-lā-tor). Apparatus ranging from what is virtually a large plastic bag in which a patient can be nursed to that in which an operation can be performed. It aims to prevent bacterial entry to or exit from the enclosed space.

isoleucine (ī'-sō-lū-sēn). One of the essential amino acids (q.v.).

Isolevin (ī-so-lev'-in). Isoprenaline sulphate (q.v.).

isometric (ī-sō-met'-rik). Of equal proportions. **isometric exercises**, carried out without movement; maintain muscle tone.

isoniazid (ī-so-nī'-az-id). A derivative of isonicotinic acid. It has a specific action against the tubercle bacillus, and is widely employed in the treatment of tuberculosis. Combined treatment with other tuberculostatic drugs such as streptomycin and PAS is not only more effective than any drug alone, but the risk of bacterial resistance is also reduced. Can be neurotoxic.

isoprenaline sulphate (ī-so-pren'-a-lēn). An adrenaline derivative with similar bronchodilator properties. Given in asthma, etc., as sublingual tablets of 20 mg; also by spray inhalation. Speeds up the heart in heart block (Stokes-Adams syndrome).

isotonic (ī-sō-ton'-ik) [G. *isos*, equal; *tonos*, tension]. Equal tension; applied to any solution which has the same osmotic pressure as blood. **isotonic saline** (syn., normal saline), 0.9 per cent solution of salt in water.

isotopes (ī'-sō-tōpz) [G. *iso*, equal; *topos*, place]. Two or more forms of the same element having identical chemical, but differing physical properties. Those isotopes with radioactive properties are used in medicine for research, diagnosis and treatment of disease.

isoxazole penicillins (i-soks'-a-zol). Can be taken orally. Give high blood levels of penicillin in a freely available form to act against staphylococci, after absorption. Particularly effective for boils and carbuncles.

isoxuprine (is-oks'-ū-prēn). Peripheral vasodilator, and spasmolytic. Acts on myometrium preventing contractions, thus useful in premature labour.

isoxyl (īs-oks'-il). New drug used for tuberculosis, in conjunction with other antituberculous drugs.

itch. See SCABIES. **itch mite**, *Sarcoptes scabiei* (q.v.).

IUCD. Intrauterine contraceptive device. See IUD.

IUD. Intrauterine device. Over 60 different forms known by the International Planning Parenthood Federation.

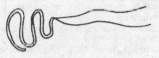

Birnberg bow (top)
Margulies spiral (centre)
Lippes loop (bottom)

Types of IUD

Izal (ī-zal). An emulsion of tar oils, widely used as a general disinfectant and deodorant for drains, skins, floors, etc. 'White fluid.'

J

Jacksonian epilepsy. See EPILEPSY. [John Hughlings Jackson, English neurologist, 1835–1911.]

Jacquemier's sign (zhak'-mē-ās). Blueness of the vaginal mucosa seen in early pregnancy. [Jean Marie Jacquemier, French obstetrician, 1806–79.]

jaundice (jawn'-dis). Syn., icterus. A condition characterized by a raised bilirubin level in the blood (hyperbilirubinaemia). Minor degrees are only detectable chemically—latent j.; major degrees are visible in the yellow skin, sclerae and mucosae—overt or clinical j. Jaundice may be due to (1) obstruction anywhere in the biliary tract (obstructive j), (2) excessive haemolysis of red blood cells (haemolytic j.), (3) toxic or infective damage of liver cells (hepatocellular j.), (4) bile stasis (cholestatic j.). **acholuric j.,** jaundice without bile in the urine; usually reserved for a familial disease—congenital haemolytic anaemia—characterized by abnormally fragile, small, spheroidal, red

blood cells which haemolyse readily. Spherocytosis (q.v.). **infective j.,** most commonly due to a virus; infective hepatitis (q.v.). **leptospiral j.,** See WEIL'S DISEASE. **malignant j.,** acute yellow atrophy of the liver. See ACUTE. **jaundice of the newborn,** icterus neonatorum (q.v.).

jaw-bone. Either the maxilla (upper jaw) or mandible (lower jaw).

Jectofer. An iron-sorbitol citric acid complex used for parenteral iron therapy.

jejunostomy (je-joon-os'-to-mi) [L. *jejunus*, empty; G. *stoma*, mouth]. A surgically made fistula between the jejunum and the anterior abdominal wall; used temporarily for feeding in cases where passage of food through the stomach is impossible or undesirable.

jejunum (je-joo'-num) [L. *jejunus*, empty]. That part of the small intestine between the duodenum and the ileum. It is about 2.438 m in length—jejunal, adj.

Jelonet (jel-on-et'). Paraffin gauze dressing consisting of specially woven (interlock) gauze impregnated with a soft paraffin mass for burns and wounds, etc.

jigger (jī' gēr) (*Tunga penetrans*). A flea, prevalent in the tropics. It burrows under the skin to lay its eggs, causing intense irritation. Secondary infection is usual.

joint. The articulation of two or more bones (arthrosis). There are three main classes: (1) fibrous (synarthrosis), e.g. the sutures of the skull; (2) cartilaginous (synchondrosis), e.g. between the manubrium and the body of the sternum; and (3) synovial, e.g. elbow or hip. **charcot's j.,** syphilitic degeneration of joint surfaces and surrounding structures. See CHARCOT.

joint-breaker fever. Syn., o'nyong-nyong fever (q.v.).

joule. The SI (International System, of Units) unit for measuring energy, work and quantity of heat. The unit (J) is the energy expended when 1 kg (kilogram) is moved 1 m (metre) by a force of 1 N (newton). The kilojoule (kJ = 10^3 J) and the megajoule (MJ = 10^6 J) is used by physiologists and nutritionists for large amounts of energy.

jugular (jug'-ū-lar) [L. *jugulum*, collarbone]. Pertaining to the throat. **j. veins,**

two veins passing down either side of the neck.

junket (jun'-ket). Milk predigested by the addition of rennet. Curds and whey.

juxtaposition (juks'-ta pō-zish-un) [L. near; *position,* a placing]. The act of placing side by side.

K

K285. A processed starch powder used as an alternative to talc for rubber gloves. Unlike talc, it does not cause granuloma.

kala-azar (ká-lá-áz'-ár). A generalized form of leishmaniasis occurring in the tropics. There is anaemia, fever, splenomegaly and wasting. It is caused by the parasite *Leishmania donovani* and is spread by sandflies.

kanamycin (kan-a-mī'-sin). Similar to neomycin and is a streptomycin-like antibiotic with basically similar neurotoxic properties but nonetheless useful in severe infections. Can be used for tuberculosis.

Kanner's syndrome. Autism (q.v.) described in 1944.

kaolin (kā'-ō-lin). Natural aluminium silicate. When given orally it absorbs toxic substances, hence useful in diarrhoea, colitis and food poisoning. Also used as a dusting powder; when mixed with glycerin, boric acid, etc. it is used as a poultice.

kaomycin (kā-ō-mī'-sin). Neomycin (q.v.) and kaolin (q.v.).

Kapilon (kap'-il-on). Acetomenaphthone (q.v.).

Kaposi's varicelliform eruption. Occurs in eczematous children. Generalized bullous eczema; formerly fatal. [Moritz K. Kaposi, Austrian dermatologist, 1837–1902.]

katabolism. See CATABOLISM.

Katonium (ka-tō'-ni-um). A synthetic resin that can bring about changes in the electrolyte balance by removing sodium from the body. Used in oedema due to sodium retention in congestive heart failure, and hypertension.

Keflex (kef'-leks). Cephalexin monohydrate (q.v.).

Keflin (kef'-lin). Cephalothin sodium (q.v.).

Kelfizine (kel'-fiz-ēn). Sulfametopyrazine (q.v.).

Keller's operation. For hallux valgus or rigidus. Excision of the proximal half of the proximal phalanx, plus any osteophytes and exostoses on the metatarsal head. The toe is fixed in the corrected position; after healing a fibrous arthroplasty results. [William Lordan Keller, US Army surgeon (retired) of Washington, 1874–1959.]

Kelly-Paterson syndrome. Also called 'Plummer-Vinson syndrome' (q.v.).

kellin (kel'-lin). Has properties similar to glyceryl trinitrate, and is given in angina pectoris.

Kelocyanor (kel-ō-sī'-an-or). See COBALT EDETATE.

keloid(kē'-loid) [G. *kelis,* spot; *eidos,* form]. An overgrowth of scar tissue, which may produce a contraction deformity.

Kemadrin (ke'-ma-drin). Procyclidine (q.v.).

Kemithal (ke'-mi-thal). Thialbarbitone (q.v.).

keratectomy (ke-ra-tek'-to-mi)[G. *keras,* horn; *ektome,* excision]. Removal of a portion of the cornea.

keratitic precipitates (KP) (ker-a-ti'-tik pre-sip'-i-tāz). Large cells adherent to posterior surface of cornea; present in inflammation of iris, ciliary body and choroid.

keratin (ker'-a-tin) [G. *keras,* horn]. A protein found in all horny tissue. Used to coat pills given for their intestinal effect, since k. can withstand gastric juice.

keratinization (ker-at-in-īz-ā'-shun) [G. *keras,* horn]. Conversion into horny tissue. Occurs as a pathological process in vitamin A deficiency.

keratitis (ke-ra-tī'-tis) [G. *keras,* horn; *-itis,* inflammation]. Inflammation of the cornea.

keratoconjunctivitis (ker-a-tō-konjungk-tiv-ī'-tis) [G. *keras,* horn; L. *conjunctivus,* serving to connect; G. *-itis,* inflammation]. Inflammation of the cornea and conjunctiva. **epidemic k.,** due to an adenovirus (q.v.). Presents as an acute follicular conjunctivitis with pre-auricular and submaxillary adenitis. **keratoconjunctivitis sicca,** see SJÖGREN'S SYNDROME.

keratoconus (ke-ra-tō-kō'-nus) [G. *keras,* horn; *konos,* cone]. A cone-like protrusion of the cornea, usually due to a non-inflammatory thinning.

keratoiritis (ke-ra-tō-ī-rī'-tis) [G. *keras,* horn; L. *iris,* rainbow; G. *-itis,* inflammation]. Inflammation of the cornea and iris.

keratolytic (ke-ra-tol'-i-tic). Having the property of breaking down keratinized epidermis.

keratoma (ke-ra-tō'-má) [G. keras, horn; -oma, tumour]. An overgrowth of horny tissue. Callosity—keratomata, pl.

keratomalacia (ke-ra-tō-mal-ā'-sē-à) [G. keras, horn; malakia, softness]. Softening of the cornea; ulcerationmay occur; frequently caused by lack of vitamin A.

keratome (ker'-a-tōm) [G. keras, horn; tomos, cutting]. A special knife with a trowel-like blade for incising the cornea.

keratomileusis (ker-a-to-mil-ū'-sis) [G. keras, horn; mileusis, to carve]. Surgical treatment for correction of myopia.

keratopathy (ke-ra-top'-a-thi) [G. keras, horn; pathos, disease]. Any disease of the cornea—keratopathic, adj.

keratophakia (ker-a-to-fāk'-i-à) [G. keras, horn; phakos, lentil (lens)]. Surgical treatment for correction of hypermetropia.

keratoplasty (ke-ra-tō-plas'-ti) [G. keras, horn; plassein, to form]. Corneal grafting. Replacing of unhealthy tissue with healthy tissue obtained from a donor—keratoplastic, adj.

keratosis (ke-ra-tō'-sis) [G. keras, horn; -osis, condition]. Thickening of the horny layer of the skin. Also referred to as 'hyperkeratosis.' Has appearance of warty excrescences. keratosis palmaris et plantaris (or tylosis) is a congenital thickening of the horny layer of the palms and soles. splar k. (Peasant's neck) is a form of chronic dermatitis on exposed areas and is a reaction to excessive sunlight.

Kerecid (ker'-e-sid). Idoxuridine (q.v.).

kerion (kē'-ri-on) [G. kerion, honeycomb]. A boggy suppurative mass of the scalp associated with ringworm of the hair.

kernicterus (ker-nik'-ter-us). Bile staining of the basal ganglia in the brain which may result in mental deficiency, and occurring in icterus gravis neonatorum (q.v.).

Kernig's sign (ker'-nigs). Inability to straighten the leg at the knee joint when the thigh is flexed at right angles to the trunk. Occurs in meningitis. [Vladimir Kernig, Russian physician, 1840–1917.]

Ketalar (ket'-al-ar). Ketamine hydrochloride (q.v.).

ketamine hydrochloride (ket'-a-mēn-hī-drō-klor'-īd). Intravenous or intramuscular anaesthetic agent. Initial dose determined by patient's weight. Does not have muscular relaxation properties and is therefore unsuitable for intra-abdominal procedures.

ketogenic diet (kē-tō-jen'-ik). A high fat content producing ketosis (acidosis).

ketonaemia (kē-tōn-ē'-mi-à) [Ger: keton; G. haima, blood]. Ketone bodies in the blood   ketonaemic, adj.

ketone (kē-tōn). k. bodies in ketosis (q.v.). Also used of the CO group (carbonyl) in the structural formulae of organic compounds, e.g. ketosteroids (q.v.).

ketonuria (kē-tōn-ū'-ri-à) [Ger. keton; G. ouron, urine]. Ketone bodies in the urine—ketonuric, adj.

ketosis (kē-tō'-sis) [Ger. keton; G. -osis, condition]. Clinical picture arises from accumulation in blood stream of ketone bodies, β-hydroxybutyric acid, acetoacetic acid and acetone. Syndrome includes drowsiness, headache and deep respiration—ketotic, adj.

ketosteroids (kē-tō-ste'-roids). Steroid hormones which contain a keto group, formed by the addition of an oxygen molecule to the basic ring structure. The 17-ketosteroids (which have this oxygen at carbon 17) are excreted in normal urine, and are present in excess in overactivity of the adrenal glands and the gonads.

Ketovite (ket'-o-vīt). Tablets and liquid. Contains vitamins A, D, C, B_{12}, B_6, B_2, B_1, folic acid, nicotinamide, calcium pantothenate, inositol, biotin, acetomenaphthone, tocopheryl acetate and choline chloride.

kidneys (kid-niz). Two glands situated in the upper, posterior abdominal cavity, one on either side of the vertebral column. Their function is to secrete urine.

Killian's operation. Curetting of the frontal sinus, leaving the supraorbital ridge intact to reduce deformity. [Gustav Killian, German laryngologist and rhinologist, 1860–1921.]

Kimmelstiel-Wilson syndrome. Intercapillary glomerulosclerosis present in diabetics, with hypertension, albuminuria and oedema. [Paul Kimmelstiel, German pathologist, 1900–   . Clifford Wilson, English physician, 1906- .]

kinaesthesis (kī-nes-thē'-sis) [G. *kinein*, to move; *aisthesis*, sensation]. Muscle sense; perception of movement—kinaesthetic, adj.

kinase (kī'-nās). An enzyme-activator. Syn., co-enzyme. See ENTEROKINASE, THROMBOKINASE.

kineplastic surgery (kī-nē-plas'-tik sur'-jer-i). Operative measures, whereby certain muscle groups are isolated, and utilized to work certain modified prostheses.

kinetic (kin'-et-ik). Pertaining to, or producing motion.

Kirschner wire (kirsch'-ner). A wire drilled into a bone to apply skeletal traction. A hand or electric drill is used, a stirrup attached and the wire rendered taut by means of a special wire-tightener. [Martin Kirschner, German surgeon, 1879–1942.]

kiss of life. Method of artificial respiration. Exhaled breath of operator inflates the patient's lungs. Routes: (1) mouth to mouth; (2) mouth to nose; (3) mouth to nose and mouth.

Klebsiella Genus of bacteria. *Klebsiella pneumoniae* is the cause of a rare form of pneumonia. See FRIEDLÄNDER'S BACILLUS.

Klebs-Loeffler bacillus (syn., *Corynebacterium diphtheriae*). A clinicolaboratory term for the diphtheria bacillus named after the discoverers of the organism. [Theodor Klebs, German bacteriologist, 1834–1913. Friedrich A. J. Loeffler, German bacteriologist, 1852–1915.]

kleptomania (klep-to-mā'-ni-à) [G. *kleptein*, to steal; *mania*, madness]. Compulsive stealing due to mental disturbance, usually of the obsessional neurosis type.

Klinefelter's syndrome. A person with 44 autosomes and XXY sex chromosomes, making a total complement of 47. Individual appears to be male, but he has large breasts, small genitalia, atrophied testes and is sterile. Genetic female, pragmatic male. Increased height apparent before puberty. It is possible that the violence and aggression have an organic basis which may be reflected in the EEG. Commonly recognized only in adult life in sterility clinic. [Harry F. Klinefelter, Jr, American physician, 1912- .]

Klumpke's paralysis. Paralysis and atrophy of muscles of forearm and hand, with sensory and pupillary disturbances due to injury to cervical sympathetic nerves. Clawhand results. [Madame Klumpke, French neurologist, 1859–1927.]

knee. The hinge joint formed by the lower end of the femur and the head of the tibia. knee cap, the patella. knee jerk, a reflex contraction of the relaxed quadriceps muscle elicited by a tap on the patellar tendon: usually performed with the lower femur supported behind, the knee bent and the leg limp. Persistent variation from normal usually signifies organic nervous disorder.

knuckles (nuk'-ls). The dorsal aspect of any of the joints between the phalanges and the metacarpal bones, or between the phalanges.

Koch's bacillus (syn., *Mycobacterium tuberculosis*). A term used for the tubercle bacillus in clinicolaboratory parlance and named after Koch, who first described the bacillus. [Robert Koch, German bacteriologist, 1843–1910.]

Koch-Weeks bacillus (syn., *Haemophilus aegyptius*). A small Gram-negative rod, characteristically intracellular in polymorphs in exudate. The cause of a form of acute infectious conjunctivitis. [Robert Koch, German bacteriologist, 1843–1910. John E. Weeks, American ophthalmologist, 1853–1949.]

Köhler's disease (kė'-lers). Osteochondritis of the navicular bone. Confined to children of 3 to 5 years. [Alban Köhler, German physician, 1874–1947.]

koilonychia (koil-o-nik'-i-à) [G. *koilos*, hollow; *onyx*, nail]. Spoon-shaped nails, characteristic of iron deficiency anaemia.

Konakion. Phytomenadione. Vitamin K. Can be given intravenously.

Koplik's spots. Small white spots inside the mouth, during the first few days of the invasion (prodromal) stage of measles. [Henry Koplik, New York paediatrician, 1858–1927.]

Korsakoff's psychosis or syndrome. A condition which follows delirium and toxic states. Often due to alcoholism. The consciousness is clear and alert, but the patient is disorientated for time and place. His memory is grossly impaired, especially for recent events. Often he confabulates to fill the gaps in his memory. Alcoholic dementia. Polyneuritic psychosis. Afflicts more men than women in the 45–55 age group. [Sergei S. Korsakoff, Russian neurologist, 1854–1900.]

Krabbe's disease. Genetically determined degenerative disease associated with mental subnormality. [Knud H. Krabbe, Danish neurologist, 1885–1961.]

kraurosis vulvae (kraw-rō'-sis vul'-vē). A degenerative condition of the vaginal introitus associated with postmenopausal lack of oestrogen.

Krukenberg tumour (kroo'-ken-berg). A secondary malignant tumour of the ovary. The primary growth is usually in the stomach. [Friedrich Ernst Krukenberg, German pathologist, 1871–1946.]

Küntscher nail. Used for intramedullary fixation of fractures of long bones, especially the femur. The nail has a 'clover-leaf' cross section. [Gerhard Küntscher, orthopaedic surgeon of Kiel, 1902-   .]

kuru (koo'-roo). Slow virus disease of central nervous system. Probably transmitted by cannibalism. Rare and declining in incidence. Occurred exclusively among New Guinea highlanders.

kwashiorkor (kwash-ē-or'-kor). A nutritional disorder of infants and young children when the diet is persistently deficient in essential protein; commonest in primitive tropical races where maize is the staple diet. Characteristic features are anaemia, wasting, dependent oedema and a fatty liver. Untreated, it progresses to death.

KY jelly. A mucilaginous lubricating jelly.

kymograph (kī' mō graf) [G. *kyma* wave; *graphein*, to write]. An apparatus for recording movements, e.g. of muscles, columns of blood. Used in physiological experiments—kymographic, adj.; kymographically, adv.

kypholordosis (ki-fō-lor-dō'-sis). Coexistence of kyphosis and lordosis (q.v.).

kyphoscoliosis (kī-fō-skōl'-i-ō-sis). Coexistence of kyphosis and scoliosis (q.v.).

kyphosis (kī-fō'-sis) [G. hunch-backed]. As in Pott's disease, an excessive backward curvature of the dorsal spine.

L

labetalol (lab-et'-al-ol). New combined alpha- beta-blocking drug useful in the acute control of severe hypertension; given by i.v. infusion.

labia (lā'-bi-á) [L.]. Lips. **labia majora**, two large lip-like folds extending from the mons veneris to encircle the vagina. **labia minora**, two smaller folds lying within the l. majora—labium, sing.; labial, adj.

labile (lā'-bīl) [L. *labilis*, apt to slip]. Unstable; readily changed, as many drugs when in solution.

lability (la-bil'-i-ti). Instability. **emotional l.**, rapid change in mood. Occurs especially in the mental disorders of old age.

labioglossolaryngeal (lā-bi-ō-glos-ō-lar-in-jē'-al) [L. *labium*, lip; G. *glossa*, tongue; *larygx*, larynx]. Relating to the lips, tongue and larynx **labioglossolaryngeal paralysis**, a nervous disease characterized by progressive paralysis of the lips, tongue and larynx.

labioglossopharyngeal (lā-bi-ō-glos-ō-far-in-jē'-al) [L. *labium*, lip; G. *glosso*, tongue; *pharygx*, pharynx]. Relating to the lips, tongue and pharynx.

labour (lā'-bor) [L. *labor*, toil]. The act of giving birth to a child; parturition. The first stage lasts from onset until there is full dilation of the cervical os; the second stage lasts until the baby is delivered; the third stage until the placenta is expelled.

labyrinth (lab'-i-rinth) [G. *labyrinthos*, labyrinth]. The tortuous cavities of the internal ear. **bony l.**, that part which is directly hollowed out of the temporal bone. **membranous l.**, the membrane which loosely lines the bony labyrinth—labyrinthine, adj.

labyrinthectomy (lab-i-rinth-ek'-to-mi) [G. *labyrinthos*, labyrinth; *ektome*, excision]. Surgical removal of part or the whole of the membranous labyrinth of the internal ear.

labyrinthitis (lab-ir-in-thī'-tis) [G. *labyrinthos*, labyrinth; *-itis*, inflammation]. Inflammation of the internal ear. Syn., otitis interna.

laceration (las-er-ā'-shun) [L. *lacerare*, to tear]. A wound with torn and ragged edges—lacerate, v.t.

lachesine (lash'-es-ēn). E₃. An alternative mydriatic in atropine sensitivity.

lachrymal (lak'-ri-mal). Also spelt lacrymal. See LACRIMAL.

lacrimal (lak'-ri-mal) [L. *lacrima*, a tear]. Pertaining to tears. **lacrimal bone**, a tiny bone at the inner side of the orbital cavity. **lacrimal duct**, connects l. gland to upper conjunctival sac. **lacrimal gland**, situated above the upper, outer canthus of the eye.

lacrimation (lak-ri-mā'-shun). An outflow of tears; weeping.

lacrimonasal (lak-ri-mō-nā'-zal) [L. *lacrima*, tear; *nasus*, nose]. Pertaining to the lacrimal and nasal bones and ducts.

lactagogue (lak'-ta-gog) [L. *lac*, milk; G. *agogos*, leading]. Any substance to stimulate lactation; none are very effective as yet.

lactalbumin (lakt-al-bū'-min) [L. *lac*, milk; *albumen*, egg-white]. The more easily digested of the two milk proteins. See CASEINOGEN.

lactase (lak'-tās). A saccharolytic enzyme of intestinal juice; it splits lactose into glucose (dextrose) and galactose.

lactase deficiency. Clinical syndrome of milk intolerance. In severe intolerance the infant may pass a litre or more of fluid stool per day. Temporary intolerance can follow neonatal alimentary tract obstructions, but rarely gives long-term problems.

lactate dehydrogenase (lak'-tāt de-hīd-roj'-en-ās). An enzyme of which there are five versions (isozymes) in the body. LDH-1 is the one in the heart; its blood level rises rapidly when heart tissue dies. After heart transplant, rejection is imminent when the LDH-1 activity is greater than that of its isozyme LDH-2 during the first 4 post-operative weeks. After 6 months this diagnostic indication disappears.

lactation (lak-tā'-shun) [L. *lactare*, to suckle]. Secretion of milk. Suckling; the period during which the child is nourished from the breast.

lacteals (lak'-tē-als) [L. *lac*, milk]. The commencing lymphatic ducts in the intestinal villi; they absorb split fats and convey them to the receptaculum chyli.

lactic acid (lak'-tik as'-id). The acid that causes the souring of milk. It is obtained by the fermentation of lactose; used as a vaginal douche, 1 per cent. Sometimes added to milk (1 drachm to 1 pint) to produce fine curds for the treatment of gastroenteritis in infants.

lactiferous (lak-tif'-er-us) [L. *lac*, milk; *ferre*, to carry]. Conveying or secreting milk.

lactifuge (lak'-tē-fūj) [L. *lac*, milk; *fugare*, to put to flight]. Any agent which suppresses milk secretion.

Lactobacillus (lak-tō-bas-il'-us). A genus of bacteria. A large Gram-postive rod which is active in fermenting carbohydrates, producing acid. No members are pathogenic.

lactoflavin (lakL-to-flā-vin). Riboflavin (q.v.)

lactogenic (lak'-tō-jen-ik) [L. *lac*, milk; G. *genesthai*, to be produced]. Stimulating milk production. See LUTEOTROPHIN.

lactometer (lak-tom'-et-ėr) [L. *lac*, milk; G. *metron*, a measure]. An instrument for measuring the specific gravity of milk.

lactose (lak'-tōs). Milk sugar. Less soluble and less sweet than ordinary sugar. Used in infant feeding to increase the carbohydrate content of diluted cow's milk. In some infants the gut is intolerant to lactose. See LACTASE. In severe intolerance the infant may pass a litre or more of fluid stool per day. Temporary intolerance can follow neonatal alimentary tract obstructions, but rarely gives long-term problems.

lactosuria (lak-tō-sū'-ri-á) [L. *lac*, milk; G. *ouron*, urine]. Lactose in the urine—lactosuric, adj.

lacuna (la-kū'-ná) [L. cavity]. A space between cells; sinus—lacunae, pl.; lacunar, adj.

laevulose (lev'-ū-lōs). Fructose or fruit sugar; sweeter and more easily digested than ordinary sugar, and is useful for diabetics. Also used as a test for hepatic function, as it does not normally increase the blood sugar level, except in hepatic damage.

lambliasis (lam-blī'a-sis). Giardiasis (q.v.).

lamella (la-mel'-á) [L. small plate]. A thin plate-like scale or partition. A gelatine-coated disc containing a drug; it is inserted under the eyelid—lamellae, pl.; lamellar, adj.

lamina (lam'-in-á) [L.]. A thin plate or layer, usually of bone—laminae, pl.

laminectomy (lam-in-ek'-to-mi) [L. *lamina*, a thin plate; G. *ektome*, excision]. Removal of laminae of vertebrae—to expose the spinal cord and meninges. Most often performed in lumbar region, for removal of degenerated invertebral disc.

Lamprene (lam'-prēn). Clofazimine (q.v.).

lanatoside C. (lan-at'-ō-sīd). A glycoside of the Austrian foxglove, usually employed by intravenous injection when rapid digitalization is required. Oral therapy is less reliable.

Lancefield's groups. Subdivision of the genus Streptococcus on the basis of antigenic structure. The members of each group have a characteristic capsular polysaccharide. The majority of streptococci of epidemiological importance to man belong to Group A. [Rebecca Lancefield, New York bacteriologist, 1895– .]

lanolin(e) (lan'-ō-lēn). Wool fat containing 30 per cent water. **anhydrous l.** is the fat obtained from sheep's wool. They are used in ointment bases, as such bases can form water-in-oil emulsions with aqueous constituents, and are readily absorbed by the skin. Adeps lanae hydrosus.

Lanoxin (lan-oks'-in). Digoxin (q.v.).

lanugo (lan ū' gō) [L. down]. Soft, downy hair often present on newborn infants, especially when they are premature.

laparoscopy (lap-ar-os'-ko-pi) [G. *lapara,* soft part of flank; *skopein,* to examine]. Endoscopic examination of the pelvic organs by the transperitoneal route. Laparoscope introduced through the abdominal wall after induction of a pneumoperitoneum. For biopsy, aspiration of cysts and division of adhesions. Tubal ligation for sterilization and even ventrosuspension can be performed via the laparoscope—laparoscopic, adj.; laparoscopically, adv.

laparotomy (lap-ar-ot'-o-mi) [G. *lapara,* soft part of flank; *tome,* a cutting]. Incision of abdominal wall. (Usually reserved for exploratory operation.)

Largactil (lar-gak'-til). Chlorpromazine (q.v.).

Laroxyl. Amitriptyline (q.v.). See ANTIDEPRESSANT.

larva (làr'-và) [L. *larva,* ghost]. An embryo which is independent before it has assumed the characteristic features of its parents. **larva migrans,** itching tracks in the skin with formation of blisters caused by the burrowing of larvae of some species of fly and normally animal-infesting Ancylostoma—larvae, pl.; larval, adj.

larvicide (làr'-vi-sīd) [L. *larva,* ghost; L. *caedere,* to kill]. Any agent which destroys larvae—larvicidal, adj.

laryngeal (lar'-in-jēl) [G. *larygx.*] Pertaining to the larynx.

laryngectomy (lar-in-jek'-to-mi) [G. *larygx,* larynx; *ektome,* excision]. Excision of the larynx.

laryngismus stridulus (lar-in-jis'-mus strid'-ū-lus). Momentary attack of laryngeal spasm as in infantile tetany associated with rickets.

laryngitis (lar-in-jī'-tis) [G. *larygx,* larynx; *-itis.* inflammation]. Inflammation of the larynx.

laryngofissure (lar-in-gō-fish'-ūr) [G. *larygx,* larynx; L. *fissura,* fissure]. The operation of opening the larynx in midline.

laryngologist ((lar-in-gol'-oj-ist) [G. *larygx,* larynx; *logos,* discourse]. A specialist in laryngeal diseases.

laryngology (lar-in-gol'-o-ji) [G. *larygx,* larynx; *logis,* discourse]. The study of diseases affecting the larynx.

laryngoparalysis (lar-in'-gō-par-al'-is-is) [G. *larygx,* larynx; G. *paralysis*]. Paralysis of the larynx.

laryngopharyngectomy (lar-in-gō-far-in-jek'-to-mi) [G. *larygx*; *pharygx*; *ektome,* excision]. Excision of the larynx and lower part of pharynx.

laryngopharynx (lar-in'-gō-far'-ingks) [G. *larygx,* larynx; *pharygx,* pharynx]. The lower portion of the pharynx—laryngopharyngeal, adj.

laryngoscope (lar-in'-gō-skōp) [G. *larygx,* larynx; *skopein,* to examine]. Instrument for exposure and visualization of larynx—laryngoscopy, n.; laryngoscopic, adj.

laryngospasm (lar'-in-gō-spazm). Convulsive involuntary muscular contraction of the larynx, usually accompanied by spasmodic closure of the glottis.

laryngostenosis (lar-in-gō-sta-nō'-sis) [G. *larygx,* larynx; *stenosis,* straitened]. Narrowing of the glottic aperture.

laryngotomy (lar-in-got'-o-mi) [G. *larygx,* larynx; *tome,* a cutting]. The operation of opening the larynx.

laryngotracheal (lar-in'-gō-tra-kē'-al) [G. *larygx,* larynx; *trachus,* rough]. Pertaining to the larynx and trachea.

laryngotracheitis (lar-in-gō-trak-ē-ī'-tis) [G. *larygx*; *trachus,* rough; *-itis,* inflammation]. Inflammation of the larynx and trachea.

laryngotracheobronchitis (lar-in-gō-trak'-ē-ō-brong-kī'-tis) [G. *larygx,* larynx; *trachus,* rough; *brogchos,* windpipe; *-itis,* inflammation]. Inflammation of the larynx, trachea and bronchi.

larynx (lar'-ingks) [G. *larygx*]. The organ of voice situated below and in front of the pharynx and at the upper end of the trachea—laryngeal, adj.

laser beam (lā-ser). Light Amplification by Stimulated Emission of Radiation. Energy transmitted as heat that can coagulate tissue. Has been used for detached retina and cancer.

Lassa fever. Previously an African malady diagnosed first in 1969; human beings ingest food or water contaminated by rat excrement containing the arenavirus which can then be transmitted from person to person. Strongly suspected that primary cases are more highly contagious than secondary ones. Incubation period 3 to 16 days, early symptoms resemble typhoid and septicaemia. By the sixth day ulcers develop in the mouth and throat; fever is variable, sometimes being very high. Fatality rate in some areas is as high as 67 per cent. Infected people must be nursed in strict isolation.

Lassar's paste (las'-sars). Contains zinc oxide, starch and salicylic acid in soft paraffin. Used in eczema and similar conditions as an antiseptic protective. [Oskar Lassar, German dermatologist, 1849–1907.]

latent heat (lā'-tent) [L. *latens*, lying hidden]. That heat which is used to bring about a change in state, not in temperature.

lateral (lat'-e-ral). [L. *latus*, side]. At or belonging to the side; away from the median line—laterally, adv.

laudanum (lawd'-num). Old name for tincture of opium.

laughing gas. Nitrous oxide.

lavage (láv-ázh') [F.]. Irrigation of or washing out a body cavity.

laxative (laks'-a-tiv). A mild aperient.

LDH. Lactate dehydrogenase (q.v.).

L-dopa (el-dō'-pa). Levodopa (q.v.).

lead (led). A metal, the salts of which are astringent when applied externally.

Leadbetter-Politano operation. An antireflux measure by tunnel reimplantation of ureter into urinary bladder.

lead lotion (led lō'-shun). A weak solution of lead subacetate used as a soothing astringent lotion for sprains and bruises.

lead poisoning (led). Acute poisoning is unusual, but chronic poisoning due to absorption of small amounts over a period, is less uncommon. This can occur in young children by sucking articles made of lead alloys, or painted with lead paint. In spite of legislation and safety precautions, industrial poisoning is still the commonest cause. Anaemia, loss of appetite, and the formation of a blue line round the gums are characteristic.

LE cells. Characteristic cells found in patients with lupus erythematosus.

lecithin (les'-i-thin) [G. *lekithos*, egg yolk]. A nitrogenous, fatty substance in cell protoplasm.

Ledermycin (led-er-mī'-sin). Demethylchlortetracycline. One of the tetracyclines (q.v.).

leech (lēch). *Hirudo medicinalis.* An aquatic worm which can be applied to the human body to suck blood. Its saliva contains hirudin, an anticoagulant.

legumen (leg-ū'-men). The protein present in pulses—peas, beans and lentils.

Leishman-Donovan bodies (lēsh'-man don'-ov-an). The rounded forms of the protozoa Leishmania found in the endothelial cells and macrophages of patients suffering from leishmaniasis (q.v.).

Leishmania (lēsh-mā'-ni-á). Genus of flagellated protozoon. *Leishmania donovani* is responsible for disease of kala-azar, or leishmaniasis (q.v.).

leishmaniasis (lēsh-man-ī'-a-sis). Infestation by Leishmania, spread by sand-flies. Generalized manifestation is kala-azar (q.v.). Cutaneous manifestation is such as Aleppo or Delhi boil (oriental sore) (q.v.). Nasopharyngeal manifestation is espundia (q.v.).

lens (lenz). 1. The small biconvex crystalline body which is supported in the suspensory ligament immediately behind the iris of the eye. On account of its elasticity, the lens can alter in shape, enabling light rays to focus exactly on the retina. 2. A piece of transparent material, usually glass, with a regular curvature of one or both surfaces, used for conveying or diffusing light rays.

lenticular (len-tik'-ū-lar) [L. *lenticula*, lentil]. Pertaining to or resembling a lens.

lentigo (len-tī'-gō) [L.]. A freckle—lentigines, pl.

lentil (len'-til). A cheap and nutritious legumen containing a large amount of protein.

Lentizol (len'-tiz-ol). A tricyclic antidepressant. Useful for depression when accompanied by agitation. Amitriptyline hydrochloride (q.v.).

leontiasis (lē-on-tī'-a-sis) [G. *leon,* lion; N.L. *-iasis,* condition]. Enlargement of face and head giving a lion-like appearance; most often caused by fibrous dysplasia of bone.

leprologist (lep-rol'-oj-ist) [G. *lepros,* scaly; *logos,* discourse]. One who specializes in the study and treatment of leprosy—leprology, n.

lepromata (lep-rō'-ma-tà) [G. *lepros,* scaly; *-oma,* tumour]. The granulomatous cutaneous eruption of leprosy leproma, sing., lepromatous, adj.

leprosy (lep'-ro-si) [G. *lepros,* scaly]. A progressive and contagious disease, endemic in warmer climates, and characterized by granulomatous formation in the nerves or on the skin. Caused by *Mycobacterium leprae* (Hansen's bacillus). BCG vaccination conferred 87 per cent protection in one large-scale trial—leprous, adj.

leptazol (lep'-ta-zol). Powerful central stimulant.

leptocytosis (lep-tō-sī-tō'-sis) [G. *leptos,* thin; *-osis,* condition]. Thin, flattened, circulating red blood cells (leptocytes). Characteristic of Cooley's anaemia (q.v.). Also seen in jaundice, hepatic disease and sometimes after splenectomy.

leptomeningitis (lep-tō-men-in-jī'-tis) [G. *leptos,* thin; *menigx,* membrane; *-itis,* inflammation]. Inflammation of the inner covering membranes (meninges) of brain or spinal cord.

Leptospira (lep-tō-spī'-rà) [G. *leptos,* thin; *speira,* coil]. A genus of bacteria. Very thin, finely coiled bacteria which require dark ground microscopy for visualization. Common in water as saprophytes; pathogenic species are numerous in many animals and may infect man. *Leptospira icterohaemorrhagiae* causes Weil's disease in man; *Leptospira canicola,* 'yellows' in dogs and pigs, transmissible to man. See CANICOLA FEVER.

leptospirosis (lep-tō-spī-rō'-sis) [G. *leptos,* thin; *speira,* coil; *-osis,* condition]. Spirochaetal disease. Leptospirosis haemorrhagica, Weil's disease (q.v.).

Leptothrix (lep'-tō-thriks) [G. *leptos,* fine; *thrix,* hair]. A genus of bacteria. Gram-negative; found in water; non-pathogenic. A term also used in medical bacteriology to describe filamentous bacteria resembling actinomycetes.

lesbianism (les'-bi-an-izm). Sexual attraction of one woman to another.

Lesch-Nyhan disease (lesh-nī'-àn). Described in 1965; transmitted via mother to only male children. Overproduction of uric acid, associated with brain damage resulting in cerebral palsy and mental retardation. Victims are compelled, by a self-destructive urge, to bite away the sides of their mouth, lips and fingers.

lesion (lē'-zhun) [L. *laesio,* a hurting]. Pathological change in a bodily tissue.

lethane (lē-thān). A mixture of thiocyanate derivatives with insecticidal properties; used for pediculosis capitis.

Lethidrone (leth'-i-drōn). Nalorphine (q.v.).

Leucarsone (lū'-kar-sōn). Carbarsome (q.v.).

leucine (lū'-sēn). One of the essential amino acids (q.v.).

leucocytes (lū'-ko-sīts) [G. *leukos,* white; *kytos,* cell]. The white corpuscles of the blood. In the blood stream they are colourless, nucleated masses, and some are motile and phagocytic. See BASOPHIL, EOSINOPHIL, LYMPHOCYTE, MONONUCLEAR, POLYMORPHONUCLEAR—leucocytic, adj.

leucocytolysis (lū-kō-sī-tol'-is-is) [G. *leukos,* white; *kytos,* cell; *lysis,* a loosening]. Destruction and disintegration of white blood cells—leucocytolytic, adj.

leucocytosis (lū-kō-sī-tō'-sis) [G. *leukos,* white; *kytos,* cell; *-osis,* condition]. Increased number of leucocytes in the blood. Often a response to infection—leucocytotic, adj.

leucoderma (lū-kō-der'-mà) [G. *leukos,* white; *derma,* skin]. Defective skin pigmentation, especially when it occurs in patches or bands.

leucoma (lū-kō'-mà) [G. white spot on the eye]. White opaque spot on the cornea—leucomata, pl.; leucomatous, adj.

leuconychia (lū-kon-ik'-i-à) [G. *leukos,* white; *onyx,* nail]. White spots on the nails.

leucopenia (lū-kō-pē'-ni-à) [G. *leukos,* white; *penia,* want]. Decreased number of leucocytes in the blood—leucopenic, adj.

leucopoiesis (lū-kō-poi-ē'-sis) [G. *leukos,* white; *poiesis,* making]. The formation of white blood cells—leucopoietic, adj.

leucorrhoea (lū-kō-rē'-á) [G. *leukos,* white; *rheein,* to flow]. A sticky, whitish vaginal discharge—leucorrhoeal, adj.

leucotomy (lū-kot'-o-mi) [G. *leukos,* white; *tome,* cutting]. **prefrontal l.,** an operation devised by Moniz (1936) for the treatment of certain forms of chronic insanity by cutting the fronto-thalamic connection fibres in the brain. Moniz's original method was to inject alcohol into the prefrontal white matter. Freeman, Watts and others (1946) introduced surgical cutting of the fibres and other modifications.

Leucovorin (lu-kov'-or-in). Folinic acid or Citrorovam Factor given by mouth, i.m. or i.v. as an antidote to methotrexate. Used to 'rescue' patients from high dose methotrexate therapy for malignant disease.

leukaemia (lū-kē'-mi-á) [G. *leukos,* white; *haima,* blood]. A malignant proliferation of the leucopoietic tissues usually producing an abnormal increase in leucocytes in the blood, with immature cells among them. The varieties are **acute lymphatic, myeloid** or **monocytic l.** and **chronic lymphatic** or **myeloid l.** Acute leukaemia rapidly results in infection, haemorrhage and anaemia. The process is slower in the chronic types, with splenomegaly and lymph node enlargement in the lymphatic variety. The term **aleukaemic l.** is used when the leucocyte count remains normal or below.

Leukeran (lū'-ker-an). Chlorambucil (q.v.).

leukoplakia (lū-kō-plā'-ki-á) [G. *leukos,* white; *plax,* flat and broad]. White, thickened patch occurring on mucous membranes. Occurs on lips, inside mouth or on genitalia. Sometimes denotes precancerous change. Sometimes due to syphilis. See KRAUROSIS VALVAE.

levallorphan tartrate. Narcotic antagonist.

levamisole (lev-a-mī'-sol). Synthetic anthelmintic. Better tolerated than piperazine citrate and virtually free of toxic effects. Currently being used for treatment of rheumatoid arthritis as an immunostimulant.

levator (le-vā'-tor) [L. *levare,* to lift up]. A muscle which acts by raising a part.

An instrument for lifting a depressed part.

Levin's tube. Used in gastric acid tests.

levodopa (lev-ō-dō'-pá). L-dopa. Synthetic anti-Parkinson drug. In Parkinson's disease there is inadequate dopamine (a transmitter substance), in the basal ganglia. In these ganglia l. is converted into dopamine and replenishes the stores. Unlike dopamine levodopa can cross the blood-brain barrier. See CARBIDOPA.

Levophed (lev'-ō-fed). Noradrenaline (q.v.).

levorphanol (lev-or'-fan-ol). A synthetic substitute for morphine. It is less hypnotic than morphine but has a more extended action. Almost as effective by mouth as by injection.

levulose (lev'-ū-lōs). Fruit sugar; fructose. Also LAEVULOSE (q.v.).

L-form. A bacterium whose cell wall has been destroyed. In this condition it can survive harmlessly for months. Under certain conditions it can quickly change into a pathogenic bacterium.

LGVCFT. Lymphogranuloma venereum complement fixation test.

libido (li-bī'-dō) [L. longing]. Freud's name for the urge to obtain sensual satisfaction which he believed to be the mainspring of human behaviour. Sometimes more loosely used with the meaning of sexual urge. Freud's meaning was satisfaction through all the senses.

Librium (lib'-ri-um). Chlordiazepoxide (q.v.).

lice (līs'). See PEDICULUS.

lichen (lī'-ken) [G. *leichen,* lichen]. Aggregations of papular skin lesions. **lichen nitidus,** characterized by minute, shiny, flat-topped, pink papules of pinhead size. **lichen planus,** aggregates of small papules, polygonal in shape, flat-topped, and of violaceous hue. **lichen scrofulosorum,** a form of tuberculide. **lichen simplex,** a psychosomatic condition which produces areas of irritating, leathery, shiny papules (lichenification). Syn., neurodermatitis. **lichen spinulosus,** a disease of children characterized by very small spines protruding from the follicular openings of the skin and resulting from vitamin A deficiency. **lichen urticatus,** papular urticaria (q.v.)—lichenoid, adj.

lichenification (lī-ken-i-fik-ā'-shun) [G. *leichen,* lichen; L. *facere,* to make].

Thickening of the skin, usually secondary to scratching. Striae become more prominent and the area affected appears to be composed of small, shiny rhomboids.

Lidocaine (lid'-ō-kān). Lignocaine (q.v.).

Lidothesin. Lignocaine (q.v.).

lien (lī'-en) [L.]. The spleen.

lienculus (lī-eng'-kū-lus) [L. *lien,* spleen]. A small accessory spleen.

lienitis (lī-en-ī'-tis) [L. *lien,* spleen; G. *itis,* inflammation]. Inflammation of the spleen.

lienorenal (lī-en-ō-rē'-nal) [L. *lien,* spleen; *ren,* kidney]. Pertaining to the spleen and kidney. In 1 shunt, the splenic vein is anastomosed to the left renal vein to relieve portal hypertension.

ligament (lig'-a-ment) [L. *ligamentum,* band]. A strong band of fibrous tissue serving to bind bones or other parts together, or to support an organ—ligamentous, adj.

ligate (lī-gāt') [L. *ligare,* to bind]. To tie off blood vessels, etc. at operation—ligation, n.

ligature (lig'-a-tūr) [L. *ligatura,* a band]. The material used for tying vessels or sewing the tissues. Silk, horse-hair, catgut, kangaroo tendon, silver wire, nylon, linen and fascia can be used.

lightening (lī'-ten-ing). Term used to denote the relief of pressure on the diaphragm by the abdominal viscera, when the presenting part of the fetus descends into the pelvis in the last 3 weeks of a primigravida's pregnancy.

lightning pains. Symptomatic of tabes dorsalis. Occur as paroxysms of swift-cutting (lightning) stabs in the lower limbs.

lignocaine (lig'-nō-kān). A local anaesthetic with a more powerful and prolonged action than procaine. The strength of solution varies from 0.5 per cent for infiltration anaesthesia to 2 per cent for nerve block. Adrenaline is usually added to delay absorption. Also effective for surface anaesthesia as ointment (2 per cent) and for urethral anaesthesia as a 2 per cent gel. Now widely accepted as an antiarhythmic agent, especially in the management of ventricular tachycardia and ventricular ectopic beats occurring as complications of acute myocardial infarction.

lime water. Solution of calcium hydroxide (about 0.15 per cent). It is used in a number of skin lotions, and with an equal volume of linseed or olive oil it forms a soothing application. It is also used in infant feeding as it hinders the formation of large curds.

liminal (lim'-in-al) [L. *limen,* threshold]. The lowest intensity of a stimulus which can be perceived by the human senses. See SUBLIMINAL.

Lincocin (lin'-kō-sin). Lincomycin (q.v.).

lincomycin (lin-kō-mī'-sin). Antibiotic for infections caused by Gram-positive pathogens.

linctus (ling'-tus) [L. *linctus,* a licking] A sweet, syrupy liquid; it should be slowly sipped. See GEE'S L.

linea (lin'-i-á). A line. **linea alba,** the white line visible after removal of the skin in the centre of the abdomen, stretching from the ensiform cartilage to the pubis, its position on the surface being indicated by a slight depression. **linea nigra,** pigmented line from umbilicus to pubis which appears in pregnancy. **lineae albicantes,** white lines which appear on the abdomen after reduction of tension as after childbirth, tapping of the abdomen, etc.

lingua (ling'-gwá) [L.]. The tongue—lingual, adj.

liniment (lin'-i-ment) [L. *linire,* to smear]. A liquid to be applied to the skin by gentle friction.

linolenic acid (lin-ō-lē'-nik). An unsaturated, essential fatty acid. Found in vegetable fats.

Lioresal (lī'-ō-rē-sal). Baclofen (q.v.).

liothyronine (lī-ō-thī'-ron-in). Secretion of thyroid gland. Together with thyroxine stimulates metabolism in body tissues.

lipaemia (lī-pē'-mi-á) [G. *lipos,* fat; *haima,* blood]. Increased lipoids (especially cholesterol) in the blood—lipaemic, adj.

lipase (lī'-pāz). Any fat-splitting enzyme. **pancreatic l.,** steapsin (q.v.).

Lipiodol (lip-i'-o-dol). Iodized oil (q.v.).

Lipiphysan. Kilocalorie provision in parenteral feeding. Ten per cent emulsion gives 1240 kcal and 15 per cent gives 1780 kcal per litre.

lipoid (lī'-poid) [G. *lipos,* fat; *eidos,* form]. Resembling fat or oil. Serum lipoids raised in thyroid deficiency.

lipoidosis (lī-poid-ō'-sis) [G. *lipos,* fat; *eidos,* form; *-osis,* condition]. Disease due to disorder of fat metabolism—lipoidoses, pl.

lipolysis (lī-pol′-i-sis) [G. *lipos*, fat; *lysis*, a loosening]. The chemical breaking down of fat. The lipolytic enzymes are responsible.

lipoma (lī-pō′-mà) [G. *lipos*, fat; *-oma*, tumour]. A benign tumour containing fatty tissue— lipomata, pl.; lipomatous, adj.

lipotrophic substances (lī-pō-trō′-fik). Factors which cause the removal of fat from the liver by transmethylation.

lipuria (lī-pū′-ri-à) [G. *lipos*, fat; *ouron*, urine]. Fat in the urine. Adiposuria— lipuric, adj.

Liquemin (lik′-wē-min). Heparin (q.v.).

liquor (lik-êr) [L. liquid]. A solution. **l. amni**, the fluid surrounding the fetus. **liquor epispasticus**, a blistering fluid. **liquor folliculi**, the fluid surrounging a developing ovum in a Graafian follicle. **liquor picis carb.**, an alcoholic extract of coal tar. Used in eczema and other conditions requiring mild tar treatment. **liquor sanguinis**, the fluid part of blood (plasma).

liquorice (lik′-or-is). Glycyrrhiza (q.v.).

Lisidonil (li-sid′-on-il). Has a relaxing effect on the neurogenic bladder.

lithiasis (lith-ī′-a-sis) [G. *lithos*, stone; N.L. *-iasis*, condition]. Formation of calculi.

lithium carbonate (li′-thi-um kar′-bon-āt). Used in manic depressive illness. Possible side effects include diarrhoea, vomiting, drowsiness, ataxia, coarse tremor. Contraindicated in cardiac or renal disease. Regular blood serum levels necessary and thyroid function should be assessed before and at regular intervals during treatment.

litholapaxy (lith-ol-a-pak′-si) [G. *lithos*, stone; *lapaxis*, evacuation]. Crushing a stone within the urinary bladder and removing the fragments by irrigation. Syn. lithopaxy.

lithopaedion (lith-ō-pē′-di-on). A dead fetus retained in the uterus, e.g. in the case of one dead twin, which becomes mummified and sometimes impregnated with lime salts.

lithotrite (lith′-ō-trīt) [G. *lithos*, stone; L. *terere*, to wear]. An instrument for crushing a stone in the urinary bladder.

lithuresis (lith-ū-rē′-sis) [G. *lithos*, stone; *ouron*, urine]. Voiding of gravel in the urine.

litmus (lit′-mus). A vegetable pigment used as an indicator of acidity or alkalinity. Blue l. paper turns red when in contact with an acid. Red l. paper turns blue when in contact with an alkali.

Little's disease. Diplegia of spastic type causing 'scissor leg' deformity. Congenital disease in which there is cerebral atrophy or agenesis [William John Little, English surgeon, 1810–94.]

liver (liv′-êr). The largest organ in the body, varying in weight in the adult from 13.59 to 18.12 hg or about one-thirtieth of body weight. It is relatively much larger in the fetus. It is situated in the right upper section of the abdominal cavity. It secretes bile, forms and stores glycogen and plays an important part in the metabolism of proteins and fats.

livid (liv′-id) [L. *lividus*, of a leaden, bluish colour]. Blue discolouration due to bruising, congestion or insufficient oxygenation.

L-lytic compound (el-lit′-ik). Isoxuprine (q.v.).

LOA. Midwifery. Left occipitoanterior presentation.

lobe (lōb) [G. *lobos*, lobe]. A rounded section of an organ, separated from neighbouring sections by a fissure or septum, etc.—lobar, adj.

lobectomy (lōb-ek′-to-mi) [G. *lobos*, lobe; *ektome*, excision]. Excision of a lobe, as of the lung.

lobeline (lob′-el-ēn). Occasionally used for resuscitation of the newborn by injection into the umbilical cord.

lobotomy (lōb-o′-to-mi) [G. *lobos*, lobe; *tome*, a cutting]. Section of brain tissue. Used in surgical treatment of emotional disease.

lobule (lob′-ūl) [G. *lobos*, lobe]. A small lobe or a subdivision of a lobe—lobular, lobulated, adj.

localize (lō′-kal-īz) [L. *localis*, place]. To limit the spread; to determine the site of a lesion—localization, n.

lochia (lō′-ki-à) [G. discharge after childbirth]. The vaginal discharge which occurs during the puerperium. At first pure blood, it later becomes paler, diminishes in quantity and finally ceases— lochial, adj.

lockjaw. Tetanus (q.v.).

locomotor (lō-kō-mō′-tor). Can be applied to any tissue or system used in human movement. Most usually refers to nerves and muscles. Sometimes includes the bones and joints. **locomotor ataxia**, the disordered gait and loss of sense of position in the lower limbs, which occurs in tabes dorsalis (q.v.). Tabes dorsalis is sometimes referred to, still, as 'locomotor ataxia.'

loculated (lok'-ū-lā-ted) [L. *loculus*, little place]. Divided into numerous cavities.

loiasis (loi'-as-is). Special form of filariasis (Filaria *Loa loa*) which occurs in West Africa, Nigeria and the Cameroons. The vector, a large horse-fly, Chrysops, bites in the daytime. Larvae take 3 years to develop and may live in a man for 17. They creep about and cause intense itching. Accompanied by eosinophilia.

loin [L. *lumbus*]. That part of the back, between the lower ribs and the iliac crest; the area immediately above the buttocks.

Lomotil (lō'-mō-til). Diphenoxylate hydrochloride and atropine sulphate. Useful for loose colostomy and postvagotomy diarrhoea. Reduces motility of gut and allows time for absorption of water from faeces. Single dose lessens desire to defaecate after one hour and is effective for 6 hours.

lomulizer (lom'ūl-ī-zer). Device which disperses fine powder (contained in a tiny plastic cartridge) through a mouthpiece.

long-sighted. Hypermetropic. See HYPERMETROPIA.

lorazepam (lor-az'-ē-pam). Tranquillizer (q.v.).

lordosis (lor-dō'-sis) [G. a spinal curvature]. An exaggerated forward, convex curve of the lumbar spine.

Lorexane (lor'-eks-ān). Gamma benzene hydrochloride (q.v.).

Lorfan. Levallorphan tartrate (q.v.).

lotio rubra. See RED LOTION.

loupe (loop) [F.]. A magnifying lens used in ophthalmology.

louping ill. Tick-borne virus meningoencephalitis in sheep. Antibodies have been found in human serum.

louse (lows). A small parasitic insect; there are three varieties affecting man — lice. pl. See PEDICULUS.

low birth-weight. Term used to indicate a weight of 2.5 kg or less at birth, whether or not gestation was below 37 weeks.

LSD. Lysergic acid diethylamide, q.v.

L-tryptophan (l-trip'-tō'-fan). See TRYPTOPHANE.

lubb-dupp. Words descriptive of the heart sounds as appreciated in auscultation.

lucanthone (lū-kan-thōn). Synthetic oral drug for the treatment of schistosomiasis.

lucid (loo'-sid) [L. *lucidus*, clear]. Clear; mental clarity

lues (lū'-ēz) [L. pestilence]. Syphilis luetic, adj.

Lugol's solution (loo'-gols). An aqueous solution of iodine and potassium iodide. Used in the pre-operative stabilization of thyrotoxic patients. It has been given by slow intravenous injection in thyrotoxic crisis. [Antoine Lugol, physician in Paris, 1786–1851.]

lumbago (lum-bā'-gō) [L.]. Incapacitating pain low down in the back A symptom of fibrositis of lumbar muscles, spondylitis, prolapsed intervertebral disc, etc.

lumbar [L. *lumbus*, loin]. Pertaining to the loins. **Lumbar sympathectomy**, surgical removal of the sympathetic chain in the lumbar region; used to improve the blood supply to the lower limbs by allowing the blood vessels to dilate.

lumbocostal (lum-bō-kos'-tal) [L. *lumbus*, loin; *costa*, rib]. Pertaining to the loin and ribs.

lumbosacral (lum-bō-sā'-kral) [L. *lumbus*, loin; *sacrum*, sacred]. Pertaining to the loin or lumbar vertebrae and the sacrum.

Lumbricus (lum'-brik-us) [L.]. A genus of earthworms. See ASCARIDES.

lumen (loo'-men) [L. light]. The space inside a tubular structure—lumina, pl.; luminal, adj.

Luminal (loo'-min-al). Phenobarbitone (q.v.).

lungs. The two main organs of respiration which occupy the greater part of the thoracic cavity; they are separated from each other by the heart and other contents of the mediastinum. Together they weigh about 11.88 hg and they are concerned with the oxygenation of the blood.

lunula (loo'-nū-lá) [L. little moon]. The semilunar pale area at the root of the nail.

lupus (loo'-pus) [L. wolf]. A nodular skin condition, with many manifestations. **lupus erythematosus**, see COLLAGEN, LE CELLS. The discoid variety is characterized by patulous follicles, adherent scales, telangiectasis and atrophy: commonest on nose, malar regions, scalp and fingers (chilblain l.). The disseminated or systemic variety is characterized by large areas of erythema on the skin, pyrexia, toxaemia, involvement of serous membranes (pleurisy, pericarditis) and renal damage. Is an autoimmune process. A syndrome closely resembling lupus erythematosus has been associated with ingestion of hydrallazine, hydantoin derivatives, griseofulvin, sulphonamides, penicillin, carbamazepine and guanoxan. **lupus pernio**, a form of sarcoidosis (q.v.). **lupus vulgaris**, the commonest variety of skin tuberculosis; ulceration occurs over cartilage (nose or ear) with necrosis and facial disfigurement.

luteotrophin (loo'-tē-ō-trō'-fin). Secreted by the anterior pituitary gland; it assists the formation of the corpus luteum in the ovary.

luteum (loo'-tē-um) [L. *luteus*, yellow]. Yellow. **corpus l.**, a yellow mass which forms in the ovary after rupture of a Graafian follicle. It secretes progesterone and persists and enlarges if pregnancy supervenes.

luxation (luks-ā'-shun). Dislocation.

lycopodium (lī-kō-pō'-di-um). A light, dry powder; it is adsorbent and can be used for dusting the skin and excoriated surfaces, and as a coating for pills.

lying-in period. Early postnatal period, not less than 10 days after the end of labour, during which the continued attendance of a midwife on the mother and/or infant is requisite.

lymecycline (līm-sī'-klin). A complex of tetracycline, formaldehyde and lysine that provides a higher blood level than that given by tetracycline alone.

lymph (limf) [L. *lympha*, water]. The fluid contained in the lymphatic vessels. It is transparent, colourless or slightly yellow. Unlike blood, lymph contains only one type of cell, the lymphocyte.

lymphadenectomy (limf-ad-en-ek'-to-mi) [L. *lympha*, water; G. *aden*, gland; *ektome*, excision]. Excision of one or more lymph nodes.

lymphadenitis (limf-ad-en-ī'-tis) [L. *lympha*, water; G. *aden*, gland; -*itis*, inflammation]. Inflammation of a lymph node.

lymphadenoma (limf-ad-en-ō'-má). Hodgkin's disease (q.v.).

lymphadenopathy (limf-ad-en-op'-ath-i) [L. *lympha*, water; G. *aden*, gland; *pathos*, disease]. Any disease of the lymph nodes—lymphadenopathic, adj.

lymphangiectasis (limf-an-ji-ek'-ta-sis) [L. *lympha*, water; G. *aggeion*, vessel; *ektasis*, extension]. Dilation of the lymph vessels—lymphangiectatic, adj.

lymphangiogram (limf-an'-ji-ō-gram) [L. *lympha*, water; G. *aggeion*, vessel; *gramma*, letter]. Radiograph demonstrating the lymphatic system after injection of an opaque medium—lymphangiography, n.; lymphangiographical, adj.; lymphangiographically, adv.

lymphangioma (limf-an-ji-ō'-má) [L. *lympha*, water; G. *aggeion*, vessel; -*oma*, tumour]. A simple tumour of lymph vessels frequently associated with similar formations of blood vessels—lymphangiomata, pl.; lymphangiomatous, adj.

lymphangioplasty (limf-an'-ji-ō-plas-ti) [L. *lympha*, water. G. *aggeion*, vessel; *plassein*, to form]. Replacement of lymphatics by artificial channels (buried silk threads) to drain the tissues. Relieves the 'brawny arm' after radical mastectomy—lymphangioplastic, adj.

lymphangitis (limf-an-jī'-tis) [L. *lympha*, water; G. *aggeion*, vessel; -*itis*, inflammation]. Inflammation of a lymph vessel.

lymphatic (limf-at'-ik) [L. *lympha*, water]. Pertaining to, conveying or containing lymph.

lymphaticovenous (limf-at-ik-ō-vēn'-us) [L. *lympha*, water; *vena*, vein]. Implies the presence of both lymphatic vessels and veins to increase drainage from the area.

lymphoblastoma (limf-ō-blas-tō'-má) [L. *lympha*, water; G. *blastos*, germ; -*oma*, tumour]. Malignant lymphoma in which single or multiple tumours arise from lymphoblasts in lymph nodes. Sometimes associated with acute lymphatic leukaemia. **lymphoblastoma malignum**, Hodgkin's disease (q.v.).

lymphocyte (limf'-ō-sīt) [L. *lympha*, water; G. *kytos*, cell]. One variety of white blood cell. The lymphocytic stem cells undergo transformation to T-lymphocytes (in the thymus) which provide cellular immunity; and B-lymphocytes (in a site as yet unknown) which form antibodies and provide humoral immunity. The transformation is usually complete a few months after birth.— lymphocytic, adj.

lymphocytosis (limf-ō-sī-tō'-sis). An increase in lymphocytes in the blood.

lymphoedema (limf-ē-dē'-má) [L. *lympha*, water; G. *oidema*, swelling]. Excess of fluid in the tissues from obstruction of lymph vessels. See ELEPHANTIASIS and FILARIASIS.

lymphoepithelioma (limf-ō-ep-i-thēl-i-ō'-má) [L. *lympha*, water; G. *epi*, on; *thele*, nipple; -*oma*, tumour]. Rapidly growing malignant pharyngeal tumour. May involve the tonsil. Often has metastases in cervical lymph nodes—lymphoepitheliomata, pl.

lymphogranuloma inguinale (lim-fō-gran-ū-lō'-má in-gwin-á'-lē) [L. *lympha*, water; *granulum*, grain; G. -*oma*, tumour; L. *inguinalis*, of the groin]. Called 'l. venereum' in USA. Tropical venereal disease caused by a virus. Primary lesion on the genitalia may be an ulcer or herpetiform eruption and is usually evanescent. Soon buboes (q.v.) appear in regional lymph nodes. They form a painful mass called 'poradenitis' and commonly produce sinuses. Further spread by lymphatics may cause severe periproctitis or rectal stricture in women. Patch skin test (lygranum) and a complement-fixation test of patient's serum are used in diagnosis.

lymphography (limf-og'-ra-fi) [L. *lympha*, water; G. *graphein*, to write]. X-ray examination of the lymphatic system after it has been rendered radio-opaque. **therapeutic l.**, endolymphatic radiotherapy. See RADIOTHERAPY—lymphographical, adj.; lymphographically, adv.

lymphoid (limf'-oid) [L. *lympha*, water; G. *eidos*, form] Pertaining to lymph

lymphoma (limf-ō'-má) [L. *lympha*, water; G. -*oma*, tumour]. A benign tumour of lymphatic tissue. **malignant l.**, term now applied to include malignant tumours arising from reticuloendothelial tissues. Previously called malignant reticulosis—lymphomata, pl.; lymphomatous, adj.

lymphorrhagia (limf-or-āj'-ē-á) [L. *lympha*, water; G. *rhegnynai*, to burst forth]. An outpouring of lymph from a severed lymphatic vessel.

lymphosarcoma (limf-ō-sár-kō'-má) [L. *lympha*, water; G. *sarkoma*, fleshly overgrowth]. A malignant tumour arising from lymphatic tissue—lymphosarcomata, pl.; lymphosarcomatous, adj.

Lyophrin (lī-of'-rin). Adrenaline preparation. Should be used only in open angle glaucoma.

lyophilization (lī-of-il-īz-ā'-shun). A special method of preserving such biological substances as plasma, sera, bacteria and tissue.

lyophilized skin (lī-of'-il-īzd). Skin which has been subjected to lyophilization. It is reconstituted and used for temporary skin replacement.

lypressin (lī-press'-in). Antidiuretic. See VASOPRESSIN.

lysergic acid diethylamide (lī-ser'-gik as'-id dī-eth-il-á-mīd). Potent hallucinogenic agent. An amino oxidase inhibitor. See MAOI.

lysin (lī'-sin). A cell dissolving substance in blood. See BACTERIOLYSIN, HAEMOLYSIN.

lysine (lī'-sēn). An essential amino acid necessary for growth. Deficiency may cause nausea, dizziness and anaemia. It is destroyed by dry heating, e.g. toasted bread and cereals such as puffed wheat.

lysis (lī'-sis) [G.]. 1. A gradual return to normal, used especially in relation to pyrexia. Opp. crisis. 2. Dissolution and disintegration of bacteria and cells by the action of a lysin.

Lysivane (lī'-si-vān) Ethopropazine (q.v.).

lysol (lī'-sol). Well known disinfectant containing 50 per cent cresol in soap solution. It has a wide range of activity, but the preparation is caustic, and this limits its use.

lysozyme (lī'-so-zim) [G. *lysis*, dissolution; *zyme*, leaven]. A bacteriolytic enzyme. See TEARS

lytic cocktail. Consists of promethazine (Phenergan), meperidine (pethidine) and chlorpromazine (Largactil) diluted in normal saline solution. Used during the induction and maintenance of hypothermia. Abolishes shivering and convulsions.

M

maceration (mas-e-rā'-shun) [L. *macerare*, to make soft]. Softening of the horny layer of the skin by moisture, e.g. in and below the toes (in tinea pedis), or in perianal area (in pruritus ani). Maceration reduces the protective quality of the integument and so predisposes to penetration by bacteria or fungi.

Mackenrodt's ligaments. The transverse cervical or cardinal ligaments, chief uterine supports. [Alwin K. Mackenrodt, German gynaecologist, 1859–1925.]

macrisalb (mac'-ri-salb). Suspension of iodinated human albumin in the form of insoluble aggregates. After i.v. injection these aggregates are normally trapped by blood capillaries in lungs, thus their presence can be detected by their radioactivity. Absence of such activity is an indication of reduced blood supply.

macrocephalous (mak-rō-kef'-a-lus) [G. makros, large; kephale, head]. Excessive development of the head—macrocephalic, adj.

macrocheilia (mak-rō-kil'-i-á) [G. makros, large; cheilos, lip]. Excessive development of the lips.

macrocyte (mak'-rō-sīt) [G. makros, large; kytos, cell]. A large red blood cell, found in association with a megaloblastic anaemia (q.v.), e.g. in pernicious anaemia. macrocytosis, an increased number of macrocytes—macrocytic, adj.

macrodactyly (mak-rō-dak'-ti-li) [G. makros, large; daktylos, finger]. Excessive development of the fingers or toes.

Macrodex (mak'-rō-deks). High molecular weight dextran for plasma volume replacement in hypovolaemic shock. Can be used as an anticoagulant when patients have to assume a particular position which increases the risk of DVT.

macroglossia (mak-rō-glos'-i-á) [G. makros, large; glossa, tongue]. Abnormally large tongue.

macromastia (mak-rō-mas'-ti-á) [G. makros, large; mastos, breast]. Abnormally large breast.

macrophage (mak'-rō-fāj) [G. makros, large; phagein, to eat]. A phagocytic cell, which plays an important part in organization and repair of tissue.

macroscopic (mak-rō-skop'-ik) [G. makros, large; skopein, to examine]. Visible to the naked eye; gross. Opp. microscopic.

macula (mak'-ū-lá) [L.]. A spot—macular, adj. macula lutea, the yellow spot on the retina, the area of clearest vision. macula solaris, a sunspot, a freckle.

macule (mak'-ūl) [L. macula, spot]. A discoloured spot, not raised above the skin's surface—macular, adj.

maculopapular (mak'-ū-lō-pap'-ū-lar) [L. macula, spot; papula, pustule]. The presence of macules and raised palpable spots (papules) on the skin.

Madecassol (mad-ek'-as-ol). Ointment with 1 per cent plant extract from Centella asiatica. Promotes healing due to stimulation of collagen formation and fibroblastin proliferation.

madribon (mad'-rib-on). A sulphonamide, useful as a prophylactic of urinary infection as resistance does not occur.

madura foot (ma-dū'-rá). Mycetoma. Fungus disease of the foot found in India and the tropics. Characterized by swelling and the development of nodules and sinuses. May terminate in death from sepsis.

magnesium carbonate (mag-nē'-zi-um). A powder widely used as an antacid in peptic ulcer and as a laxative.

magnesium hydroxide. A valuable antacid and laxative, usually given as an aqueous suspension referred to as cream of magnesia or mist. mag. hydrox. It is sometimes preferred to magnesium and other carbonates, as it does not liberate carbon dioxide in the stomach. Also used as an antidote in poisoning by mineral acids.

magnesium sulphate. Epsom salts; an effective rapid-acting laxative, especially when given in dilute solution on an empty stomach. It is used as a 25 per cent solution as a wet dressing for inflamed conditions of the skin, and as a paste with glycerin for the treatment of boils and carbuncles.

magnesium trisilicate. Tasteless white powder with a mild but prolonged antacid action. It is therefore used extensively in peptic ulcer, often combined with more rapidly acting antacids. It does not cause alkalosis, and large doses can be given without side effects.

magnum (mag'-num) [L. magnus, large]. Large or great, as foramen m. in occipital bone.

Majeptil (ma-jep'-til). Closely resembles chlorpromazine (q.v.).

mal [F.]. Disease. mal de mer, seasickness. grand m., major epilepsy. petit m., minor epilepsy.

malabsorption (mal-ab-sorb'-shun). Poor or disordered absorption. malabsorption syndrome, loss of weight and steatorrhoea, varying from mild to severe. Caused by: (1) lesions of the small intestine; (2) lack of digestive enzymes or bile salts; (3) surgical operations.

malacia (mal-ā′-si-à) [G. *malakia*, softness]. Softening of a part. See KERATOMALACIA, OSTEOMALACIA.

maladjustment (mal-ad-just′-ment) [L. *malus*, bad; *a*, to; *justus*, right]. Bad or poor adaptation to environment, socially, mentally or physically.

malaise (mal′-āz) [F.]. A feeling of illness and discomfort.

malalignment (mal-al-īn′-ment) [L. *malus*, bad; *linea*, line]. Faulty alignment—as of the teeth, or fracture.

malar (māl′-ár) [L. *mala*, cheek]. Relating to the cheek.

malaria (mal-ār′-i-à) [It. *malaria*, bad air]. A tropical disease caused by one of the genus Plasmodium and carried by infected mosquitoes of the genus Anopheles. *Plasmodium falciparum* causes malignant tertian m.; *Plasmodium vivax* causes benign tertian m.; and *Plasmodium malariae* causes quartan m. Signs and symptoms are caused by the presence in the red blood cells of the erythrocytic (E) stages of the parasite. In the falciparum malaria *only* the blood-forms of the parasite exist. There is an additional persistent infection in the liver (the extraerythrocytic or EE form) in all other forms of malaria and it is the factor responsible for relapses. Clinical picture is one of recurring rigors, anaemia, toxaemia and splenomegaly—malarial, adj.

malarial therapy. Induction of hyperpyrexia by inoculation with benign form of malaria. Used in the treatment of neurosyphilis

malariologist (mal-ār-ī-ol′-o-jist) [It. *malaria*, bad air; G. *logos*, discourse]. An expert in the study of malaria.

malassimilation (mal-a-sim-il-ā′-shun). Poor or disordered assimilation.

malathion (mal-ath-ī′-on). Organophosphorus compound, used as insecticide in agriculture. Powerful and irreversible anticholinesterase action following excessive inhalation. Potentially dangerous to man for this reason. Currently being used for treatment of head lice.

male fern. Filix mas (q.v.).

malformation (mal-for-mā′-shun) [L. *malus*, bad; *formare*, to form]. Abnormal shape or structure; deformity.

malignant (mal-ig′-nant) [L. *malignus*, wicked]. Virulent and dangerous; that which is likely to have a fatal termination. **malignant growth** or **tumour**, cancer or sarcoma. **malignant pustule**, anthrax malignancy, n.

malingering (mal-ing′-er-ing). Deliberate (volitional) production of symptoms to evade an unpleasant situation.

malleolus (mal-lē′-o-lus) [L. hammer]. A part or process of a bone shaped like a hammer. **external m.**, at the lower end of the fibula. **internal m.**, situated at the lower end of the tibia -malleoli, pl.; malleolar, adj.

malleus (mal′-i-us) [L.]. The hammer-shaped lateral bone of the middle ear.

malnutrition (mal-nu-trish′-un) [L. *malus*, bad; *nutrire*, to nourish]. The state of being poorly nourished. May be caused by inadequate intake of one or more of the essential nutrients or by malassimilation.

malocclusion (mal-ok-klū′-shun) [L. *malus*, bad; *occludere*, to close]. Failure of the upper and lower teeth to meet properly when the jaws are closed.

malposition (mal-pō-zi′-shun)[L. *malus*, bad; *positio*, place]. Any abnormal position of a part.

malpractice (mal-prak′-tis) [L. *malus*, bad; G. *praktikos*, fit for doing]. Malpraxia. Unethical, improper or injurious treatment.

malpresentation (mal-prez-en-tā′-shun) [L. *malus*, bad; *proesentere*, to present]. Any unusual presentation of the fetus in the pelvis.

Malta fever. See BRUCELLA, BRUCELLOSIS. The condition is also called 'abortus f.', 'Mediterranean f.' and 'undulant f.'

maltase (mawl′-tas). A sugar splitting (saccharolytic) enzyme found in the body, especially in intestinal juice.

maltose (mawl′-tōs). Malt sugar a disaccharide; produced by the hydrolysis of starch during digestion.

malunion (mal-ūn′-yon) [L. *malus*, bad; *unite*, to unite]. Union of a fracture in bad position.

mamma (ma′-mà) [L. breast]. The breast; milk-secreting gland -mammae, pl.; mammary, adj.

mammaplasty (ma′-ma-plas-ti) [L. *mamma*, breast; G. *plassein*, to form]. Any plastic operation on the breast—mammaplastic, adj.

mammilla (mam-il′-à) [L. nipple]. The nipple; a small papilla—mammillae, pl.

mammography (mam-og′-ra-fi) [L.

mamma, breast; G. *graphein*, to write]. X-ray examination of the breast after injection of an opaque agent. Syn. mastography—mammographic, adj.; mammographically, adv.

mammotrophic (mam-o-trō'-fik) [L. *mamma*, breast; G. *trephein*, to nourish]. Having an effect upon the breast.

Manchester operation. See FOTHERGILL'S OPERATION.

Mandelamine (man-del'-a-mēn). See MANDELIC ACID.

mandelic acid (man-del'-ik as'-id). A urinary antiseptic used mainly as the calcium or ammonium salts. A high degree of urinary acidity is essential for activity, and supplementary administration of ammonium chloride may be required. Limitation of fluids is also desirable.

Mandrax (man'-draks). Methaqualone (q.v.). and diphenhydramine (q.v.).

mania (mā'-ni-á) [G. madness]. One phase of manic depressive psychoses in which the prevailing mood is one of undue elation and there is pronounced psychomotor overactivity and often pathological excitement—maniac, adj.

manic depressive psychosis (man'-ik dēpres'-iv sī-kō'-siz). A type of mental disorder which alternates between phases of excitement and phases of depression. Often between these phases there are periods of complete normality.

manipulation (man-ip-ū-lā'-shun). Using the hands skilfully as in reducing a fracture or hernia, or changing the fetal position.

mannitol (man'-i-tol). A natural sugar that is not metabolized in the body and acts as an osmotic diuretic. When the renal blood flow is low, mannitol probably exerts a direct action on the renal vessels and restores the flow with a rapid improvement in renal function. Mannitol-induced diuresis used in tranquillizer and barbiturate poisoning, and in head injuries to shrink brain.

mannityl hexanitrate (man'-i-til heks-anīt'-rāt). A long-acting vasodilator, used mainly for the prophylactic treatment of angina pectoris. Prolonged administration may cause methaemoglobinaemia.

mannomustine (man-o-mus'-tēn). Antimitotic agent useful in cancer.

mannose (man'-ōs). A fermentable monosaccharide.

manometer (man-om'-et-ér) [G. *manos*,

rare; *metron*, a measure]. An instrument for measuring the pressure exerted by liquids or gases. See SPHYGMOMANOMETER.

Mantoux reaction (man'-too). An intradermal method of determining the degree of sensitivity of a patient to old tuberculin by using serial dilutions 1:10 000, 1:1000 and 1:100. Purified protein derivative (PPD) is a purified type of tuberculin. [Charles Mantoux, French physician, 1877–1947.]

manubrium (man-ū'-bri-um) [L. handle]. A handle-shaped structure; the upper part of the breast bone or sternum.

MAOI. Monoamine oxidase inhibitor (q.v.)

maple syrup urine disease. Genetic disorder of recessive familial type. Leucine, isoleucine and valine are excreted in excess in urine giving the smell of maple syrup. Symptoms include spasticity, feeding and respiratory difficulties; severe damage to the CNS may occur. A diet low in the three amino acids may be effective if started early enough, otherwise the disorder is fatal. Genetic counselling may be indicated. In the pregnant woman, examination may reveal evidence of the disorder and in such cases it may be wise to advise termination of pregnancy.

marasmus (mar-az'-mus) [G. a withering]. Wasting away of the body, especially that of a baby, without apparent cause. The currently preferred term is failure to thrive (q.v.)—marasmic, adj.

Marboran (mar'-bor-an). Methisazone (q.v.).

marburg disease. Syn., 'green monkey' disease. Highly infectious viral disease characterized by a sudden onset of fever, malaise, headache and myalgia—especially in the lumbar region. Between days 5 and 7, a rash appears on the buttocks, trunk, outer aspects of arms and around the hair roots. Treatment is symptomatic. Virus can persist in the body for 2 to 3 months after the initial attack. Cross infection probably occurs by the aerosol route. Incubation period believed to be 4 to 9 days and mortality rate in previous outbreaks has been approximately 30 per cent.

Marcain (már'-kān). Bupivacaine (q.v.).

Marevan (mar'-e-van). Slow-acting anticoagulant. Warfarin (q.v.).

Marfan's syndrome. Hereditary genetic disorder of unknown cause. There is dislocation of the lens, congenital heart disease and arachnodactyly with hypotonic musculature and lax ligaments, occasionally excessive height and abnormalities of the iris. [B.J.A. Marfan, Paris physician, 1858–1942.]

marihuana. Indian hemp (q.v.). Hashish.

Marion's disease. Hypertrophic stenosis of the internal urinary meatus.

Marmite. A proprietary concentrated extract obtained from yeast by autolysis with salt and flavoured with vegetables and spices. It contains vitamins of the B₂ complex (riboflavin, 1.5 mg per g; niacin (nicotinic acid), 16.5 mg per g).

Marplan. Isocarboxozid (q.v.).

marrow (mar'-ō) [A.S. *mearg*, pith]. The soft, pulpy substance present in bones. **red m.** is present in the cancellous tissue of bones, and is concerned with blood formation. **yellow m.** is a fatty substance, present in the shafts of long bones.

Marshal-Marchetti-Krantz operation. For stress incontinence. Usually undertaken in patients who have not been controlled by a colporrphaphy. 85 per cent success rate.

Marsilid. A monoamine oxidase inhibitor (q.v.).

marsupialization (mar-sūp-i-al-iz-ā'-shun) [G. *marsippion*, bag]: An operation for cystic abdominal swellings, which entails stitching the margins of an opening made into the cyst, to the edges of the abdominal wound, thus forming a pouch.

Marzine (mar'-zēn). Cyclizine. Action quick and short. Should not be given in pregnancy. See ANTIHISTAMINES

masochism (mas'-o-kizm). Punishing the self. It may be a conscious or unconscious process. Opp., sadism. [Leopold von Sacher-Masoch, Austrian historian, 1836–95.]

mastalgia (mas-tal'-ji-á) [G. *mastos*, breast; *algos*, pain]. Pain in the breast.

mastectomy (mas-tek'-to-mi) [G. *mastos*, breast; *ektome*, excision]. Surgical removal of the breast. **simple m.**, removal of the breast with the overlying skin. Combined with radiotherapy this operation is the usual treatment for carcinoma of the breast. **radical m.**, removal of the breast with the skin and underlying pectoral muscle together with all the lymphatic tissue of the axilla.

Masteril (mas'-ter-il). Drostanolone (q.v.).

mastication (mas-tik-ā'-shun) [L. *masticare*, to chew]. The act of chewing.

mastitis (mas-tī'-tis) [G. *mastos*, breast; *-itis*, inflammation]. Inflammation of the breast. **chronic m.**, the name formerly applied to the nodular changes in the breasts now usually called 'fibrocystic disease'.

mastography (mas-tog'-ra-fi). See **mammography**—mastographic, adj., mastographically, adv.

mastoid (mas'-toid) [G. *mastos*, breast; *eidos*, form]. Nipple-shaped. **mastoid air cells** extended in a backward and downward direction from the antrum. **mastoid antrum**, the air space within the mastoid process, lined by mucous membrane continuous with that of the tympanum and mastoid cells. **mastoid process**, the prominence of the mastoid portion of the temporal bone just behind the ear.

mastoidectomy (mas-toid-ek'-to-mi) [G. *mastos*, breast; *eidos*, form; *ektome*, excision]. Drainage of the mastoid aircells and excision of diseased tissue. **cortical m.**, all the mastoid cells are removed making one cavity which drains through an opening (aditus) into the middle ear. The external meatus and middle ear are untouched. **radical m.**, the mastoid antrum, and middle ear are made into one continuous cavity for drainage of infection. Loss of hearing is inevitable.

mastoiditis (mas-toid-i'-tis) [G. *mastos*, breast; *eidos*, form; *-itis*, inflammation]. Inflammation of the mastoid air-cells.

mastoidotomy (mas-toid-o'-to-mi) [G. *mastos*, breast; *eidos*, form; *stoma*, mouth]. Incision into the mastoid process of temporal bone.

masturbation (mas-tur-bā'-shun) [L. *masturbari*, to defile oneself]. The production of sexual excitement by friction of the genitals.

materia medica (mat-ē'-ri-á med'-i-ká) [L.]. The science dealing with the origin, action and dosage of drugs.

matrix (mā'-triks) [L.]. The foundation substance in which the tissue cells are embedded.

Matromycin (mat-rō-mi'-sin). Oleandomycin (q.v.).

maturation (mat-ū-rā'-shun) [L. *maturare*, to make ripe]. The process of attaining full development.

Maurice Lee tube. Combine nasogastric aspiration and jejunal feeding.

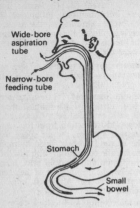

Wide-bore
aspiration
tube

Narrow-bore
feeding tube

Stomach

Small
bowel

Maurice Lee tube

Maxidex (mak'-si-deks). Dexamethasone (q.v.). Steroid drops for eyes to counteract inflammatory condition.

maxilla (maks-il'-a) [L. jaw]. The jawbone; in particular the upper jaw—maxillary, adj.

maxillofacial (maks-il-ō-fā'-shal) [L. *maxilla*, jaw; *facies*, face]. Pertaining to the maxilla and face. A subdivision in plastic surgery.

meatotomy (mē-at-ot'-o-mi) [L.; G. *tome*, a cutting]. Surgery to urinary meatus for meatal ulcer and stricture in men.

M and B 7714 (3-methyl-4-bromo-5-formylisothiazole thiosemicarbazone). Smallpox prophylactic agent.

McBurney's point. A point one-third of the way between the anterior superior iliac spine and the umbilicus, the site of maximum tenderness in cases of acute appendicitis [Charles McBurney, New York surgeon, 1845–1913.]

measles (mēz'-lz). Morbilli. An acute infectious disease caused by a virus. Characterized by fever, a blotchy rash and catarrh of mucous membranes. Endemic and worldwide in distribution.

Maxolon (maks'-o-lon). Metoclopramide (q.v.).

meatus (mē-ā'-tus) [L.]. An opening or channel—meatal, adj.

mebanazine (meb-an'-a-zēn). A monoamine oxidase inhibitor (q.v.).

mecamylamine (me-ka-mī'-la-min). An orally effective ganglionic blocking agent used in the treatment of hypertension. It is much more potent than hexamethonium, and the response is smoother and more predictable. Like similar drugs, it may cause severe constipation, but this does not interfere significantly with absorption. The action lasts over 6 to 12 hours, and three doses daily afford adequate control.

mechanism of labour. The forces which extrude the fetus through the birth canal together with the opposing, resisting forces which affect its position. [See diagram on opposite page.]

mechlorethamine hydrochloride (mē-klor-eth'-a-mēn). Cytotoxic agent.

Mecholyl. Cholinergic agent.

Meckel's diverticulum (mek'-els dī-ver-tik'-ū-lum). A blind, pouch-like sac sometimes arising from the free border of the ileum. Occurs in 2 per cent of population: usually symptomless. May cause GI bleeding; may intussuscept or obstruct. [Johann Friedrich Meckel, German anatomist and gynaecologist, 1714–74.]

meclozine (mek'-lō-zēn). Antihistamine (q.v.).

meconium (me-kōn'-i-um) [G. *mekonion*]. The discharge from the bowel of a newly born baby. It is a greenish-black, viscid substance. **meconium ileus,** impaction of m. in bowel. Associated with smelly, fatty stools and chest infection. Earliest sign of mucoviscidosis.

Medetron (med'-ē-tron). Stethoscope (q.v.) that can be used over clothing.

media (mē'-di-á) [L. *medius*, middle]. The middle coat of a vessel. Nutritive jelly used for culturing bacteria.

medial (mē-di-al) [L. *medius*, middle]. Pertaining to or near the middle—medially, adv.

median (mēd'-i-an) [L. *medius*, middle]. The middle. **median line,** an imaginary line passing through the centre of the body from a point between the eyes to between the closed feet.

mediastinum (mēd-i-as-tī'-num) [L. *medius*, middle]. The space between the lungs—mediastinal, adj.

mediastinoscopy (mēd-i-as'-tin-os'-ko-pi) [L. *medius*, middle; G. *skopein*, to examine]. Minor surgical procedure for visual inspection of the mediastinom. May be combined with biopsy of lymph nodes for histological examination.

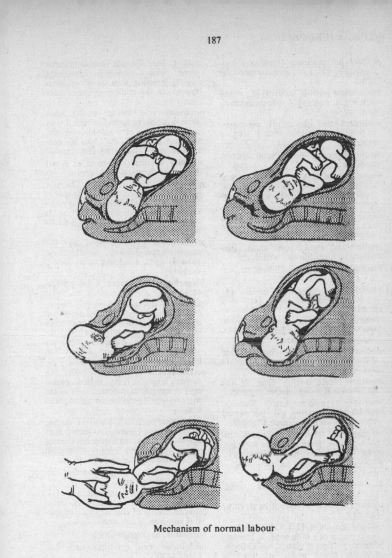

Mechanism of normal labour

medical jurisprudence (med'-ik-al-joo-ris-proo'-dens). Syn., forensic medicine (q.v.)

medicament (med-ik'-a-ment) [L. *medicamentum*, remedy]. A remedy or medicine.

medicated (med'-i-kā-ted) [L. *medicare*, to heal]. Impregnated with a drug or medicine.

medicinal (med-is'-in-al). Pertaining to a medicine.

medicine (med'-sin). 1. Science or art of healing, especially as distinguished from surgery and obstetrics. 2. A therapeutic substance.

medicochirurgical (med-i-kō-kī-rur'-ji-kal). Pertaining to both medicine and surgery.

medicosocial (med-i-kō-sō'-shal). Pertaining to medicine and sociology.

Medinal (med'-in-al). Barbitone sodium (q.v.)

mediolateral (mē-di-ō-lat'-er-al) [L. *medius*, middle; *latus*, side]. Term used in midwifery.

Mediterranean fever. See BRUCELLA, BRUCELLOSIS. Also called 'abortus f.', 'Malta f.' and 'undulant f.'

medium (mē'-di-um). A substance used in bacteriology for the growth of organisms—media, pl.

Medomin (med'-ō-min). One of the barbitones. Hypno/sedative capsules.

Medresco (med-res'-ko). National Health issue hearing aid. So named after the Medical Research Council.

medrogestone (med-rō-jes'-tōn). A female hormone, given orally or by injection. Shrinks diseased prostate gland.

Medrone (med'-rōn). Methylprednisolone (q.v.).

medroxyprogesterone acetate (med-oks'-i-prō-jes-ter-ōn as'-ē-tāt). Long-acting (90 days) contraceptive given by injection.

medulla (me-dul'-á) [L.]. 1. The marrow in the centre of a long bone. 2. The soft internal portion of glands, e.g. kidneys, adrenals, lymph nodes, etc. medulla oblongata, the upper part of the spinal cord between the foramen magnum of the occipital bone and the pons cerebri—medullary, adj.

medullated (med'-ul-ā-ted). Containing or surrounded by a medulla or marrow, particularly referring to nerve fibres.

medulloblastoma (med-ul'-ō-blas-tō'-

má) [L. *medulla*, marrow; G. *blastos*, germ; *-oma*, tumour]. Malignant, rapidly growing tumour of children: appears in the midline of the cerebellum.

mefenamic acid (mef-en-am'-ik). Analgesic that does not interfere with uricosuric action of sulphinpyrazone, therefore useful in gout. Also has anti-inflammatory and antipyretic actions.

mefenide acetate (mef'-en-īd as'-ē-tat). Antiseptic dermatological cream.

mefruside (mef-rū'-sīd). Diuretic. Smooth prolonged action, maximal in first 12 hours, produces salt and water loss with little potassium depletion. In hypertensive patients m. has a useful hypotensive action.

megacephalic (me-ga-kef-al'-ik) [G. *megas*, large; *kephale*, head]. Large headed. Syn., macrocephalic, megalocephalic.

Megaclor (meg'-a-klor). Clomocycline (q.v.).

megacolon (me-ga-kō'-lon) [G. *megas*, large; *kolon*, colon]. Condition of dilated and elongated colon. In an adult the cause is unknown. In a child the parasympathetic ganglion cells are absent in the distal part of the colon (Hirschsprung's disease (q.v.).

megakaryocyte (mega-kar'-i-ō-sīt) [G. *megas*, large; *karyon*, kernal; *kytos*, cell]. Large multinucleated cells of the marrow which produce the blood platelets.

megaloblast (meg'-a-lō-blast) [G. *megas*, large; *blastos*, germ]. A large, nucleated, primitive red blood cell formed where there is a deficiency of vitamin B_{12} or folic acid—megaloblastic, adj.

megalocephalic (meg-al-ō-kef-al'-ik). See MEGACEPHALIC.

megalomania (meg-a-lō-mān'-i-á) [G. *megas*, large; *mania*, madness]. Delusion of grandeur, characteristic of general paralysis of the insane (q.v.).

Megimide, Bemegride (q.v.).

meibomian cyst (mī-bōm'-i-an). See CHALAZION.

Meibomian glands (mī-bōm'-i-an). Sebaceous glands lying in grooves on the inner surface of the eyelids, their ducts opening on the free margins of the lids. [Heinrich Meibom, German anatomist, 1638–1700.]

Meigs's syndrome (megz). Benign, solid ovarian tumour associated with hydroperitoneum and hydrothorax. [Joe V. Meigs, American surgeon, 1892–   .]

meiosis (mē-ī-ō'-sis). Miosis (q.v.). Also **myosis.**

melaena (mel-ē'-nȧ) [G. *melas,* black]. Black, tar-like stools. Evidence of intestinal bleeding.

melancholia (mel-an-kō'-li-ȧ) [G. *melagcholia*]. Term reserved in psychiatry to mean severe forms of depression—melancholic, adj.

melanin (mel'-an-in) [G. *melas,* black]. A black pigment found in hair, skin and the choroid of the eye.

melanoma (mel-an-ō'-mȧ) [G. *melas,* black; *-oma,* tumour]. A tumour arising from the pigment-producing cells of the deeper layers in the skin, or of the eye—melanomata, pl.; melanomatous, adj.

melanosarcoma (mel-an-ō-sȧr-kō'-mȧ) [G. *melas,* black; *sarkoma,* fleshy overgrowth]. One form of malignant melanoma—melanosarcomata, pl.; melanosarcomatous, adj.

melanosis (mel-an-ō'-sis) [G. *melas,* black; *-osis,* condition]. Dark pigmentation of surfaces as in sunburn, Addison's disease, etc.—melanotic, adj.

melanuria (mel-an-ūr'-i-ȧ) [G. *melas,* black; *ouron,* urine]. Melanin in the urine—melanuric, adj.

melarsoprol (mel-ar'-sō-prol). Organic arsenical given i.v. in trypanosomiasis.

melarsonyl potassium (mel-ar'-son-il). Organic arsenical given i.v. in trypanosomiasis. Less toxic than melarsoprol.

melitensis. See BRUCELLOSIS.

Melleril. Thioridazine (q.v.).

Melphalan (mel'-fa-lan). Alkylating cytotoxic agent.

membrane (mem'-brān). A thin lining or covering substance. **basement m.,** a thin layer beneath the epithelium of mucous surfaces. **hyaloid m.,** that surrounding the vitreous humor of the eye. **mucous m.,** contains glands which secrete mucus. It lines the cavities and passages that communicate with the exterior of the body. **serous m.,** a lubricating membrane lining the closed cavities, and reflected over their enclosed organs. **synovial m.,** that lining the intra-articular parts of bones and ligaments. **tympanic m.,** the eardrum—membranous, adj.

menadione (men-ȧ-dī'-ōn). Chemical name for vitamin K (q.v.).

menaphthone (men-af'-thōn). Vitamin K is an essential factor in blood coagulation, and menaphthone is a synthetic oil-soluble compound with similar activity. Used in haemorrhage and obstructive jaundice. Given intramuscularly.

menarche (men-ar'-kē) [G. *men,* month; *arche,* beginning]. When the menstrual periods commence and other bodily changes occur.

Mendel's law. A theory of heredity, evolved by an Austrian monk, which deals with the interaction of dominant and recessive characters in cross-breeding. [Gregor Johann Mendel, 1822–84.]

Mendelson's syndrome. Inhalation of regurgitated stomach contents, which can cause immediate death from anoxia, or it may produce extensive lung damage or pulmonary oedema with severe bronchospasm.

Ménière's disease (Mān-yers). Distension of membranous labyrinth of middle ear from excess fluid. Pressure causes ischaemia and failure of function of nerve of hearing and balance, thus there is fluctuating deafness, tinnitus and repeated attacks of vertigo. [Prosper Ménière, French otologist, 1799–1862]

meninges (men-in'-jēs) [G. *menigx,* membrane]. The surrounding membranes of the brain and spinal cord. They are three in number: (1) the dura mater (outer); (2) arachnoid membrane (middle); (3) pia mater (inner)—meninx (mē'-ningks), sing.; meningeal, adj.

meningioma (men-in-ji-ō'-mȧ) [G. *menigx,* membrane; *-oma,* tumour]. A slowly growing fibrous tumour arising in the meninges—meningiomata, pl.; meningiomatous, adj.

meningism, meningismus (men'-in-jism or men-in-jis'-mus). Condition presenting with signs and symptoms of meningitis (e.g. neck stiffness); meningitis does not develop.

meningitis (men-in-jī'-tis) [G. *menigx,* membrane; *-itis,* inflammation]. Inflammation of the meninges. An epidemic form is known as cerebrospinal fever, the infecting organism is *Neisseria meningitidis* (meningococcus). The term meningococcal meningitis is now preferred. See LEPTOMENINGITIS, PACHYMENINGITIS —meningitides, pl.

meningocele (men-ing'-gō-sēl) [G. *menigx,* membrane; *kele,* hernia]. Protrusion of the meninges through a bony defect. It forms a cyst filled with cerebrospinal fluid. See SPINA BIFIDA.

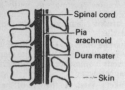

Spinal cord

Pia arachnoid

Dura mater

Skin

Meningocele   Meningo-myelocele

meningococcus (men-ing-gō-ko′-kus). Syn., *Neisseria meningitidis* meningococcal, adj.

meningoencephalitis (mening′-gō-en-kef-al-ī′-tis). Inflammation of the brain and the meninges—meningoencephalitic, adj.

meningomyelocele (men-ing′-gō-mī′-el-ō-sēl) [G. *menigx,* membrane; *myelos,* marrow; *kele,* hernia]. Protrusion of a portion of the spinal cord and its enclosing membranes through a bony defect. Syn., myelomeningocele.

meniscectomy (men-i-sek′-to-mi) [G. *meniskos,* crescent-shaped; *ektome,* excision]. The removal of a semilunar cartilage of the knee joint, following injury and displacement. The medial cartilage is damaged most commonly.

meniscus (men-is′-kus) [G. *meniskos,* crescent]. 1. semilunar cartilage, particularly in the knee joint. 2. The curved upper surface of a column of liquid-menisci, pl.

menopause (men′-ō-pawz) [G. *men,* month; *pausis,* stopping]. The cessation of menstruation; occurring normally between the ages of 45 and 50. The change of life. Climacteric. **artificial m.,** an earlier menopause induced by radiotherapy or surgery for some pathological condition menopausal, adj.

menorrhagia (men-or-ā′-ji-a) [G. *men,* month; *rhegnynai,* to burst forth]. An excessive regular menstrual flow.

menses (men′-sēz) [L. months]. The sanguineous fluid discharged from the uterus during menstruation; menstrual flow.

menstrual (men′-stroo-al). Relating to the menses. **menstrual cycle,** the cyclical chain of events that occurs in the uterus in which a flow of blood occurs for 4 to 5 days every 28 days. The cycle is governed by hormones from the anterior pituitary gland and the ovaries.

menstruation (men-stroo-ā′-shun) [L. *menstruare,* to menstruate]. The flow of blood from the uterus once a month in the female. It commences about the age of 13 and ceases about 45.

mental (men′-tal) [L. *mentum,* chin]. Pertaining to the chin.

mental disorder. Mental illness, arrested or incomplete development of mind, psychopathic disorder and any other disorder or disability of mind, and 'mentally disordered' shall be construed accordingly. **mental subnormality,** see SUBNORMALITY.

Mental Health Review Tribunal. A body set up in each Regional Health Administration area to deal with patients' applications for discharge or alteration of their conditions of detention in hospital.

Mental Welfare Officer. Appointed by the Local Health Authority to deal with: (1) applications for compulsory or emergency admission to hospital, or for conveyance of patients there; (2) applications concerning guardianship, the functions of the nearest relative, or acting as nearest relative if so appointed; (3) returning patients absent without leave, or apprehending patients escaped from legal custody. In addition, the MWO may have a wide range of functions in the care and aftercare of the mentally disordered in the community. This includes home visiting, training centres, clubs and general supervision of the discharged patient.

menthol (men′-thol). Mild analgesic obtained from oil of peppermint. Used in liniments and ointments for rheumatism, and as an inhalation or drops for nasal catarrh.

mentoanterior (men-to-an-tē′-ri-or). Forward position of the fetal chin in the maternal pelvis in a face presentation.

mentoposterior (men-to-pos-tē′-ri-or). Backward position of the fetal chin in the maternal pelvis in a face presentation.

mepacrine (me′-pa-krēn). Synthetic antimalarial substance, more effective than quinine, and better tolerated. Occasionally used against tapeworm, and in lupus erythematosus.

Mepazine (mep′-a-zēn). Similar to chlorpromazine (q.v.). Useful in midwifery.

mephenesin elixir. Mild muscle relaxant. Can be given through stomach tube.

Mephine (mef′-ēn). A sympathomimetic hypertensive agent.

Mephyton (me′-fi-ton). Phytomenadione. An emulsion of vitamin K for oral administration.

Mepilin (mep′-il-in). Androgen-oestrogen mixture, useful at the menopause. Theoretically the oestrogens give relief and prevent masculinization by the androgens, while the latter prevent undue stimulation of the breasts and of the endometrium, and also by their anabolic effects promote a feeling of well-being.

meprobamate (mep-rō′-bam-āt). One of the carbamates. A tranquillizer which, by central nervous action, produces mental relaxation. For poisoning, see p. 337.

mepyramine (me-pir′-a-mēn). An effective antihistamine, useful in allergic skin conditions. The sedative side effects may cause drowsiness in some patients.

Merbentyl (mer-ben′-til). Dicyclomine (q.v.).

mercaptopurine (mer-kap′-to-pūr-in). Used in the treatment of acute leukaemia in children. Prevents synthesis of nucleic acid.

mercurialism (mer-kū′-ri-al-izm). Toxic effects on human body of mercury—the ancient cure for syphilis. May result from use of teething powders (cf. pink disease) or calomel (as an abortifacient). Symptomatology includes stomatitis, loosening of teeth, gastroenteritis and skin eruptions.

mercuric oxide (mer-kū′-rik oks′-īd). A bright yellow powder, used mainly as oculent hydrarg. ox. flav (golden eye ointment). It is antiseptic and is used in conjunctivitis and other eye conditions.

mercurochrome (mer-kū′-rō-krōm). Red dye containing mercury in combination. Has antiseptic properties, and is sometimes used for skin sterilization as a 2 per cent solution in a mixture of acetone, alcohol and water.

Merthiolate (mer-thī′-ō-lāt). Thiomersalate (q.v.). Used in bone bank (1 in 1000 to 1 in 3000). Organic iodine solution. Useful for preparation of skin prior to surgery.

mesateritis (mes-árt-ér-ī′-tis) [G. *mesos,* middle; *arteria,* artery; *-itis,* inflammation]. Inflammation of the middle coat of an artery.

mescaline (mes′-kal-ēn). A hallucinogenic agent. Can be used to produce abreaction.

mesencephalon (mes-en-kef′-a-lon) [G. *mesos,* middle; *egkephalos,* brain]. The midbrain.

mesentery (mes′-en-te-ri) [G. *mesos,* middle; *enteron,* intestine]. A large fold of peritoneum passing between a portion of intestine and the posterior abdominal wall—mesenteric, adj.

Mesontoin (mes′-on-toin). Methoin (q.v.).

mesothelioma (mes-ō-thē-li-ō′-ma). A rapidly fatal tumour that spreads over the pleural covering of the lung. Of current interest because of its association with the asbestos industry.

Mestinon (mes′-tin-on). Pyridostigmine (q.v.).

metabolic (met-ab-ol′-ik) [G. *metabole,* change]. Pertaining to metabolism. **basal m. rate (BMR),** the expression of basal metabolism in terms of kcal per sq.m of body surface per hour—metabolically, adv

metabolism (met-ab′-ol-izm) [G. *metabole,* change]. The series of chemical changes in the living body by which life is maintained. The tissues are broken down by wear and tear (catabolism) and rebuilt (anabolism) continuously, **basal m.,** the energy used by a body at complete rest, being the minimum necessary to maintain life. See ADENOSINE DIPHOSPHATE and TRIPHOSPATE—metabolic, adj.

metabolite (met-ab′-ol-īt) [G. *metabole,* change]. Any product of metabolism, **essential m.,** a substance necessary for proper metabolism, e.g. vitamins.

metacarpophalangeal (met-a-kár′-pō-fal-an′-jē-al) [G. *meta,* after; *karpos,* wrist; *phalagx,* series]. Pertaining to the metacarpus and the phalanges.

metacarpus (met-ak-ár′-pus) [G. *meta,* after; *karpos,* wrist]. The five bones which form that part of the hand between the wrist and fingers—metacarpal, adj.

metaraminol (met-ar-a-mín'-ol). Vaso-pressor agent used in hypotensive shock.

Metastab (met'-a-stab). Methylprednis-olone (q.v.).

metastasis (me-tas'-ta-sis) [G. removal]. The transference of disease from one part of the body to another, usually by blood or lymph. A secondary growth—metastases, pl.; metastatic, adj.; metastasize, v.

metatarsalgia (met-a-tár-sal'-ji-á) [G. meta, after; L. tarsus, ankle; G. algos, pain]. Pain under the metatarsal heads.

metatarsophalangeal (met-a-tár'-só-fal-an'-jē-al) [G. meta, after; L. tarsus, ankle; phalagx, series]. Pertaining to the metatarsus and the phalanges.

metatarsus (met-a-tár'-sus) [G. meta, after; L. tarsus, ankle]. The five bones of the foot between the ankle and the toes—metatarsal, adj.

metatone (met'-a-tōn). Glycerophos-phates (q.v.).

metazoa (met-á-zō-á) [G. meta, after; zoion, living being]. Multicellular ani-mal organisms with differentiation of cells to form tissues—metazoal, adj.

meteorism (mē'-tē-or-izm) [G. meteoros, lofty]. Excessive accumulation of gas in the intestines. Tympanites.

metformin (met-form'-in). One of the diaguanides. Antidiabetic agent.

methacycline (meth-á-sī'-klin). Antibi-otic particularly useful in exacerbations of chronic bronchitis.

methadone (me'-tha-dōn). A synthetic morphine-like analgesic, but with a reduced sedative action. Can be given orally or by injection. Particularly valu-able in visceral pain, and useful in the treatment of useless cough. May cause addiction if treatment is prolonged. Can be used in withdrawal programmes for heroin addicts.

methaemalbumin (met-hēm-al-bū'-min). Abnormal compound in blood from combination of haem with plasma albu-men.

methaemoglobin (met-hēm-ō-glōb'-in). A form of haemoglobin consisting of a combination of globin with an oxidized haem, containing ferric iron. This pig-ment is unable to transport oxygen. May be formed following the adminis-tration of a wide variety of drugs, including the sulphonamides. May be present in the blood as a result of a congenital abnormality.

methaemoglobinaemia (met-hēm-ō-glōb-in-ē'-mi-á). Methaemoglobin in the blood. If large quantities are pres-ent, individuals may show cyanosis, but otherwise no abnormality except, in severe cases, breathlessness on exertion, because the methaemoglobin cannot transport oxygen—methaemoglobin-aemic, adj.

methaemoglobinuria (met-hēm-ō-glōb-in-ūr'-i-á). Methaemoglobin in the urine—methaemoglobinuric, adj.

methandienone (meth-an'-di-en-ōn). Anticatabolic agent, useful in muscle wasting occurring as a result of the body's attempt to restore nitrogen bal-ance, as when protein nitrogen is lost in serum from a large wound or pressure sore, and in senile debility.

methane (mēth'-ān). Most important component of natural gas. See BENZ-TROPINE and THAM.

methaqualone (meth-a-qwal'-ōn). Oral hypnotic; useful alternative to the bar-biturates. Has been used i.v. to produce loss of consciousness as an alternative to thiopentone. For poisoning, see p. 342.

Methedrine (meth'-i-drin). See METHYL-AMPHETAMINE.

methenolone enanthate (meth-en'-ō-lōn en-an'-thāt). Anabolic steroid.

methicillin (meth-i-sil'-lin). A semisyn-thetic penicillin active against penicillin-resistant staphylococci. Destroyed by gastric juice. Given by injection.

methionine (meth'-i-o-nēn). One of the essential sulphur-containing amino acids. Occasionally used in hepatitis and other conditions associated with liver damage.

methohexitone (methohexital) sodium (meth-ō-heks'-i-tōn). Ultrashort-acting barbiturate given i.v. pre-operatively.

methoin (meth'-oin). Anticonvulsant used for major, focal and psychomotor epilepsy.

methotrexate (meth-ō-treks'-āt). Ameth-opterin (q.v.).

methotrimeprazine (meth-ō-trī-mep'-ra-zēn). Useful for pain in paralysed limbs.

methoxamine (meth-oks'-a-mēn). A pressor drug used to restore blood pres-sure. It has few side effects on the heart or central nervous system. Given intrav-enously or intramuscularly.

methoxyflurane (meth-oks-i-flūr'-ān). Obstetric inhalational analgesic.

methsuximide (meth-suks'-i-mīd). For

control of temporal lobe epilepsy and petit mal.

methyclothiazide (meth-i-klō-thī'-az-īd). See CHLOROTHIAZIDE.

methylamphetamine hydrochloride (meth-il-am-fet'-a-mēn hī-drō-klōr'-īd). A central nervous system stimulant similar to amphetamine (q.v.). Produces a marked and prolonged rise in blood pressure if injected. Can be given orally, intramuscularly or intravenously. Dependence on drug is a danger.

methylated spirit. Alcohol containing 5 per cent of wood naphtha to make it non-potable. The methylated spirit used for spirit stoves, etc. is less pure, and is coloured to distinguish it from the above.

methyldopa (meth-il-dō'-pa). Causes decarboxylase inhibition. Hypotensive agent. Action increased with thiazide diuretics.

methylene blue (meth'-i-lēn). Antiseptic dye sometimes used in urinary infections, often with hexamine (q.v.). The intramuscular injection of a 2.5 per cent solution has been used as a renal function test.

methylpentynol (meth-il-pen'-tin-ol). A short-acting mild sedative. One of the carbamates. It reduces apprehension in some cases, and is useful in conditions of emotional stress.

methyl phenidate (meth'-il fen'-i-dāt). Antidepressant. Acts by stimulation of central nervous system.

methylphenobarbitone (meth-il-fē-nō-bár'-bit-ōn). Greater anticonvulsant action than phenobarbitone. Useful in epilepsy, anxiety states and for senile tremor.

methylprednisolone (meth-il-pred-nis'-ō-lōn). Steroid suitable for rheumatoid arthritis, inflamatory and allergic conditions. Sometimes injected locally for exophthalmos.

methylsalicylate (meth-il-sal-is'-il-āt). Wintergreen. Used externally as a mild counterirritant and analgesic in rheumatic and similar conditions. Supplied as ointment or liniment.

methylscopolamine (meth-il-sko-pol'-a-min). Antispasmodic, especially useful for relaxing gastric and intestinal muscle.

methyltestosterone (meth-il-tes-tos'-ter-ōn). An orally active form of testosterone (q.v.). Given as sublingual tablets.

methylthiouracil (meth-il-thī'-ō-ū'-ra-

sil). An antithyroid compound used in thyrotoxicosis. It inhibits the formation of thyroxine. Reactions have followed its use, and carbimazole (q.v.) is often preferred.

methyprylone (meth-ip'-ril-ōn). Non-barbiturate hypno-sedative.

methysergide (meth-i-ser'-jīd). Used for migraine. Can cause retroperitoneal fibrosis.

metiamide (met'-i-á-mīd). Gastric secretory inhibitor thus encouraging healing of peptic ulcers.

metoclopramide (met-ō-klō'-pra-mīd). Gastric sedative. Antiemetic that can be given orally or by injection. Not so effective in vomiting of labyrinthine origin.

metritis (me-trī'-tis) [G. *metra*, womb; *-itis*, inflammation]. Inflammation of the uterus.

metronidazole (met-rō-ni-dā'-zol). Antimicrobial agent especially useful for treating severe anaerobic sepsis. Can be given intravenously and orally. Drug of choice for amoebiasis, Trichomonas, bacteroides and Vincent's infection.

metropathia haemorrhagica (met-rō-path'-i-á hem-or-aj'-ik-á). Irregular episodes of uterine bleeding due to excessive and unopposed oestrin in the blood stream. Usually associated with a follicular cyst in the ovary.

metorrhagia (met-rō-rā'-ji-á) [G. *metra*, womb; *rhegnynai*, to burst forth]. Uterine bleeding between the menstrual periods.

Metrulen (met-rū'-len). Ethynodiol diacetate (q.v.).

Metycaine (me'-ti-kān). A local anaesthetic of the cocaine type, used for infiltration, spinal anaesthesia, and as eye drops.

mexiteline hydrochloride. Antiarrhythmic agent. Controls existing ventricular arrhythmia and can be used as a prophylactic.

Mexitil. Mexiteline hydrochloride (q.v.).

Michel's clips (mi'-shels). Small metal clips used instead of sutures for the closure of a wound. [Gaston Michel, French surgeon in Nancy, 1875–1937.]

microangiopathy (mī-krō-an-ji-op'-ath-i). Thickening and reduplication of basement membrane in blood vessels. Occurs in diabetes mellitus.

microbe (mī'-krōb) [G. *mikros*, small; *bios*, life]. A microscopic organism (syn., micro-organism) microbial, microbic, adj.

microbiology (mī-krō-bī-ol'-o-ji) [G. *mikros,* small; *bios,* life; *logos,* discourse]. The science of micro-organisms.

microcephalic (mī-krō-kef-al'-ik) [G. *mikros,* small; *kephale,* head]. Pertaining to an abnormally small head.

Micrococcus (mī-krō-kok'-us) [G. *mikros,* small; *coccus,* a berry]. A genus of bacteria. Gram-positive spherical bacteria occurring in irregular masses. They comprise saprophytes, parasites and pathogens.

microcyte (mī'-krō-sīt) [G. *mikros,* small; *kytos,* cell]. An undersized red blood cell found especially in iron deficiency anaemia. **microcytosis,** an increased number of microcytes—microcytic, adj.

Microfilaria. Tiny worms, Cause filariasis (q.v.).

micrognathia (mī-krō-nath'-i-á) [G. *mikros,* small; *gnathos,* jaw]. Small jaw, especially the lower one.

Microgynon (mī-krō-gī'-non). Low oestrogen oral contraceptive.

micron (mī'-kron) [G. *mikros,* small]. A millionth part of a metre, represented by the Greek letter mu (μ).

micro-organism (mī-krō-or'-gan-izm). A microscopic cell. (Often synonymous with bacterium but includes virus, protozoon, rickettsia, fungus, alga and lichen.)

microscopic (mī-krō-skop'-ik) [G. *mikros,* small; *skopein,* to examine]. Extremely small; visible only with the aid of a microscope.

Microsporum (mī-krō-spō'-rum) [G. *mikros,* small; *sporos,* seed]. A genus of fungi. Parasitic, living in keratin-containing tissues of man and animals. Cause of ringworm. *Microsporum audouini* is the commonest cause of scalp ringworm.

microsurgery (mī-krō-sur'-je-ri). Use of the binocular operating microscope during the performance of operations, usually aural—microsurgical, adj.

micturition (mik-tū-rish'-un). [L. *micturire,* to make water]. The act of passing urine.

Midamor (mid'-a-mor). Amiloride (q.v.).

midbrain. The mesencephalon (q.v.).

midriff. The diaphragm (q.v.).

migraine (mē'-gren). Hemicrania. Periodic throbbing headache, unilateral initially, with at least three of the following features: (*a*) sensory prodromata; (*b*) photophobia; (*c*) nausea or vomiting; (*d*) family history of m., and (*e*) fluid retention before or diuresis during the attack. Tyramine in food has been investigated as a cause migrainous, adj.

Mikulicz's disease. Chronic hypertrophic enlargement of the lacrimal and salivary glands. Now thought to be an autoimmune process. [Johannes von Mikulicz-Radecki, Rumanian surgeon, 1850–1905.]

miliaria (mil-i-ėr'-i-á) [L. *miliarius,* millet]. Prickly heat. Common in the tropics, and affects waistline, cubital fossae, and the chest. Vesicular and erythematous eruption, caused by blocking of sweat ducts, and their subsequent rupture, or their infection by fungi or bacteria.

miliary (mil'-i-a-ri) [L. *miliarius,* millet]. Resembling a millet seed. **miliary tuberculosis,** a form in which tuberculous nodules are widely disseminated throughout the organs and tissues of the body.

milium (mil'-ē-um) [L. millet]. Condition in which tiny, white, cystic excrescences appear on the face, especially about the eyelids; associated with seborrhoea.

milk sugar. Lactose.

Miller-Abbot tube. A double lumen rubber tube used for intestinal suction. The second channel leads to a balloon near the tip of the tube. This balloon is inflated when the tube reaches the duodenum and it is then carried down the intestine by peristaltic activity.[Thomas Grier Miller, consultant physician of Philadelphia, Emeritus Professor of Medicine, 1886– ; William Osler Abbot, Assistant Professor of Medicine and Lecturer in Pharmacology in the University of Pennsylvania, 1902–43 (he died of leukaemia.)]

Milontin (mil'-on-tin). Phensuximide (q.v.).

Miltherex (mil'-thėr-eks). Chlorine preparation, for safe disposal of tuberculous sputum.

Milton. A stabilized solution of sodium hypochlorite. Used as 2.5 to 5 per cent solution for wounds and other antiseptic purposes, as 1 per cent solution for sterilizing babies' feeding bottles.

Miltown. Meprobamate (q.v.).

Minadex (min'-a-deks). General tonic in convalescence.

mineralocorticoid (min-er-al-ō-kor'-ti-koid). See ALDOSTERONE.

miner's anaemia. Hookworm disease. See ANKYLOSTOMIASIS.

miner's elbow. Inflammation of the bursa over the point of the elbow. Syn., student's elbow.

Minovlar (min-ov'-lár). Oral contraceptive.

Mintezol (min'-tez-ol). Thiabendazole (q.v.).

miosis (mī-ōs'-is) [G. *meiosis*, diminution]. Excessive contraction of the pupil of the eye. Also MYOSIS.

miotic (mī-ot'-ik). Pertaining to or producing miosis. Also MYOTIC.

Miracil D. Lucanthone (q.v.).

miscarriage (Mis-kar'-ij). The lay term for an abortion.

mistura (mis-tū'-rá). A mixture.

Misuse of Drugs Act 1971. Combines and extends the Dangerous Drugs Acts 1965 and 1967 and the Drugs (Prevention of Misuse) Act 1964, which have been repealed. The Act is designed to control the manufacture, sale, prescribing and dispensing of certain habit-forming drugs, to which an addiction may arise; these are now called 'controlled' drugs and are available to the public by medical prescription only, and heavy penalties may follow any illegal sale or supply. The principal drugs concerned are opium, morphine, cocaine, diamorphine, cannabis indica, and the many synthetic morphine substitutes as exemplified by pethidine.

mithramycin (mith-ra-mī'-sin). Antitumour compound. Derived from a micro-organism of the Streptomyces genus. Has been used for Paget's disease. It probably acts directly on osteoclasts.

mitosis (mītō'-sis) [G. *mitos*, thread; *-osis*, condition]. A complicated method of cell division occurring in specialized cells.

mitral (mī'-tral) [G. *mitra*, turban]. Mitre-shaped, as the valve between the left atrium and ventricle of the heart (bicuspid valve). **mitral incompetence,** a defect in the closure of the m. valve whereby blood tends to flow backwards into the left atrium from the left ventricle. **mitral stenosis,** narrowing of the m. orifice, usually due to rheumatic fever.

mitral valvulotomy (valvotomy), an operation for splitting the cusps of a stenosed m. valve.

Mixogen (miks'-ō-jen). Androgenoestrogen mixture. See MEPILIN.

MK-870. A potassium-sparing diuretic.

MLNS. Mucocutaneous lymph node syndrome.

Modecate (mod'-ē-kāt). Fluphenazine. (q.v.)

Moditen. Fluphenazine (q.v.).

Moduretic (mod-ūr-et'-ik). Amiloride (q.v.) and hydrochlorothiazide (q.v.).

Mogadon (mog'-a-don). Nitrazepam (q.v.).

molar teeth (mol'-lár). The double teeth or grinders, three on either side of each jaw.

mole (mōl) [A.S., *mal*, spot]. See NAEVUS. **carneous m.,** the result of a missed abortion, i.e. the uterus retains the dead and organized products of conception. **hydatidiform m.,** a condition in which the chorionic villi of the placenta undergo cystic degeneration and the fetus is absorbed. A proportion of the moles are active and if remnants are left in the uterus after abortion of the mole, malignant changes may ensue, giving rise to a chorionepithelioma (q.v.).

molecule (mol'-ē-kūl). The smallest particle into which matter can be divided and still retain its identity—molecular, adj.

mollities (mol-ish'-i-ēz) [L.] Softness. **mollities ossium,** osteomalacia (q.v.).

molluscum (mol-us'-lum) [L. *molluscus,* soft]. A soft tumour. **molluscum contagiousum,** an infectious type of wart which appears on the skin as a waxy papule, often umbilicated; spread is by autoinoculation. **molluscum fibrosum,** the superficial tumours of Recklinghausen's disease (q.v.).

monarticular (mon-ar-tik'-ū-lar) [G. *monos,* single; L. *articulus,* joint]. Relating to one joint.

Mönckeberg's sclerosis. Senile degenerative change resulting in calcification of the media in arteries, especially of the limbs; leads to intermittent claudication or gangrene. [Johann Georg Mönckeberg, German pathologist, 1877-1925.]

mongol mong'-gol). Preferred term is Down's syndrome. Refers to a type of congenital mentally subnormal child, with facial characteristics resembling the Mongolian races. Stigmata include oval tilted eyes, squint and a flattened occiput. Increased susceptibility to leukaemia. Abnormality of chromosome 21. Two types: 1. Failure of division of chromosome 21 results in an extra chromosome instead of the normal pair. The infant has 47 chromosomes. Usually born of elderly mothers. 2. Abnormality of chromosome 21, total number of 46 being normal. Usually born of young mothers. Higher risk of recurrence in subsequent pregnancies.

Monilia. Syn., Candida (q.v.).

moniliasis (mon-il-ī-a-sis). Disease caused by infection with species of Monilia (Candida). Candidiasis (q.v.).

moniliform (mo-nil'-i-form) [L. *monile*, necklace; *forma*, form]. Like a string of beads. Used to describe the arrangement of micro-organisms, or clinical features such as a skin rash.

monitoring (mon'-it-or-ing). Sequential recording. Term usually reserved for automatic visual display of such measurements as temperature, pulse, respiration and blood pressure.

Monitron (mon'-i-tron) An apparatus for the automatic recording of temperature, pulse, respiration, and systolic and diastolic blood pressures.

monoamine oxidase (mon-ō-ā'-mēn oks'-i-dās). An enzyme which inhibits the breakdown of serotonin and catecholamines in the brain.

monoamine oxidase inhibitor (mon-ō-ā'-mēn oks'-i-dās in-hib'-it-or). MOAI. A substance which, by inhibiting the action of monoamine oxidase, increases the level of serotonin and catecholamines in the brain; useful for relief of exogenous or reactive depression. Increases the effects of barbiturates and alcohol. Patients advised to abstain from cheese, Marmite, Bovril, broadbeans (because of episodic hypertension and possibility of subarachnoid haemorrhage) and any drug not ordered by the doctor.

monocular (mon-ok'-ū-lar) [G. *monos*, single; L. *oculus*, eye]. Pertaining to one eye.

monocyte (mon'-o-sīt) [G. *monos*, single; *kytos*, cell]. A mononuclear cell—monocytic, adj.

monomania (mon-ō-mā'-ni-ȧ) [G. *monos*. one; *mania*, madness]. Obsessed with a single idea.

mononuclear (mon-ō-nū'-klē-ar) [G. *monos*, one; L. *nucleus*, kernel]. With a single nucleus. Usually refers to a type of blood cell (monocyte), the largest of the cells in the normal blood with a round, oval or indented nucleus.

mononucleosis (mon-ō-nū-klē-ō'-sis) [G. *monos*, one; L. *nucleus*, kernal; G. *-osis*, condition]. An increase in the number of circulating monocytes (mononuclear cells) in the blood. **infectious m.,** syn. glandular fever (q.v.).

monoplegia (mon-ō-plē'-ji-ȧ) [G. *monos*, single; *plege*, a stroke]. Paralysis of only one limb—monoplegic, adj.

monosaccharide (mon-ō-sak'-a-rīd). A simple sugar ($C_6H_{12}O_6$). Examples are glucose, fructose and galactose.

monosomy (mon'-o-sō-mi). 'Nondisjunction' autosomal anomaly when one cell is left without one particular chromosome.

monosulfiram (mon-o-sul-fīr'-am). Lotion for topical application in scabies. 25 per cent alcoholic solution which is diluted with 3 parts of water immediately before use. Chemically similar to disulfiram. Systemic toxic effects occur if alcohol is taken.

monovular (mon-ov'-ū-lar). Uniovular (q.v.).

mons veneris (mons ven'-er-is) [L. *mons*, mountain]. The eminence formed by the pad of fat which lies over the pubic bone in the female.

Mooren's ulcer. Corneal rodent ulcer (q.v.). [Albert Mooren, German ophthalmologist, 1828–99.]

morbilli (mor-bil'-li). Measles (q.v.).

morbilliform (mor-bil'-i-form). Describes a rash resembling that of measles.

moribund (mor'-i-bund) [L. *moribundus*, dying]. In a dying state.

moron (mōr'-on) [G. *moros*, stupid]. American term. Syn., ESN (q.v.).

Moro reflex (mor'-o). Contraction of an infant's limb and neck when he is allowed to drop a short distance through the air or is startled by a sudden noise. [Ernst Moro, German physician, 1874–1951.]

morphine (mor'-fēn). The active principle of opium and a most valuable analgesic. Widely used in pain due to spasm, in haemorrhage, shock, and in useless cough. May cause some respiratory depression, especially in full doses.

morphology (mor-fol'-oj-i) [G. *morphe*, form; *logos*, discourse]. The science which deals with the form and structure of living things—morphological, adj. morphologically, adv.

mortality (mor-tal'-i-ti)[L. *mors*, death]. The death-rate; the ratio of the total number of deaths to the total population.

Mortha (mor'-thá). Analgesic with morphine as a base. Is not a respiratory depressant. Can be given orally and by injection.

mortification (mor-ti-fik-ā'-shun) [L. *mors*, death]. Death of tissue. See GANGRENE.

Moryl (mor'-il). Carbachol (q.v.).

motile (mō'-til) [L. *movere*, to move]. Capable of spontaneous movement—motility, n.

motion (mō'-shun). An evacuation of the bowel.

motor (mō'-tėr) [L. *movere*, to move]. Pertaining to action. See NEURONE.

mould (mōld). Multicellular fungus. Often used synonymously with fungus. Member of the plant kingdom with no differentiation into root, stem or leaf, and without chlorophyll. Structurally consists of filaments or hyphae, which aggregate into a mycelium. Propagation is by means of spores. Occurs in infinite variety, as common saprophytes contaminating foodstuffs, and more rarely as pathogens.

moulding (mōld'-ing). The compression of the fetal head during its passage through the genital tract in labour.

mountain sickness. Symptoms of sickness, tachycardia and dyspnoea, due to low oxygen content of rarefied air at a high altitude.

mucilage (mū'-sil-áj). The solution of a gum in water—mucilaginous, adj.

mucin (mū'-sin) [L. *mucus*, mucus]. A mixture of glycoproteins found in or secreted by many cells and glands—mucinous, adj.

mucinase (mū'-sin-ās). A specific mucin-dissolving substance contained in some aerosols. Useful in fibrocystic disease.

mucinolysis (mū-sin-ol'-i-sis) [L. *mucus*; G. *lysis*, a loosening]. Dissolution of mucin—mucinolytic, adj.

mucocele (mū'-ko-sēl)[L. *mucus*, mucus; G. *kele*, tumour]. Distension of a cavity with mucus.

mucocutaneous (mū-kō-kū-tān'-ē-us). Pertaining to mucous membrane and skin.

mucocutaneous lymph node syndrome. MLNS. A disease affecting mainly babies and children; first noticed in Japan in the late 1960s. Characterized by fever, dry lips, red mouth and strawberry-like tongue. A rash is in a glove-and-stocking distribution and is followed by desquamation. There is cervical adenitis, polymorphonuclear leucocytosis and a raised ESR.

mucoid (mū'-koid). Resembling mucus.

mucolytics (mū-kō-lit'-iks)[L.*mucus*; G. lysis, a loosening]. Drugs which soften mucus and so reduce viscosity of secretion from the respiratory tract.

mucopurulent (mū-kō-pū'-rū-lent) [L. *mucus*, mucus; *pus*, pus]. Containing mucus and pus.

mucopus (mū-kō-pus') [L. *mucus*, mucus; *pus*, pus]. Mucus containing pus.

mucosa (mū-kō'-sa) [L. *mucus*, mucus]. A mucous membrane (q.v.)—mucosal, adj.; mucosae, pl.

mucous (mū'-kus). Pertaining to or containing mucus. mucous colitis, mucomembranous colitis. Possibly a functional disorder, manifested by passage of mucus in the stool, obstinate constipation and occasional colic. mucous polypus, a growth (adenoma) of m. membrane which becomes pedunculated. See MEMBRANE.

mucoviscidosis (mū-kō-vis-kid-ō'-sis) [L. *mucus*, mucus; *viscidus*, sticky; G. *-osis*, condition] A congenital hereditary disease with failure of development of normal mucus-secreting glands, sweat glands and pancreas. May present in a baby as meconium ileus; in infancy with septic bronchitis and steatorrhoea. Stools contain excess fat; trypsin is absent from stool and duodenal juice. See CYSTIC.

mucus (mū'-kus) [L.]. The viscid fluid secreted by mucous glands—mucous mucoid, adj.

multicellular (mul-ti-sel'-ū-lar) [L. *multus*, many; *cellula*, small cell]. Constructed of many cells.

multigravida (mul-ti-grav'-id-á) [L.*multus*, many; *gravidus*, pregnant]. A woman who has borne many children—multigravidae, pl.

multilobular (mul-ti-lob'-ū-lar) [L. *multus*, many; G. *lobos*, lobe]. Possessing many lobes.

multilocular (mul-ti-lok'-ū-lar) [L. *multus*, many; *loculus*, compartment]. Possessing many small cysts, loculi or pockets.

multinuclear (mul-tin-nū'-klē-ár) [L. *multus*, many; *nucleus*, nut]. Possessing many nuclei—multinucleate, adj.

multipara (mul-tip'-a-rà). See MULTI-GRAVIDA—multiparae, pl

multiple sclerosis. See SCLEROSIS.

Multivite (mul'-ti-vīt). Tablets containing vitamin A 2500 units, aneurine hydrochloride 0.5 mg, ascorbic acid 12.5 mg and calciferol 6.25 µg.

mumps. An acute, specific inflammation of the parotid glands, caused by a virus. Syn., infectious parotitis.

mural (mūr'-al) [L. *murus* wall]. Pertaining to the wall of a cavity, organ or vessel.

murmur. Abnormal sound heard on auscultation of heart or great vessels. **presystolic m.**, characteristic of mitral stenosis in regular rhythm.

Musca (mus'-kà). Genus of the common house-fly, capable of transmitting many enteric infections.

muscle (mus'-l) [L. *musculus*, muscle]. Strong, contractile tissue which produces movement in the body. **cardiac m.** makes up the middle wall of the heart; it is involuntary, striated and innervated by autonomic nerves. **skeletal m.** surrounds the skeleton; it is voluntary, striated and innervated by the peripheral nerves of the central nervous system. **visceral (internal) m.** is nonstriated and involuntary and is innervated by the autonomic nerves. **muscle relaxants**, widely used in surgery, in tetanus to prevent spasm, in mechanically aided respiration and in the convulsive shock therapy for mental disorder muscular, adj.

muscular dystrophies (mus'-kū-lar dis'-trō-fēz) [L. *musculus*, muscle; G. *dys-* faulty; *trophe*, nourishment]. Pseudohypertrophic or Duchenne type is the most severe. Presents in early childhood. Runs a malignant course—there is a saying, off his feet by 10, dead by 20. A clue to future treatment lies in recent advances in biochemical knowledge of the condition.

musculature (mus'-kū-lat-ūr) [L. *musculus*, muscle]. The muscular system or any part of it.

musculocutaneous (mus'-kū-lō-kū-tā'-nē-us) [L. *musculus*, muscle; *cutis*, skin]. Pertaining to muscle and skin.

musculoskeletal (mus-kū-lō-skel-ēt'-al) [L. *musculus*, muscle; G. *skeletos*, dried]. Pertaining to the muscular and skeletal systems. Diseases of the musculoskeletal system is now a preferred term to rheumatism.

Mustagen (mus'-ta-jen). Mechlorethamine hydrochloride (q.v.).

mustard. Crushed seeds of the m. plant which can be used orally as an emetic, or externally as a counterirritant.

mustine (mus'-tēn). Nitrogen mustard, a cytotoxic alkylating agent (q.v.).

mutagenesis (mū-ta-jen'-e-sis) [L. *mutare*, to change; G. *genesis*, descent]. The production of mutations—mutagenic, mutagenetic, adj.; mutagenetically, adv.

mutagenicity (mū-ta-jen-is'-i-ti) [L. *mutare*, to change; G. *genes*, producing]. The capacity to produce gene mutations or chromosome aberrations.

mutant (mū'-tant). A cell which is the result of a genetic change.

mutation (mū-tā'-shun) [L. *mutare*, to change]. A change. An alteration in the genes of a living cell gives rise to genetic mutation, as a result of which the characters of the cell change. This change is heritable, remaining until a further mutation occurs. **induced m.**, a gene mutation produced by a known agent outside the cell, e.g. ultraviolet radiation. **spontaneous m.**, a gene mutation taking place without apparent influence from outside the cell.

myalgia (mī-al'-ji-à) [G. *mys.*, muscle; *algos*, pain]. Pain in the muscles—myalgic, adj.

Myambutol (mī-am-bū'-tol). Ethambutol (q.v.).

Myanesin (mī-an-ēs'-in). Mephenesin (q.v.).

myasthenia (mī-as-thē'-ni-à) [G. *mys*, muscle; *astheneia*, weakness]. Muscular weakness **myasthenia gravis**, a disorder characterized by marked fatiguability of voluntary muscles, especially those of the eye. Due to a biochemical defect associated with abnormal behaviour of acetylcholine at neuromuscular junctions. There is considerable evidence for an autoimmune process. Patient forms antibody (to his own striated muscle fibres) which competes with acetylcholine and prevents it from carrying out its transmission duties especially when only small quantities are available. Heredity, infections, environmental influences or a combination of these factors are all possible causes. Research on twins suggests that a rare recessive trait may be instrumental in causing the disease. See CRISIS.—myasthenic, adj.

myatonia (mī-a-tō'-ni-á) [G. *mys*, muscle; *a-*, not; *tonos*, tone]. Absence of tone in muscle. **myatonia congenita,** a form of congenital muscular dystrophy in infancy. Child is unable to bear the weight of the head on the shoulders—myatonic, adj.

Mycardol (mī-kar'-dol). Pentaerythrityl tetranitrate (q.v.).

mycelium (mī-sē'-li-um) [G. *mykes*, fungus]. A mass of branching filaments of moulds or fungi (hyphae)—mycelial, adj.

mycetoma (mī-sē-tō'-má) [G. *mykes*, fungus; *-oma*, tumour]. A fungus infection, usually of the feet, occurring in tropical and subtropical regions. Similar to actinomycosis (q.v.) and aspergillosis. Syn., Madura foot.

Mycifradin (mī-si-frá'-din). Neomycin (q.v.).

Mycobacterium (mī-kō-bak-tē'-ri-um) [G. *mykes*, fungus; *bacterium*, small rod]. Small slender rod bacteria. Grampositive and acid-fast, both to a varying degree. Saprophytic, commensal and pathogenic species. *Mycobacterium tuberculosis* causes tuberculosis; *M. leprae*, leprosy. 'Anonymous' mycobacteria are acid-fast bacilli with bacteriological differences from *M. tuberculosis* and have been subclassified. The pathogenic varieties, *M. kansassi* and the Battey bacillus are elective human pathogens causing pulmonary and cervical 'tuberculosis'.

mycology (mī-kol'-o-ji) [G. *mykes*, fungus; *logos*, discourse]. The study of fungi—mycologist, n.; mycological, adj.; mycologically, adv.

Mycoplasma (mī-kō-plaz'-má) [G. *mykes*, fungus; *plasma*, form]. A small organism intermediate in size between viruses and bacteria. *Mycoplasma pneumoniae* proposed as syn. for Eaton agent (q.v.). One type of Mycoplasma associated with acute leukaemia. Now believed to play a significant role in reproductive failure. Published evidence now associating m. with various infections—pneumonia, bronchitis, and even NSU.

mycosis (mī-kō'-sis) [G. *mykes*, fungus; *-osis*, condition]. Disease caused by any fungus—mycotic, adj. **mycosis fungoides** is a chronic and usually fatal disease, not fungal in origin. It is manifested by generalized pruritis, followed by skin eruptions of diverse character which become infiltrated and finally develop into granulomatous ulcerating tumours. A form of reticuloendothelial disease.

Mydriacyl (mid'-ri-á-sil). Mydriatic and cycloplegic.

mydriasis (mid-rī'-a-sis) [G. dilation of the pupil]. Abnormal dilation of the pupil of the eye.

mydriatics (mid-ri-at'-iks). Drugs which cause mydriasis.

mydricaine (mid'-ri-kān). Atropine, cocaine and adrenaline for ophthalmic work.

Mydrilate (mid'-ril-āt). Cyclopentolate. Mydriatic. Useful prior to examining the optic fundus.

myelin (mī'-e-lin) [G. *myelos*, marrow]. The white, fatty substance constituting the medullary sheath of a nerve.

myelitis (mī-e-lī'-tis) [G. *myelos*, marrow; *-itis*, inflammation]. Inflammation of the spinal cord.

myelocele (mī'-el-ō-sēl) [G. *myelos*, marrow; *kele*, hernia]. An accompaniment of spina bifida (q.v.) wherein development of the spinal cord itself has been arrested, and the central canal of the cord opens on the skin surface discharging cerebrospinal fluid. Incompatible with life.

myelocytes (mī'-el-ō-sīts) [G. *myelos*, marrow; *kytos*, cell]. Precursor cells of granulocytic white blood cells normally present only in bone marrow—myelocytic, adj.

myelofibrosis (mī-el-ō-fi-brō'-sis). Formation of fibrous tissue within the bone marrow cavity. Interferes with the formation of blood cells.

myelogenous (mī-el-oj'-en-us) [G. *myelos*, marrow; *genesthai*, to be produced]. Produced in or by the bone marrow.

myelogram (mī'-el-ō-gram) [G. *myelos*, marrow; *gramma*, letter]. Radiograph of spinal canal.

myelography (mī-el-og'-ra-fi) [G. *myelos*, marrow; *graphein*, to write]. Radiographic examination of the spinal canal by injection of a contrast medium into the subarachnoid space— myelographic, adj.; myelographically, adv.

myeloid (mī'-e-loid) [G. *myelos*, marrow; *eidos*, form]. Relating to the granulocyte precursor cells in the bone marrow. See LEUKAEMIA.

myeloma (mī-el-ō'-má) [G. *myelos*, marrow; *-oma*, tumour]. A malignant condition arising from plasma cells, usually in the bone marrow. **multiple m.**, the formation of a number of myeloma tumours in bones—myelomatous, adj.

myelomatosis (mī-el-ō-ma-tō'-sis). Plasma cells neoplasia which can manifest as myeloma tumours in bones, a diffuse change throughout the marrow or as extramedullary lesions. May produce changes in serum globulins (q.v.) and Bence-Jones proteinuria (q.v.).

myelomeningocele (mī-el-ō-men-ing'-gō-sēl) [G. *myelos*, marrow; *menigx*, membrane; *kele*, hernia]. Differs from a meningocele in being covered with a thin, transparent membrane which may be granular and moist. Syn., meningomyelocele (q.v.).

myelopathy (mī-el-op'-ath-i) [G. *myelos*, marrow; *pathos*, disease]. Disease of the spinal cord. Can be a serious complication of cervical spondylosis—myelopathic, adj.

Myleran (mī'-ler-an). Busulphan (q.v.).

myocarditis (mī-ō-kár-dī'-tis) [G. *mys*, muscle; *kardia*, heart; *-itis*, inflammation]. Inflammation of the myocardium.

myocardium (mī-ō-kár'-di-um) [G. *mys*, muscle; *kardia*, heart]. The middle layer of the heart wall. See MUSCLE—myocardial, adj.

myocele (mī'-ō-sēl) [G. *mys*, muscle; *kele*, tumour]. Protrusion of a muscle through its ruptured sheath.

myoclonus (mī-ō-klō'-nus) [G. *mys*, muscle; *klonos*, confused movement]. Clonic contractions of individual or groups of muscles.

Myocrisin (mī-ō-krī'-sin). Aurothiomalate (q.v.).

Myodil (mī'-ō-dil). An oily liquid used as a contrast agent in myelography. Given by intrathecal injection.

myoelectric (mī-ō-ē-lek'-trik). Pertaining to the electrical properties of muscle.

myofibrosis (mī-ō-fī-brō'-sis). Excessive connective tissue in muscle. Leads to inadequate functioning of part—myofibroses, pl.

myogenic (mī-ō-jen'-ik) [G. *mys*, muscle; *genesis*, descent]. Originating in, starting from, muscle.

myoglobin (mī-ō-glō'-bin) [G. *mys*, muscle; L. *globus*, ball]. Oxygen-transporting muscle protein. Syn., myohaemoglobin.

myoglobinuria (mī-ō-glō-bin-ū'-ri-á) [G. *mys*, muscle; L. *globus*, ball; G. *ouron*, urine]. Excretion of myoglobin in the urine as in crush syndrome. Syn., myohaemoglobinúria.

myohaemoglobin (mī'-ō-hēm-ō-glōb'-in). A haemoglobin present in muscle; of much lower molecular weight than blood haemoglobin. It is liberated from muscle and appears in the urine in the 'crush syndrome.'

myohaemoglobinuria (mī'-ō-hēm-ō-glōb'-in-ūr'-i-á). Myohaemoglobin in the urine. See CRUSH SYNDROME.

myokymia (mī-ō-kī'-mi-á) [G. *mys*, muscle; *kyma*, wave]. Muscle twitching. In the lower eyelid it is benign. **facial m.**, may result from long use of phenothiazine drugs; has also been observed in patients with disseminated sclerosis.

myoma (mī-ō'-má) [G. *mys*, muscle; *-oma*, tumour]. A tumour of muscle tissue—myomata, pl.; myomatous, adj.

myomalacia (mī-ō-mal-ā'-si-á) [G. *mys*, muscle; *malakia*, softness]. Softening of muscle, as occurs in the myocardium after coronary occlusion.

myomectomy (mī-om-ek'-to-mi) [G. *mys*, muscle; *-oma*, tumour; *ektome*, excision]. Enucleation of uterine fibroid(s).

myometrium (mī-ō-mē'-tri-um) [G. *mys*, muscle; *metra*, womb]. The thick muscular wall of the uterus.

myoneural (mī-ō-nūr'-ál) [G. *mys*, muscle; *neuron*, nerve]. Pertaining to muscle and nerve.

myopathy (mī-ō-op'-ath-i) [G. *mys*, muscle; *pathos*, disease]. Any disease of the muscles—myopathic, adj. See GLYCOGENOSIS.

myope (mī'-ōp) [G. *myein*, to close; *ops*, eye]. A shortsighted person—myopic, adj.

myopia (mī-ō'-pi-á) [G. *myein*, to close; *ops*, eye]. Shortsightedness. The light rays come to a focus in front instead of on, the retina—myopic, adj.

myoplasty (mī'-ō-plas-ti) [G. *mys*, muscle; *plassein*, to form]. Plastic surgery of muscles—myoplastic, adj.

myosarcoma (mī-ō-sár-kō'má) [G. *mys*,

muscle; *sarkoma*, fleshy overgrowth]. A malignant tumour derived from muscle—myosarcomata, pl.; myosarcomatous, adj.

myosin (mī'-ō-sin) [G. *mys*, muscle]. The main protein of muscle.

myosis (mī-ō'-sis). Excessive contraction of the pupil of the eye. Also **miosis** myotic. adj.

myositis (mī-ō-sī'-tis) [G. *mys*, muscle; *-itis*, inflammation]. Inflammation of a muscle. **myositis ossificans**, deposition of active bone cells in muscle, resulting in hard swellings.

myotics (mī-ot'-iks). Drugs which cause myosis (q.v.). Also **miotics**.

myotomy (mī-ot'-om-i) [G. *mys*, muscle; *tome*, a cutting]. Cutting or dissection of muscle tissue.

myringa (mi-ring'-gá) [L. *miringa;* G. *menigx*, membrane]. The eardrum or tympanic membrane.

myringitis (mir-in-jī'-tis) [G. *menigx*, membrane; *-itis*, inflammation]. Inflammation of the eardrum (tympanic membrane).

myringoplasty (mir-ing'-ō-plas'-ti) [G. *menigx*, membrane; *plassein*, to form]. This operation is designed to close a defect in the tympanic membrane. Grafts from a suitable vein, perichondrium of the tragus or temporalis fascia, have been used—myringoplastic, adj.

myringotome (mir-ing'-ot-ōm) [G. *menigx*, membrane; *tomos*, a cutting]. A delicate instrument for incising the eardrum (tympanic membrane).

myringotomy (mir-ing-ot'-o-mi) [G. *menigx*, membrane; *tome*, a cutting]. Incision into the eardrum (tympanic membrane). Done previously to drain pus from the middle ear. Now done for aspiration of non-suppurative exudates or transudates of the middle ear cleft. Middle ear ventilation maintained by insertion of teflon tube so that the fluid can drain down narrowed or malfunctioning pharyngotympanic tube; teflon tube removed when pharyngotympanic tube functioning normally.

Mysoline (mī'-sō-lēn). Primidone (q.v.).

Mysteclin F. Tetracycline, a broad-spectrum antibiotic combined with an antifungal powder.

myxoedema (miks-ē-dē'-má) [G. *myxa*, mucus; *oidema*, swelling]. Clinical syndrome of hypothyroidism (q.v.). Patient becomes slow in movement and dull mentally; there is bradycardia, low temperature, dry skin and swelling of limbs and face. the BMR (q.v.) is low, and the blood cholesterol is raised. No enlargement of gland as in Hashimoto's disease. **pretibial m.**, unsightly thickening of skin over shins and feet which occurs rarely in patients with hyperthyroidism. Cause unknown; condition persists in spite of antithyroid treatment. **myxoedema coma**, impaired level of consciousness in severe m. Mortality rate high from hypothermia. heart failure, cardiac arrhythmias or bronchopneumonia—myxoedematous, adj.

myxoma (miks-ō'-má) [G. *myxa*, mucus; *oma*, tumour]. A connective tissue tumour composed largely of mucoid material—myxomata, pl.; myxomatous, adj.

myxosarcoma (miks-ō-sár-kō'-má) [G. *myxa*, mucus; *sarkoma*, fleshy overgrowth]. A malignant tumour of connective tissue with a soft, mucoid consistence—myxosarcomata, pl.; myxosarcomatous, adj.

myxoviruses ((miks-ō-vī'-rus). Name for the influenza group of viruses.

N

NAB. See NEOARSPHENAMINE.

Nabothian follicles. Cystic distension of chronically inflamed cervical glands of uterus, where the duct of the gland has become obliterated by a healing epithelial covering, and the normal mucus cannot escape. [Martin Naboth, German anatomist, 1675–1721.]

NAC. *N*-Acetylcysteine. Mucolytic agent.

Naclex (nā'-kleks). Hydroflumethiazide (q.v.).

Nacton (nak'-ton). Poldine methylsulphate (q.v.).

Naegele's obliquity. Tilting of the fetal head to one or other side to decrease the transverse diameter presented to the pelvic brim.

naevus (nē'-vus) [L. mole]. A mole; a circumscribed lesion of the skin arising from pigment-producing cells (melanoma), or due to a developmental abnormality of blood vessels (angioma)—naevi, pl.; naevoid, adj.

naftidrofuryl oxalate (naf-tid-rō-fūr'-il oks-al-at). Increases blood flow without altering blood pressure. Used for both cerebral and peripheral disorders. Side effects said to be headache, nausea, diarrhoea and dizziness.

nalidixic acid (nal-i-diks'-ik). For urinary infection.

nalorphine (nal-or'-fēn). Neutralizes the action of morphine, pethidine and similar drugs. Following injection, respiration and blood pressure are dramatically improved. Very useful in morphine overdosage, and in the prevention of neonatal respiratory depression. Given intravenously or intramuscularly.

naloxone (nal-oks'-ōn). Re-establishes normal respiration and conscious level.

nape. The back of the neck; the nucha.

naphazoline (naf-az'-o-lēn). Decongestive substance used in allergic nasal conditions, and in rhinitis; 1 in 2000 to 1 in 1000 solution as spray or drops.

napkin rash. An erythema of the napkin area. Usual cause is ammoniacal decomposition of urine.

Naprosyn (nap'-rō-sin). Naproxen q.v.).

naproxen (nap-roks'-en). Relieves pain, reduces inflammation and eases joint stiffness without causing gastric bleeding.

narcissism (nár-sis'-izm) [G. *Narkissos,* a beautiful youth who fell in love with his own reflection]. Self-love. In psychiatry the narcissistic type of personality is one where the sexual love-object is the self.

narcoanalysis (nár-kō-an-al'-i-sis) [G. *narco,* stupor; *analysis,* a loosening]. Analysis of mental content under light anaesthesia, usually an intravenous barbiturate—narcoanalytic, adj.; narcoanalytically, adv.

narcolepsy (nár'-kō-lep-si) [G. *narco,* stupor; *lepsis,* a seizing]. An irresistible tendency to go to sleep. It is more usual to speak of the narcolepsies rather than of narcolepsy, for sudden, repetitive attacks of sleep occurring in the daytime arise in diverse clinical conditions—narcoleptic, adj.

narcosis (nár-kō'-sis) [G. *narco,* stupor]. Unconsciousness produced by a drug. **basal n.,** a state of unconsciousness produced by drugs prior to an anaesthetic or operation. The drugs most commonly used for this purpose were avertin, paraldehyde or a barbiturate. Not so widely used as formerly. **carbon dioxide n.,** full bounding pulse, muscular twitchings, mental confusion and eventuatl coma due to increased CO_2 in the blood. **continuous n.,** treatment by prolonged sleep by spaced administra-

tion of narcotics. Introduced by Woolf in 1901. Used occasionally in mental illness to cut short attacks of excitement or for severe emotional upset.

narcosynthesis (nár-kō-sin'-thē-sis) [G. *narco,* stupor; *synthesis,* putting together]. The building up of a clearer mental picture of an incident involving the patient by reviving memories of it, under light anaesthesia, so that both he and the therapist can examine the incident in clearer perspective.

narcotherapy (nar-ko-ther'-á-pi). See NARCOSIS.

narcotic (nár-kot'-ik) [G. *narkotikos,* narcotic]. A drug which produces abnormally deep sleep.

Nardil. Phenelzine (q.v.).

nares (nār'-ēz) [L.]. The nostrils. **anterior n.,** the pair of openings from the exterior into the nasal cavities. **posterior n.,** the pair of openings from the nasal cavities into the nasopharynx. Syn., choanae—naris, sing.

Narphen (nar'-fen). Phenazocine (q.v.).

nasal (nā'-zal) [L. *nasus,* nose]. Pertaining to the nose.

Naseptin (nā-sep'-tin). Cream containing chlorhexidine hydrochloride 0.1 per cent and neomycin sulphate 0.5 per cent for nasal carriers of staphylococci.

nasogastric (nā-sō-gas'-trik) [L. *nasus,* nose; G. *gaster,* belly]. Pertaining to the nose and stomach, as passing a **n. tube** via this route usually for suction, lavage or feeding.

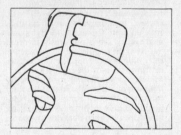

Disposable nasogastric tube holding device

nasolacrimal (nā-zō-lak'-ri-mal) [L. *nasus,* nose; *lacrima,* tear]. Pertaining to the nose and lacrimal apparatus.

naso-oesopageal (nā'-zō-ēs-of-a-jē'-al) [L. *nasus,* nose; G. *oisophagos,* gullet].

Pertaining to the nose and the oesophagus, as passing a tube via this route.

nasopharyngitis (nā-zō-far-in-jī'-tis) [L. *nasus*, nose; G. *pharygx*, pharynx; *-itis*, inflammation]. Inflammation of the nasopharynx.

nasopharyngoscope (nā-zō-far-in'-gō-skōp) [L. *nasus*, nose; G. *pharygx*, pharynx; *skopein*, to examine]. An endoscope for viewing the nasal passages and postnasal space nasopharyngoscopic, adj.

nasopharynx (nā-zō-far'-inks) [L. *nasus*, nose; G. *pharygx*, pharynx]. The portion of the pharynx above the soft palate—nasopharyngeal, adj.

nasosinusitis (nā-zō-sī-nus-ī'-tis) [L. *nasus*, nose; *sinus*, curve; G. *-itis*, inflammation]. Inflammation of the nose and adjacent sinuses.

Natulan (nat'-ū-lan). Procarbazine (q.v.).

nausea (naw'-sē-á) [G. *nausia*, sea-sickness]. A feeling of sickness without actual vomiting nauseate, v.t., v.i.

Navane (na'-vān). Thiothixine (q.v.).

navel (nā'-vl). The umbilicus.

navicular (nav-ik'-ū-lar) [L. *navicula*, small boat]. Shaped like a canoe. The scaphoid bone of the tarsus and carpus.

Navidrex (nav'-i-dreks). Cyclopenthiazide (q.v.).

Navidrex-K (nav'-i-dreks). Cyclopenthiazide with potassium.

Nebcin (neb'-sin). Tobramycin (q.v.).

nebula (neb'-ū-lá) [L. mist]. A greyish, corneal opacity.

nebulizer (neb-ūl-īz'-ér). An apparatus for converting a liquid into a fine spray. Syn., atomizer.

Necator (nēk-āt'-or). A genus of hookworms. See ANCYLOSTOMA.

necropsy (ne-krop'-si) [G. *nekros*, corpse; *opsis*, sight]. The examination of a dead body.

necrosis (ne-krō'-sis) [G. mortification]. Localized death of tissue—necrotic, adj.

needling (nēd'-ling). Puncturing with a needle, especially of lens capsule to allow entry of aqueous humor which will absorb the lens or remnants thereof. Discission.

Nefrolan (nef'-rō-lan). Clorexolone (q.v.).

negativism (neg'-at-iv-izm) [L. *negati-*

vus, negative]. Active refusal to co-operate, usually shown by the patient consistently doing the exact opposite of what he is asked. Common in schizophrenia.

Negram (nā'-gram). Nalidixic acid.

Neisseria. A genus of bacteria. Gram-negative diplococci which are found as commensals of man and animals, e.g. *Neisseria catarrhalis*. Some are pathogenic to man. *Neisseria gonorrhoeae* causes gonorrhoea and *N. meningitidis* causes meningitis.

Nelaton's line. An imaginary line joining the anterior superior iliac spine to the ischial tuberosity. In coxa vara and upward dislocation of the hip joint, the great trochanter of the femur lies above this line. [Auguste Nélaton, French surgeon, 1807–73.]

nematodes (nē'-ma-tōdz). Wormlike creatures that have two sexes and an intestinal canal. Various species are parasitic to man and can be divided into two groups: (1) those that mainly live in the intestine, e.g. hookworms and whipworms; (2) those that are mainly tissue parasites, e.g. guinea worms, filarial worms.

Nembutal (nem'-bū-tal). Pentobarbitone (q.v.).

neoarsphenamine (nē-ō-árs-fen'-a-mēn). An organic arsenic compound, and one of the first chemotherapeutic drugs. Once widely used in the treatment of syphilis by intravenous injection. Occasionally used for Vincent's angina as a 5 per cent paint.

neoarthrosis (nē-ō-ár-thrō'-sis) [G. *neos*, new; *arthrosis*, articulation]. Abnormal articulation: a false joint as at the site of a fracture.

Neo-Cytamen (nē-o-sīt'-a-men). Hydroxocobalamin (q.v.).

Neo-epinine (nē-ō-ep'-in-nēn). Tablets and spray solutions containing isoprenaline (q.v.).

neologism (nē-ol'-oj-izm) [G. *neos*, new; *logos*, discourse]. A specially coined word, often nonsensical; may express a thought disorder.

Neo-Mercazole. Carbimazole (q.v.).

Neomin (nē'-o-min). Streptomycin and neomycin.

neomycin (nē-ō-mī'-sin). An antibiotic frequently used with corticosteroids in the treatment of inflamed and infected skin conditions. Sometimes given orally for intestinal infections. See FRAMY-CETIN SULPHATE.

Neo Naclex (nē-ō-nā'-kleks). Bendroflu-azide (q.v.).

neonatal period (nē-ō-nā'-tal). The first month of life in a baby. **neonatal mortality,** the death-rate of babies in the first month of life.

neonate (nē'-ō-nāt) [L. *natus,* birth]. A newborn baby up to one month old.

neonatology (nē-ō-nāt-ol'-o-ji) [G. *neos,* new; L. *natus,* birth; G. *logos,* discourse]. The scientific study of the new-born.

neonatorum (nē-ō nat-ōr'-um) [G. *neos,* new; L. *natus,* birth]. Pertaining to the newborn.

neoplasia (nē-ō-plā'-zi-à) [G. *neos,* new; *plassein,* to form]. Literally the formation of new tissue. By custom refers to the pathological process in tumour formation—neoplastic, adj.

neoplasm (nē'-ō-plazm) [G. *neos,* new; *plasma,* form]. A new growth; a tumour—neoplastic, adj.

Neosporin (nē-ō-spor'-in). Ophthalmic drops containing polymixin, neomycin and gramicidin.

neostigmine (nē-os-tig'-mēn). Synthetic compound used in myasthenia gravis; as a curarine antagonist, and in postoperative intestinal atony. Given orally and by injection. Can cause excess bronchial secretion.

Neothyl (nē'-ō-thil). An inhalation anaesthetic similar to ether.

Nepenthe (ne-pen'-thē). an opium preparation resembling tincture of opium.

nephralgia (nef-ral'-ji-à) [G. *nephros,* kidney; *algos,* pain]. Pain in the kidney. See DIETL'S CRISIS.

nephrectomy (nef-rek'-to-mi) [G. *nephros,* kidney; *ektome,* excision]. Removal of a kidney.

Nephril (nef'-ril). Polythiazide. See CHLOROTHIAZIDE.

nephritis (nef-rī'-tis) [G. *nephros,* kidney; *-itis,* inflammation]. A term embracing a group of conditions in which there is either an inflammatory, or an inflammatory-like reaction, focal or diffuse, in the kidneys. **acute glomerulo n.,** Syn., acute n., Bright's disease, Type I n. A diffuse inflammatory reaction of both kidneys, usually following a streptococcal infection, and classically manifest by puffiness of the face and scanty blood-stained urine. **chronic**

n. syn., Type III n. A chronic condition, sometimes the sequel to Type I or Type II n. in which there is a widespread fibrous replacement of functioning kidney tissue, resulting in progressive renal failure and an arterial hypertension and teminating ultimately in death. **nephrotic n.** syn., Type II n. A chronic condition of unknown cause characterized by massive oedema and heavy proteinuria. See NEPHROTIC SYNDROME—nephritic, adj.

nephrocalcinosis (nef-rō-kal-sin-ō-'sis) [G. *nephros,* kidney; L. *calx,* lime; G. *-osis,* condition]. Multiple areas of calcification within the kidney substance.

nephrocapsulectomy (nef-rō-kap-sūl-ek'-to-mi) [G. *nephros,* kidney; L. *capsula,* small box; G. *ektome,* excision]. Surgical removal of the kidney capsule. Usually done for chronic nephritis.

nephrogenic (nef-rō-jen'-ik) [G. *nephros,* kidney; *gignesthai,* to be produced]. Arising in or produced by the kidney.

nephrogram (nef'-rō-gram) [G. *nephros,* kidney; *gramma,* letter]. Renogram (q.v.).

nephrolithiasis (nef-rō-lith-ī'-a-sis) [G. *nephros,* kidney; *lithos,* stone; N.L. *-iasis,* condition]. The presence of stones in the kidney.

nephrolithotomy (nef-rō-lith-ot'-o-mi) [G. *nephros,* kidney; *lithos,* stone; *tome,* a cutting]. Removal of a stone from the kidney by an incision through the kidney substance.

nephrology (nef-rol'-o-ji) [G. *nephros,* kidney; *logos,* discourse]. Special study of the kidneys and the diseases which afflict them.

nephron (nef'-ron) [G. *nephros,* kidney]. The basic unit of the kidney, comprising a glomerulus, Bowman's capsule, proximal and distal convoluted tubules, with loop of Henle connecting them; a straight collecting tubule follows via which urine is conveyed to the renal pelvis.

nephropathy (nef-ro'-path-i) [G. *nephros,* kidney; *pathos,* disease]. Kidney disease—nephropathic, adj.

nephropexy (nef'-rō-peks-i) [G. *nephros,* kidney; *pexis,* a fixing]. Surgical fixation of a floating kidney.

nephroplasty (nef-rō-plas'-ti) [G. *nephros,* kidney; *plassein,* to form]. Any plastic operation on the kidney, especially for large aberrant renal vessels that are dissected off the urinary tract

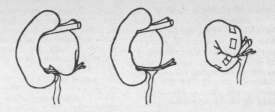

Hamilton-Stewart nephroplasty

and the kidney folded laterally upon itself. See HYDRONEPHROSIS.

nephroptosis (nef-rop-tō'-sis) [G. *nephros*, kidney; *ptosis*, a falling]. Downward displacement of the kidney.

nephropyosis (nef-rō-pī'-ō-sis) [G. *nephros*, kidney; *pyon*, pus; *-osis*, condition]. Pus formation in the kidney.

nephrosclerosis (nef-rō-skler-ō'-sis) [G. *nephros*, kidney; *sklerosis*, a hardening]. Renal insufficiency from hypertensive vascular disease, developing into picture identical with that of chronic nephritis—nephrosclerotic, adj.

nephrosis (nef-rō'-sis) [G. *nephros*, kidney; *-osis*, condition]. Any degenerative, non-inflammatory change in the kidney—nephrotic, adj.

nephrostomy (nef-ros'-to-mi) [G. *nephros*, kidney; *stoma*, mouth]. A surgically established fistula from the pelvis of the kidney to the body surface.

nephrotic syndrome. Used as synonym for Type II nephritis (q.v.) Characteristics are reduction in blood plasma albumen, albuminuria and oedema, usually with hyperlipaemia. May occur in other conditions such as amyloid disease and glomerulosclerosis (q.v.) of diabetes.

nephrotomy (nef-rot'-o-mi) [G. *nephros*, kidney; *tomos*, a cutting]. An incision into the kidney substance.

nephrotoxic (nef-rō-toks'-ik) [G. *nephros*, kidney; *toxikon*, poison]. Any substance which inhibits or prevents the functions of kidney cells, or causes their destruction—nephrotoxin, n.

nephroureterectomy (nef-rō-ūr-ēt-er-ek'-to-mi) [G. *nephros*, kidney; *oureter*, ureter; *ektome*, excision]. Removal of the kidney along with a part or the whole of the ureter.

nerve. An elongated bundle of fibres which serves for the transmission of impulses between the periphery and the nerve centres. **afferent n.**, one conveying impulses from the tissues to the n. centres; also known as 'receptor' and 'sensory' nerves. **efferent n.**, one which conveys impulses outwards from the n. centres; also known as 'effector', 'motor', 'secretory,' 'trophic,' 'vasoconstrictor,' 'vasodilator', etc., according to function and location. See GANGLION, NEURONE, PLEXUS.

nervous (nér'-vus). 1. Relating to nerves or nerve tissue. 2. Referring to a state of restlessness or timidity. **nervous system,** the structures controlling the actions and functions of the body; it comprises the brain and spinal cord and their nerves, and the ganglia and fibres forming the autonomic system.

Nethaprin Dospan (neth'-a-prin dos'-pan). Bronchial relaxant, useful in asthma. Available as syrup, which is particularly useful for elderly patients.

nettlerash (net'-tl). Popular term to describe urticaria; weals of the skin.

Neulactil (nū-lak'-til). Pericyazine (q.v.).

neural (nūr'-al) [G. *neuron*, nerve]. Pertaining to nerves.

neuralgia (nū-ral'-ji-á) [G. *neuron*, nerve; *algos*, pain]. Pain in the distribution of a nerve—neuralgic, adj.

neurapraxia (nū-ra-praks'-i-á) [G. *neuron*, nerve; *apraxia*, nonaction]. Temporary loss of function in peripheral nerve fibres. Most commonly due to crushing or prolonged pressure. See AXONOTMESIS.

neurasthenia (nū-ras-thē'-ni-á) [G. *neuron*, nerve; *asthenia*, weakness]. A frequently misused term, the precise meaning of which is an uncommon nervous condition consisting of lassitude, inertia, fatigue and loss of initiative.   Restless   fidgeting, over-sensitivity, undue irritability and often an asthenic physique are also present—neurasthenic, adj.

neurectomy (nū-rek'-to-mi) [G. *neuron*, nerve; *ektome*, excision]. Excision of part of a nerve.

neurilemma (nūr-i-lem'-a) [G. *neuron*, nerve; *lemma*, sheath]. The thin membranous outer covering of a nerve fibre surrounding the myelin sheath.

neuritis (nū-rī'-tis) [G. *neuron*, nerve; *-itis*, inflammation]. Inflammation of a nerve—neuritic, adj.

neuroblast (nūr'-ō-blast) [G. *neuron*, nerve; *blastos*, germ]. A primitive nerve cell.

neuroblastoma (nū-rō-blas-tō'-má) [G. *neuron*, nerve; *blastos*, germ; *-oma*, tumour]. Malignant tumour arising in adrenal medulla from tissue of sympathetic origin. Most cases show a raised urinary catecholamine excretion—neuroblastomata, pl.; neuroblastomatous, adj.

neurodermatitis (nū-rō-dėr-ma-tī'-tis) [G. *neuron*, nerve; *derma*, skin; *-itis*, inflammation]. Lichen simplex (q.v.) Leathery, thickened patches of skin secondary to pruritus and scratching. As the skin thickens, irritation increases, scratching causes further thickening and so a vicious circle is set up. The appearance of the patch develops characteristically as a thickened sheet dissected into small, shiny, flat-topped papules.

neurofibroma (nū-rō-fi-brō'-má) [G. *neuron*, nerve; L. *fibra*, fibre; G. *-oma*, tumour]. A tumour arising from the connective tissue of nerves. A generalized form of neurofibromatosis (Recklinghausen's disease) is recognized: multiple tumours occur in the skin but may also be associated with visceral branches of the sympathetic nervous system—neurofibromata, pl.; neurofibromatous, adj.

neurogenic (nū-rō-jen'-ik) [G. *neuron*, nerve; *gignesthai*, to be formed]. Originating within or forming nervous tissue. **neurogenic bladder**, see BLADDER.

neuroglia (nū-rog'-li-á) [G. *neuron*, nerve; *glia*, glue]. The supporting tissue of the brain and cord—neuroglial, adj.

neuroglycopaenia (nū-ro-glī'-kō-pēn'-i-á). Shortage of glucose in nerve cells, which is the immediate cause of brain dysfunction when it occur in hypoglycaemia.

neuroleptanalgesia (nū-rō-lept-an-al-jē'-zi-á) [G. *neuron*, nerve; *lepsis*, seizing; *a-*, not; *algos*, pain]. Anaesthetic technique in which the major agents are a neuroleptic and an analgesic drug, allowing patient to retain ability to cooperate.

neuroleptics (nū-rō-lep'-tiks) [G. *neuron*, nerve; *lepsis*, seizing]. Drugs acting on the nervous system. Includes the major antipsychotic tranquillizers.

neurologist (nū-rol'-o-jist) [G. *neuron*, nerve; *logos*, word]. A specialist in neurology.

neurology (nū-rol'-o-ji). The science and study of nerves—their structure, function and pathology; the branch of medicine dealing with diseases of the nervous system—neurological, adj.

neuromuscular (nū-rō-mus'-kūl-er) [G. *neuron*, nerve; L. *musculus*, muscle]. Pertaining to nerves and muscles.

neuron(e) (nū'-ron) [G. *neuron*, nerve]. The structural unit of the nervous system comprising fibres (dendrites) which convey impulses to the nerve cell; the nerve cell itself, and the fibres (axons) which convey impulses from the cell. **lower motor n.**, the cell is in the spinal cord and the axon passes to skeletal muscle. **upper motor n.**, the cell is in the cerebral cortex and the axon passes down the spinal cord to arborize with a lower motor n.—neuronal, neural, adj.

neuronotmesis (nū-ron-ot-mēs'-is). Syn. neurotmesis, axonotmesis. Total severence of a nerve.

neuropathic (nū-rō-path'-ik) [G. *neuron*, nerve; *pathos*, disease]. Relating to disease of the nervous system—neuropathy, n.

neuropathology (nū-rō-path-ol'-oj-i) [G. *neuron*, nerve; *pathos*, disease; *logos*, discourage]. A branch of medicine dealing with diseases of the nervous system.

neuropharmacology (nū-rō-far-ma-kol'-o-ji) [G. *neuron*, nerve; *pharmakon*, drug; *logos*, discourse]. The branch of pharmacology dealing with drugs that affect the nervous system.

neuroplasty (nū'-rō-plas-ti) [G. *neuron*, nerve; *plassein*, to form]. Surgical repair of nerves—neuroplastic, adj.

neuropsychiatry (nū-rō-sik-ī'-a-tri). The combination of neurology and psychiatry. Speciality dealing with organic and functional disease—neuropsychiatric, adj.

neurorrhaphy (nū-ror'-a-fi) [G. *neuron*,

nerve; *raphe*, a suture]. Suturing the ends of a divided nerve.

neurosis (nū-rō'-sis) [G. *neuron*, nerve; *-osis*, condition]. A functional (i.e. psychogenic) disorder consisting of a symptom or symptoms caused, though usually unknown to the patient, by mental disorder. The four commonest are anxiety state, reactive depression, hysteria and obsessional neurosis. (q.v.). Distinguished from a psychosis (q.v.) by the fact that a neurosis arises as a result of stresses and anxieties in the patient's environment. **institutional n.**, apathy, withdrawal and non-participation occurring in long-stay patients as a result of the environment. May be indistinguishable from the signs and symptoms for which the patient was admitted to the institution—neurotic, adj.

neurosurgery (nū-rō-sur'-jer-i) [G. *neuron*, nerve; *cheirourgos*, working by hand]. Surgery of the nervous system—neurosurgical, adj.

neurosyphilis (nū-rō-si'-fi-lis) [G. *neuron*, nerve; N.L. *syphilis*]. Infection of brain or spinal cord, or both, by *Treponema pallidum*. The variety of clinical pictures produced is large, but the two common syndromes encountered are tabes dorsalis and general paralysis of the insane (GPI). The basic pathology is disease of the blood vessels, with later development of pathological changes in the meninges and the underlying nervous tissue. Very often symptoms of the disease do not arise until 20 years or more after the date of primary infection. See ARGYLL ROBERTSON PUPIL—neurosyphilitic, adj.

neurotomy (nū-rot'-o-mi) [G. *neuron*, nerve; *tome*, cutting]. Surgical cutting of a nerve.

neurotoxic (nū-rō-toks'-ik)[G. *neuron*, nerve; *toxikon*, poison]. Poisonous or destructive to nervous tissue—neurotoxin, n.

neurotropic (nū-rō-trō'-pik) [G. *neuron*, nerve; *trepein*, to turn]. With predilection for the nervous system, used especially of *Treponema pallidum*, some forms of which seem always to produce neurosyphilitic complications. **n.** viruses (rabies, poliomyelitis, etc.) make their major attack on the cells of the nervous system.

neutron capture therapy. A new concept of treatment for carcinoma.

neutropenia (nū-trō-pē'-ni-à) [L. *neuter*, neither; G. *penia*, want]. Shortage of

neutrophils, not sufficient to warrant the term 'agranulocytosis' neutropenic, adj.

neutrophil (nū'-trō-fil) [L. *neuter*, neither; G. *philein*, to love]. The most common form of granulocyte (q.v.) in the blood, in which the granules are neither strongly basophilic or eosinophilic.

Neutrophylline (nū-trō-fil'-in). Diprophylline (q.v.).

NGU. Non-gonococcal urethritis. See NSU.

nialamide (ni-al'-à-mīd). A monoamine oxidase inhibitor.

Niamid. A monoamine oxidase inhibitor.

Nicetal (nik'-ē-tal). See ISONIAZIDE.

niclosamide (nī-klō'-sà-mīd). Causes expulsion of adult tapeworm. Given in a single dose of 2 g. No starvation or purgation necessary.

nicotinamide (ni-kō-tin'-a-mīd). A derivative of nicotinic acid and useful when the vasodilator action of that drug is not desired as in treatment of pellagra.

nicotinic acid (nik-ō-tin'-ik as'-id). One of the essential food factors of the vitamin B complex. The vasodilator action of the compound is useful in chilblains, migraine, etc.

nictitation (nik-ti-tā'-shun)[L. *nictare*, to wink]. Rapid and involuntary blinking of the eyelids.

nidation (nī-dā'-shun) [L. *nidus*, nest]. Implantation of the early embryo in the uterine mucosa.

nidus (nī'-dus) [L. nest]. The focus of an infection. Septic focus.

Niemann-Pick disease. A lipoid metabolic disturbance, chiefly in female Jewish infants. Now thought to be due to absence or inadequacy of enzyme sphingomyelinase. There is enlargement of the liver, spleen and lymph nodes with mental subnormality. Now classified as a lipid reticulosis. [Albert Niemann, German paediatrician, 1880–1921. Ludwig Pick, German paediatrician, 1868–1935.]

nifenazone (nī-fen'-a-zōn). Antiarthritic drug.

night blindness. Nyctalopia. Sometimes occurs in vitamin A deficiency and is a maladaptation of vision to darkness.

night cry. A shrill noise, uttered during sleep. May be of significance in hip disease when pain occurs in the relaxed joint.

night sweat. Profuse sweating, usually during sleep; typical of tuberculosis.

nihilistic (nī-hil-is′-tik) [L. *nihil*, nothing]. Delusions and ideas of unreality; of not existing.

nikethamide (ni-keth′-a-mīd). Central nervous system (CNS) stimulant used in respiratory depression and collapse. Given intravenously or intramuscularly.

Nikolsky's sign. Slight pressure on skin causes 'slipping' of apparently normal epidermis, in the way that a rubber glove can be moved on a wet hand. Characteristic of pemphigus. [Pyotr V. Nickolsky, Russian dermatologist, 1858–1940.]

Nilodin (nil′-o-din). Lucanthone (q.v.).

nipple (nip′-l). The conical eminence in the centre of each breast, containing the outlets of the milk ducts.

niridazole (ni-ri-dāz′-ol). The drug of choice for *Schistosoma haematobium* infestation. Given orally in two divided doses, preferably at 12-hourly intervals; can be used as outpatient treatment if patient warned that urine will be dark brown. Can also be used for *S. mansoni* and *S. japonicum* infestations, but patient should be in hospital and outpatient treatment is not recommended. Toxic symptoms may be severe especially in patients with hepatosplenic disease.

nit. The egg of the head louse (*Pediculus capitis*). It is firmly cemented to the hair.

Nitoman. Tetrabenazine (q.v.).

nitrazepam (nī-traz′-ē-pam). A benzodiazepine hypnotic and as such drug of first choice. Is known to cause vivid dreams of a grandiose, futuristic nature in some people.

nitric acid (nī′-trik as′-id). Dangerous caustic. Occasionally used in testing urine for albumen.

nitrofurantoin (nī-trō-fūr′-an-toin). Urinary antiseptic, of great value in Grampositive and Gram-negative infections. Unrelated to sulphonamides or antibiotics.

nitrofurazone (nī-trō-fū′-ra-zōn). Not for systemic administration by any route. Available as ointment and solution for topical application.

nitrogen (nīt′-rō-jen). A gaseous element;

chief constituent of the atmosphere; essential constituent of protein foods **nitrogen balance** is when a person's daily protein n. intake equals the daily excretion of n.: a negative balance occurs when excretion of n. exceeds the daily intake. Nitrogen is excreted mainly as urea in the urine: ammonia, creatinine and uric acid account for a further small amount. Less than 10 per cent total n. excreted in faeces. **nonprotein n. (NPN)**, nitrogen derived from all nitrogenous substances other than protein, i.e. urea, uric acid, creatinine, creatine, amino acids, ammonia. **nitrogen mustards**, a group of cytotoxic drugs, derivatives of mustard gas— nitrogenous, adj.

nitrous oxide. Widely used inhalation anaesthetic, especially for induction. Supplied in blue cylinders.

Nivaquine (niv′-a-kwin). Chloroquine (q.v.).

NMR. Nuclear magnetic resonance (q.v.).

Nobecutane (nōb′-e-kū-tān). A soluble acrylic resin, which is sprayed over a wound and forms a transparent, noninflammable elastic film. This permits the passage of air and water vapour but is impervious to bacteria. **Nobecutane marking ink**, a blue surgical marking ink. **Nobecutane remover**, a solvent for removal of n. plastic dressing and marking ink.

nocturia (nok-tū′-ri-â) [L. *nox*, night; G. *oiron*, urine]. Passing urine at night.

nocturnal (nok-tur′-nal)[L. *nocturnalis*]. Nightly; during the night. **nocturnal enuresis,** bed wetting during sleep.

node (nōd) [L. *nodus*, knot]. A protuberance or swelling. A constriction. **atrioventricular n.,** the commencement of the bundle of His in the right atrium of the heart. [Wilhelm His, jun., German physician, 1863–1934.]. **node of Ranvier,** the constriction in the neurilemma of a nerve fibre. [Louis Antoine Ranvier, French pathologist, 1835–1922.] **sinoatrial n.,** situated at the opening of the superior vena cava into the right atrium; the wave of contraction begins here, then spreads over the heart.

nodule (nod′-ūl) [L. *nodulus*, knot]. A small node—nodular, adj.

Noludar (nol′-ū-da). Methyprylone (q.v.).

non compos mentis (non kom′-pos men′-tis) [L.]. Of unsound mind.

noradrenaline (nor-ad-ren'-a-lēn). Endogenous noradrenaline is a neuro-humoral transmitter which is released from adrenergic nerve endings. Although small amounts are associated with adrenalin in the adrenal medulla, its role as a hormone is a secondary one. It has an intense vasoconstrictor action, and is given by slow intravenous injection in shock and peripheral failure.

norethisterone (nor-eth-is-tēr'-ōn). Progestogen, said to suppress the gonadotrophin production by the pituitary. Given by tablet for irregular bleeding, dysmenorrhoea and premenstrual tension.

Norflex (nor-fleks). Orphenadrine (q.v.).

normoblast (nor'-mō-blast) [L. *norma*, rule; G. *blastos*, germ]. A normal sized nucleated red blood cell, the precursor of the erythrocyte—normoblastic, adj.

normocyte (nor'-mō-sit) [L. *norma*, rule; G. *kytos*, cell]. A red blood cell of normal size—normocytic, adj.

normoglycaemic (nor-mō-glī-sē-mik). A normal amount of glucose in the blood normoglycaemia, n.

normotension (nor-mō-ten'-shun) [G. *norma*, rule; *tendere*, to stretch]. Normal tension by current custom alluding to blood pressure normotensive, adj.

normothermia (nor-mō-ther'-mi-á) [G. *norma*, rule; *therme*, heat]. Normal body temperature, as opposed to hyperthermia and hypothermia—normothermic, adj.

normotonic (nor-mō-ton'-ik) [G. *norma*, rule; *tonos*, tension]. Normal strength, tension, tone, by current custom referring to muscle tissue. Spasmolytic drugs induce normotonicity in muscle, and can be used before radiography normotonicity, n.

nortriptyline (nor-trip'-til-ēn). Similar to amitriptyline (q.v.).

nosocomial (nō-sō-kōm'-i-al) [G. *nosos*, disease; *komeo*, to take care of]. A n. infection is one which occurs in a patient who has been in hospital for at least 72 hours and did not have signs and symptoms of such infection on admission.

nostalgia (nos-tal'-ji-á) [G. *nostos*, return home; *algos*, pain]. Homesickness nostalgic, adj.

nostrils (nos'-trils). The anterior openings in the nose: the anterior nares; choanae.

novobiocin (nō-vō-bī'-ō-sin). An orally active antibiotic. It should be reserved for use in infections resistant to other drugs.

Novocaine (nō'-vō-kān). Procaine (q.v.).

Novutox (nō'-vū-toks). Procaine (q.v.)

Noxylflex (nok'-zi-fleks). An anti-infective agent used for irrigation of a wound or bladder.

NSU. Non-specific urethritis. Medically but not legally classified as a venereal disease. Now firmly linked with a viruslike organism similar to that responsible for trachoma. See MYCOPLASMA.

nucha (nū'-ká). The nape of the neck—nuchal, adj.

nuclear magnetic resonance. NMR. Non-surgical technique for cancer detection and the analysis of cancer growth rates.

nucleated (nūk'-li-āt-ed) [L. *nucleatus*, having a kernel]. Possessing one or more nuclei.

nucleoproteins (nū'-klē-ō-prō'-tēnz). Proteins found especially in the nuclei of cells. They consist of a protein conjugated with nucleic acid and are broken down during digestion. Among the products are the purine and pyrimidine bases. An end product of nucleoprotein metabolism is uric acid which is excreted in the urine.

nucleotoxic (nū-klē-ō-toks'-ik) [L. *nucleus*, kernal; G. *toxikon*, poison]. Poisonous to cell nuclei as some drugs, toxins and viruses—nucleotoxin, n.

nucleus (nūk'-li-us) [L.]. 1. The inner essential part of a tissue cell, being necessary for the growth, nourishment and reproduction of the cell. 2. A circumscribed accumulation of nerve cells in the central nervous system associated with a particular function. **nucleus pulposus**, the soft core of an intervertebral disc which can prolapse (q.v.) into the spinal cord and cause sciatica—nuclei, pl.; nuclear, adj.

nullipara (nul-lip'-a-rá) [L. *nullus*, none; *parere*, to bring forth]. A woman who has not borne a child—nulliparous, adj.; nulliparity, n.

nummular (num'-ū-lar) [L. *nummularis*, of money]. Coin shaped; resembling rolls of coins, as the sputum in phthisis.

Nupercaine (nū'-pêr-kān). See CINCHOCAINE.

nutation (nū-tā'-shun) [L. *nutare*, to

nod]. Nodding; applied to uncontrollable head shaking.

nutrient (nū'-tri-ent) [L. *nutrire*, to nourish]. Serving as or providing nourishment. **nutrient artery**, one which enters a long bone. **nutrient foramen**, hole in a long bone which admits the n. artery.

nutrition (nū-tri'-shun). The sum total of the processes by which the living organism receives and utilizes the materials necessary for survival, growth and repair of worn-out tissues.

nux vomica (nuks vom'-ik-à). The nuts from which strychnine is obtained. Occasionally used with other bitters as a gastric stimulant.

nyctalgia (nik-tal'-ji-à) [G. *nyx*, night; *algos*, pain]. Pain occurring during the night.

nyctalopia (nik-tal-ō'-pi-à) [G. *nyx*, night; *alaos*, blind; *ops*, eye]. Night blindness (q.v.).

nyctophobia (nik-tō-fō'-bi-à) [G. *nyx*, night; *phobos*, fear]. Abnormal fear of the night and darkness.

nycturia (nik-tū'-ri-à) [G. *nyx*, night; *ouron*, urine]. Incontinence of urine at night.

nymphae (nim'-fē) [G.]. The labia minora.

nymphomania (nim-fō-mā'-ni-à) [G. *nymphe*, a bride, nymph; *mania*, madness]. Excessive sexual desire in a female—**nymphomaniac**, adj.

Nystaform (nīs'-ta-form). Fungicidal cream of nystatin with cortisone, in a water miscible base. Cortisone relieves the fungal irritation.

nystagmus (nis-tag'-mus) [G. *nystagmus*, nodding]. Involuntary and jerky repetitive movement of the eyeballs.

Nystan betnovate (nis'-tan bet'-nō-vāt). Nystatin (q.v.) and betamethasone (q.v.).

nystatin. An antifungal antibiotic effective in the treatment of candidiasis (moniliasis). Prevents intestinal fungal overgrowth during broad spectrum antibiotic treatment.

O

Obin (ō'-bin). Metformin (q.v.).

objective (ob-jek'-tiv) [L. *obicere*, to throw before]. Pertaining to things external to one's self. Opp. subjective (q.v.). **objective signs**, those which the observer notes, as distinct from the symptoms of which the patient complains.

obligate (ob'-li-gāt) [L. *obligatus*, bound]. No alternative. Used to describe functions of cells which are essential, e.g. o. parasite, cannot exist other than as a parasite.

Oblivon (ob-liv-on'). Methylpentynol (q.v.).

obracin (ob'-rà-sin). Tobramycin (q.v.).

obsessional neurosis (ob-sesh'-on-al nū-rō'-sis). Two types. 1. Obsessive compulsive thoughts: constant preoccupation with a constantly recurring morbid thought which cannot be kept out of the mind, and enters against the wishes of the patient who tries to eliminate it. The thought is almost always painful and out of keeping with the person's normal personality. 2. Obsessive compulsive actions: consists of a feeling of compulsion to perform repeatedly a simple act, e.g. handwashing, touching door knobs, etc. Ideas of guilt frequently form the basis of an obsessional state.

obstetrician (ob-stet-rish'-n) [L. *obstetrix*, midwife]. A qualified doctor who practises the science and art of obstetrics.

obstetrics (ob-stet'-riks) [L. *obstetrix*, midwife]. The science dealing with the care of the pregnant woman during the antenatal, parturient and puerperal stages; midwifery.

obturator (ob'-tū-rāt-or) [L. *obturare*, to close]. That which closes an aperture. **obturator foramen**, the opening in the innominate bone which is closed by muscles and fascia.

occipital (ok-sip'-it-al) [L. *occiput*, back part of head]. Pertaining to the back of the head. **occipital bone**, characterized by large hole through which spinal cord passes.

occipito-anterior (ok-sip'-it-ō-an-tē'-ri-or) [L. *occiput*, back of head; *anterior*, foremost]. When the fetal occiput lies in the anterior half of the maternal pelvis.

occipitofrontal (ok-sip'-it-ō-fron'-tal) [L. *occiput*, back of head; *frons*, forehead]. Pertaining to the occiput and forehead.

occipitoposterior (ok-sip'-it-ō-pos-tē'-ri-or) [L. *occiput*, back of head; *posterior*, posterior]. When the fetal occiput is in the posterior half of the maternal pelvis.

occiput (ok'-si-put) [L.]. The posterior region of the skull.

occlusion (ok-kloo'-zhun) [L. *occludere*, to close up]. The closure of an opening, especially of ducts or blood vessels. In dentistry, the fit of the teeth as the two jaws meet.

occult blood (ok'-ul-t). Blood which is not visible to the naked eye but the presence of which can be detected by chemical means.

occupational delirium. A psychiatric term for a condition which occurs in many cases of dementia consisting of purposeless overactivity relating to patient's occupation.

occupational disease. See INDUSTRIAL DISEASE.

occupational therapy. The use of occupations, usually manual, for therapeutic or remedial purposes in mental and physical disorders.

Ochsner-Sherran treatment. Conservative measures sometimes used for patients with acute appendicitis. [Albert John Ochsner, American surgeon, 1858–1925.]

Octapressin (ok ta pres'-sin). Prilocaine with felypressin.

octyl nitrite (ok'-til-nīt-rīt). Vasodilator similar to amyl nitrate (q.v.). Given by inhalation.

ocular (ok'-ū-lar) [L. *ocularis*, of the eyes]. Pertaining to the eye.

oculentum (ok'-ū-len-tum). Eye ointment—oculenta, pl.

oculist (ok'-ū-list). Medically qualified person who refracts and treats eye disease.

oculogenital (ok-ū-lo-jen'-it-al) [L. *oculus*, eye; G. *genesis*, descent]. Pertaining to the eye and genital region, as the virus TRIC. It is found in the male and female genital canals and in the conjunctival sacs of the newborn.

oculogyric (ok-ū-lō-jī'-rik) [L. *oculus*, eye; G. *gyros*, circle]. Referring to movements of the eyeball. **oculogyric crises**, occur in Parkinsonism.

oculomotor (ok-ū-lō-mōt'-or) [L. *oculus*, eye; *movere*, to move]. The third cranial nerve which moves the eye and supplies the upper eye lid.

odontalgia (ō-don-tal'-ji-á) [G.]. Toothache.

odontic (ō-don'-tik) [G. *odous*, tooth]. Pertaining to the teeth.

odontitis (ō-don-tī'-tis) [G. *odous*, tooth; *-itis*, inflammation]. Inflammation of the teeth.

odontoid (ō-don'-toid) [G. *odous*, tooth; *eidos*, form]. Resembling a tooth. **odontoid peg or process**, the toothlike projection of the body of the second cervical vertebra or axis.

odontolith (ō-don'-to-lith) [G. *odous*, tooth; *lithos*, stone]. Tartar; the concretions which are deposited around teeth.

odontology (ō-don-tol'-o-ji) [G. *odous*, tooth; *logos*, discourse]. Dentistry.

odontoma (ō-don-tō'-má) [G. *odous*, tooth; *-oma*, tumour]. A tumour developing from or containing tooth structures—odontomata, pl.; odontomatous, adj.

odontoprisis (ō-don-to-prī'-sis) [G. *odous*, tooth; *prisis*, sawing]. Grinding of the teeth.

odontotherapy (ō-don-tō-ther'-a-pi) [G. *odous*, tooth; *therapeia*, treatment]. The treatement given for diseases of the teeth.

oedema (ē-dē'-má) [G. *oidema*, swelling]. Dropsy. Abnormal infiltration of tissues with fluid. **cardiac o.**, a dependent oedema of subcutaneous tissues in cardiac failure. **hepatic o.** is caused by osmotic pressure changes in the blood. **hunger (famine) o.** results from reduced osmotic pressure of blood, secondary to protein starvation. **pulmonary o.** is a form of waterlogging of the lungs because of left ventricular failure or mitral stenosis. **renal o.** results from disturbed kidney filtration in nephritis. **subcutaneous o.** is demonstrable by the 'pitting' produced by pressure of the finger. See ANGIONEUROTIC O.— oedematous, adj.

Oedipus complex (ēd'-i-pus kom'-pleks) [Oedipus, King of Thebes, who unwittingly killed his father and married his mother]. An unconscious attachment of a son to his mother resulting in a feeling of jealousy towards the father and then guilt, producing emotional conflict. This process was described by Freud as part of his theory of infantile sexuality and considered to be normal in male infants.

oesophageal (ē-sof-a-jē'-al) [G. *oisophagos*, gullet]. Pertaining to the oesophagus (q.v.).

oesophagectasis (ē-sof-a-jek'-tā-sis) [G. *oisophagos*, gullet; *ektasis*, extension]. A dilated gullet (oesophagus).

oesophagectomy (ē-sof-a-jek'-to-mi) [G. *oisophagos*, gullet; *ektome*, excision]. Excision of part or the whole of the oesophagus.

oesophagitis (ē-sof-a-jī'-tis) [G. *oisophagos*, gullet; *-itis*, inflammation]. Inflammation of the oesophagus.

oesophagoscope (ē-sof'-a-gos-kōp) [G. *oisophagos*, gullet; *skopein*, to examine]. See ENDOSCOPE—oesophagoscopy, n.; oesophagoscopic, adj.

oesophagostomy (ē-sof-a-gos'-to-mi) [G. *oisophagos*, gullet; *stoma*, mouth]. A surgically established fistula between the oesophagus and the skin in the root of the neck. Used temporarily for feeding after excision of the pharynx for malignant disease.

oesophagotomy (ē-sof-a-got'-o-mi) [G. *oisophagos*, gullet; *tome*, a cutting]. An incision into the oesophagus.

oesophagus (ē-sof'-ā-gus) [G. *oisophagos*, gullet]. The musculomembranous canal, 22.86 cm in length, extending from the pharynx to the stomach—oesophageal, adj.

oestradiol (ēs-trad'-i-ol). Synthetic oestrogen. Given in amenorrhoea, kraurosis, menopause and other conditions of oestrogen deficiency. Given orally and by injection.

oestriol (ēs'-tri-ol). An oestrogen metabolite present in the urine of pregnant women. Fetus and placenta concerned in production. Oestriol excretion is an indicator of fetal well-being.

Oestroform (ēs'-trō-form). Oestradiol (q.v.).

oestrogen (ēs'-trō-jen). A generic term referring to ovarian hormones. Three 'classical' ones: oestriol, oestrone and oestradiol. Urinary excretion of these substances increases throughout normal pregnancy—oestrogenic, adj.

oestrone (ēs'-trōn). A hormone similar to oestradiol, used mainly in local applications.

Oidium (ō-id'-i-um) Syn., Candida (q.v.).

oleandomycin (ol-ē-an-dō-mī'-sin). An antibiotic with a range of activity similar to that of penicillin. Should be reserved for infections resistant to other antibiotics.

olecranon (ō-lek'-ra-non) [G. *olekranon*, point of elbow]. The large process at the upper end of the ulna; it forms the tip of the elbow when the arm is flexed.

oleum olivae. Olive oil (q.v.).

oleum ricini (ol'-ē-um ri-si'-ni). Castor oil (q.v.).

olfactory (ol-fak'-to-ri) [L. *olfacere*, to smell]. Pertaining to the sense of smell. **olfactory nerve,** the nerve supplying the nose; the first cranial nerve. **olfactory organ,** the nose—olfaction, n.

oligaemia (ol-i-gē'-mi-à) [G. *oligos*, little; *haima,* blood]. Diminished total quantity of blood—oligaemic, adj.

oligohydramnios (ol-i-gō-hid-ram'-ni-os) [G. *oligos*, little; *hydor*, water; *amnion*, fetal membrane]. Deficient amniotic fluid.

oligomenorrhoea (ol-ig-ō-men-or-rē'-à) [G. *oligos*, little; *men*, month; *rheein*, to flow]. Infrequent menstruation, normal cycle is prolonged beyond 35 days.

oligophrenia (ol-ig-ō-frē'-ni-à) Mental deficiency. 'Subnormality' and 'severe subnormality' are now the official terms—oligophrenic, adj.

oligospermia (ol-i-gō-spėr'-mi-à) [G. *oligos*, little; *sperma*, seed]. Deficiency of spermatozoa in the semen.

oliguria (ol-ig-ū'-ri-à) [G. *oligos*, little; *ouron*, urine]. Deficient urine secretion—oliguric, adj.

olive oil. Used in gastric ulcer and as a laxative. Useful externally as emollient.

omentum (ō-men'-tum) [L. apron]. A fold of peritoneum. **gastrosplenic o.** connects the stomach and spleen. The functions of the o. are protection, repair and fat storage. **greater o.,** the fold which hangs from the lower border of the stomach and covers the front of the intestines. **lesser o.,** a smaller fold, passing between the transverse fissure of the liver and the lesser curvature of the stomach—omental, adj.

Omnopon (om'-nō-pon). A preparation of opium alkaloids.

omphalitis (om-fa-ī'-tis) [G. *omphalos,* navel; *-itis,* inflammation]. Inflammation of the umbilicus.

omphalocele (om'-fal-ō-sēl) [G. *omphalos*, navel; *kele*, hernia]. Umbilical hernia.

Onchocerca (on-kō-ser'-ka). Genus of filarial worms.

onchocerciasis (on-kō-ser-kī-a'-sis). Infestation of man with Onchocerca. Adult worms encapsulated in subcutaneous connective tissue. Can cause 'river blindness'.

oncogenic (on-kō-jen'-ik) [G. *onkos,* bulk; *genesis,* descent]. 1. Capable of tumour production. 2. The process of tumour formation. Currently used to describe the carcinogenic viruses.

oncology (on-kol'-o-ji) [G. *onkos*, bulk; *logos*, discourse]. The scientific study of neoplasms—oncological, adj.; oncologically, adv.

oncolysis (on-kol'-i-sis) [G. *onkos*, bulk; *lysis*, a loosening]. Destruction of a neoplasm. Sometimes used to describe reduction in size of tumour—oncolytic, adj.

Oncovin (onk'-o-vin). Vincristine (q.v.).

onychia (ō-nik'-i-á) [G. *onyx*, nail]. Acute inflammation of the nail matrix; suppuration may spread beneath the nail, causing it to become detached and fall off.

onychocryptosis (on-ik-ō krip-tō'-sis) [G. *onyx*, nail; *kryptos*, hidden; *-osis*, condition]. Ingrowing of the nail.

onychogryphosis (on-ik-o-grī-fō'-sis) [G. *onyx*, nail; *griphos*, fishing net]. A ridged, thickened deformity of the nails. Also ONYCHOGRYPOSIS

onycholysis (on-ik-ol'-i-sis) [G. *onyx*, nail; *lysis*, a loosening]. Loosening of toe or finger nail—onycholytic, adj.

onychomycosis (on-ik-ō-mī-kō sis) [G. *onyx*, nail; *mykes*, fungus; *-osis*, condition]. A fungal infection of the nails.

o'nyong-nyong fever (on-i'-ong-ni'-ong fē-vér). Syn., joint-breaker fever. Caused by virus transmitted by mosquitoes in East Africa. First noted in 1959 in north-west Uganda.

oocyte (ō-o-sīt) [G. *oion*, egg; *kytos*, cell]. An immature ovum.

oogenesis (ō-ō-jen'-e-sis) [G. *oion*, egg; *genesis*, production]. The production and formation of ova in the ovary—oogenetic, adj.

oophorectomy (ō-ō-for-ek'-to-mi) [G. *oion*, egg; *ektome*, excision]. Excision of an ovary.

oophoritis (ō-ō-for-ī' tis) [G. *oion*, egg; *-itis*, inflammation]. Inflammation of an ovary.

oophoron (ō-of'-ér-on) [G. *oion*, egg; *pherein*, to bear]. The ovary.

oophorosalpingectomy (ō-ō-for-ō-sal-pin-jek'-to-mi) [G. *oion*, egg; *pherein*, to bear; *salpigx*, tube; *ektome*, excision]. Excision of an ovary and its associated Fallopian tube.

oosperm (ō'-ō-spérm) [G. *oion*, egg; *sperma*, seed]. A fertilized ovum.

opacity (ō-pas'-i-ti) [L. *opacus*, shaded]. Non-transparency; cloudiness; an opaque spot, as on the cornea or lens.

Operidine (o-pér'-i-dēn). A mixture of curare and phenoperidine. Useful prior to use of ventilator for gravely ill asthmatic patients.

ophthalmia (of-thal'-mi-á) [G.]. Inflammation of the eye. **ophthalmia neonatorum**, defined by law in 1914 as a 'purulent discharge from the eyes of an infant commencing within 21 days of birth'. Only 6 per cent of total cases are gonorrhoeal, but all are notifiable. **sympathetic o.**, iridocyclitis of one eye secondary to injury or disease of the other.

ophthalmic (of-thal'-mik) [G. *ophthalmos*, eye]. Pertaining to the eye.

ophthalmitis (of-thal-mī' tis) [G. *ophthalmos*, eye; *-itis*, inflammation]. Syn., ophthalmia (q.v.).

ophthalmologist (of-thal-mol'-o-jist). One who studies ophthalmology.

ophthalmology (of-thal-mol'-o-ji) [G. *ophthalmos*, eye; *logos*, discourse]. The science which deals with the structure, function and diseases of the eye—ophthalmological, adj.; ophthalmologically, adv.

ophthalmoplegia (of-thal-mō-plē'-ji-á) [G. *ophthalmos*, eye; *plege*, stroke]. Paralysis of the eye muscles—ophthalmoplegic, adj.

ophthalmoscope (of-thal'-mō-skōp) [G. *ophthalmos*, eye; *skopein*, to examine]. An instrument fitted with a lens and illumination for examining the interior of the eye—ophthalmoscopic, adj.

ophthalmotonometer (of thal'-mo-tonom'-eter). Instrument for determining the intraocular pressure.

opisthotonos (op-is-thot'-on-os) [G. *opisthen*, behind; *tonos*, tension]. Extreme extension of the body occurring in tetanic spasm. Patient may be supported on his heels and his head alone—opisthotonic, adj.

opium (ō'-pi-um). Dried juice of o. poppy capsules. Contains morphine, codeine and other alkaloids. Valuable analgesic, but more constipating than morphine (q.v.). Also used as tincture of o. and as paregoric (camphorated tincture of o.).

Opoidine (op-oy'-din). Papaveretum (q.v.).

opportunistic infection. A serious infection with a micro-organism which normally has little or no pathogenic activity but which has been activated by a serious disease or by a modern method of treatment.

opsonic index (op-son'-ik in'-deks) [G. *opsonion*, provisions; L. *index*, a pointer]. A figure obtained by experiment which indicates the ability of phagocytes to ingest foreign bodies such as bacteria.

opsonin (op'-son-in) [G. *opsonion*, provisions]. An antibody which unites with antigen, usually part of intact cells, and renders the cells more susceptible to phagocytosis. See ANTIBODIES opsonic, adj.

optic (op'-tik) [G. *optikos*, of sight]. Pertaining to sight. **optic chiasma**, the X-shaped crossing of the fibres of the o. nerve. **optic disc**, the point where the o. nerve enters the eyeball.

optician (op-ti'-shun) [G. *optikos*, of sight]. One who prescribes glasses to correct refractive errors.

optics (op'-tiks) [G. *optikos*, of sight]. The branch of physics which deals with light rays and their relation to vision.

optimax (op'-ti-maks). L-tryptophan with pyridoxine and ascorbic acid. Amino acid and vitamin preparation.

optimum (op'-tim-um) [L. *optimus*, best]. Most favourable. **optimum position**, that which will be least awkward and most useful should a limb remain permanently paralysed.

optometry (op-tom'-et-ri) [G. *optikos*, of sight; *metron*, a measure]. Measurement of visual acuity.

orabase (or'-a-bās). Ointment; protects lesions on mucous membranes. **adcortyl in o.** (triamcinalone emollient), useful for mouth ulcers.

oral (ō'-ral) [L. *os*, mouth]. Pertaining to the mouth. orally, adv.

Oratrol (or'-à-trol). Dichlorphenamide (q.v.).

Orbenin. Cloxacillin (q.v.).

orbicular (or-bik'-ū-lar) [L. *orbicularis*, circular]. Resembling a globe; spherical or circular.

orbit (or'-bit) [L. *orbita*, circuit]. The bony socket containing the eyeball and its appendages —orbital, adj.

orchidectomy (or-ki-dek'-to-mi) [G. *orchis*, testis; *ektome*, excision]. Excision of a testicle.

orchidopexy (or-ki-dō-pek'-si) [G. *orchis*, testicle; *pexis*, a fixing]. The operation of bringing an undescended testicle into the scrotum, and fixing it in this position.

orchis (or'-kis) [G.]. The testicle.

orchitis (or-kī'-tis) [G. *orchis*, testicle; -*itis*, inflammation]. Inflammation of the testicle.

orciprenaline sulphate (or-si-pren'-à-lin-sul'-fāte). Relaxant for relief of bronchospasm. A derivative of adrenaline. Available as tablets or aerosol.

orf. Skin lesions caused by a virus of sheep.

organic (or-gan'-ik). Pertaining to an organ. Associated with life. **organic disease**, one in which there is structural change.

organism (or'-gan-izm) [G. *organon*, tool]. A living cell or group of cells differentiated into functionally distinct parts which are interdependent.

orgasm (or'-gazm) [G. *orgasmos*]. The crisis of sexual excitement.

oriental sore (o-ri-en'-tal sōr'). Delhi boil. A form of cutaneous leishmaniasis producing papular, crusted, granulomatous eruptions of the skin. A disease of the tropics and subtropics.

orientation (or-i-en-tā'-shun). Clear awareness of one's position relative to the environment. In mental conditions o. 'in space and time' means that the patient knows where he is and recognizes the passage of time, i.e. can give the correct date. Disorientation means the reverse.

orifice (or'-i-fis) [L. *orificium*, opening]. A mouth or opening.

origin (or'-i-jin) [L. *origo*]. The commencement or source of anything. **origin of a muscle**, the end that remains relatively fixed during contraction of the muscle.

Orinase (o'-rin-āz). Tolbutamide (q.v.).

ornithine (or'-ni-thēn). An amino acid, obtained from arginine, by splitting off urea.

ornithosis (or-ni-thō'-sis) [G. *ornis*, bird; -*osis*, condition]. Human illness resulting from disease of birds.

orogenital (or-ō-jen-'it-al) [L. *os*, mouth; G. *genesis*, descent]. Pertaining to the mouth and the external genital area.

oropharynx (or-ō-far'-inks) [L. *os*, mouth; G. *pharygx*, pharynx]. 1. That portion of the pharynx which is below the level of the soft palate and above the level of the hyoid bone. 2. Pertaining to the mouth and pharynx—oropharyngeal, adj.

Oroya fever. See BARTONELLA FEVER.

orphenadrine (or-fen'-a-drēn). Tablets

which counteract any tendency to Parkinsonism produced by tranquillizers. Sometimes useful in incontinence of urine.

orthocaine (or'-thō-kān). Local anaesthetic similar to benzocaine (q.v.).

orthodontic (or-thō-don'-tik) [G. orthos, straight; odous, tooth]. A branch of dentistry dealing with prevention and correction of irregularities of the teeth.

orthopaedics (or-thō-pē'-diks) [G. orthos, straight; pais, child]. Formerly devoted to the correction of deformities in children. It is now a branch of surgery dealing with all conditions affecting the locomotor system, whether by apparatus, manipulation or operation.

orthopnoea (or-thop-nē'-ā) [G. orthos, straight; pnoe, breath]. Breathlessness necessitating an upright, sitting position for its relief—orthopnoeic, adj.

orthoptics (or-thop'-tiks) [G. orthos, straight; optikos, optic]. Study and treatment of muscle imbalances of eye (squint).

orthostatic (or-thō-stat'-ik) [G. orthos, straight; statikos, causing to stand]. Caused by the upright stance. **orthostatic albuminuria**, occurs in some healthy subjects only when they take the upright position. When lying in bed the urine is normal.

orthotic (or-thot'-ik) [G. orthos, straight]. Any device applied to or around the body in the care of physical impairment or disability.

Ortolani's sign (or-to-lan'-iz). Test performed shortly after birth to discern dislocation of the hip.

os [L.]. A mouth. **external o.**, the opening of the cervix into the vagina. **internal o.**, the opening of the cervix into the uterine cavity—ora, pl.

oscillation (os-il-ā'-shun) [L. oscillare, to swing]. A swinging or moving to and fro; a vibration.

oscillometry (os-il-om'-et-ri) [L. oscillare, to swing; G. metron, a measure]. Measurement of vibration, using a special apparatus (oscillometer, oscilloscope). Measures the magnitude of the pulse wave more precisely than palpation.

Osler's nodes. Small painful areas (due to emboli) in pulp of fingers or toes, or palms and soles, occurring in subacute bacterial endocarditis. [William Osler, English physician (Canadian birth), 1849–1919.]

osmolarity (os-mō-lar'-i-ti) [G. osmos, impulse]. The osmotic pressure exerted by a substance in aqueous solution, defined in terms of the number of active particles per unit volume.

osmosis (os-mō'-sis) [G. osmos, impulse]. The passage of water across a membrane under the influence of osmotic pressure.

osmotic pressure (os-mot'-ik). The pressure with which sodium chloride, sugars, urea and many other substances in solution draw water across a membrane, which allows the molecules of water to pass through, but which is relatively impermeable or semipermeable to other molecules.

Ospolot (os'-pol-ot). Sulthiame (q.v.)

osseous (os'-ē-us) [L. osseus, of bone]. Pertaining to or resembling bone.

ossicles (os'-ik-ls) [L. os, bone]. Small bones, particularly those contained in the middle ear: the malleus, incus and stapes.

ossification (os-if-i-kā'-shun) [L. os, bone; facere, to make]. The conversion of cartilage, etc. into bone—ossify, v.t., v.i.

osteitis (os-tē-ī'-tis) [G. osteon, bone; -itis, inflammation]. Inflammation of bone. **osteitis deformans**, Paget's disease (q.v.). **osteitis fibrosa**, cavities form in the interior of bone. Cysts may be solitary or the disease generalized. This second condition is the result of excessive parathyroid secretion and absorption of calcium from bone.

osteoarthritis (os-tē-ō-arth-rī'-tis) [G. osteon, bone; arthron, joint; -itis, inflammation]. Degenerative arthritis; may be primary, or may follow injury or disease involving the articular surfaces of synovial joints. The articular cartilage becomes worn, osteophytes form at the periphery of the joint surface and loose bodies may result—osteoarthritic, adj.

osteoblast (os'-tē-ō-blast) [G. osteon, bone; blastos, germ]. A bone-forming cell—osteoblastic, adj.

osteochondritis (os-tē-ō-kon-drī'-tis) [G. osteon, bone; chondros, cartilage; -itis, inflammation]. Originally an inflammation of bone cartilage. Usually applied to non-septic conditions, especially avascular necrosis involving joint surfaces, e.g. osteochondritis dissecans in which a portion of joint surface may separate to form a loose body in the joint. See SCHEUERMAN'S DISEASE.

osteochondroma (os-tē-ō-kon-drō'-má) [G. *osteon*, bone; *chondros*, cartilage; *-oma*, tumour]. A benign bony and cartilaginous tumour.

osteoclasis (os-tē-ō-klā'-sis) [G. *osteon*, bone; *klasis*, a breaking]. The therapeutic fracture of a bone.

osteoclast (os'-tē-ō-klast) [G. *osteon*, bone; *klastos*, broken]. Bone destroyer; the cell which dissolves or removes unwanted bone.

osteoclastoma (os-tē-ō-klas-tō'-má) [G. *osteon*, bone; *klastos*, broken; *-oma*, tumour]. A tumour of the osteoclasts. May be benign, locally recurrent, or frankly malignant. The usual site is near the end of a long bone. See MYELOMA.

osteocyte (os'-tē-ō-sīt) [G. *osteon*, bone; *kytos*, cell]. A bone cell.

osteodystrophy (os-tē-ō-dis'-tro-fi) [G. *osteon*, bone; *dys*, bad; *trophe*, nourishment]. Faulty growth of bone.

osteogenic (os-tē-ō-jen'-ik) [G. *osteon*, bone; *genesis*, descent]. Bone-producing. **osteogenic sarcoma**, malignant tumour originating in cells which normally produce bone.

osteolytic (os-tē-ō-lit'-ik) [G. *osteon*, bone; *lysis*, a loosening]. Destructive of bone, e.g. osteolytic malignant deposits in bone.

osteoma (os-tē-ō'-má) [G. *osteon*, bone; *-oma*, tumour]. A bony tumour. (1) compact (ivory o.). (2) cancellous. May be single or multiple.

osteomalacia (os-tē-ō-mal-ā'-sē-á) [G. *osteon*, bone; *malakia*, softness]. Infectious mineralization of the mature skeleton, with softening and bone pain. It is commonly caused by insufficient dietary intake of vitamin D.

osteomyelitis (os-tē-ō-mī-el-ī'-tis) [G. *osteon*, bone; *myelos*, marrow; *-itis*, inflammation]. Inflammation commencing in the marrow of bone—osteomyelitic, adj.

osteopath (os'-tē-ō-path) [G. *osteon*, bone; *pathos*, disease]. One who practises osteopathy.

osteopathy (os-tē-op'-a-thi) [G. *osteon*, bone; *pathos*, disease]. 1. Any disease of bone. 2. A theory which attributes a wide range of disorders to mechanical derangements of the skeletal system, which it is claimed can be rectified by suitable manipulations. Usually practised by medically unqualified persons —osteopathic, adj.

osteopetrosis (os-tē-ō-pet-rō'-sis) [G. *osteon*, bone; *petros*, stone; *-osis*, condition]. See ALBERS–SCHÖNBERG DISEASE.

osteophony (os-tē-of'-on-i) [G. *osteon*, bone; *phone*, sound]. The conduction of sound waves to the inner ear by bone.

osteophyte (os'-tē-ō-fīt) [G. *osteon*, bone; *phyton*, plant]. A bony outgrowth or spur, usually at the margins of joint surfaces, e.g. in osteoarthritis —osteophytic, adj.

osteoplasty (os'-tē-ō-plas-ti) [G. *osteon*, bone; *plassein*, to form]. Any plastic operation on bone—osteoplastic, adj.

osteoporosis (os-tē-ō-por-ō'-sis) [G. *osteon*, bone; *poros*, passage; *-osis*, condition]. Loss of bone density due to excessive absorption of calcium and phosphorus from the bone, due to progressive loss of the protein matrix of bone which normally carries the calcium deposits—osteoporotic, adj.

osteosarcoma (os-tē-ō-sár-kō'-má) [G. *osteon*, bone; *sarkoma*, fleshly overgrowth]. A sarcomatous tumour growing from bone—osteosarcomata, pl.; osteosarcomatous, adj.

osteosclerosis (os-tē-ō-skle-rō'-sis) [G. *osteon*, bone; *sklerosis*, hardening]. Increased density or hardness of bone—osteosclerotic, adj.

osteotome (os'-tē-ot-ōm) [G. *osteon*, bone; *tomos*, cutting]. An instrument for cutting bone; it is similar to a chisel, but it is bevelled on both sides of its cutting edge.

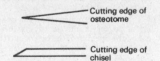

Cutting edge of osteotome

Cutting edge of chisel

Osteotome

osteotomy (os-tē-ot'-om-i) [G. *osteon*, bone; *tome*, a cutting]. Division of bone. **McMurray's o.**, division of femur between lesser and greater trochanter. Shaft displaced inwards beneath the head and abducted. This position maintained by a nail plate. Restores painless weight bearing. In congenital dislocation of hip, deliberate pelvic o. renders the outer part of the socket (acetabulum) more horizontal. Pelvic o. now preferred to the shelf operation to provide a better roof at the acetabulum.

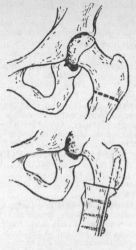

Osteotomy

ostium (os'-ti-um) [L.]. The opening or mouth of any tubular passage—ostial, adj.; ostia, pl.

otalgia (ō-tal'-ji-á) [G. *ous*, ear; *algos*, pain]. Earache.

otitis (ō-tī'-tis) [G. *ous*, ear; *-itis*, inflammation]. Inflammation of the ear. **otitis externa**, inflammation of the skin of the external auditory canal. **otitis interna**, see LABYRINTHITIS. otitis media, inflammation of the middle ear cavity. The effusion tends to be of a serious nature in adults; and of a mucous nature in children, giving rise to the label 'glue ear'—otitic, adj.

otolaryngology (ō-tō-lar-in-gol'-o-ji) [G. *ous*, ear; *larygx*, larynx; *logos*, discourse]. The science which deals with the structure, function and diseases of the ear and larynx.

otoliths (ō'-tō-liths) [G. *ous*, ear; *lithos*, stone]. Tiny calcareous deposits within the membranous labyrinth of the internal ear.

otologist (ō-tol'-oj-ist) [G. *ous*, ear; *logos*, discourse]. One specializing in the functions and diseases of the ear.

otology (ō-tol'-o-ji) [G. *ous*, ear; *logos*, discourse]. The science which deals with the structure, function and diseases of the ear.

otomycosis (ō-tō-mī-kō'-sis) [G. *ous*, ear;

mykes, fungus; *-osis*, condition]. A fungal (Aspergillus, Candida) infection of the external auditory meatus—otomycotic, adj.

otorhinolaryngology (ō-tō-rī-nō-lar-in-gol'-o-ji) [G. *ous*, ear; *rhis*, nose; *larygx*, larynx; *logos*, discourse]. The science which deals with the structure, function and diseases of the ear, nose and throat.

otorrhoea (ō-tō-rē'-á([G. *out*, ear; *rheein*, to flow]. A discharge from the external auditory meatus.

otosclerosis (ō-tō-skler-ō-sis) [G. *out*, ear; *sklerosis*, hardening]. New bone formation affecting primarily the labyrinth of the inner ear and a common cause of progressive deafness—otosclerotic, adj.

ototoxic (ō-tō-tok'-sik) [G. *ous*, ear; *toxikon*, poison]. Having a toxic action on the ear.

ouabaine (oo'-á-bān). A cardiac glycoside. Like digoxin, it has a steadying effect on the heart.

ova (ō'-vá) [L.]. The female reproductive cells—ovum, sing.

ovabain (ō'-va-bān). Glycoside of digitalis.

ovarian (ō-vā'-ri-an) [N.L. *ovarium*, egg]. Pertaining to the ovaries, **ovarian** cyst, an ovarian tumour containing fluid—may be benign or malignant.

ovariectomy (ō-vē-ri-ek'-to-mi) [N.L. *ovarium*, egg; *ektome*, excision]. Excision of an ovary. Oopherectomy.

ovariotomy (ō-vē-ri-ot'-om-i) [N.L. *ovarium*, egg; G. *tome*, cutting]. Literally means incision of an ovary, but is the term usually applied to the removal of an ovary. Also OOPHORECTOMY.

ovaritis (ō-vē-rī'-tis). Oophoritis (q.v.).

ovary (ō'-vér-i) [N.L. *ovarium*, egg]. One of two small oval bodies situated on either side of the uterus on the posterior surface of the broad ligament. The structures in which the ova are developed—ovarian, adj. **cystic o.**, retention cysts in ovarian follicles; o. rarely larger than a plum. Cysts contain oestrogen-rich fluid. Causes menorrhagia.

overcompensation (ō-vér-kom-pen-sā'-shun). Name given to any type of behaviour which a person adopts in order to cover up a deficiency in his personality, of which he is aware. Thus a person who is afraid may react by becoming arrogant or boastful or quarrelsome.

oviduct (ō'-vi-dukt). Syn., Fallopian tube (q.v.).

ovulation (ov-ū-lā'-shun) [L. *ovum*, egg]. The maturation and rupture of a Graafian follicle (q.v.) with the discharge of an ovum.

oxacillin (oks'-á-sil-in). See FLUCLOXA-CILLIN.

oxalate (oks'-al-āt). Any salt of oxalic acid.

oxaluria (oks-al-ū'-ri-á) [G. *oxalis*, garden sorrel; *ouron*, urine]. Excretion of urine containing calcium oxalate crystals; associated often with dyspepsia.

oxazepam (oks-az'-e-pam). Mild tranquillizer.

ox bile. Fel bovinum (q.v.).

Oxford inflator. A hand-operated bellows attached to a face mask for emergency artificial respiration.

oxidase (oks'-i-dās). Any enzyme which promotes oxidation.

oxidation (oks-i-dā'-shun). The process of converting a substance into an oxide by the addition of oxygen. The carbon in organic compounds undergoes oxidation with the formation of carbon dioxide when they are combusted in air, or when they are metabolized in living material in the presence of oxygen. Also used in biochemistry for the process of the removal of hydrogen from a molecule (e.g. in the presence of air ascorbic acid undergoes o. with the formation of dehydroascorbic acid). The loss of an electron with an increase in valency (e.g. the conversion of ferrous to ferric iron) is also an oxidation. The greater part of the energy present in foods is made available to the body by the processes of o. in the tissues.

Oxycel (oks'-i-sel). This is oxidized cellulose, and is a useful haemostatic for plugging wounds when suturing is difficult. The material is subsequently absorbed by the tissues.

oxygen (oks'-i-jen). A colourless, odourless, gaseous element; necessary for life and combustion. Used medicinally as an inhalation. Supplied in cylinders (black with a white top) in which the gas is at a high pressure. See HYPERBARIC.

oxygenation (oks-i-jen-ā'-shun). The saturation of a substance (particularly blood) with oxygen—oxygenated, adj.

oxygenator (oks-ij'-jen-ā-tor). Artificial 'lung' as used in heart surgery.

oxyhaemoglobin (oks-i-hē-mō-glō'-bin). Oxygenated haemoglobin, an unstable compound.

oxyntic (oks-in'-tik) [G. *oxynein*, to make acid]. Producing acid. oxyntic cells, the cells in the gastric mucosa which produce hydrochloric acid.

oxypertine (oks-i-per'-tēn). Tranquillizer, useful in anxiety neuroses.

oxyphenbutazone (oks-i-fen-bū'-tá-zōn). Anti-inflammatory, analgesic, anti-arthritic drug. Available as suppositories.

oxytetracycline (oks-i-tet-ra-sī'-klin). An orally effective antibiotic with a wide range of activity. May be given by slow intravenous injection in severe infections. Prolonged use may cause monilial overgrowth in the intestinal tract.

oxytocic (oks-i-tō'-sik) [G. *oxys*, sharp; *tokos*, childbirth]. Hastening parturition; an agent promoting uterine contractions.

oxytocin (oks-i-tō'-sin). One of the posterior pituitary hormones. Contracts muscle in milk ducts and hence causes milk ejection. A preparation of pituitary extract that can cause uterine contractions, and so is useful in postpartum haemorrhage. Given intramuscularly, subcutaneously, orally, nasally, or intravenously in titration method with a positive pressure peristaltic pump.

Oxyuris (ok-si-ūr'-is). Nematodes, commonly called threadworms (q.v.).

ozaena (ō-zē'-ná) [G. *ozein*, to smell]. Atrophic condition of the nasal mucous membrane with associated crusting and foetor.

ozone (ō'-zōn). An allotropic form of oxygen, O_2. Has powerful oxidizing properties and is therefore a disinfectant.

P

^{32}P. Radioactive phosphorus.

pacemaker. Sinoatrial node. See node. artifical p., an electrode can be fitted on the epicarium and attached to a p. implanted in the rectus sheath or worn externally. An electrode catheter can be introduced via the jugular vein with its tip wedged at the apex of the right ventricle. This electrode may be connected to an implanted p., or by leads brought out from a neck vein to an external p.

pachyblepharon (pak-i-blef'-a-ron) [G. *pachys*, thick; *blepharon*, eyelid]. Thick eyelids.

pachycephalia (pak-i-kef-ā-li-á) [G.

pachys, thick; *kephale,* head]. A thick skull.

pachychilia (pak-i-kī'-li-à) [G. *pachys,* thick; *cheilos,* lip]. Thick lip(s).

pachydermia (pak-i-dèrm'-i-á) [G. *pachys,* thick; *derma,* skin]. Thick skin. See ELEPHANTIASIS.

pachymeningitis (pak-i-men-in-jī'-tis) [G. *pachys,* thick; *meninx,* membrane; *-itis,* inflammation]. Inflammation of the dura mater (or pachymeninx).

paediatrician (pē-dē-at-ri'-shun) [G. *pais,* child; *iatros,* physician]. A specialist in children's diseases.

paediatrics (pē-dē-at'-riks) [G. *pais,* child]. The branch of medicine dealing with children.

Paget-Schroetter syndrome. Axillary or subclavian vein thrombosis, often associated with effort, in fit young persons.

Paget's disease. 1. Osteitis deformans. Excess of the enzyme alkaline phosphatase causes too rapid bone formation; consequently bone is thin. There is loss of stature, crippling deformity, abnormality enlarged head, collapse of vertebrae and nervous complications can result. Sufferers are particularly susceptible to sarcoma of bone. If the auditory nerve is involved, there is impairment of hearing. 2. Carcinoma of the nipple. [James Paget, English surgeon, 1814–99.]

painter's colic. Lead colic (q.v.). See LEAD POISONING.

palate (pal'-lat) [L. *palatum*]. The roof of the mouth. **artificial p.,** prosthesis for use in cleft palate. **cleft p.,** a congenital cleft between the palatal bones, which leaves a gap in the roof of the mouth, opening directly into the nose. **hard p.,** the front part of the roof of the mouth formed by the two palatal bones. **soft p.,** situated at the posterior end of the p. and consisting of muscle covered by mucous membrane—palatal, palatine, adj.

palatine (pal'-a-tīn). Pertaining to the palate. **palatine arches,** the bilateral double pillars or arch-like folds formed by the descent of the soft palate as it meets the pharynx.

palatoplegia (pal-at-ō-plē'-ji-à) [L. *palatum,* palate; *plege,* stroke]. Paralysis of the soft palate—palatoplegic, adj.

palliative (pal'-i-a-tiv) [L. *palliatus,* cloaked]. Anything which serves to alleviate but cannot cure a disease.

pallidectomy (pal-id-ek'-to-mi). Destruction of a predetermined section of globus pallidus. See CHEMOPALLIDECTOMY and STEREOTAXIS.

pallidotomy (pal-id-ot'-o-mil) [L. *pallidus,* pale; G. *tome,* a cutting]. Surgical severance of the fibres from the cerebral cortex to the corpus striatum. Done to relieve the tremor in Parkinson's disease. Less common now.

palm (pám) [L. *palma*]. The anterior or flexor surface of the hand.

palmar (pal'-mar) [L. *palmaris*]. Pertaining to the palm of the hand. **palmar arches,** superficial and deep, are formed by the anastomosis of the radial and ulnar arteries.

palpable (pal'-pa-bl) [L. *palpare,* to touch softly]. Capable of being palpated.

palpation (pal-pā'-shun) [L. *palpare,* to touch softly]. The act of manual examination—palpate, v.t.

palpebra (pal-pē'-bra) [L.]. The eyelid—palpebral, adj.; palpebrae, pl.

palpitation (pal-pit-a'-shun) [L. *palpitare,* to palpitate]. Rapid forceful beating of the heart of which the patient is conscious.

palsy (pawl'-zi). See PARALYSIS. **Bell's p.,** facial hemiparesis from oedema of the seventh (facial) cranial nerve. Cause unknown. [Charles Bell, Scottish physician, 1774–1842.] **Erb's p.,** involves the shoulder and arm muscles from a lesion of the fifth and sixth cervical nerve roots. The arm hangs loosely at the side, with the forearm pronated ('waiter's tip position'). Most commonly a birth injury. [Wilhelm Heinrich Erb, German neurologist, 1840–1921.]

Paludrine (pal'-ū-drin). Proguanil (q.v.).

pamaquin (pa'-ma-kwin). Synthetic antimalarial, used mainly in association with quinine or chloroquine.

Pamergan. Pethidine and promethazine, with or without atropine. Used mainly as premedication.

Panadol (pan'-a-dol). Paracetamol (q.v.).

panarthritis (pan-àrth-rī'-tis) [G. *pas,* whole; *arthron,* joint; *-itis,* inflammation]. Inflammation of all the structures of a joint.

pancarditis (pan-kár-dī'-tis) [G. *pas,* whole; *kardia,* heart; *-itis,* inflammation]. Inflammation of all the structures of the heart.

pancreas (pan'-kri-as) [G. *pagkreas*]. A

tongue-shaped glandular organ lying below and behind the stomach. Its head is encircled by the duodenum and its tail touches the spleen. It is about 17.78 cm long and weighs about 98 g. It secretes the hormone insulin, and also pancreatic juice which contains enzymes involved in the digestion of fats and proteins in the small intestine.

pancreatectomy (pan-krē-at-ek'-to-mi) [G. *pagkreas*, pancreas; *ektome*, excision]. Excision of part or the whole of the pancreas.

pancreatin (pan'-krē-a-tin). A mixture of enzymes obtained from the pancreas. Used in pancreatic diseases and deficiency. Standard and triple-strength products are available.

pancreatitis (pan-krē-a-tī'-tis) [G. *pagkreas*, pancreas; *-itis*, inflammation]. Inflammation of the pancreas. Lipase level of blood and urine used as indicator of p. See DIASTASE.

pancreatrophic (pān-krē'-a-trōf'-ik). Stimulating the pancreas. Some of the anterior pituitary hormones have a p. action.

pancreozymin (pan-krē-ō-zī'-min). A hormone secreted in the small intestine; stimulates flow of pancreatic enzymes.

Pancrex (pan'-kreks). Supplements deficient digestive enzymes in fibrocystic disease.

pancuronium bromide (pan-kū-rō'-ni-um). Muscle relaxant (q.v.).

pancytopenia (pan-sī-tō-pēn'-i-a). Describes peripheral blood picture when red cells, granular white cells and platelets are reduced as occurs in suppression of bone marrow function.

pandemic (pan-dem'-ik) [G. *pandemia*, the whole people]. An infection spreading over a whole country or the world.

panhysterectomy (pan-his-tėr-ek'-to-mi). An old term for the removal of the uterus and adnexa; more accurately described as a total hysterectomy (q.v.) with bilateral salpingo-oophorectomy (q.v.).

pannus (pan'-us) [L. cloth]. Corneal vascularization, often caused by conjunctival irritation.

panophthalmitis (pan-of-thal-mī'-tis) [G. *pas*, whole; *ophthalmos*, eye; *-itis*, inflammation]. Inflammation of all the tissues of the eyeball.

panosteitis (pan-os-tē-ī'-tis) [G. *pas*, whole; *osteon*, bone; *-itis*, inflammation]. Inflammation of all

constituents of a bone—medulla, bony tissue and periosteum.

pantie-girdle syndrome. The ankles of women of sedentary occupation, wearing a pantie-type of foundation garment, become swollen by night.

Pantocaine. Amethocaine (q.v.).

pantothenic acid (pan-to-thē'-nik as'-id). A constituent of the vitamin B complex. Therapeutic value is uncertain.

PAO Peak acid output. See PENTAGASTRIN TEST.

papaveretum (pa-pa-ver'-ē-tum) [L. *papaver*, poppy]. A mixture of opium alkaloids containing 50 per cent of morphine.

papaverine (pa-pav'-ėr-ēn). One of the less important alkaloids of opium, used mainly as a relaxant in spasm, asthma and peripheral vascular disorders.

papilla (pa-pil'-à). A minute nipple-shaped eminence, i.e. eminence. **anal p.**, epithelial projections on the edges of the anal valves. **circumvallate p.**, the large papillae found at the base of the tongue. **filiform p.**, the fine hair-like papillae at the tip of the tongue. **fungiform p.**, papillae shaped like a fungus, found chiefly on the dorsocentral area of the tongue. **renal p.**, the summit of one of the renal pyramids—papillae, pl.; papillary, adj.

papillitis (pap-il-ī'-tis) [L.*papilla*, nipple; G. *-itis*, inflammation]. Most usually inflammation of the optic disc. Otherwise inflammation of a papilla. Can arise in the kidney after excessive phenacetin intake.

papilloedema (pap-il-ē-dē'-mà) [L. *papilla*, nipple; *oidema*, swelling]. Oedema of the optic disc; indicative of increased intracranial pressure. Choked disc (q.v.).

papilloma (pap-i-lō'-mà) [L.*papilla*, nipple; G. *-oma*, tumour]. A simple tumour arising from a non-glandular epithelial surface—papillomatous, adj.; papillomata, pl.

papule (pa'-pūl) [L. *papula*, pimple]. A small circumscribed elevation of the skin—papular, adj.

papulopustular (pa-pū-lō-pus'-tūl-ar) [L. *papula*, pimple; *pustula*, blister]. Pertaining to both papules and pustules (q.v.).

para-aminobenzoic acid (par-a a-mī'-nō-ben-zō-ik as'-id). An acid which acts as an essential metabolite for many bacteria. Sulphonamide drugs prevent some bacteria from using PA and so stop their growth.

para-aminosalicylic acid (par-a a-mīn-ō-sal-is-il'-ik as'-id). Widely used antitubercular drug, usually in association with isoniazid or streptomycin. Has nauseous taste, so is usually given as cachets or granules.

para-aortic (par-a ā-or'-tik) [G. *para*, beside; *aorte*, aorta]. Near the aorta.

paracentesis (par-a-sen-tē'-sis) [G. *parakentesis*, a tapping]. The withdrawal of fluid from its containing, closed cavity by insertion of a hollow needle or cannula. Aspiration—paracenteses, pl.

paracetamol (par-a-sē'-ta-mol). An analgesic resembling phenacetin in effect, but less liable to cause side effects in those patients sensitive to phenacetin.

Paracodol (par-a-kō'-dol). Soluble tablets of paracetamol with codeine.

Paradione (par-a-dī'ōn). An anticonvulsant compound, useful in petit mal resistant to trioxidione therapy.

paraesthesia (par-es-thē'-zi-a) [G. *para*, beside; *aisthesis*, perception]. Any abnormality of sensation.

paraffin (par'-af-in). Medicinal paraffins are: liquid paraffin, used as a laxative; soft paraffin, the familiar ointment base; and hard paraffin, used in wax baths for rheumatic conditions.

paraformaldehyde (par-a-form-al'-dē-hī-d). A solid modification of formaldehyde (q.v.), used for sterilizing catheters and disinfecting rooms.

paraganglioma. See PHAEOCHROMO-CYTOMA.

Paragesic (par-a-gēz'-ik). Analgesic relaxant, useful for painful upper respiratory infection and migraine.

parainfluenza virus. Causes acute upper respiratory infection.

paraldehyde (par-al'-dē-hīd). Liquid with characteristic odour. Has sedative properties similar to chloral. Given orally or by intramuscular injection, or rectally as a solution in olive oil. Now rarely used.

paralysis (par-al'-i-sis) [G.]. Complete or incomplete loss of nervous function to a part of the body. This may be sensory or motor or both. **paralysis agitans**, Parkinson's disease (q.v.). **bulbar p.**, involves the labioglossopharyngeal region and results from degeneration of motor nuclei in the medulla oblongata. **diver's p.**, see CAISSON DISEASE. **infantile p.**, see POLIOMYELITIS. **flaccid p.**

results mainly from lower motor neurone lesions. There are diminished or absent tendon reflexes. **Landry's (acute ascending) p.** is accompanied by fever and may terminate in respiratory stasis and death. **pseudo p. of parrot**, there is inability to move upper limb because of syphilitic osteochondritis; found in neonatal congenital syphilis. **pseudobulbar p**, there is gross disturbance in control of tongue, bilateral hemiplegia and mental changes following on a succession of 'strokes'. **spastic p.** results mainly from upper motor neurone lesions. There are exaggerated tendon reflexes. See PALSY.

paralytic (par al it'-ik) [G. *paralytikos*]. Pertaining to paralysis. **paralytic ileus**, paralysis of the intestinal muscle so that the bowel content cannot pass onwards even though there is no mechanical obstruction. See APERISTALSIS.

paramedian (par-a-mē'-di-an) [G. *para*, beside; L. *medianus*, middle]. Near the middle.

paramedical (par-a-mēd'-ik-al) Associated with the medical profession. The p. services include occupational, physical and speech therapy, and medical social work.

paramenstruum (par-a-men'-stroo-um) [G. *para*, beside; L. *menstruare*, to menstruate]. The four days before the start of menstruation and the first four days of the period itself.

Paramethasone (para-a-meth'-a-zōn). One of the corticosteroids.

parametritis (par-a-met-rī'-tis) [G. *para*, beside; *metra*, womb; *-itis*, inflammation]. Inflammation of the pelvic connective tissue.

parametrium (par-a-met'-ri-um) [G. *para*, beside; *metra*, womb]. The connective tissues immediately surrounding the uterus—parametrial, adj.

paranasal (par-a-nā'-zal) [G. *para*, beside; L. *nasus*, nose]. Near the nasal cavities, as the various sinuses.

paraneoplastic (par-a-nē-o-plas'-tik) [G. *para*, beside; *neos*, new; *plasma*, form]. Paraneoplastic disease describes syndromes associated with malignancy but not caused by the primary growth or its metastases.

paranoia (par-a-noi'-a) [G. *para*, beyond; *noos*, mind]. Delusions of persecution—paranoic, adj.

paranoic behaviour. Acts denoting suspicion of others.

paraoesophageal (par-a-ē-sof'-a-jēl) [G. *para*, beside; *oisophagos*. gullet]. Near the oesophagus.

paraphimosis (par-a-fī-mō'-sis) [G. *para*, beside: *phimosis*, a stopping up]. Retraction of the prepuce behind the glans penis so that the tight ring of skin interferes with the flood flow in the glans.

paraphrenia (par-a-frē'-ni-á) [G. *para*, beyond: *phren*, mind]. A psychiatric illness in the elderly characterized by well-circumscribed delusions, usually of a persecutory nature.—paraphrenic, adj.

paraplegia (par-a-plē'-ji-á) [G. *para*, beyond; *plege*, stroke]. Paralysis of the lower limbs, usually including the bladder and rectum—paraplegic, adj.

pararectal (par-a-rĕk'-tal) [G. *para*, beside; I. *rectus*, straight]. Near the rectum.

parasitaemia (par-a-sit-ē'-mi-á) [G. *parasitos*, parasite; *haima*, blood]. Parasites in the blood—parasitaemic, adj.

parasite (par-a-sīt) [G. *parasitos*]. An organism which contains food or shelter from another host organism—parasitic, adj.

parasiticide (par-a-sit'-i-sīd) [G. *parasitos*, parasite: L. *caedere*, to kill]. An agent which will kill parasites.

parasympathetic (par-a-sim-path-et'-ik) [G. *para*, beside; *sympathes*, sympathetic]. A portion of the autonomic nervous system, derived from some of the cranial and sacral nerves belonging to the central nervous system.

parasympatholytic (par-a-sim'-path-ō-lit'-ik). Capable of neutralizing the effect of parasympathetic stimulation, e.g. atropine and hyoscine.

parathion (par-a-thī'-on). Organophosphorus compound used as insecticide in agriculture. Powerful and irreversible anticholinesterase action. Potentially dangerous to man for this reason.

parathormone (par-a-thor'-mōn). A hormone secreted by the parathyroid glands, which controls the calcium content of bone. Excess hormone causes mobilization of calcium from the bones, which become rarefied.

parathyroid (par-a-thī'-roid) [G. *para*, beside: *thureieudes*, shield-shaped]. Four small endocrine glands lying close to or embedded in the posterior surface of the thyroid gland. They secrete a hormone, parathormone.

parathyroidectomy (par-a-thī-roid-ek'-to-mi) [G. *para*, beside: *thureoeides*, shield-shaped; *ektome*, excision]. Excision of one or more parathyroid glands.

paratracheal (par-a-trak-ē'-al) [G. *para*, beside: *trachus*, rough]. Near the trachea.

paratyphoid fever (par-a-tī'-foid fē'-vèr) [G. *para*, near; *typhodes*, delirious]. A variety of enteric fever, but less severe and prolonged than typhoid fever. Caused by *Salmonella paratyphi A* and *B*, and more rarely *C*. See TAB.

paraurethral (par-a-ū-rēth'-ral) [G. *para*, beside; *ourethra*, urethra]. Near the urethra.

paravaginal (par-a-va-jī'-nal) [G. *para*, beside: L. *vagina*]. Near the vagina.

paravertebral (par-a-vèr'-te-bral) [G. *para*, beside: L. *vertebra*, joint]. Near the spinal column. **paravertebral block anaesthesia** (more correctly, 'analgesia') is induced by infiltration of local anaesthetic around the spinal nerve roots as they emerge from the intervertebral foramina. **paravertebral injection** of local anaesthetic into sympathetic chain. Can be used as a test in ischaemic limbs to see if sympathectomy will be of value.

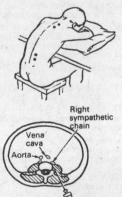

Right sympathetic chain

Vena cava

Aorta

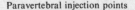

Paravertebral injection points

parenchyma (par-eng-kī'-má) [G. *para*, beside: *engchyma*, infusion]. The parts of an organ which, in contradistinction to its interstitial tissue, are concerned with its function parenchymal, parenchymatous, adj.

parenteral (par-en'-tĕr-al) [G. *para*, beyond; *enteron*, intestine]. Not via the alimentary tract.

paresis (par-ē'-sis) [G. a letting go]. Partial or slight paralysis; weakness of a limb—paretic, adj.

pareunia (par-ūn'-i-à) [G. *pareunos*, lying beside]. Coitus. See DYSPAREUNIA.

pargyline. A monoamine oxidase inhibitor.

parietal (par-ī'-et-al) [L. *paries*, an enveloping structure]. Pertaining to a wall. **parietal bones**, the two bones which form the sides and vault of the skull.

parity (par-i-ti) [L. *parere*, to bring forth]. Condition of a woman with regard to the number of children she has borne.

Parkinsonism. A syndrome of mask-like expression, shuffling gait, tremor of the limbs and pill-rolling movements of the fingers. Can be drug-induced. The post-encephalitic type comes on in the 30 to 40 age group and there may or may not be a clear history of encephalitis (sporadic type). Degenerative type of P. (paralysis agitans) comes on during middle life; arteriosclerotic type comes on in the elderly. Characterized by a distinctive clinical pattern of tremor and rigidity.

Parnate. Tranylcypromine. A monoamine oxidase inhibitor.

paromomycin (par-ōm-ō-mī'-sin). Only administered orally. Useful for temporary or long-term suppression of bowel flora; treatment of various forms of acute enteritis.

paronychia (par-on-ik'-i-à) [G. *para*, beside; *onyx*, nail]. A whitlow. Suppurative inflammation around a finger-nail. The virus of herpes simplex can cause multiple vesicles over inflamed skin—herpetic p.

parosmia (par-os'-mi-à) [G. *para*, beside; *osme*, smell]. Perverted sense of smell, usually of an hallucinatory nature.

parotidectomy (par-ot-id-ek'-to-mi) [G. *para*, beside; *ous*, ear; *ektome*, excision]. Excision of the parotid salivary gland.

parotid gland (par-o'-tid) [G. *para*, beside; *ous*, ear]. The salivary gland situated in front of and below the ear.

parotitis (par-ō-tī'-tis) [G. *para*, beside; *ous*, ear; *-itis*, inflammation]. Inflammation of parotid gland. **infectious (specific) p.**, mumps (q.v.). **septic p.**

refers to ascending infection from the mouth via the parotid duct, when a parotid abscess may result.

parous (par'-us) [L. *parere*, to bring forth]. Having borne a child or children.

paroxysm (par'-oks-izm) [G. *paroxysmos*, irritation]. A sudden, temporary attack.

paroxysmal (par-oks-iz'-mal). Coming on in attacks or paroxysms. **paroxysmal dyspnoea**, occurs mostly at night in patients with cardiac disease. **paroxysmal fibrillation** occurs in the atrium of the heart and is associated with a ventricular tachycardia and total irregularity of the pulse rhythm. **paroxysmal tachycardia** may result from ectopic impulses arising in the atrium or in the ventricle itself.

parrot disease. Psittacosis (q.v.).

Parrot's nodes. Bossing of frontal bones in the congenital syphilitic. [Joseph Parrot, French physician, 1829–83.]

Parstelin (pars'-tel-in). Tranylcypromine (q.v.) and trifluoperazine (q v)

parturient (pár-tūr'-i-ent) [L. *parturure*, to bring forth]. Pertaining to childbirth.

parturition (pár-tūr-i'-shun) [L. *parturire* to bring forth]. The act of bearing a child; labour.

PAS. Para-aminosalicyclic acid. See AMINOSALICYCLIC ACID.

Pasinah (pas'-in-à). Antitubercular drug.

passive (pas'iv). Inactive. Opp. active. **passive hyperaemia**, see HYPERAEMIA. **passive immunity**, see IMMUNITY. **passive movement**, performed by the physiotherapist, the patient being relaxed.

Pasteurella (pas-tūr-el'-là). A genus of bacteria. Short Gram-negative rods, staining more deeply at the poles (bipolar staining). Pathogenic in man and animals. *Pasteurella pestis* is the causative organism of classical plague. Currently preferred name is Yersinia. [Louis Pasteur, French scientist and bacteriologist, 1822–95.]

pasteurization (pas-tūr-īz-ā-shun). A process whereby pathogenic organisms in fluid (especially milk) are killed by heat. **flash method of p.** (H.T., S.T—high temperature, short time), the fluid is heated to 72°C, maintained at this temperature for 15 s, then rapidly cooled. **holder method of p.**, the fluid is heated to 63 to 65.5°C maintained at this temperature for 30 min then rapidly cooled. [Louis Pasteur, French scientist and bacteriologist, 1822–95.]

Patau's (13-15) syndrome. Autosomal trisomy. Closely associated with mental subnormality. Cells have 47 chromosomes.

patella (pat-el'-á) [L. small pan]. The knee-cap; a triangular, sesamoid bone—patellar, adj.; patellae, pl.

patellectomy (pat-el-ek'-to-mi) [L. *patella*, small pan G. *ektome*, excision]. Excision of the patella.

patent (pā'-tent) [L. *patens*, open]. Open; not closed or occluded. **patent ductus arteriosus**, failure of ductus arteriosus to close soon after birth, so that the abnormal shunt between the pulmonary artery and the aorta is preserved. **patent interventricular septum**, a congenital defect in the dividing wall between the right and left ventricle of the heart—patency, n.

pathogen (path'-o-jen) [G. *pathos*, disease; *genes*, producing]. A disease-producing agent, usually restricted to a living agent—pathogenic, adj.; pathogenicity, n.

pathogenesis (path-ō-jen'-e-sis) [G. *pathos*, disease; *genes*, producing]. The origin and development of disease—pathogenetic, adj.

pathogenicity (path-ō-jen-is'-i-ti). The capacity to produce disease.

pathognomonic (path-og-nō-mon'-ik) [G. *pathos*, disease; *gnomonikos*, skilled in one thing]. Characteristic of or peculiar to a disease.

pathology (path-ol'-o-ji) [G. *pathos*, disease; *logos*, discourse]. The science which deals with the cause and nature of disease—pathological, adj.; pathologically, adv.

pathophobia (path-ō-fō'-bi-á) [G. *pathos*, disease; *phobos*, fear]. A morbid dread of disease.

Patterson-Kelly syndrome. See PLUMMER-VINSON SYNDROME.

patulous (pat'-ū-lus) [L. *patulus*, standing open]. Opened out; expanded.

Paul-Mikulicz operation (pawl mik'-u-litsh). A method for excision of a portion of the colon whereby the two cut ends of the bowel are kept out on the surface of the abdomen, and are joined at a later date without entering the peritoneal cavity. The method was designed to lessen the risk of peritonitis from leakage at the suture line. [Frank Thomas Paul, English surgeon, 1851–1941. Johann von Mikulicz-Rad-

ecki, Rumanian surgeon (in Poland), 1850–1905.]

Paul's tube. A flanged glass tube used to collect the contents after the bowel has been opened on the surface of the abdomen. [Frank Thomas Paul, English surgeon, 1851–1941.]

Pavulon (pav'-ū-lon). Pancuronium bromide (q.v.).

Pawlik's grip. A method of determining the engagement or otherwise of the fetal head in the maternal pelvic brim. [Karel Pawlik, Czechoslovakian surgeon, 1849–1914.]

PBI (protein bound iodine). Iodine combined with protein as part of the thyroid hormone. Low in thyroid deficiency.

Pearson bed. A special type of hospital bed used for fractures. It is higher and narrower than the usual type. Instead of springs there are tight strips of webbing. The mattress is in three or four sections. A Balkan beam is attached to the bed frame.

peau d'orange (pō-dor-ongzh') [F.]. Term applied to the appearance of the skin over the breast in acute inflammation or in advanced carcinoma, when lymphoedema causes the orifices of the hair follicles to appear as dimples, resembling the pits in the skin of an orange.

pecazine (pek'-a-zēn). A phenothiazine derivative very similar to chlorpromazine, and with similar therapeutic applications.

pectoral (pek'-tor-al) [L. *pectoralis*, of the breast]. Pertaining to the breast.

pectus (pek'-tus) [L.]. The chest. **pectus carinatum**, pigeon chest. **pectus excavatum**, funnel chest.

pedal (ped'-al) [L. *pes*, foot]. Pertaining to the foot.

pedascope (ped'-a-skōp). Allows shoe fitting under fluoroscopy.

pediatrician. See PAEDIATRICIAN.

pediatrics. See PAEDIATRICS.

pedicle (ped'-ik-l) [L. *pediculus*, little foot]. A stalk, e.g. the narrow part by which a tumour is attached to the surrounding structures.

pediculosis (ped-ik-ū-lō'-sis) [L. *pediculus*, little foot; G. *-osis*, condition]. Infestation with lice (pediculi).

Pediculus (ped-ik'-ū-lus) [L.]. A genus of parasitic insects (lice) important as vectors of disease. *Pediculus capitis,* the head louse. *Pediculus corporis,* the body louse. *Pediculus* (more correctly, *Phthirius*) *pubis,* the pubic louse.

ped-o-jet. Apparatus for introduction of vaccines under pressure into the skin. Avoids the use of a needle with consequent danger of spreading serum hepatitis.

pedopompholyx (pē-dō-pom'-fo-liks). See CHEIROPOMPHOLYX.

peduncle (ped-ungk'-l) [L. *pedunculus,* little foot]. A stalk-like structure, often acting as a support—peduncular, pedunculated, adj.

peeling. Desquamation (q.v.).

Peganone (peg'-a-nōn). Ethotoin (q.v.).

Pel-Ebstein fever. Recurring bouts of pyrexia in regular subsequence found in lymphadenoma (Hodgkin's disease). Less frequent manifestation with improving treatment. [Pieter Klazes Pel, Dutch physician, 1852–1919. Wilhelm Ebstein, German physician, 1836–1912.]

Pelizaeus-Merzbacher disease. Genetically determined degenerative disease associated with mental subnormality. [Friedrich Pelizaeus, German neurologist, 1850– . Ludwig Merzbacher, German physician in Argentina, 1875–].

pellagra (pel-a'-grá) A deficiency disease caused by lack of vitamin B complex and protein. Syndrome includes glossitis, dermatitis, peripheral neuritis and spinal cord changes (even producing ataxia), anaemia and mental confusion.

pellet (pel'-et) [L. *pila,* ball]. A little pill. See IMPLANT.

pelvic floor repair. See FOTHERGILL'S OPERATION.

pelvimeter (pel-vim'-et-ér) [L. *pelvis,* basin; G. *metron,* a measure]. An instrument especially devised to measure the pelvic diameters.

pelvimetry (pel-vim'-et-ri) [L. *pelvis,* basin; G. *metron,* a measure]. The measurement of the dimensions of the pelvis.

pelvis (pel'-vis) [L.]. 1. A basin-shaped cavity, e.g. pelvis of the kidney. 2. The large bony basin-shaped cavity formed by the innominate bones and sacrum, containing and protecting the bladder, rectum and organs of generation. **contracted p.,** one in which one or more diameters are smaller than normal and

this may result in difficulties in childbirth. **false p.,** the wide expanded part of the pelvis above the brim. **true p.,** that part of the pelvis below the brim—pelvic, adj.; pelves, pl.

pemphigoid (pem'-fi-goid) [G. *pemphix,* pustule]. Allied to pemphigus. A bullous eruption in the latter half of life. Of unknown cause. Histological examination of the base of a blister differentiates it from pemphigus.

pemphigus (pem'-fig-us) [G. *pemphix,* pustule]. Skin conditions with bullous (blister) eruptions, but more correctly used of a group of dangerous diseases called 'p. vulgaris,' 'p. vegetans' and 'p. erythematosus'. The latter two are rare. **pemphigus neonatorum;** (1) a dangerous form of impetigo occurring as an epidemic in the hospital nursery; (2) bullous eruption in congenital syphilis of the newborn. **pemphigus vulgaris** is a bullous disease of middle-age and later, of unknown aetiology. Oedema of the skin results in blister formation in the epidermis, with resulting secondary infection and rupture, so that large raw areas develop. Bullae develop also on mucous membranes. Death is from malnutrition or intercurrent disease.

pempidine (pem'-pi-dēn). A blocking agent used for the treatment of hypertension. It is active orally and the response is reliable and consistent in effect. Side effects are fewer than those experienced with other drugs of this type.

Penbritin. Ampicillin (q.v.).

pendulous (pen'-dū-lus) [L. *pendere,* to hang]. Hanging down.

penethamate hydriodide (pe-nē-tham'-āt hīd ri ō-dīd). An iodine-containing form of penicillin. Said to be absorbed by lung tissue, and is therefore used in respiratory infections.

penicillamine (pen-i-sil'-a-mēn). A degradation product of penicillin used in the treatment of heavy mental intoxication, Wilson's disease, lead poisoning, cystinuria and rheumatoid arthritis.

penicillin (pen-i-sil'-in). The first antibiotic, also known as 'p. G' or 'benzyl p.' Widely used by injection in many infections due to Gram-positive bacteria, some cocci, and spirochaetes. High blood levels are obtained rapidly, and can be supplemented by injections of the slower acting procaine-p. **fortified p.** is a mixture of p. G and procaine-p. p. V is an orally active form, as ordinary p. is rapidly destroyed by the gastric juice. The dose of penicillin varies widely according to the severity of infection, the largest being given in bacterial endocarditis (2 000 000 units).

penicillinase (pen-i-sil'-in-āz). An enzyme which destroys penicillin.

Penicillium (pe-ni-sil'-i-um) [L. *penicillus,* brush]. A genus of moulds. The hyphae bear spores characteristically arranged like a brush. Common contaminant of food. *Penicillium chrysogenum* is now used for the commercial production of the antibiotic. *P. notatum* is a species shown by Fleming (1928) to produce penicillin.

Penidural (pen-i-dū'-ral). Benzathine penicillin.

penis (pē'-nis) [L.]. The male organ of copulation—penile, adj.

Penofome (pen'-ō-fōm). Mild detergent for therapeutic application to the skin and vagina.

Penotrane (pen'-ō-trān). Effective against Candida and pyogenic organisms.

pentaerythrityl tetranitrate. Coronary vasodilator in tablet form.

Pentacynium (pen-ta-sin'-i-um). Ganglion blocking agent. Anti-hypertensive.

pentagastrin (pen-ta-gas'-trin). A synthetic hormone which has largely replaced older drugs as the stimulant of choice for evoking maximal acid secretion.

pentamidine (pen-tam'-i-dēn). Synthetic compound used in trypanosomiasis, kala-azar and leishmaniasis. Has also been used in moniliasis.

pentazocine (pen-taz'-o-sēn). Relief of severe pain in the presence of bradycardia or hypertension pentazocine is better than morphine. Can be given orally, intramuscularly, intravenously.

Penthrane (pen'-thrān). Methoxyflurane (q.v.).

pentobarbitone (pen-tō-bàr'-bit-ōn). One of the short-acting barbiturates. Often used for premedication in children.

pentolinium (pen-tō-lin'-i-um). A ganglionic blocking agent used in hypertension; active orally. Can be given by injection.

pentose (pen'-tōs). A class of monosaccharides with five carbon atoms in their molecule.

pentosuria (pen-tos-ū'-ri-á). [G. *pente,* five; *ouron,* urine]. Pentose in the urine. Can be due to a metabolic disorder—pentosuric, adj.

Pentothal (pen'-tō-thal). Thiopentone (q.v.).

peppermint (pep'-ér-mint). An aromatic carminative and stimulant. Also used as a flavouring agent.

pepsin (pep'-sin). A proteolytic enzyme of the gastric juice.

pepsinogen (pep-sin'-ō-jen). Secreted by the peptic cells in the gastric mucosa and converted into pepsin by contact with hydrochloric acid.

peptic (pep'-tik) [G. *peptikos,* helping digestion]. Pertaining to pepsin or to digestion generally. **peptic ulcer,** a nonmalignant ulcer in those parts of the digestive tract which are exposed to the gastric secretions; hence usually in stomach or duodenum.

peptides (pep'-tīdz). Chemical combinations of one or more amino acids, i.e. dipeptides, tripeptides or polypeptides.

peptone (pep'-tōn). Substance produced when the enzyme pepsin acts upon the acid metaproteins produced in the first stage of digestion of proteins.

peptonuria (pep-tōn-ū'-ri-á). [G. *peptos,* cooked; *ouron,* urine]. Peptones in the urine.

percept (pēr'-sept). The mental product of a sensation; a sensation plus memories of similar sensations and their relationships.

perception (pér-sep'-shun) [L. *perceptio*]. The reception of a conscious impression through the senses by which we distinguish objects one from another and recognize their qualities according to the different sensations they produce.

percolation (pér-kō-lā'-shun) [L. *percolare,* to strain through]. The process by which fluid slowly passes through a hard but porous substance.

Percorten (per-kor'-ten). De-oxycortone (q.v.).

percussion (pér-kush'-un) [L. *percussio,* a striking]. Tapping to determine the resonance or dullness of the area examined. Normally a finger of the left hand is laid on the patient's skin and the middle finger of the right hand (plexor) is used to strike the left finger.

percutaneous (pér-kū-tā'-nē-us) [L. *per,* through; *cutis,* skin]. Through unbroken skin. See CHOLANGIOGRAPHY.

perforation (pêr-forā'-shun) [L. *perforare*, to pierce through]. A hole in an intact sheet of tissue. Used in reference to p. of the tympanic membrane, or the wall of the stomach or gut, constituting a surgical emergency.

perhexiline (per-heks'-ī-lēn). Antianginal drug. Coronary vasodilator.

periadenitis (per-i-ad-en-ī'-tis) [G. *peri*, around; *aden*, gland; *-itis*, inflammation]. Inflammation in soft tissues surrounding glands. Responsible for the 'bull' neck in German measles.

perianal (per-i-ān'-al) [G. *peri*, around; L. *anus*, anus]. Surrounding the anus.

periarterial (per-i-árt-ē'-rial) [G. *peri*, around; *arteria*, artery]. Surrounding an artery.

periarteritis (per-i-árt-e-rī'-tis) [G. *peri*, around; *arteria*, artery; *-itis*, inflammation]. Inflammation of the outer sheath of an artery and the periarterial tissue. **periarteritis nodosa.** see COLLAGEN and POLYARTERITIS.

periarthritis (per-i-árth-rī'-tis) [G. *peri*, around; *arthron*, joint; *-itis*, inflammation]. Inflammation of the structures surrounding a joint. Sometimes applied to frozen shoulder (q.v.).

periarticular (per-i-árt-ik'-ū-lar) [G.*peri*, around; L. *articulus*, joint]. Surrounding a joint.

pericardectomy (per-i-kárd-ek'-to-mi) [G.*peri*, around; *kardia*, heart; *ektome*, excision]. Surgical removal of pericardium, thickened from chronic inflammation and embarrassing the heart's action.

pericardiocentesis (per-i-kar-di-ō-sentē'-sis) [G. *peri*, around; *kardia*, heart; *kentesis*, puncture]. The withdrawal of fluid from the pericardial sac by insertion of a hollow needle or cannula.

pericarditis (per-i-kár-dī'-tis) [G. *peri*, around; *kardia*, heart; *-itis*, inflammation]. Inflammation of the outer, serous covering the heart. It may or may not be accompanied by an effusion and formation of adhesions between the two layers. See BROADBENT'S SIGN and PERICARDECTOMY.

pericardium (per-i-kárd'-i-um). The double membranous sac which envelops the heart. The layer in contact with the heart is called 'visceral'; that reflected to from the sac is called 'parietal'. Between the two is the pericardial cavity, which normally contains a small amount of serous fluid—pericardial, adj.

perichondrium (per-i-kond'-ri-um) [G. *peri*, around; *chondros*, cartilage]. The membranous covering of cartilage— perichondrial, adj.

pericolic (per-i-kol'-ik) [G. *peri*, around; *kolikos*, suffering in the colon]. Around the colon.

pericranium (per-i-krān'-i-um) [G. *peri*, around; *kranion*, skull]. The periosteal covering of the cranium—pericranial, adj.

pericyazine (per-i-sī'-a-zēn). Phenothiazine derivative; much stronger than chlorpromazine.

perifollicular (per-i-fol-ik'-ū-lar) [G. *peri*, around; L. *folliculus*, small sac]. Around a follicle.

perilymph (per-i-limf) [G. *peri*, around; L. *lympha*, water]. The fluid contained in the internal ear, between the bony and membranous labyrinth.

perimetrium (per-i-mēt'-ri-um) [G. *peri*, around; *metra*, womb]. The peritoneal covering of the uterus—perimetrial, adj.

perinatal (per-i-nā'-tal) [G. *peri*, around; L. *natus*, birth]. Occurring at, or pertaining to, the time of birth.

perineorrhaphy (per-i-nē-or'-raf-i) [G. *perineos*, space between anus and scrotum]. The operation for the repair of a torn perineum.

perineotomy. Episiotomy (q.v.).

perinephric (per-i-nef'-rik) [G. *peri*, around; *nephros*, kidney]. Surrounding the kidney.

perineum (per-i-nē'-um) [G. *perineos*, space between anus and scrotum]. The portion of the body included in the outlet of the pelvis—perineal, adj.

perionychia (per-i-ōn-ik-i-a) [G. *peri*, around; *onyx*, nail]. Red and painful swelling around nail fold. Common in hands that are much in water or have poor circulation. Due to infection from the fungus Candida, more common now because of the use of antibiotics which subdue organisms which previously curtailed the activity of Candida. Secondary infection can occur.

periosteum (per-i-ost'-i-um). The membrane which covers a bone. In long bones only the shaft as far as the epiphysis is covered. It is protective and essential for regeneration—periosteal, adj.

periostitis (per-i-os-tī'-tis), **periosteitis** [G. *periosteos*, around bone; *-itis*, inflammation]. Inflammation of the periosteum. **periostitis diffuse,** that involving the periosteum of long bones. **periostitis haemorrhagic,** that accompanied by bleeding between the periosteum and the bone.

periostosis (per-i-os-tō'-sis) [G. *periosteos*, around bone; *-osis*, condition]. Inflammatory hypertrophy of bone.

periportal (per-i-por'-tal) [G. *peri*, around; L. *portia*, gate]. Surrounding the portal vein.

periproctitis (per-i-prok-tī'-tis) [G. *peri*, around; *proktos*, anus; *-itis*, inflammation]. Inflammation around the rectum and anus.

perirenal (per-i-rēn'-al) [G. *peri*, around; L. *renes*, kidneys]. Around the kidney.

perisplenitis (per-i-splen-ī'-tis) [G. *peri*, around; *splen*, spleen; *-itis*, inflammation]. Inflammation of the peritoneal coat of the spleen and of the adjacent structures.

peristalsis (per-i-stal'-sis) [G. *peri*, around; *stellein*, to draw in]. The characteristic movement of the intestines by which the contents are moved along the lumen. It consists of a wave of contraction preceded by a wave of relaxation—peristaltic, adj.

peritomy (per-it'-o-mi) [G. *peri*, around; *tome*, a cutting]. Excision of a portion of conjunctiva at the edge of cornea to prevent vascularization of a corneal ulcer.

peritoneoscopy (per-it-on-ē-os'-ko-pi) [G. *peri*, around; *teinein*, to stretch; *skopein*, to examine]. Laparoscopy (q.v.).

peritoneum (per-i-to-nē'-um) [G. *peri*, around; *teinein*, to stretch]. The delicate serous membrane which lines the abdominal and pelvic cavities and also covers the organs contained in them—peritoneal, adj.

peritonitis (per-i-ton-ī'-tis) [G. *peri*, around; *teinein*, to stretch; *-itis*, inflammation]. Inflammation of the peritoneum, usually secondary to disease of one of the abdominal organs.

peritonsillar abscess. Quinsy (q.v.).

peritrichous (per-i-trī'-kus) [G. *peri*, around; *thrix*, hair]. Applied to bacteria which possess flagella on all sides of the cell. See BACILLUS.

periumbilical (per-i-um-bil-īk'-al) [G. *peri*, around; L. *umbilicus*, middle]. Surrounding the umbilicus.

periurethral (per-i-ū-rē'-thral) [G. *peri*, around; *ourethra*, urethra]. Surrounding the urethra, as a p.u. abscess.

perivascular (per-i-vas'-kū-lar) [G. *peri*, around; L. *vasculum*, vessel]. Around a blood vessel.

perlèche (per-lesh') Lip licking. An intertrigo at the angles of the mouth with maceration, fissuring, or crust formation. May result from use of poorly fitting dentures, bacterial infection, thrush infestation, vitamin deficiency, drooling or thumb-sucking.

permeability (per-mē-a-bil'-it-i) [L. *permeabilis*, that can be passed through]. In physiology, the ability of cell membranes to allow salts, glucose, urea and other soluble substances to pass into and out of the cells from the body fluids.

pernicious (per-nish'-us) [L. *perniciosus*, destructive]. Deadly, noxious.

pernicious anaemia. Results from the inability of the bone marrow to produce normal red cells because of the deprivation of a protein released by gastric glands, previously called the intrinsic factor which is necessary for the absorption of vitamin B_{12}. An autoimmune mechanism may be responsible.

perniosis (per-ni-ō'-sis) [L. *chilblain*]. Chronic chilblains. The smaller arterioles go into spasm readily from exposure to cold.

Peroidin (per-ō'-i-din). Potassium perchlorate (q.v.).

Perolysen (per-ō-lī'-sen). Pempidine (q.v.).

peromelia (per-ō-mē'-li-á) [G. *peros*, maimed; *melos*, limb]. Teratogenic malformation of a limb.

peroral (per-or'-al) [L. *per*, through; *os*, mouth]. Through the mouth, as p. biopsy of the small bowel.

peroxide. See HYDROGEN.

perphenzine (per-fen'-a-zēn). Antiemetic and tranquillizing agent.

perseveration (per-sev-er-ā'-shun) [L. *perseverare*, to persist]. A mental symptom consisting of an apparent inability for the patient's mind to detach itself from one idea to another with normal speed. Thus shown a picture of a cow, the patient repeats 'cow' when shown further pictures of different objects. Common in senile dementia, schizophrenia.

personality (per-son-al'-i-ti) [L. *personalis*, of a person]. The various mental attitudes and characteristics which distinguish a person. The sum total of the mental make-up. **psychopathic p.**, a persistent disorder or disability of mind (whether or not including subnormality of intelligence) which results in abnormally aggressive or seriously irresponsible conduct that requires, or is susceptible to, medical treatment.

perspiration (pėr-spi-rā′-shun) [L. *per*, through; *spirare*, to breathe]. The excretion of the sweat glands through the skin pores. **insensible p.**, invisible, the perspiration is evaporated immediately it reaches the skin surface. **sensible p.**, visible drops of sweat on the skin.

Perthes' disease (Legg-Perthes-Calvé's disease). Syn., pseudocoxalgia. A vascular degeneration of the upper femoral epiphysis; revascularization occurs, but residual deformity of the femoral head may subsequently lead to arthritic changes. [Georg Clemens Perthes, German surgeon, 1869–1927.]

Pertofran. Desipramine. See ANTIPRESSANT

pertussis (pėr-tus′-ls). Whooping cough. An infectious disease of children with attacks of coughing which reach a peak of violence ending in an inspiratory whoop. The basis of the condition is respiratory catarrh and the organism responsible is *Bordetella pertussis*. Prophylactic vaccination is responsible for a decrease in case incidence.

pes [L.]. A foot or foot-like structure. **pes cavus**, 'hollow' foot when the longitudinal arch of the foot is accentuated. Claw-foot is accentuated. Claw-foot. **pes planus**, valgus-foot, flat-foot.

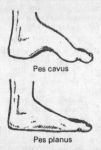

Pes cavus

Pes planus

pessary (pes′-a-ri) [L. *pessarium*]. 1. An instrument inserted into the vagina to correct uterine displacements. A ring or shelf p. is used to support a prolapse. A Hodge p. is used to correct a retroversion. 2. A medicated suppository used to treat vaginal infections, or as a contraceptive.

pesticides (pes-ti-sīdz). Substances which kill pests.

petechia (pe-tē′-ki-á). A small, haemorrhagic spot—petechiae, pl., petechial, adj.

pethidine (peth′-i-din). Synthetic analgesic and spasmolytic. Widely used for both pre-operative and postoperative analgesia instead of morphine. Can be given orally, intramuscularly or intravenously.

Pethilorfan (peth-il-or′-fan). Pethidine and levallorphan tartrate, a narcotic antagonist that reduces respiratory depression without affecting analgesia.

petit mal (pet′-ė mal). Minor epilepsy (q.v.). Momentary loss of consciousness is characteristic.

petrous (pē′-trus) [G. *petros*, stone]. Resembling stone.

Peyer's patches (pī′-ers). Flat patches of lymphatic tissue situated in the small intestine but mainly in the ileum; they are the seat of infection in typhoid fever; also known as 'aggregated lymph nodules.' [Johann Conrad Peyer, Swiss anatomist, 1653–1712.]

Peyronie's disease. Deformity and painful erection of penis due to fibrous tissue formation from unknown cause. Often associated with Dupuytren's contracture. [François de la Peyronie, French surgeon, 1678–1747.]

pH. The concentration of hydrogen ions expressed as a logarithm. A neutral solution has a pH 7.0. With increasing acidity the pH falls and with increasing alkalinity it rises.

phaeochromocytoma (fē-ō-krō-mō-sī-tō′-má). A condition in which there is a tumour of the adrenal medulla, or of the structurally similar tissues associated with the sympathetic chain. It secretes adrenaline and allied hormones and the symptoms are due to the excess of these substances. Aetiology unknown. See TEST: ROGITINE.

phagocyte (fag′-ō-sit) [G. *phagein*, to eat; *kytos*, cell]. A cell capable of engulfing other cells and debris in the tissues—phagocytic, adj.

phagocytosis (fag-ō-sī-tō′-sis) [G. *phagein*, to eat; *kytos*, cell; -*osis*, condition]. The engulfment by phagocytes of foreign or other particles, or cells harmful to the body.

phako-emulsification (fā-kō-ēm-uls-i-fik-ā'-shun). Ultrasonic vibration is used to liquefy mature lens fibres. The liquid lens matter is then sucked out in an action similar to that of a vacuum cleaner.

phalanges (fal-an'jēz). The small bones of the fingers and toes—phalanx, sing; phalangeal, adj.

phallus (fal'-us) [G.*phallos*]. The penis—phallic, adj.

phanquone (fan'-qwōn). Antidysentery drug.

phantasy. See FANTASY.

pharmaceutical (far-ma-sū'-tik-al) [G. *pharmakeutikos*]. Relating to drugs.

pharmacogenetic (far-ma-kō'-jen-et'-ik) [G.*pharmakon*, drug; *genesis*, descent]. Produced by drugs, usually referring to side effects.

pharmacology (far-ma-kol'-o-ji) [G. *pharmakon*, drug; *logos*, discourse]. The science dealing with drugs.

pharyngectomy (far-in-jek'-to-mi) [G. *pharygx*, ,pharynx; *ektome*, excision]. Removal of part of the pharynx.

pharyngismus (far-in-jis'-mus). Spasm of the pharynx.

pharyngitis (far-in-jī'-tis) [G. *pharygx*, pharynx; *-itis*, inflammation]. Inflammation of the pharynx.

pharyngolaryngeal (far-ing'-gō-lar-in-jē'-al) [G. *pharygx*, pharynx; *larygx*, larynx]. Pertaining to the pharynx and larynx.

pharyngolaryngectomy (far-ing-gō-lar-in-jek'-to-mi) [G. *pharygx*, pharynx; *larygx*, larynx; *tome*, a cutting). Surgical removal of the pharynx and larynx.

pharyngoplasty (far-ing'-go-plas-ti) [G. *pharygx*;*plassein*, to form]. Any plastic operation to the pharynx.

pharyngotomy (far-in-got'-o-mi) [G. *pharygx*, pharynx; *tome*, a cutting]. The operation of opening into the pharynx.

pharyngotympanic tube (far-ing'-gō-tim-pan'-ik). See EUSTACHIAN TUBE.

pharynx (far'-ingks) [G. *pharygx*]. The cavity at the back of the mouth. It is cone shaped, varies in length (average 76 mm), and is lined with mucous membrane; at the lower end it opens into the oesophagus. The Eustachian tubes pierce its lateral walls and the posterior nares pierce its anterior wall. The larynx lies immediately below it and in front of the oesophagus—pharyngeal, adj.

phemitone (fem'-i-ton). Barbiturate very similar to phenobarbitone, but with greater anticonvulsant action. Used in epilepsy.

phenacemide (fen-as'-ē-mīd). Anticonvulsant useful in temporal lobe epilepsy.

phenacetin (fen-as'-et-in). Analgesic of great usefulness and low toxicity.Constituent of many analgesic preparations.

phenadoxone (fen-a-doks'-ōn). Analgesic with considerable spasmolytic action, useful in severe pain. Can be given orally or intramuscularly.

phenazone (fen'-a-zōn). An analgesic resembling phenacetin in effect, but is more toxic. Soluble in water.

phenazocine (fen-az'-o-sēn). Potent analgesic for severe acute or chronic pain.

phenazopyridine hydrochloride (fen-az-ō-pir'-i-dēn). Urinary tract sedative, especially useful in cystitis.

phenelzine (fen'-el-zēn). Antidepressant drug; a monoamine oxide inhibitor.

Phenergan (fen'-er-gan). Promethazine (q.v.).

phenethicillin (fen-eth-i-sil'-in). Acid stable and can be given by mouth. Alternative to penicillin but contraindicated in penicillin sensitivity.

pheneturide (fen-et-ūr'-īd). Used in major epilepsy, especially of temporal lobe type.

phenformin (fen'-for-min). Antidiabetic agent. One of the diaguanides. Said to reduce weight and blood cholesterol thus possibly preventing blood vessel complications. Has an insulin-like action, stimulates the uptake of glucose by cells.

phenindamine (fen-ind-ā'-mēn). An antihistamine free from sedative side effects.

phenindione (fen-in-dī'-on). An orally active anticoagulant with an intermediate action. Widely used in thromboembolic disorders, often after initial heparin therapy. Maintenance doses regulated according to prothrombin time.

pheniodol (fen-ī'-o-dol). An iodine compound used as a contrast agent in cholecystography.

phenmetrazine hydrochloride (fen-met'-rā-zēn-hī-drō-klor'-īd).   Appetite depressant. Danger of addiction and psychosis of a paranoid nature.

pheniprazine (fen-ip'-rá-zēn). A monoamine oxidase inhibitor.

phenobarbitone (fē-nō-bár'-bit-ōn). Long-acting barbiturate and anticonvulsant. Used as general sedative, and in epilepsy.

phenol (fē'-nol). Carbolic acid. Powerful antiseptic, widely used as a 1 in 20 solution. Weaker solutions occasionally used for application. Strong solutions are caustic—phenolic, adj.

phenolphthalein (fēn-olf-tha'-lē-in). Powerful non-toxic purgative, often given with liquid paraffin.

phenoperidine. Powerful analgesic that is a respiratory centre depressant. Useful where breathing is controlled by mechanical ventilation.

phenothiazines (fen-ō-thī'-a-zēns). Tranquillizing compounds. Chlorpromazine and promazine belong to this group.

phenoxybenzamine (fen-oks-i-ben'-za-min). Peripheral vasodilator used in Raynaud's disease and as an antihypertensive agent.

phenoxymethylpenicillin (fen-oks-i-meth'-il-pen-i-sil-in). Oral penicillin (q v.)

phenoxypropazine. A monoamine oxidase inhibitor.

phensuximide (fen-suks'-i-mīd). For petit mal.

phentolamine (fen-tol-a'-mēn) An adrenaline antagonist, used mainly by injection in the diagnosis and surgery of phaeochromocytoma, to control excessive variation of blood pressure. Occasionally used orally in vasospasm.

Phenurone (fen'-ū-rōn). Phenylacetylurea (q.v.).

phenylacetylurea (fen'-īl-as-et'-īl-ur-ē'-a). A powerful but toxic anticonvulsant. Used in epilepsy resistant to other therapy.

phenylalanine (fē-nīl'-āl-a-nin). An essential amino acid associated with thyroxine and adrenaline, **phenylalanine mustard (PAM)**, cytotoxic, alkylating agent.

phenylbutazone (fen-īl-bū'-ta-zōn). Analgesic with powerful and prolonged action. Used mainly in rheumatic disorders. Toxic reactions are common and minimum maintenance doses are essential. Occasionally causes salivary gland enlargement.

phenylephrine (fēn-īl-ef'-rin). Vasoconstrictor and pressor drug similar to adrenaline, but more stable. Phenylephrine administrated simultaneously with isoprenaline appreciably reduces the effect on blood pressure and heart rate of isoprenaline alone. Can be given intramuscularly or subcutaneously. Used as eyedrops (0.5 to 10 per cent) and as nasal spray (0.25 per cent).

phenylethylacetylurea (fen'-īl-eth'-īl-as-et'-īl-ur-ē'-a). See PHENYLACETYLUREA.

phenylketonuria (fē-nīl-kē-tōn-ūr'-i-á) Metabolites of phenylalanine (the best known being the phenylketones) in urine. Occurs in hyperphenylalaninaemia, owing to the lack of inactivity of the phenylalanine hydroxylase enzyme in the liver which converts dietary phenylalanine into tyrosine. Autosomal recessive disease, resulting in mental subnormality—phenylketonuric, adj.

phenylpyruvic oligophrenia (fē-nil-pī-rū'-vik ol-ig-ō-frē' nī á). See PHENYLKETONURIA.

phenytoin (fen'-i-toin). Anticonvulsant used in grand mal epilepsy, sometimes in association with phenobarbitone.

phimosis (fī-mō'-sis) [G.]. Tightness of the prepuce so that it cannot be retracted over the glans penis.

pHisoHex (fī'-sō-heks). Antiseptic and antibacterial skin cleansing agent combining a detergent—Entsufon, 3 per cent hexachlorophane, lanolin, cholesterols and petrolatum, in an emulsion with the same pH as skin.

phlebectomy (flē-bek'-to-mi). [G. *phleps*, vein; *ektome*, excision]. Excision of a vein. **multiple cosmetic p.**, (MCP), removal of varicose veins through little stab incisions which heal without scarring.

phlebitis (flē-bi'-tis) [G. *phleps*, vein; *-itis*, inflammation]. Inflammation of a vein—phlebitic, adj.

phlebogram (flē'-bō-gram) [G. *phleps*, vein; *gramma*, letter]. See VENOGRAM.

phlebography (flē-bog'-ra-fi). See VENOGRAPHY.

phlebolith (flē'-bō-lith) [G. *phelps*, vein; *lithos*, stone]. A concretion which forms in a vein.

phlebothrombosis (flē-bō-throm-bō'-sis) [G. *phleps*, vein; *thrombosis*, curdling]. Thrombosis in a vein due to sluggish flow of blood rather than to inflammation in the vein wall, occurring chiefly in bedridden patients and affecting the deep veins of the lower limbs or pelvis. The loosely attached thrombus is liable to break off and lodge in the lungs as an embolus.

phlebotomy (flē-bot'-o-mi). Venesection (q.v.).

phlegm (flem) [G. *phlegma*]. The secretion of mucus expectorated from the bronchi.

phlegmatic (fleg-mat'-ik). Emotionally stable. Not easily excited.

phlyctenule (flik-ten'-ūl) [G.*phlyktaina*, blister]. A minute blister (vesicle) usually occuring on the conjunctiva or cornea—phlyctenular, adj.

phobia (fō'-bi-à) [G.*phobos*, fear]. Morbid fear, e.g. cardiac p., fear of heart disease, cancer p., etc.—phobic, adj.

phocomelia (fō-kō-mē'-li-à) [G.*phoke*, a seal; *melos*, limb]. Teratogenic malformation. Arms and feet attached directly to trunk giving a seal-like appearance.

pholcodine (fol'-ko-dēn). Cough centre depressant similar to codeine. Useful in unproductive cough, and is well tolerated.

phonocardiogram (fō-nō-kàr'-di-ō-gram) [G. *phone*, voice; *kardia*, heart; *gramma*, letter]. A graphic record of heart sounds.

phonocardiography (fō-nō-kàr-di-og'-ra-fi)[G. *phone*, voice; *kardia*, heart; *graphein*, to write]. The graphic recording of heart sounds and murmurs by electric reproduction. The fetal heart rate and its relation to uterine contraction can be measured continuously—phonocardiographic adj.; phonocardiographically, adv.

phosphaturia (fos-fa-tū'-ri-à) [G. *phosphoros*, light-bringer; *ouron*, urine]. Excess of phosphates in the urine—phosphaturic, adj.

phospholine iodide (fos'-fō-līn ī'-ō-dīd). Anticholinesterase drug; powerful miotic.

phosphonates (fos'-fon-āts). Chemical; when deposited in bone makes it harder for osteoclasts to reabsorb that bone. Being tried for Paget's disease.

phosphonecrosis (fos-fō-nē-krō'-sis). 'Fossy-jaw' occurring in workers engaged in the manufacture of matches made with white phosphorus: necrosis of the jaw with loosening of the teeth.

phosphorus (fos'-for-us). A non-metallic element forming an important constituent of bone and nerve tissue. Radioactive p. used in treatment of thrombocythaemia.

photalgia (fō-tal'-ji-à) [G. *phos*, light; *algos*, pain]. Pain in the eyes from exposure to intense light.

photochemical (fō-tō-kem'-ik-al). Chemical changes brought about by light.

photocoagulation (fō-tō-kō-ag-ū-lā'-shun). See LASER BEAM.

photo-endoscope (fō-tō-end'-ō-skōp). An endoscope to which a camera is attached for the purpose of making a permanent record—photoendoscopy, n.; photoendoscopic, adj.; photoendoscopically, adv.

photophia (fō-tō-fō'-bi-à) [G. *phos*, light; *phobia*, fear]. Inability to expose the eyes to light—photophobic, adj.

photosensitive (fō-tō-sen'-sit-iv). Sensitive to light as the pigments in the eye.

phototherapy (fō-tō-ther'-à-pi) [G.*phos*, light; *therapeia*, treatment]. Exposure to artificial blue light. In hyperbilirubinaemia it appears to dehydrogenate the bilirubin to biliverdin. Used for mild neonatal jaundice and to prevent jaundice in premature infants.

phren (fren) [G. midriff]. The diaphragm—phrenic, adj.

phrenic avulsion. See AVULSION.

phrenicotomy (fre-ni-ko'-to-mi) [G. *phren*, midriff; *tome*, cutting]. Division of the phrenic nerve to paralyse one-half of the diaphragm

phrenoplegia (fren-ō-plē'-ji-à) [G.*phren*, midriff; *plege*, stroke]. Paralysis of the diaphragm.

phrenotropic (fren-ō-trō'-pik). Having an effect upon the mind.

phthalylsulphathiazole (thā-līl-sul-fa-thī'-a-zol). A sulphonamide poorly absorbed from the alimentary tract, hence useful in intestinal infections, and before abdominal surgery.

phthisis (thī'-sis). Old term for pulmonary tuberculosis.

Physeptone (fī-sep'-tōn). Methadone (q.v.).

physicochemical (fiz-i-kō-kem'-ik-al). Pertaining to physics and chemistry.

physiological (fiz-i-ō-loj'-ik-al). In accordance with natural processes of the body. Adjective often used to describe a normal process or structure, to distinguish it from an abnormal or pathological feature (e.g. the p. level of glucose in the blood is from 3.0 to 5.0 mmol per litre; higher and lower levels are pathological and indicative of disease). **physiological saline** (normal or isotonic), a 0.9 per cent solution of sodium chloride in water. **physiological solution**, a fluid isotonic with the body fluids and containing similar salts.

physiology (fiz-i-ol'-o-ji). The science which deals with the normal functions of the body.

physostigmine (fi-so-stig'-min). An alkaloid used in glaucoma as drops (0.25 to 1 per cent) and to reverse the action of atropine. Occasionally used in paralytic ileus.

phytomenadione. Intravenous vitamin K.

phytomitogens (fīt-ō-mīt'-ō-jens). Agents that appear to enhance immunity in vitro, and perhaps in vivo.

pia or **pia mater** (pē-a mā'-ter). The innermost of the meninges; the vascular membrane which lies in close contact with the substance of the brain and spinal cord.

pica (pī'-ká) [L. magpie]. Desire for extraordinary articles of food.

Pick's disease. 1. Syndrome of ascites, hepatic enlargement, oedema, and pleural effusion occurring in constrictive pericarditis. [Friedel Pick, German physician, 1867–1926.]. 2. A type of cerebral atrophy which produces mental changes similar to senescence (q.v.). [Arnold Pick, Czechoslovakian physician, 1851–1924.]

picorna virus. Pico (very small) and RNA (ribonucleic acid). Small RNA viruses. The group includes poliomyelitis virus, Coxsackie, ECHO and rhinoviruses. See VIRUS.

picrotoxin (pik-rō-toks'-in). Central nervous system stimulant used in barbiturate poisoning.

pigeon chest. A narrow chest, bulging anteriorly in the breast bone region. (Pectus carinatum.)

pigment (pig'-ment) [L. *pigmentum*]. Any colouring matter of the body.

pigmentation (pig-men-tā'-shun) [L. *pigmentum*, pigment]. The deposit of pigment, especially when abnormal or excessive.

piles. See HAEMORRHOIDS.

pilocarpine (pī-lō-kár'-pin). An alkaloid

used in a 0.5 to 1 per cent solution as a miotic in glaucoma. Stimulates the salivary glands, and is occasionally used in high dose atropine therapy.

pilomotor nerves (pī-lō-mō'-tor) [L. *pilus*, hair; *movere*, to move]. Tiny nerves attached to the hair follicle; innervation causes the hair to stand upright and give the appearance of 'goose flesh.'

pilonidal (pī-lō-nī'-dal) [L. *pilus*, hair; *nidus*, nest]. Hair containing. **pilonidal sinus**, a sinus containing hairs and which is usually found in hirsute people in the cleft between the buttocks. In this situation it is liable to infection.

pilosebaceous (pī-lō-sē-bā'-shus) [L. *pilus*, a hair; *sebaceus*, tallow candle]. Pertaining to the hair follicle and the sebaceous gland opening into it.

pilosis (pī-lō'-sis) [L. *pilus*, hair; G. *-osis*, condition]. An abnormal growth of hair.

Pimafucin. (pim-á-fū-sin). Antifungal antibiotic, active against monilial infection.

pimozide (pim'-oz-īd). A long-acting neuroleptic which can be used to overcome the problem of a patient's non-compliance. Used only where there can be supervision for side effects.

pimple (pim'-pl). See PAPULE.

pineal body (pin'-e-al) [L. *ptnea*, pine cone]. A small reddish-grey conical structure on the dorsal surface of the midbrain. Its functions are not fully understood but there is some evidence that it is an endocrine gland concerned with growth.

pinguecula (pin-gwek'-ū-lá) [1 *pinguiculus*, fattish]. A yellowish, slightly elevated thickening of the bulbar conjunctiva near the lid aperture. Associated with the ageing eye.

pink disease. Acrodynia. Disease of infants thought to be the result of mercury poisoning. (The sale of mercury-containing teething powders is now prohibited.) Child presents the picture of misery, with photophobia, restlessness and wasting. The extremities are swollen, and blue if child is cold, pink if he is warm. There is marked perspiration and generalized pruritis. See ERYTHROEDEMA.

pink-eye. Popular name for acute contagious conjunctivitis.

pinna (pin'-á) [L. feather]. That part of

the ear which is external to the head; the auricle

pinta (pin'-ta). Colour changes in patches of skin due to *Treponema pinta,* identical with the spirochaete of syphilis and yaws (q.v.).

Pipanol. Benzhexol (q.v.).

piperazine (pi-per'-a-zēn). A highly effective anthelmintic against threadworms and roundworms. Piperazine therapy can be followed by incidents of unsteadiness and falling; 'worm wobble'.

pipobromen (pip-ō-brō'-men). Alkylating agent; given orally. Used for chronic myeloid leukaemia.

piposulfan (pip-ō-sul'-fan). Similar structure to alkylating agents but its exact mode of action is unknown. Given orally. Used in chronic myeloid leukaemia.

Piracetam (pir-a-sēt'-am). For senile dementia.

Piriton (pi'-ri-ton). An antihistamine of high potency and of value in the treatment of transfusion reactions. Can be given orally or by injection.

Pitressin (pit-res'-in). Vasopressin (q.v.).

pitting (pit'-ting). 1. Making an indentation in dropsical tissues. 2. Depressed scars left on the skin, especially after smallpox.

pituitary extract (pi-tū'-it-a-ri). Vasopressin (q.v.).

pituitary gland. A small oval endocrine gland lying in the p. fossa of the sphenoid bone; the hypophysis cerebri. The anterior lobe secretes several hormones, having an effect upon other endocrine glands. Their general overall function is to regulate growth and metabolism.

pityriasis (pit-i-rī'-ā-sis) [G.]. Scaly (branny) eruption of the skin. **pityriasis capitis,** dandruff. **pityriasis rosea,** a slightly scaly eruption of ovoid erythematous lesions which are widespread over the trunk and proximal parts of the limbs. There may be mild itching. It is a self-limiting condition. **pityriasis rubra,** a form of exfoliative dermatitis. **pityriasis rubra pilaris,** a chronic skin disease characterized by tiny red papules of perifollicular distribution. **pityriasis versicolor,** called also 'tinea versicolor,' is a fungus infection which causes the appearance of buff-coloured patches on the chest.

Pityrosporum (pit-i-rō-spōr'-um). A fungus associated with dandruff.

pivhydrazine (piv-hīd'-ra-zēn). A monoamine oxidase inhibitor.

PKU. Phenylketonuria (q.v.).

placebo (plas-ē'-bō). A harmless substance given as medicine. In experimental research an inert substance, identical in appearance with the material being tested. Neither the physician nor the patient know which is which.

placenta (pla-sen'-ta) [L. cake]. Afterbirth. A vascular structure developed about the third month of pregnancy and attached to the inner wall of the uterus. Through it the fetus is supplied with nourishment and oxygen and through it the fetus gets rid of its waste products. In normal labour it is expelled within an hour of the birth of the child. When this does not occur it is termed a **retained p.** and may be an **adherent p.** The placenta is usually attached to the upper segment of the uterus; where it lies in the lower uterine segment it is called a **p. praevia,** and usually causes antepartum haemorrhage (now called placental abruption). See HAEMORRHAGE—placental, adj.

placental insufficiency. Inefficiency of the placenta. Can occur due to maternal disease or postmaturity of fetus giving rise to a 'small for dates' baby.

placentography (pla-sen-tog'-ra-fi). X-ray examination of the placenta by injection of opaque substance.

plague (plāg) [L. *plaga*]. Very contagious epidemic disease caused by *Pasteurella pestis,* and spread by infected rats. Transfer of infection from rat to man is through the agency of fleas. The main clinical types are bubonic, septicaemic or pneumonic.

plantar (plan'-tar). Pertaining to the sole of the foot. **plantar arch,** the union of the plantar and dorsalis pedis arteries in the sole of the foot. **plantar flexion,** downward movement of the big toe.

Plaquenil (pla'-qwan-il). Hydroxychloroquine. See CHLOROQUINE.

plasma (plaz'-ma) [G.]. The fluid fraction of blood. Blood p. is used for infusion in cases of haemoconcentration of the patient's blood, as in severe burns. Dried p. is in the form of a yellow powder which must be 'reconstituted' before being used for infusion. Various plasma substitutes are available, e.g. dextran, plasmosan. **plasma cell,** a normal cell with an eccentric nucleus produced in the bone marrow and retiuloendothelial system, and concerned with the production of antibodies; abnormally produced in myelomatosis (q.v.).

plasmapherisis (plas-má-fer-ēs'-is). Taking blood from a donor, removing some desired fraction then returning the red cells and repeating the whole process.

plasmin (plaz'-min). A fibrinolysin (q.v.).

plasminogen (plaz-min'-ō-jen). Precursor of plasmin. Release of activators from damaged tissue promotes the conversion of plasminogen into plasmin.

Plasmodium (plaz-mō'-di-um) [G. *plasma*, form; *eidos*, form]. A genus of protozoa. Parasites in the blood of warm-blooded animals which complete their sexual cycle in blood-sucking arthropods. Four species cause malaria in man—plasmodial, adj.

plasmoquine. See PAMAQUIN.

Plastazote (plas'-tá-zōt). New lightweight thermoplastic material used for splints, supports and appliances.

plastic (plas'-tik). Capable of taking a form or mould. **plastic surgery,** transfer of healthy tissue to repair damaged area and restore form.

platelet (plāt'-let). Syn., thrombocyte (q.v.).

Platyhelminth (plat-i-hel'-minth) [G. *platys*, broad; *helmins*, worm]. Flat worm; fluke. See SCHISTOSOMIASIS.

pleomorphism (plē-ō-mor'-fizm) [G. *pleon*, more; *morphe*, form]. Denotes a wide range in shape and size of individuals in a bacterial population—pleomorphic, adj.

plethora (pleth'-o-rá) [G.]. Fullness; overloading—plethoric, adj.

plethysmograph (pleth-is'-mo-graf). An instrument which measures accurately the blood flow in a limb.

pleura (ploo'-ra) [G. rib]. A thin serous membrane covering the surface of the lung and reflecting at the root of the lung, on to the chest wall. That portion lining the chest wall is termed 'parietal p.'; that closely adherent to lung tissue is 'visceral p.'—pleural, adj.

pleurisy (ploo'-ri-si) [G. *pleuritis*]. Inflammation of the pleura. Pleuritis. May be fibrinous (dry), or be associated with an effusion (wet), or be complicated by empyema—pleuritic, adj.

pleurodesis (ploo-rō-dē'-sis) [G. *pleura*, rib; *desis*, a binding together]. Adherence of the visceral to the parietal pleura. Can be achieved therapeutically by using iodized talc.

pleurodynia (ploo-rō-din'-i-á) [G. *pleura*, rib; *odyne*, pain]. Intercostal myalgia or muscular rheumatism (fibrositis). Is a feature of Bornholm disease (q.v.).

pleuropulmonary (ploo-rō-pul'-mon-a-ri) [G. *pleura*, rib; L. *pulmo*, lung]. Pertaining to the pleura and lung.

plexus (pleks'-us) [L. a twining]. A network of vessels or nerves.

plica (plī'-ká) [L. *plicare*, to fold]. A fold—plicate, adj.; plication, n.

plombage. Extrapleural compression of the tuberculous lung cavity.

plumbism. Lead poisoning (q.v.).

plumbum (plum'-bum) [L.]. Lead.

Plummer-Vinson syndrome. Also Kelly-Paterson syndrome. Combination of severe glossitis with dysphagia and nutritional iron deficiency anaemia. [Henry Stanley Plummer, American physician, 1874–1936. Porter Paisley Vinson, American physician, 1890– .]

pluriglandular (plū-ri-gland'-ū-lár). Pertaining to several glands as mucoviscidosis.

pneumaturia (nū-mat-ū'-ri-á) [G. *pneuma*, wind; *ouron*, urine]. The passage of flatus with urine, usually as a result of a bladder-bowel fistula.

pneumococcus (nū-mō-kok'-us) [G. *pneumon*, lung; *kokkos*, berry]. (*Streptococcus pneumoniae*.) A coccal bacterium arranged characteristically in pairs. A common cause of lobar pneumonia and other infections—pneumococcal, adj.

pneumoconiosis (nū-mō-kō-ni-ō'-sis). Dust disease. Fibrosis of the lung caused by long continued inhalation of dust in industrial occupations. The most important complication is the occasional superinfection with tuberculosis. Examples are silicosis, coal workers' p., asbestosis, sideriosis grinders' lung and byssinosis, described elsewhere. **rheumatoid p.,** fibrosing alveolitis occurring in patients suffering from rheumatoid arthritis—pneumoconioses, pl.

pneumoencephalogram (nū-mō-en-kef'-al-ō-gram) [F. *pneuma*, wind; *egkephalos*, brain; *gramma*, letter]. X-ray picture of cerebral ventricles after injection of air.

pneumoencephalography (nū-mō-en-kef-al-og'-ra-fi) [G. *neuma*, wind; *egkephalos*, brain; *raphein*, to write]. Radiographic examination of cerebral ventricles after injection of air by means of a lumbar or cisternal puncture.

pneumogastric (nū-mō-gas'-trik). Pertaining to the lungs and stomach. See VAGUS.

pneumokoniosis. See PNEUMOCONIOSIS.

pneumolysis (nū-mol'-i-sis) [G. *pneuma*, air; *lysis*, a loosening]. Separation of the two pleural layers, or the outer pleural layer from the chest wall to collapse the lung.

pneumomediastinogram (nū-mō-mēd-i-as-tī-nō-gram). X-ray of the mediastinum after rendering opaque with air.

pneumomycosis (nū-mō-mī-kō'-sis) [G. *pneuma*, air; *mykes*, fungus; *-osis*, condition]. Fungus infection of the lung such as aspergillosis, actinomycosis, moniliasis—pneumomycotic, adj.

pneumonectomy (nū-mon-ek'-to-mi) [G. *pneumon*, lung; *ektome*, excision]. Excision of a lung.

pneumonia (nū-mō'-ni-á) [G. *pneumon*, lung]. Inflammation of the lung with production of alveolar exudate. Traditionally, two main types were recognized, on an anatomical or radiological basis, viz. lobar p. and broncho–p. The tendency these days is to classify according to the specific bacterium or virus causing the infection (specific pneumonias) on the one hand, and the aspiration or secondary pneumonias (non-specific) on the other. **hypostatic p.** is the result of stasis and occurs in the case of debilitated patients from lack of movement in the dependent part of the lung. **unresolved p.**, wherein the alveolar exudate does not liquefy but consolidation persists—pneumonic, adj.

pneumonitis (nū-mon-īt'-is) [G. *pneumon*, lung; *-itis*, inflammation]. Inflammation of lung tissue.

pneumoperitoneum (nū-mō-per-it-on-ē'-um) [G. *pneumon*, lung; *peri*, around; *teinein*, to stretch]. Air or gas in the peritoneal cavity. Can be introduced for diagnostic or therapeutic purposes.

pneumoradiography (nū-mō-rā-di-og'-ra-fi) [G. *pneuma*, wind; L. *radius*, ray; G. *graphein*, to write]. Radiographic examination after injection of air.

Pneumosol. An aerosol used in pneumonia.

pneumothorax (nū-mō-thor'-aks) [G. *pneumon*, lung; *thorax*, thorax]. Air or gas in the pleural cavity separating the visceral from the parietal pleura so that lung tissue is compressed. **artificial p.**, induced in the treatment of pulmonary tuberculosis. **spontaneous p.** occurs when an overdilated pulmonary air sac ruptures, permitting communication of respiratory passages and pleural cavity. **tension p.**, occurs where a valve-like wound allows air to enter the pleural cavity at each inspiration but not to escape on expiration, thus progressively increasing intrathoracic pressure and constituting an acute medical emergency—pneumothoraces, pl.

pneumoventriculography (nū-mō-ventrik-ū-log'-ra-fi) [G. *pneuma*, wind; L. *ventriculum*, ventricle; G. *graphein*, to write]. Examination of cerebral ventricles by X-ray after injection of air directly.

poldine methylsulphate (pol'-dēn-methil-sul'-fāt). Inhibits gastric secretion of acid in response to food.

polioencephalitis (pō-li-ō-en-kef'-a-līʹ-tis) [G. *polios*, grey; *egkephalos*, brain; *-itis*, inflammation]. Inflammation of the cerebral grey matter—this may or may not include the central nuclei—polioencephalitic, adj.

poliomyelitis (pol-i-ō-mī-el-īʹ-tis) [G. *polios*, grey; *myelos*, marrow]. Infantile paralysis. An epidemic virus infection which attacks the motor neurones of the anterior horns in brain stem (bulbar p.) and spinal cord. An attack may or may not lead to paralysis of the lower motor neurone type with loss of muscular power and flaccidity. Vaccination against the disease is desirable. When it occurs within two days of vaccination with any alum-containing prophylactic, the term 'provocative paralytic p.' is used.

polioviruses. Cause poliomyelitis (q.v.).

Politzer's bag. Rubber bag for Eustachian inflation. [Adam Politzer, Austrian otologist, 1835–1920.]

pollenosis (pol-en-ō'-sis). Allergic condition arising from sensitization to pollen.

Polya operation (pol'-i-á). Partial gastrectomy (q.v.).

polyarteritis (pol-i-árt-er-īt'-is) [G. *polys*, many; *arteria*, artery; *-itis*, inflammation]. Inflammation of many arteries. In **p. nodosa** (periarteritis nodosa) aneurysmal swellings and thrombosis occur in the affected vessels.

Further damage may lead to haemorrhage and the clinical picture presented depends upon the site affected. See COLLAGEN and PERIARTERITIS.

polyarthralgia (pol-i-ár-thral'-ji-á) [G. *polys*, many; *arthron*, joint; *algos*, pain]. Pain in several joints.

polyarthritis (pol-i-ár-thrī'-tis) [G. *polys*, many; *arthron*, joint; *-itis*, inflammation]. Inflammation of several joints at the same time. See STILL'S DISEASE.

Polybactrin. Neomycin sulphate, polymyxin B, and bacitracin. Antibiotic powder spray. Used topically in surgery, burns and wounds.

Polybrene. Protamine sulphate (q.v.).

polycystic (pol-i-sis'-tik) [G. *polys*, many; *kystos*, bladder]. Composed of many cysts. Polycystic kidney disease is congenital, and slowly fatal.

polycythaemia (pol-i-sī-thē'-mi-á) [G. *polys*, many; *kytos*, cell; *haima*, blood]. Increase in the number of circulating red blood cells. This may result from dehydration or be a compensatory phenomenon to increase the oxygen carrying capacity, as in congenital heart disease. **polycythaemia vera** (erythraemia) is an idiopathic condition in which the red cell count is very high. The patient complains of headache and lassitude, and there is danger of thrombosis and haemorrhage. See also ERYTHROCYTHAEMIA.

polydactyly (pol-i-dak'-til-i) [G. *polys*, many; *daktylos*, finger]. Having more than the normal number of fingers or toes. Also **polydactylism.**

polydipsia (pol-i-dip'-si-á) [G. *polys*, many; *dipsa*, thirst]. Excessive thirst.

polygraph (pol'-i-graf) [G. *polys*, many; *graphein*, to write]. Instrument which records pulses simultaneously.

polyhydramnios (pol-i-hī-dram'-ni-os) [G. *polys*, many; *hydor*, water; *amnion*, membrane around fetus]. An excessive amount of amniotic fluid.

poly-I-C (pol'-i-ī-sē). Polysinosinic-polycytidylic acid (q.v.).

polymyalgia rheumatica (pol-i-mī-al'-ji-á roo-mat-ik-á) [G. *polys*, many; *mys*, muscle; *algos*, pain; *rheumatismos*, that which flows]. A syndrome occurring in elderly people comprising of a sometimes crippling ache in the shoulders, pelvic girdle muscles and spine, with pronounced morning stiffness and a raised ESR. There is an association with temporal arteritis. Clinically different from rheumatoid arthritis.

polymorphonuclear (pol-i-mor-fo-nū-klē-ar) [G. *polys*, many; *morphos*, shape; L. *nucleus*, kernel]. Having a many-shaped or lobulated nucleus, usually applied to the phagocytic neutrophil leucocytes (granulocytes) which constitute 70 per cent of the total white blood cells.

polymyxin B (po-li-miks'-in). An antibiotic used in infections due to *Pseudomonas pyocyanea*. Also used in ear infections.

polyneuritis (pol-i-nū-rī'-tis) [G. *polys*, many; *neuron*, tendon; *-itis*, inflammation]. Multiple neuritis—polyneuritic, adj.

polyoma. One of the tumour-producing viruses.

polyopia (pol-i-ōp'-i-á) [G. *polys*, many; *ops*, eye]. Seeing many images of a single object.

polyp or **polypus** (pol'-ip(-us)) [G. *polypous*, many-footed]. A pedunculated tumour arising from any mucous surface, e.g. cervical, uterine, nasal, etc. Usually benign but may become malignant—polypi, pl.; polypous, adj.

polypectomy (pol-ip-ek'-to-mi) [G. *polypous*, many-footed; *ektome*, excision]. Surgical removal of a polyp.

polypeptides (pol-i-pep'-tīdz). Proteins with long chains of amino acids linked together.

polypoid (pol'-i-poid) [G. *polypous*, many-footed; *eidos*, form]. Resembling a polyp(us).

polyposis (pol-i-pō'-sis) [G. *polypous*, many-footed; *-osis*, condition]. A condition in which there are numerous polypi in an organ. **polyposis coli**, a hereditary condition in which polypi occur throughout the large bowel and which leads eventually to carcinoma of the colon.

polysaccharide (pol-i-sak'-ar-īd) [G. *polys*, many; *sakcharon*, sugar]. $(C_6H_{10}O_5)n$. Carbohydrates containing a large number of monosaccharide groups. Starch, inulin, glycogen, dextrin and cellulose are examples.

polyserositis (pol-i-sē-rō-sī'-tis) [G. *polys*, many; L. *serum*, whey; G. *-itis*, inflammation]. Inflammation of several serous membranes.

polysinosinic-polycytidylic acid (pol-i-sin-ō-sin'-ik-pol-i-sit-i-dil'-ik). An artificial nucleic acid that enhances the ability of cells to reject tumours in some way not yet understood.

polythiazide (pol-i-thī'-a-zīd). Diuretic. See CHLOROTHIAZIDE.

polyuria (pol-i-ūr'-i-á) G. *polys*, much; *ouron*, urine]. Excretion of an excessive amount of urine—polyuric, adj.

pompholyx (pom'-fol-iks) [G. bubble]. Vesicular skin eruption on hands or feet. See CHEIROPOMPHOLYX.

Ponderax (pon'-der-aks). Fenfluramine hydrochloride (q.v.).

pons [L.]. A bridge; a process of tissue joining two sections of an organ. **pons varolii**, the white convex mass of nerve tissue at the base of the brain which serves to connect the various lobes of the brain—pontine, adj. [Constantio Varoliùs, Italian anatomist, 1543–75.]

Ponstan (pon'-stan). Mefenamic acid (q.v.).

popliteal (pop-lit-ē'-al) [L. *poples*, ham]. Pertaining to the popliteus. **popliteal space**, the diamond-shaped depression at the back of the knee joint, bounded by the muscles and containing the popliteal nerve and vessels.

poradenitis (por-ad-en-ī'-tis) [G. *poros*, pore; *aden*, gland; *-itis*, inflammation]. Painful mass of iliac glands, characterized by abscess formation. Occurs in lymphogranuloma inguinale (q.v.).

pore (pōr) [G. *poros*, channel]. A minute surface opening. One of the mouths of the ducts (leading from the sweat glands) on the skin surface; they are controlled by fine papillary muscles, contracting and closing in the cold, and dilating in the presence of heat.

porphyria (por-fī'-ri-á) [G. *porphyra*, purple]. An inborn error in porphyrin metabolism, probably hereditary, causing pathological changes in nervous and muscular tissue in some cases of intermittent p., and photosensitivity in some cases of congenital p.

porphyrins (por-fī'-rins) [G. *porphyra*, purple]. Coloured organic compounds; they form the basis of respiratory pigments. Naturally occurring porphyrins are uroporphyrin and coproporphyrin. They fluoresce when exposed to Wood's light. See PORPHYRIA.

porphyrinuria (por-fī-rin-ūr'-i-á) [G. *porphyros*, purple; *ouron*, urine]. Excretion of porphyrins in the urine.

Such pigments are produced as a result of an inborn error of metabolism.

porta (por'-tá) [L. *gate*]. The depression (hilum) of an organ at which the vessels enter and leave—portal, adj. **porta hepatis**, the transverse fissure through which the portal vein, hepatic artery and bile ducts pass on the under surface of the liver.

portacaval (por-ta-kā'-val) [L. *porta*, gate; *cavum*, hollow]. Pertaining to the portal vein and inferior vena cava. **portacaval anastomosis**, a fistula made between the portal vein and the inferior vena cava with the object of reducing the pressure within the portal vein in cases of cirrhosis of the liver. Also PORTOCAVAL.

portahepatitis (por-ta-hep-at-ī'-tis) [L. *porta*, gate; G. *hepar*, liver; *-itis*, inflammation]. Inflammation around the transverse fissure of the liver.

portal hypertension. Condition when there is increased pressure in portal vein (q.v.). Usually caused by cirrhosis of liver and results in splenomegaly, with hypersplenism (q.v.) and alimentary bleeding. See also BANTI'S DISEASE.

portal vein. That conveying blood into the liver; it is about 76.2 mm long and is formed by the union of the superior mesenteric and splenic veins.

portogram (por'-to-gram). X-ray of portal vein after splenic puncture and injection of radio-opaque liquid, or after injection of radio-opaque liquid into portal vein at operation.

position (pō-zish'-un) [L. *positio*, a placing]. Posture: attitude. (See diagrams, pp. 239-240).

positive pressure breathing (PPB). Inflation of lungs to produce inspiration. Exhaled air, hand bellows or more sophisticated apparatus can be used. Elastic recoil produces expiration.

posseting (pos'-et-ing). Regurgitation of small amounts of clotted milk in infants.

possum (pos'-sum). Patient-Operated Selector Mechanism. An apparatus which can be operated by a slight touch, or by suction using the mouth if no other muscle movement possible. It may transmit messages or be adapted for typing, telephoning and other activities.

postanaesthetic (pōst-an-es-thet'-ik) [L. *post*, after; G. *anaisthesia*, loss of sensation]. After anaesthesia.

239

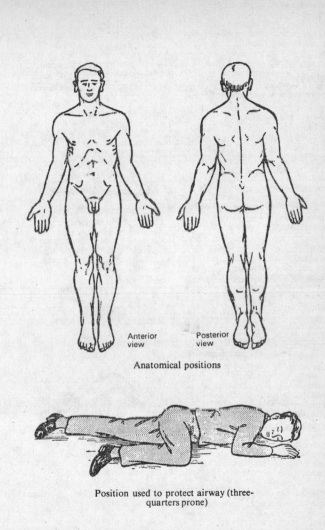

Anterior view

Posterior view

Anatomical positions

Position used to protect airway (three-quarters prone)

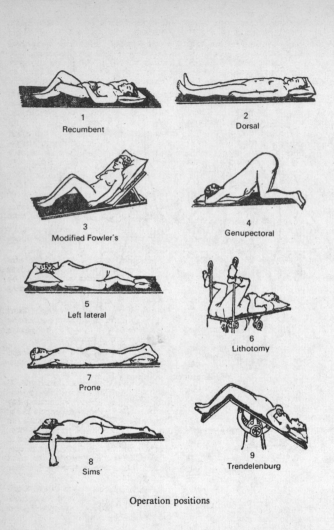

1
Recumbent

2
Dorsal

3
Modified Fowler's

4
Genupectoral

5
Left lateral

6
Lithotomy

7
Prone

8
Sims'

9
Trendelenburg

Operation positions

postanal (pōst'-ān'-al) [L. *post*, after; *anus*]. Behind the anus.

postconcussional syndrome (pōst-kon-kush'-on-al sin'-drōm). The association of headaches, giddiness and a feeling of faintness, which may persist for a considerable time after a head injury.

postdiphtheritic (pōst-dif-thèr-it'-ik) [L. *post*, after; G. *dipthera*, leather]. Following an attack of diphtheria. Refers especially to the paralysis of limbs and palate.

postencephalitic (pōst-en-kef-al-it'-ik) [L. *post*, after; G. *egkephalos*, brain; *-itis*, inflammation]. Following encephalitis lethargica. The adjective is commonly used to describe the syndrome of Parkinsonism, which so often results from an attack of this kind of encephalitis.

postepileptic (pōst-ep-il-ep'-tik) [L. *post*, after; G. *epileptikos*]. Following on an epileptic seizure. **postepileptic automatism** is a fugue state, following on a fit, when patient may undertake a course of action, even involving violence, without having any memory of this (amnesia).

posterior (pos-tē'-ri-or) [L. Situated at the back] **posterior chamber of the eye**, space between the anterior surface of lens and p. surface of iris. See AQUEOUS posteriorly, adv.

postganglionic (pōst-gang-gli-on'-ik) [L. *post*, after; G. *gagglion*, tumour]. Situated after a collection of nerve cells (ganglion) as a p. nerve fibre.

postgastrectomy syndrome. Covers two sets of symptoms, those of hypoglycaemia when the patient is hungry, and those of a vasovagal attack immediately after a meal.

postherpetic (pōst-hèr-pet'-ik) [L. *post*, behind; G. *herpein*, to creep]. After shingles.

posthitis (pos-thī'-tis) [G. *posthe*, prepuce *-itis*, inflammation]. Inflammation of the prepuce.

postmature (pōst-ma-tūr') [L. *post*, behind; *maturus*, ripe]. Past the expected date of delivery. A baby is postmature when labour is delayed beyond the usual 40 weeks postmaturity, n.

postmenopausal (pōst-men-ō-pawz'-al) [L. *post*, after; G. *men*, month; *pausis*, a stopping]. Occurring after the menopause has been established.

postmortem (pōst-mor'-tem) [L. *post*, after; *mors*, death]. After death, usually inferring dissection of the body. Autopsy.

postmyocardial infarction syndrome. Pyrexia and chest pain associated with inflammation of the pleura, lung or pericardium. Due to sensitivity to released products from dead muscle.

postnasal (pōst-nā'-zal) [L. *post*, behind; *nasus*, nose]. Situated behind the nose and in the nasopharynx—postnasally, adv.

postnatal (pōst-nā'-tal) [L. *post*, after; *natalis*, of birth]. After delivery. **postnatal examination**, routine examination 6 weeks after delivery—postnatally, adv.

postoperative (pōst-op'-er-at-iv) [L. *post*, after; *operari*, to operate]. After operation—postoperatively, adv.

postpartum (pōst-pàr'-tum) [L. *post*, after; *partus*, a birth]. After a birth (parturition).

postprandial (pōst-pran'-di-al). Following a meal.

postural (pos'-tū-ral). Pertaining to posture. **postural drainage**, usually infers drainage from the respiratory tract, by elevation of the foot of the bed or using a special frame.

posture (pos'-tūr) [L. *positura*, from *ponere*, to place]. Active or passive arrangement of the whole body, or a part, in a definite manner.

postvaccinal (pōst-vak'-sin-al) [L. *post*, after; *vaccinus*, of cows]. After vaccination.

postvagotomy diarrhoea. Three types: 1. Transient diarrhoea shortly after operation, lasting from a few hours to a day or two. These episodes disappear in 3 to 6 months. 2. If they recur later than this and the attacks last longer, the term, 'recurrent episodic diarrhoea' is used. 3. An increased daily bowel frequency; may be of disabling severity, but often acceptable in contrast to preoperative constipation.

potassium chlorate (pō-ta'-si-um klor'-āt). Mild antiseptic used in mouthwashes and gargles. Distinguish from potassium chloride.

potassium chloride (pō-ta'-si-um klor'-īd). Used in potassium replacement solutions, and as a supplement in chlorothiazide therapy.

potassium citrate (pō-ta'-si-um sit'-rāt). Alkalinizes urine; widely used in cystitis, etc. and during sulphonamide therapy to prevent renal complications.

potassium deficiency. Disturbed electrolyte balance; can occur after excessive vomiting, and/or diarrhoea; after prolonged use of diuretics, steroids, etc. Signs and symptoms variable, but nausea and muscle weakness often present. Heart failure can quickly supervene.

potassium hydroxide (pō-ta'-si-um hīdroks'-īd). Caustic potash; used as liq. potassae in urine testing.

potassium iodide (pō-ta'-si-um ī'-ō-dīd). Used as an expectorant in bronchitis and asthma; also used in the prophylaxis of simple goitre, and pre-operatively in toxic goitre.

potassium perchlorate (pō-ta'-si-um perklor'-at). Suppresses trapping of iodine in thyroid gland.

potassium permanganate (pō-ta'-si-um per-mang'-gan-āt). Purple crystals with powerful disinfectant and deodorizing properties. Used as lotion 1 in 1000; 1 in 5000 to 10 000 for baths.

Potaba+6 (pot-ō'-ba). Potassium para-aminobenzoate. Has an antifibrotic effect. Three g capsules orally four times daily with meals for several months.

potter's rot (pot'-ers rot). One of the many popular names for silicosis arising in workers in the pottery industry.

Pott's disease. Spondylitis; spinal caries; spinal tuberculosis. [Percivall Pott, English surgeon, 1714–88.]

Pott's fracture. A fracture-dislocation of the ankle joint. A fracture of the lower end of the fibula, 76 mm above the ankle joint, and a fracture of the medial malleolus of the tibia. [Percivall Pott, English surgeon, 1714–88.]

pouch (powch) [F. *poche*, pocket]. A pocket or recess. **pouch of Douglas**, recto-uterine pouch.

PPB. Positive pressure breathing (q.v.).

PPD. Purified protein derivative. See TEST: MANTOUX.

PPLO. Pleuropneumonia-like organism similar to the virus that causes contagious pleuropneumonia in cattle. See EATON AGENT.

Prader-Willi syndrome. Described in 1956. Low birth weight, hypotonia, mental retardation, acromicria and often obesity and diabetes mellitus develop during childhood or adolescence.

praecordial. See PRECODIAL.

praxilene (praks'-i-lēn). Naftidrofuryl oxalate (q.v.).

prazosin (praz'-ō-sin). Antihypertensive agent which is said to act peripherally by direct vasodilation.

pre-anaesthetic (prē-an-es-thet'-ik) [L. *prae*, before; G. *anaisthesia*, lack of sensation]. Before an anaesthetic.

precancerous (prē-kan'-sėr-us) [L. *prae*, before; *cancer*, crab]. Occurring before cancer with special reference to non-malignant pathological changes which are believed to lead on to, or to be followed by, cancer.

precipitin (prē-sip'-it-in) [L. *precipitare*, to precipitate]. An antibody which forms a specific complex with precipitinogen (antigen), and under certain physiochemical conditions this results in the formation of a precipitate. This reaction forms the basis of many delicate diagnostic serological tests for the identification of minute traces of material and bacteria. See ANTIBODIES.

precordial (prē-kor'-di-al) [L. *prae*, before; *cor*, heart]. Pertaining to the area of the chest immediately over the heart.

precursor (prē-kurs'-or). Forerunner.

prediabetes (prē-dī-a-bē'-tēz) [L. *prae*, before; G. *diabainein*, to cross through]. Potential predisposition to diabetes mellitus. Preventive mass urine testing can detect the condition. Early treatment prevents ketoacidosis and may help to prevent the more serious complications such as retinopathy and neuropathy—prediabetic, adj., n.

predigestion (prē-di-jest'-chun). Artificial digestion of protein (e.g. in peptonized foods) or amylolysis (e.g. in malt extracts or dextronized cereals) before digestion takes place in the body.

predisposition (prē-dis-pō-zi'-shun). A natural susceptibility to develop or contract certain diseases.

Prednesol (pred'-nes-ol). Prednisolone (q.v.).

prednisolone (pred-nis'-ō-lōn). A synthetic hormone with properties similar to those of cortisone (q.v.). but side effects, such as salt and water retention, are markedly reduced. Widely prescribed for connective tissue diseases, conditions involving immune reaction including autoimmune disorders.

prednisone (pred'-ni-sōn). Converted into prednisolone in the liver.

pre-eclampsia (prē-ē-klamp'-si-á) [L. *prae*, before G. *eklampsis*, a shining forth]. A condition characterized by albuminuria, hypertension and oedema, arising usually in the latter part of pregnancy—pre-eclamptic, adj.

prefrontal (prē-front'-al) [L. *prae*, before; *frons*, forehead]. Situated in the anterior portion of the frontal lobe of the cerebrum. See LEUCOTOMY.

Pregaday (preg'-á-dā). Ferrous fomarate (q.v.). and folic acid (q.v.).

Pregamal (preg'-a-mal). Folic acid (q.v.).

preganglionic (prē-gang-gli-on'-ik) [L. *prae*, before; G. *gagglion*, tumour]. Preceding or in front of a collection of nerve cells (ganglion) as a p. nerve fibre.

pregnancy (preg'-nan-si) [L. *praegnans*]. Being with child, i.e. from conception to parturition, normally 40 weeks or 280 days. **extrauterine p.,** see ECTOPIC P. **multiple p.,** more than one fetus in the uterus. **phantom p.,** see PSEUDOCYESIS.

pregnanediol. Urinary excretion product from progesterone.

Pregnyl (preg'-nil). Chorionic gonadotrophin for undescended and ectopic testes.

prehensile (prē-hen'-sīl) [L. *prehendere*, to seize]. Equipped for grasping.

Preludin (prel'-ū-din). Phenmetrazine hydrochloride (q.v.).

Premarin (pre'-mar-in). Conjugated oestrogens. Can be given orally. Useful for menopausal symptoms.

premature (pre'-mat-ūr) [L. *praematurus*, too soon]. Occurring before the proper time. **premature baby,** where the birth weight is less than 2.5 kg (5½ 1b) and therefore special treatment is needed. Current syns. are low weight or dysmature baby. Not all low birth weight babies are premature, but are included in a new category 'small for dates.' See PLACENTAL INSUFFICIENCY. **premature beat,** see EXTRASYSTOLE. **premature labour,** expulsion of the fetus before the 280th day of gestation.

premedication (prē-med-ik-ā'-shun) [L. *prae*, before; *medicare*, heal]. Drugs given before the administration of another drug, e.g. those given before an anaesthetic. The latter are of two types: (1) sedative, e.g. morphine; (2) drugs which inhibit the secretion of saliva and of mucus from the upper respiratory tract, e.g. atropine.

premenstrual (prē-men'-stroo-al) [L. *prae*, before; *menstrualis*, monthly]. Preceding menstruation. Cyclical syndrome (q.v.) now preferred for p. symptom-complex.

premolars (prē-mól'-arz) [L. *prae*, before; *molere*, grind]. The eight bicuspid teeth, two on each side of each jaw, lying between the canine and the molars.

prenatal (prē-nā'-tal) [L. *prae*, before; *natalis*, of birth]. Before birth—prenatally, adv.

pre-operative (prē-op'-er-at-iv) [L. *prae*, before; *operari*, to operate]. Before operation—pre-operatively, adv.

preparalytic (prē-par-al-it' ik) [L. *prae*, before; G. *paralytikos*]. Before the onset of paralysis, usually referring to the early stage of poliomyelitis.

prepatellar (prē-pat-el'-ar) [L. *prae*, before; *patella*, kneecap]. In front of the kneecap, as applied to a large bursa.

prepubertal (prē-pū'-bert-al) [L. *prae*, before; *pubertas*, puberty]. Before puberty.

prepuce (prē'-pūs) [L. *praeputium*, foreskin]. The foreskin of the penis.

prerenal (prē-rē'-nal) [L. *prae*, before; *renalis*, of the kidney]. Before, or in front of the kidney.

presacral air insufflation. Injection of air into retroperitoneal interstitial tissues, mainly used to demonstrate renal and adrenal outlines.

presbyopia (prez-bi-ōp'-i-á) [G. *presbys*, old man; *ops*, eye]. Long-sightedness, due to failure of accommodation in those of 45 years and onwards—presbyopic, adj.; presbyope, n.

prescription (prē-skrip' shun). A written formula, signed by a physician, directing the pharmacist to prepare a remedy.

presenility (prē-sen-il'-i-ti) [L. *prae*, before; *senilis*, aged]. A condition occurring before senility is established—presenile, adj.

presentation (prez-en-tā'-shun) [L. *presentare*, to present]. The part of the fetus which first enters the pelvic brim and will be felt by the examining finger through the cervix in labour. May be vertex, face, brow, shoulder or breech.

pressor (pres'-sor). A substance which raises the blood pressure.

pressure areas (presh'-ér). The bony prominences of the body, over which the flesh of bedridden patients is denuded of its blood supply as it is compressed between the bone and an external source of pressure; the latter is usually the bed, but may be a splint, plaster, upper bedclothes, chair, etc.

pressure point. A place at which an artery passes over a bone, against which it can be compressed, to stop bleeding.

pressure sore. A decubitus ulcer, arising from continual compression of the flesh over a bony prominence. The first sign is redness, then there is bruising of the skin, which finally breaks and sloughs before healing takes place by granulation. Skin grafting may be necessary.

presystole (prē-sis'-to-li). The period preceding the systole or contraction of the heart muscle—presystolic, adj.

preterm delivery. When the expected date of delivery (EDD) is taken as the beginning of the 40th week rather than the end, and the mother has completed 39 weeks plus 6 days from the first day of her last menstrual period before entering the 40th week of pregnancy, then 'preterm' is delivery before the onset of the 37th week or three weeks or more before the EED.

prevesical (prē-ves'-ik-al) [L. *prae,* before; *vesica,* bladder]. Anterior to the bladder.

priapism (pri'-ap-izm) [*Priapus,* the god of procreation]. Prolonged penile erection in the absence of sexual stimulation.

Priadel (pri'-a-del). Lithium carbonate (q.v.).

prickly heat. Miliaria (q.v.).

prilocaine (pril'-o-kān). Local anaesthetic containing local blood vessel constrictor; synthetic; less toxic than cocaine. Basically similar to lignocaine, but less likely to cause vasodilation.

primaquine (prim'-a-qwin). Antimalarial. Useful for eradication of *Plasmodium vivax* from the liver.

primary complex or **Ghon's focus.** The initial tuberculous infection in a person, usually in the lung, and manifest as a small focus of infection in the lung tissue and enlarged caseous, hilar glands. It usually heals spontaneously. [Anton Ghon, Austrian pathologist, 1866–1936.]

primidone (pri'-mi-dōn). An anticonvulsant used mainly in grand mal, but is sometimes effective in petit mal.

primigravida (prīm-i-grav'-i-dà) [L. *pri-*

mus, first; *gravidus,* pregnant]. A woman who is pregnant for the first time—primigravidae, pl.

primipara (prī-mip'-a-rà) [L. *primus,* first; *parere,* to bear]. A woman who is giving birth to her first child—primiparous, adj.

Primobolan (prim-ō'-bol-an). Methenolone enanthate (q.v.).

Primolut depot. Hydroxyprogesterone caproate (q.v.).

Primolut N. Norethisterone (q.v.).

primordial (prī-mor'-di-al) [L. *primordius,* original]. Primitive, original; applied to the ovarian follicles present at birth.

Primoteston depot (prī-mō-tes'-ton). Intramuscular hormone preparation for male climacteric, cancer of breast and osteoporosis.

Priscol (pris'-kol). Tolazoline (q.v.).

Pro-Banthine (prō-ban'-thin). Propantheline (q.v.).

probenecid (prō-ben'-ē-sid). A drug which inhibits the renal excretion of certain compounds, notably penicillin and paraaminosalicyclic acid, and is used to increase the blood level of such drugs. It also hinders the reabsorption of urates by the renal tubules, so increasing the excretion of uric acid, and on that account it is used in the treatment of gout.

procainamide (prō-kān-ā'-mīd). Derivative of procaine used in cardiac arrhythmias such as paroxysmal tachycardia. Also helps to relax voluntary muscle and thus overcome myotonia. Given orally or by slow intravenous injection.

procaine (prō'-kān). Widely used local anaesthetic of high potency and low toxicity. Used mainly for infiltration anaesthesia as a 0.5 to 2 per cent solution. Now tending to be replaced by lignocaine (q.v.). **procaine benzylpenicillin,** longer acting than benzylpenicillin.

procarbazine (prō-kar'-baz-ēn). Drug of the nitrogen mustard group useful in Hodgkin's disease.

process (prō'-ses) [L. *processus*]. A prominence or outgrowth of any part.

prochlorperazine (prō-klor-pêr'-a-zēn). One of the phenothiazines. Has sedative and anti-emetic properties. Useful for vertigo, migraine, Ménière's disease, severe nausea and vomiting, schizophrenia.

procidentia (prō-si-den'-shi-à) [L. falling forward]. Complete prolapse of the uterus, so that it lies within the vaginal sac but outside the contour of the body.

proctalgia (prok-tal'-ji-à) [G. *proktos*, anus; *algos*, pain]. The presence of pain in the rectal region.

proctitis (prok-tī'-tis) [G. *proktos*, anus; *-itis*, inflammation]. Inflammation of the rectum. **granular p.**, acute p.; so called because of the granular appearance of the inflamed mucous membrane.

Proctocaine (prok'-tō-kān). A solution of procaine, butyl-aminobenzoate and benzyl alcohol in almond oil. Used in pruritus ani, anal fissure, etc. Given by deep subcutaneous injection.

proctoclysis (prok-tō-klī'-sis) [G. *proktos*, anus; *klysis*, a drenching]. The administration of fluid by the rectum. See CLYSIS.

proctocolectomy (prok-tō-kol-ek'-to-mi) [G. *proktos*, anus; *kolon*, colon; *ektome*, excision]. Surgical excision of the rectum and colon.

proctocolitis (prok-tō-kol-ī'-tis) [G. *proktos*, anus; *kolon*, colon; *-itis*, inflammation]. Inflammation of the rectum and colon; usually a type of ulcerative colitis.

proctoscope (prok'-tō-skōp) [G. *proktos*, anus; *skopein*, to examine]. An instrument for examining the rectum. See ENDOSCOPE—proctoscopic, adj.; proctoscopy, n.

proctosigmoiditis (prok-tō-sig-moid'-ī-tis) [G. *proktos*, anus; letter sigma; *-itis*, inflammation]. Inflammation of the rectum and sigmoid colon.

procyclidine (prō-sīk-li-dēn). A spasmolytic drug similar in action to benzhexol, and used in the treatment of Parkinsonism. It reduces the rigidity but has little action on the tremor.

Prodexin. Antacid tablets containing aluminium glycinate and magnesium carbonate.

prodromal (prō-drō'-mal) [G. *prodromos*, running before] Preceding, as the transitory rash before the true rash of an infectious disease.

proflavine (prō-flā'-vēn). An antiseptic very similar to acriflavine (q.v.).

Progestasert (prō-jes'-tà-sert). A flexible T-shaped unit, like an IUD; contains the natural hormone progesterone, released at a continuous rate of 65 mg daily.

progestational (prō-jes-tā'-shun-al) [G. *pro*, before; L. *gestare*, to carry]. Before pregnancy. Favouring pregnancy—progestation, n.

progesterone (prō-jes'-ter-ōn). The hormone of the corpus luteum. Used in the treatment of functional uterine haemorrhage, and in threatened abortion. Given by intramuscular injection.

progestogens (prō-jes'-to-jens). Substances that have an action like progesterone.

proglottis (prō-glot'-is) [G. *pro*, before; *glotta*, tongue]. Sexually mature segment of tapeworm—proglottides, pl.

prognosis (prog-nō'-sis) [G.] A forecast of the probable course and termination of a disease—prognostic, adj.

proguanil (prō-gwan'-il). Synthetic antimalarial used in prophylaxis and suppressive treatment of malaria.

projection (prō-jck'-shun) [L. *projectio*, throwing forward]. A mental mechanism occurring in normal people unconsciously, and in exaggerated form in mental illnesses, especially paranoia, whereby the person fails to recognize certain motives and feelings in himself but attributes them to others.

prolactin (prō-lak'-tin). Hormone secreted in the anterior pituitary gland. It acts only on the pregnant woman's breasts, preparing them for milk production. Thereafter it is secreted as a reflex response to the act of suckling, which starts the flow of milk.

Proladone (prō-la-dōn). Analgesic. Given by injection and suppository. Latter can be used to supplement pethidine.

prolapse (prō-laps) [L. *prolapsus*, a falling]. Descent; the falling of a structure. **prolapse of an intervertebral disc (PID)**, protrusion of the disc nucleus (q.v.) into the spinal cord and/or nerve roots. Most common in the lumbar region where it causes low back pain and/or sciatica. **prolapse of the iris**, the iris bulges forward through a corneal wound. **prolapse of the rectum**, the lower portion of the intestinal tract descends outside the external anal sphincter. **prolapse of the uterus**, the uterus descends into the vagina and may be visible at the vaginal orifice. See PROCIDENTIA.

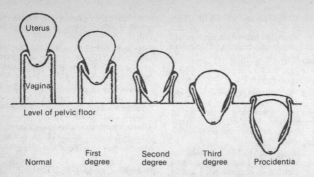

Normal — First degree — Second degree — Third degree — Procidentia

Degrees of prolapse of the uterus

proliferate (prō-lif´-er-āt) [L. *proles,* offspring; *ferre,* to bear]. Increase by cell division—proliferation, n.; proliferative, adj.

prolific (prō-lif´-ik) [L. *proles,* offspring]. Fruitful, multiplying abundantly.

promazine (prō´-ma-zēn). A tranquillizing drug similar to, but less hepatotoxic than chlorpromazine. Also useful in midwifery, treatment of alcoholism, senile agitation and for shivering attacks.

promethazine (prō-meth´-az-ēn). An antihistamine of high potency and low toxicity. Very effective in urticaria. Hypnotic side effect useful in psychiatry and midwifery. Also a useful antiemetic. Given 2 hours before journey it will last for 6 to 12 h.

Prominal (prō´-min-al). Methylphenobarbitone (q.v.).

promontory (prom´-on-to-ri) [L. *promontorium*]. A projection; a prominent part.

pronate (prō´-nāt) [L. *pronare,* to bend forward]. To turn the ventral surface downward, e.g. to lie on the face; to turn the palm of the hand downwards. Opp., supinate—pronation, n.

pronator (prō-nā´-tor) [L. *pronare,* to bend forward]. That which pronates, usually applied to a muscle. Opp. supinator.

Prondol (pron´-dol). Iprindole (q.v.).

prone (prōn) [L. *pronus*]. Face downwards. Opp. supine.

Pronestyl (pro-nes´-til). Procainamide (q.v.).

Propaderm (prop´-a-derm). Beclomethasone (q.v.).

Propamidine (prō-pam´-i-dēn). Antiseptic cream and jelly used for wounds and burns. Treatment for longer than 10 days is inadvisable owing to possible irritation.

propanidid (prō-pan´-i-did). Non-barbiturate, short-acting i.v. anaesthetic.

propantheline (prō-panth´-el-ēn). A synthetic compound with an atropine-like action. Used for its antispasmodic effects in pylorospasm, peptic ulcer, etc. Dryness of the mouth may occur in some patients.

properdin (prop-er´-din). A protein of normal blood serum. It can destroy certain bacteria, neutralize certain viruses and damage foreign red blood cells.

prophylaxis (prō-fil-aks´-is) [G. *prophylaxis,* a guarding]. Prevention—prophylactic, adj.; prophylactically, adv.

propicillin (prō-pi-sil´-in). Oral penicillin tablets and syrup.

propranolol (prō-pran´-o-lol). Effective drug in the prevention or correction of cardiac arrhythmias and dysrhythmias. It reduces frequency of anginal attacks by helping to reduce the unnecessarily high level of noradrenaline activity, thus blocking the effects of beta-receptor activation in both heart and lungs. Prepared as eye drops for glaucoma.

proptosis (prop-tō´-sis) [G.]. Forward protrusion, especially of the eyeball.

propyliodone (prō-pīl-ī´-ō-dōn). A contrast agent used like iodized oil (q.v.) in bronchography. Has the advantage of being eliminated more rapidly, but is more liable to cause coughing.

propylthiouracil (prō-pīl-thī-ō-ūr'-as-il). Inhibits thyroid activity, and is used in thyrotoxicosis as a less toxic alternative to methylthiouracil (q.v.).

proquanil (prō'-qwan-il). Antimalarial.

prostaglandins (pros-ta-glan'-dins). Share some of the properties of hormones, vitamins, enzymes and catalysts. All body tissues probably contain some p. Used to terminate early pregnancy, and prostaglandin therapy to all systems of the body is currently under investigation. Prostaglandin X (PGX) is a hormone generated in arterial walls; antithrombotic; relaxes arterial smooth muscle.

prostate (pros'-tāt) [L. *pro*, before; *stare*, to stand]. A small conical gland at the base of the male bladder and surrounding the first part of the urethra—**prostatic**, adj.

prostatectomy (pros-tat-ek'-to-mi) [L. *pro*, before; *stare*, to stand; G. *ektome*, excision]. Surgical removal of the prostate gland. **retropubic p.**, the prostate is reached through a lower abdominal (suprapubic) incision, the bladder being retracted upwards to expose the prostate behind the pubis. **transurethral p.**, the operation whereby shreds of prostatic tissue are cut from within the urethra using either a cold knife or electric cautery; usually restricted to small fibrous glands or to cases of prostatic carcinoma. **transvesical p.**, the operation in which the prostate is approached through the bladder, using a lower abdominal (suprapubic) incision. See RESECTOSCOPE

prostatism (pros'-tat-ism). General condition produced by hypertrophy or chronic disease of the prostate gland.

prostatitis (pros-ta-tī'-tis) [L. *pro*, before; *stare*, to stand; G. *-itis*, inflammation]. Inflammation of the prostate gland.

prostatocystitis (pros'-ta-tō-sis-tī'-tis)[L. *pro*, before; *stare*, to stand; G. *kystis*, bladder; *-itis*, inflammation]. Inflammation of the prostate gland and male urinary bladder.

prosthesis (pros'-thē-sis) [G. addition]. An artificial substitute for a missing part. **powered p.**, in electromyographic control, electrodes placed on opposing muscles transmit a signal to an electronic device which operates the prosthesis—**prostheses**, pl.; **prosthetic**, adj.

prosthetics (pros-thet'-iks) [G. *prosthetikos*, adding]. The branch of surgery which deals with prostheses.

prosthokeratoplasty (pros-thō-ke-ra-tō-plas'-ti) [G. *prosthetikos*, adding; *keras*, horn; *plassein*, to form]. Keratoplasty in which the corneal implant is of some material other than human or animal tissue.

Prostigmin (pros-tig'-min). Neostigmine (q.v.).

prostoglandins (pros-to-glan'-dins). Name given in 1935 to a factor in human semen which stimulated smooth muscle. Thirteen have now been isolated. Prostoglandins are secreted by a wide range of tissues and often act near the tissue producing them. They have therefore been described as 'local hormones'. They have an effect on the uterine musculature, varying with the type of prostoglandin and whether the uterus is gravid or not. Can be given by various routes—oral, intravenous, intrauterine and intra-amniotic.

protamine sulphate (prō'-ta-min-sul'-fāt). A protein of simple structure used as an antidote to heparin. One ml of 1 per cent solution will neutralize the effects of about 1000 units of heparin.

protamine zinc insulin (prō'-ta-min). An insoluble form of insulin, formed by combination with protamine (a simple protein) and a trace of zinc. It has an action lasting over 24 hours, and in association with initial doses of soluble insulin permits a wide degree of control.

protease (prō-tē'-āz). Any enzyme which digests protein: **proteolytic**, adj.

proteins (prō'-tē-inz). Highly complex, nitrogenous compounds, found in all animal and vegetable tissues. They are built up of amino acids and are essential for growth and repair of body. Those from animal sources are of high biological value since they contain the essential amino acids. Those from vegetable sources do not contain all, but some of the essential amino acids. Proteins are hydrolysed in the body to produce amino acids which are then used to build up new body proteins.

proteinuria (prō-tēn-ū'-ri-á) [G. *proteios*, primary]. Protein in the urine. Syn., albuminuria.

proteolysis (prō-tē-ol'-i-sis) [G. *proteios*, primary; *lysis*, a loosening]. The breaking down of proteins into simpler substances—**proteolytic**, adj.

proteose (prō'-tē-ōs) [G. *proteios,* primary]. The first cleavage product in the breakdown of proteins, intermediate between protein and peptone.

Proteus (prō'-tē-us) [L. *Proteus,* a Greek god who continually changed shape]. A bacterial genus. Gram-negative motile rods which swarm in culture. Found in damp surroundings. Sometimes a commensal of the intestinal tract. May be pathogenic, especially in wound and urinary tract infections as a secondary invader. Production of alkali turns infected urine alkaline.

prothionamide (prō-thī-on'-a-mīd). Synthetic antitubercular compound.

prothipendyl (prō-thī-pen'-dil). Antihistaminic, antiemetic and spasmolytic. Potentiates the effects of alcohol, analgesics, barbiturates and anaesthetics.

prothrombin (prō-throm'-bin). A precursor of thrombin formed in the liver. The p. time is a measure of its production and concentration in the blood. It is the time taken for plasma to clot after the addition of thrombokinase. It is inversely proportional to the amount of prothromin present, a normal person's plasma being used as a standard of comparison. Prothrombin time is lengthened in certain haemorrhagic conditions and in a patient on anticoagulant drugs.

protopathic (prō-tō-path'-ik) [G. *protos,* first; *pathos,* disease]. The term applied to a less sensibility, as opposed to epicritic (q.v.).

protoplasm (prō'-tō-plazm) [G. *protos,* first; *plasma,* anything formed]. The complex chemical compound constituting the main part of the tissue cells; it may be clear or granulated—protoplasmic, adj.

protozoa (prō-tō-zō'-á) [G. *protos,* first; *zoion,* living being]. The smallest type of animal life; unicellular organisms. See AMOEBA. The commonest protozoan infestation is *Trichomonas vaginalis*—protozoon, sing.; protozoal, adj.

protriptyline (prō-trip'-til-ēn). Antidepressant (q.v.).

proud flesh. Excessive granulation tissue.

provitamin (prō-vī'-ta-min) [L. *pro,* before; *vita,* life]. A vitamin precursor, e.g. carotene is converted into vitamin A.

proximal (proks'-im-al) [L. *proximus,* nearest]. Nearest to the head or source—proximally, adv.

prurigo (proo-rī'-gō) [L. itching]. A chronic, itching disease occurring most frequently in children. **prurigo aestivale,** hydroa aestivale (q.v.). **Besnier's p.,** an inherited flexural neurodermatitis with impaired peripheral circulation giving rise to dry thickened epidermis and outbreaks of eczema in childhood. Sometimes referred to as the atopic syndrome. See ECZEMA. **prurigo ferox,** a severe form. **prurigo mitis,** a mild form. **purigo nodularis,** a rare disease of the adult female in which intensely pruritic, pea-sized nodules occur on the arms and legs.

pruritus (proo-rī'-tus) [L.]. Itching. Pruritus ani and p. vulvae are considered to be psychosomatic conditions (neurodermatitis) except in the few cases where a local cause can be found, e.g. worm infestation, vaginitis, Generalized p. may be a symptom of systemic disease as in diabetes, icterus, Hodgkin's disease, carcinoma, etc. It may be psychogenic, e.g. widow's itch (q.v.)—pruritic, adj.

prussic acid (prus'-ik as'-id). A 4 per cent solution of hydrogen cyanide. Both the solution and its vapour are poisonous, and death may occur very rapidly from respiratory paralysis. Prompt treatment with intravenous injections of sodium nitrite and sodium thiosulphate may be life-saving.

pseudoangina (sū-dō-an-jī'-ná) [G. *pseudo,* false; L. *angina,* quinsy]. False angina. Sometimes referred to as 'left mammary pain', it occurs in anxious individuals. Usually there is no cardiac disease present. May be part of effort syndrome (q.v.).

pseudoarthrosis (sū-dō-árth-rō'-sis) [G. *pseudo,* false; *arthron,* joint; *-osis,* condition]. A false joint, e.g. due to ununited fracture; also congenital, e.g. in tibia.

pseudocholinesterase (soo-dō-kol-in-es'-ter-āz). A genetically inherited enzyme present in plasma and tissues (other than nerve tissue) and is synthesized in the liver. See SUXAMETHONIUM.

pseudocoxalgia (sū-dō-koks-al'-ji-á) [G. *pseudo,* false; L. *coxa,* hip; G. *algos,* pain]. See PERTHES' DISEASE.

pseudocrisis (sū-dō-krī'-sis) [G. *pseudo,* false; *krisis,* turning point]. A rapid reduction of body temperature resembling a crisis, followed by further fever.

pseudocyesis (sū-dō-sī-ē'-sis) [G. *pseudo,*

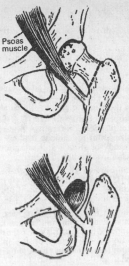

Pseudoarthrosis of hip

false; *kyesis,* pregnancy]. The existence of the signs and symptoms of pregnancy in a woman who believes that she is pregnant, when, in fact, this is not so.

pseudohermaphrodite (oū dō-her-maf-rō-dīt). A person in whom the gonads of one sex are present, whilst the external genitalia comprise those of the opposite sex.

pseudologia fantastica (sū-dō-loj'-i-á fan-tas'-ţi-ká). A constitutional tendency to tell, and defend, fantastic lies plausibly, found in some hysterics.

Pseudomonas (sū-dō-mon'-as) [G. *pseudo,* false; *monas,* unit]. A bacterial genus. Gram-negative motile rods. Found in water and decomposing vegetable matter. Some are pathogenic to plants and animals and *Pseudomonas pyocanea (aeruginosa)* is able to produce disease in men. Found commonly as a secondary invader in urinary tract infections and wound infections. Produces a blue pigment (pyocyanin) which colours the exudate or pus.

pseudomucin (sū-dō-mū'-sin) [G. *pseudo,* false; L. *mucus,* mucus]. A gelatinous substance (not mucin) found in some ovarian cysts.

pseudoparalysis (sū-dō-par-al'-i-sis) [G. *pseudo,* false; *paralysis,* paralysis]. See PSEUDOPLEGIA.

pseudo-Parkinsonism (sū-dō-park-in-son-izm). The signs and symptoms of paralysis (q.v.) agitans when they are not postencephalitic.

pseudoplegia (sū-dō-plē'-ji-á) [G. *pseudo,* false; *plege,* stroke]. Paralysis mimicking that of organic nervous disorder but usually hysterical in origin.

pseudopodia (sū-dō-pō'-di-á) [G. *pseudo,* false; *pous,* foot]. False legs; the projectile parts of an amoeba or amoeboid cell (leucocyte) which assist it in movement—pseudopodium, sing.

pseudopolyposis (sū-dō-pol-i-pōs'-is) [G. *pseudo,* false; *polypous,* many-footed; *-osis,* condition]. Widely scattered polypi, usually the result of previous inflammation—sometimes ulcerative colitis.

psittacosis (sit-a-kō'-sis) [G. *psittakos,* parrot; *-osis,* condition]. Disease of parrots, pigeons and budgerigars which is occasionally responsible for a form of pneumonia in man. Due to an organism (Bedsonia) resembling a virus. It behaves as a bacterium though multiplying intracellularly. Sensitive to sulphonamides and antibiotics.

psoas (sō'-as) [G.]. Muscles of the loin.

psoriasis (so-rī'-a-sis) [G.]. A chronic skin disease in which erythematous areas are covered with adherent scales. Although the condition may occur on any part of the body, the characteristic sites are extensor surfaces, especially over the knees and elbows. When the scales are scraped they produce a shiny, silver sheen which is diagnostic. Not infectious. Cause unknown. Psoriatic arthritis—articular symptoms similar to those of rheumatoid arthritis occur in 3 to 5 per cent of patients with psoriasis—psoriactic, adj.

Psoriderm (so-rī'-derm). Colourless preparation of lethicin and coal tar, especially for psoriasis.

psychiatry (sī-kī'-at-ri). The branch of medical study devoted to the diagnosis and treatment of mental illness—psychiatric, adj.

psychic (sī'-kik). Of the mind.

psychoanalysis (sī-kō-an-al'-i-sis). A specialized branch of psychiatry founded by Freud. It is a method of diagnosis and treatment of neuroses.

Briefly the method is to revive past forgotten emotional experiences and effect a cure of the neurosis by helping the patient readjust his attitudes to those experiences—psychoanalytic, adj.

psychochemotherapy (sī'-kō-kēm-ō-ther'-api). The use of drugs to improve or cure pathological changes in the emotional state—psychochemotherapeutic, adj.; psychochemotherapeutically, adv.

psychodrama (sī-kō-drá'-mà). A method of psychotherapy whereby patients act out their personal problems by taking roles in spontaneous dramatic performances. Group discussion aims at giving the patients a greater awareness of the problems presented and possible methods of dealing with them.

psychodynamics (sī-kō-dī-nam'-ikz) [G. *psyche*, mind; *dynamis*, power]. The science of the mental processes, especially of the causative factors in mental activity.

psychogenesis (sī-kō-jen'-e-sis) [G. *psyche*, mind; *genesis*, production]. The development of the mind.

psychogenic (sī-kō-jen'-ik) [G. *psyche*, soul; *genesis*, production]. Arising from the psyche or mind. **psychogenic symptom**, a neurotic symptom.

psychogeriatric (sī-kō-gē-ri-at'-rik) [G. *psyche*, mind; *geras*, old age; *iatrikos*, healing]. Psychology applied to geriatrics.

psychology (sī-kol'-o-ji) [G. *psyche*, mind; *logos*, discourse]. The study of the behaviour of an organism in its environment. Medically the study of human behaviour.

psychometric (sī-kō-met'-rik) [G. *psyche*, mind; *metron*, a measure]. Measurement of the duration and force of mental processes.

psychomotor (sī'-kō-mō'-ter) [G. *psyche*, mind; L. *movere*, to move]. Motor effect of psychic or cerebral activity.

psychoneurosis (sī-kō-nū-rō'-sis). Neurosis (q.v.).

psychopath (sī-kō-path) [G. *psyche*, mind; *pathos*, disease]. One who is morally irresponsible. See PERSONALITY—psychopathic, adj.

psychopathology (sī-kō-path-ol'-oj-i) [G. *psyche*, mind; *pathos*, disease; *logos*, discourse]. The pathology of abnormal mental processes—psycho-

pathological adj.; psychopathologically, adv.

psychopathy (sī-kōp'a-thi) [G. *psyche*, mind; *pathos*, disease]. Any disease of the mind. The term is used by some people to denote a marked immaturity in emotional development—psychopathic, adj.

psychopharmacology (sī-kō-far-ma-kol'-o-ji). The use of drugs which influence the affective and emotional state.

psychophysics (sī-kō-fiz'-iks) [G. *psyche*, mind; *physikos*, natural]. A branch of experimental psychology dealing with the study of stimuli and sensations—psychophysical, adj.

psychoprophylactic (sī-kō-prō-fil-ak'-tik) [G. *psyche*, mind; *prophylaxis*, a guarding]. That which aims at preventing mental disease.

psychosis (sī-kō'-sis) [G. giving life to]. A mental illness arising in the mind itself, as opposed to a neurosis where the mind is affected by factors arising in the environment—psychoses, pl.; psychotic, adj.

psychosomatic (sī-kō-sō-mat'-ik) [G. *psyche*, mind; *soma*, body]. Mind-body illness, illness where emotional factors produce physical symptoms. These arise mainly from overactivity of the autonomic nervous system which is influenced by the emotional state, e.g. chronic blushing may be due to feelings of guilt, the skin arterioles dilate as a result of autonomic overactivity, inflammation follows, death of some skin cells results in the development of a rash. The same 'blushing' can occur in the bowel; the p. process is the same, resulting in ulcerative colitis. Other p. conditions include hyperthyroidism, asthma, migraine, urticaria, hay-fever, peptic ulcer and several skin conditions.

psychosomimetic (sī-kō-sō-mim'-et-ik) [G. *psyche*, mind; *mimetikos*, imitative]. Drugs that produce psychosis-like symptoms. Hallucinogens. Also **psychotomimetic**.

psychotherapy (sī-kō-ther'-a-pi) [G. *psyche*, mind; *therapeia*, treatment]. Treatment of mental disorder, ranging from discussion, explanation, reassurance and psychoanalysis. **group p.**, a product of World War II when free discussion of 'effort syndrome' produced therapeutic results. At a meeting, the anxieties of staff and patients are discussed and everyone is enlisted in the treatment programme—psychothera-peutic, adj.

psychotropic (sī-kō-trō'-pik) [G. *psyche,* mind; *trepein,* to turn]. That which exerts its specific effect upon the brain cells.

psyllium (si'-li-um). The seeds of an Afri-can plant. They contain mucilage, which swells on contact with water; useful as a bulk-forming laxative.

pteroylglutamic acid (ter'-ō-il-gloo-tam'-ik as'-id). Folic acid (q.v.).

pterygium (te-rij'-ē-um) [G. a wing]. A degenerative condition of conjunctiva which encroaches on cornea—ptery-gial, adj.

ptosis (tō'-sis). A drooping, particularly that of the eyelid. See VISCEROPTO-SIS—ptotic, adj.

ptyalin (tī'u lin) [G. *ptyalon,* saliva]. Salivary amylase which is a slightly acid medium (pH 6.8) converts starch into dextrin and maltose.

ptyalism (tī'-a-lizm) [G. *ptyalon,* saliva]. Excessive salivation

ptyalolith (tī'-a-lo-lith) [G. *ptyalon,* saliva; *lithos,* stone]. Salivary calculus.

pubertas praecox (pū-bcr'-tas prē'-koks) [L.]. Premature (precocious) sexual development.

puberty (pū'-běr-ti) [L. *pubertas*]. The age at which the reproductive organs become functionally active. It is accom-panied by secondary characteristics—pubertal, adj.

pubes (pū'-bēz) [L. private parts]. 1. The hairy region covering the pubic bone. 2. Os pubis.

pubiotomy (pū-bi-ot'-o-mi) [L. *pubes,* private parts; G. *oktome, excision*]. Cutting the pubic bone to facilitate delivery of a live child.

pubis (pū'-bis) [N.L.]. The pubic bone or os pubis, forming the centre bone of the front of the pelvis—pubic, adj.

pudendal block. The rendering insensi-tive of the pudendum by the injection of local anaesthetic. Used mainly for episiotomy and forceps delivery. See TRANSVAGINAL.

pudendum (pū-den'-dum) [L. *pudere,* to be ashamed]. The external reproductive organs, especially of the female—pudenda, pl.; pudendal, adj.

Pudenz-Hayer valve. One-way valve implanted at operation for relief of hydrocephalus.

puerperal (pū-er'-pe-ral) [L. *puerperus,* childbearing]. Pertaining to childbirth. **puerperal sepsis,** infection of the genital tract occurring within 21 days of abor-tion or childbirth.

puerperium (pū-cr-pē'-ri-um) [L. *puer-perus,* childbearing]. The period imme-diately following childbirth to the time when involution is completed, usually 6 to 8 weeks—puerperia, pl.

pulmoflator (pul'-mo-flā-tor). Appara-tus for inflation of lungs.

pulmonary (pul'-mon-ar-ri) [L. *pulmon-arius*]. Pertaining to the lungs. **pulmon-ary distress syndrome,** see RESPIRATORY DISTRESS SYNDROME.

pulp [L. *pulpa*]. The soft, interior part of some organs and structures. **dental p.,** found in the p. cavity of teeth; carries blood, nerve and lymph vessels. **digital p.,** the tissue pad of the finger tip. Infection of this is referred to as 'p. space infection'.

pulsatile (pul'-sa-tīl) [L. *pulsare,* to beat]. Beating, throbbing.

pulsation (pul on' shun) [L. *pulsure, to* beat]. Beating or throbbing, as of the heart or arteries.

pulse [L. *pulsus,* a striking]. The impulse transmitted to arteries by contraction of the left ventricle, and customarily pal-pated in the radial artery at the wrist. The p. rate is the number of beats or impulses per minute and is about 130 in the newborn infant, 70 to 80 in the adult and 60 to 70 in old age. The p. rhythm is its regularity—can be regular or irregu-lar; the p. volume is the amplitude of expansion of the arterial wall during the passage of the wave; the p. force or tension is its strength, estimated by the force needed to obliterate it by pressure of the finger. **bounding p.,** one of large volume and force. **collapsing p.** (Corri-gan's p.), the water-hammer p. of aortic incompetence with high initial upthrust, which quickly falls away. **pulse deficit,** the difference in rate of the heart (counted by stethoscope) and the pulse (counted at the wrist). It occurs when some of the ventricular contrac-tions are too weak to open the aortic valve and hence produce a beat at the heart but not at the wrist. **pulse pressure** is the difference between the systolic and diastolic pressures. **soft p.,** one of low tension. **thready p.,** a weak, usually rapid and scarcely perceptible pulse. See BEAT.

'pulseless' disease. Progressive obliterative arteritis of the vessels arising from the aortic arch resulting in diminished or absent pulse in the neck and arms. Thromboendarterectomy or a bypass procedure may prevent blindness by improving the carotid blood-flow at its commencement in the aortic arch.

pulsus alternans (pul'-sus awl-ter'-nans). A regular pulse with alternate beats of weak and strong amplitude and of ominous import.

pulsus bigeminus (pul'-sus bī-jem'-in-us). Double pulse wave produced by interpolation of extrasystoles. A coupled beat. A heart rhythm (usually due to excessive digitalis administration) of paired beats, each pair being followed by a prolonged pause. The second weaker beat of each pair may not be strong enough to open the aortic valve, in which case it does not produce a pulse beat and the type of rhythm can then only be detected by listening at the heart.

pulsus paradoxus (pul'-sus pa-ra-doks'-us). Alteration of the volume of the pulse sometimes found, for example, in disease of the pericardium. The volume becomes greater with expiration, which is the reverse of the usual.

pulvis (pul'-vis) [L.]. A powder.

punctate (pungk'-tāt) [L. *punctum,* point]. Dotted or spotted, e.g. punctate basophilia describes the immature red cell in which there are droplets of blue-staining material in the cytoplasm—punctum, n.; puncta, pl.

puncture (pungk'-tūr) [L. *punctura,* prick]. A stab; a wound made with a sharp pointed hollow instrument for withdrawal or injection of fluid or other substance. **cisternal p.,** insertion of a special hollow needle with stylet through the atlanto-occipital ligament between the occiput and atlas, into the

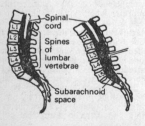

Spinal cord

Spines of lumbar vertebrae

Subarachnoid space

Diagram of lumbar vertebrae

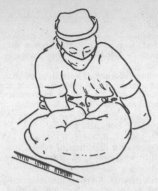

Position for lumbar puncture

cisterna magna. One method of obtaining cerebrospinal fluid. **lumbar p.,** insertion of a special hollow needle with stylet either through the space between the third and fourth lumbar vertebrae or, lower, into the subarachnoid space to obtain cerebrospinal fluid. **splenic p.,** injection of radio-opaque medium prior to portogram. **sternal p.,** insertion of a special guarded hollow needle with stylet into the body of the sternum for aspiration of a bone marrow sample. **ventricular p.,** a highly skilled method of puncturing a cerebral ventricle for a sample of cerebrospinal fluid.

pupil (pū-pil) [L. *pupilla,* pupil of eye]. The opening in the centre of the iris of the eye to allow the passage of light—pupillary, adj. .

pupillary (pū-pil'-a-ri). Pertaining to the pupil.

purgative (pur'-jat-iv). A drug causing evacuation of fluid faeces. **drastic p.,** even more severe in action, when the fluid faeces may be passed involuntarily.

purin(e)s (pū-rinz). Constituents of nucleoproteins from which uric acid is derived. Gout is thought to be associated with the disturbed metabolism and excretion of uric acid, and foods of high purine content are excluded in its treatment.

Puri-Nethol. Mercaptopurine (q.v.).

puromycin (pū-rō-mī'-sin). Antibiotic cytotoxic agent that inhibits protein formation in cells.

purpura (pur'-pū-rá) [L. purple]. A disorder characterized by spontaneous extravasation of blood from the capillaries into the skin, or into or from the mucous membranes. Manifest either by small red spots (petechiae) or large plaques (ecchymoses) or by oozing, the latter, in the absence of trauma, being confined to the mucous membranes. It is believed that the disorder can be due to impaired function of the capillary walls, or to defective quality or quantity of the blood platelets, and can be caused by many different conditions, e.g. infective, toxic allergic, etc. See SCHÖNLEIN'S DISEASE. **anaphylactoid p.,** excessive reaction between antigen and the protein globulin IgG (antibody). Antigen often unknown, but may be beta-haemolytic streptococci, or drugs such as sulphonamides may interact chemically with body proteins creating substances called haptens which are antigenic. **purpura haemorrhagica** (thrombocytopenic p) is characterized by a greatly diminished platelet count. The clotting time is normal but the bleeding time is prolonged. **Henoch's p.,** a disorder mainly affecting children; characterized by purpuric bleeding into and from the wall of the gut, resulting in abdominal colic and melaena. Skin purpura and fleeting joint pains may or may not be present. Recurrences are common. [Edward Henoch, German paediatrician, 1820–1910.]

purulent (pū-rū-lent) [L. *purulentus*]. Pertaining to or resembling pus.

pus [L.]. A liquid, usually yellowish in colour, formed in certain infections and composed of tissue fluid containing bacteria and leucocytes. Various types of bacteria are associated with pus having distinctive features, e g the faecal smell of p. due to *Bacterium coli;* the green colour of p. due to *Pseudomonas pyocyanea.*

pustule (pus'-tūl) [L. *pustula,* blister]. A small inflammatory swelling containing pus—pustular, adj. **malignant p.,** anthrax (q.v.).

putrefaction (pūt-ri-fak'-shun) [L. *putrefacere,* to rot]. The process of rotting; the destruction of organic material by bacteria—putrefactive, adj.

putrescible (pū-tres'-ib-l). Capable of undergoing putrefaction.

pyaemia (pī-ē'-mi-à) [G. *pyon,* pus; *haima,* blood]. A grave form of septicaemia (q.v.) in which blood-borne bacteria lodge and grow in distant organs, e.g. brain, kidneys, lungs, heart, to form multiple abscesses—pyaemic, adj.

pyarthrosis (pī-àrth-rō'-sis) [G. *pyon,* pus; *arthron,* joint; *-osis,* condition]. Pus in a joint cavity.

Pycazide (pik'-a-zīd). Isoniazid (q.v.).

pyelitis (pī-e-lī'-tis) [G. *pyelos,* trough; *-itis,* inflammation]. Mild form of pyelonephritis (q.v.) with pyuria but minimal involvement of renal tissue. Pyelitis on the right side is a common complication of pregnancy.

pyelography (pī-el-og'-raf-i) [G. *pylos,* trough; *graphein,* to write]. Radiographic visualization of the renal pelvis and ureter by injection of a radio-opaque liquid. The liquid may be injected into the blood stream whence it is excreted by the kidney (intravenous p.) or it may be injected directly into the renal pelvis or ureter by way of a fine catheter introduced through a cystoscope (retrograde or ascending p.)—pyelogram, n.; pyelographic, adj.; pyelographically, adv.

pyelolithotomy (pi-el-ō-lith-ot'-om-i) [G. *pyelos,* a trough; *lithos,* stone; *tome,* a cutting]. The operation for removal of a stone from the renal pelvis.

pyelonephritis (pī-e-lō-nef-rī'-tis) [G. *pyelos,* trough; *nephros,* kidney; *-itis,* inflammation]. A form of renal infection which spreads outwards from the pelvis to the cortex of the kidney. The origin of the infection is usually from the ureter and below, or from the blood stream—pyelonephritic, adj.

pyeloplasty (pī-el-ō-plas'-ti). A plastic operation on the kidney pelvis. See HYDRONEPHROSIS.

pyelostomy (pī-el-os'-to-mi) [G. *pyelos,* trough; *stoma,* mouth]. Surgical formation of an opening into the kidney pelvis.

pyknic (pik'-nik). See KRETSCHMER'S PERSONALITY TYPES.

pyknolepsy (pik'-nō-lep-si) [G. *pyknos,* thick; *lepsis,* a seizure]. A frequently recurring form of petit mal epilepsy seen in children. Attacks may number a hundred or more in a day.

pylephlebitis (pī-lē-fle-bī'-tis) [G. *pyle,* gate; *phelps,* vien; *-itis,* inflammation]. Inflammation of the veins of the portal system secondary to intra-abdominal sepsis.

pylethrombosis (pī-lē-throm-bō'-sis) [G.

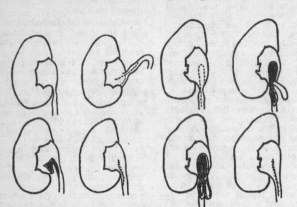

FOLEY P., narrowed segment of kidney pelvis widened by a Y-V procedure

CULP/P., pelvic-ureteric junction and upper ureter incised, narrowed segment then widened by inserting the pelvic flap into ureteric incision

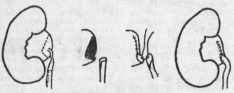

HYNES-ANDERSON P., abnormal part of ureter and adjacent pelvis excised. Enough pelvis may be removed to give appropriate reduction in size, and pelvi-ureteric junction widened with oblique anastomosis

Types of pyeloplasty

r.le, gate; *thrombos,* clot; *-osis,* condition]. Intravascular blood clot in portal vein or any of its branches.

pyloric stenosis (pī-lor'-ik sten-ō'-sis)[G. *pylouros,* gatekeeper; *stenosis,* a being straitened]. 1. Narrowing of the pylorus due to scar tissue formed during the healing of a duodenal ulcer. 2. Congenital hypertrophic p. s., due to a thickened pyloric sphincter muscle. See RAMSTEDT'S OPERATION.

pyloroduodenal (pī-lor-ō-dū-ō-dēn'-al). Pertaining to the pyloric sphincter and the duodenum.

pyloromyotomy (pī-lor-ō-mī-ot'-o-mi) [G. *pylouros,* gatekeeper; *mys,* muscle; *tome,* cutting]. Incision of pyloric sphincter muscle as in pyloroplasty and Ramstedt's operation.

pyloroplasty (pī-lor-ō-plas'-ti)[G.*pylouros,* gatekeeper; *plassein,* to form]. A plastic operation on the pylorus designed to widen the passage.

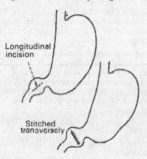

Pyloroplasty

Longitudinal incision

Stitched transversely

pylorospasm (pī-lor'-ō-spazm) [G. *pylouros,* gatekeeper; *spasmos,* spasm]. Spasm of the pyloric muscle; usually due to the presence of a duodenal ulcer.

pylorus (pī-lō'-rus) [G. *pylouros,* gatekeeper]. The opening of the stomach into the duodenum, encircled by a sphincter muscle—pyloric, adj.

Pylostrophin (pī-los-trō'-fin). Thin gelatin discs containing 1/750th g atropine methonitrate, and used in the treatment of pylorospasm in infants.

pyocolpos (pī-ō-kol'-pos). Pus in the vagina.

pyodermia: pyoderma (pī-ō-der'-má)[G. *pyon,* pus; *derma,* skin]. Chronic cellulitis of the skin, manifesting itself in granulation tissue, ulceration, colliqua-

tive necrosis or vegetative lesions—pyodermic, adj.

pyogenic (pī-ō-jen'-ik) [G. *pyon,* pus; *genesis,* production]. Pertaining to the formation of pus.

pyometra (pī-o-met'-ra) [G. *pyon,* pus; *metra,* uterus]. Pus retained in the uterus and unable to escape through the cervix, due to malignancy or atresia—pyometric, adj.

pyonephrosis (pī-ō-nef-rō'-sis) [G.*pyon,* pus; *nephros,* kidney; *-osis,* condition]. Distension of the renal pelvis with pus—pyonephrotic, adj.

Pyopen (pī'-ō-pen). Carbenicillin (q.v.).

pyopericarditis (pī-o-pe-ri-kárd-ī'-tis) [G. *pyon,* pus; *peri,* around; *kardia,* heart; *-itis,* inflammation]. Pericarditis with purulent effusion.

pyopneumothorax (pī-ō-nū-mō-thor'-aks) [G. *pyon,* pus; *pneuma,* breath; *thorax,* thorax]. Pus and gas or air within the pleural sac.

pyorrhoea (pī-or-rē'-á) [G. *pyon,* pus; *rheein,* to flow]. A flow of pus, usually referring to that from teeth sockets, p. alveolaris.

pyosalpinx (pī-ō-sal'-pingks) [G. *pyon,* pus; *salpigx,* trumpet]. A Fallopian tube containing pus.

pyothorax (pī-ō-thor'-aks) [G. *pyon,* pus; *thorax,* thorax]. Pus in the pleural cavity.

pyramidal (pi-ram'-id-al) [G. *pyramis,* pyramid]. Applied to some conical-shaped eminences in the body. **pyramidal cells,** nerve cells in the pre-Rolandic area of the cerebral cortex, from which originate impulses to voluntary muscles. **pyramidal tracts in the brain and spinal cord** transmit the fibres arising from the p. cells.

pyrazinamide (pir-az-in'-a-mīd). Expensive, oral, antituberculosis drug. Hepatotoxicity guarded against by SGOT tests twice weekly. Can produce gastrointestinal side effects.

pyrexia (pī-rek'-si-á) [G. *pyressein,* to be feverish]. Fever; elevation of the body temperature above normal—pyrexial, adj.

Pyridium (pir-id'-i-um). Phenazopyridine hydrochloride (q.v.).

pyridostigmine (pi-ri-dos-tig'-min). Inhibits breakdown of acetylcholine at neuromuscular junctions. Used in myasthenia gravis. Less toxic and potent, and has more prolonged action than neostigmine.

pyridoxin(e) (pi-ri-doks'-in). Vitamin B₆, may be connected with the utilization of unsaturated fatty acids or the synthesis of fat from proteins. Deficiency may lead to dermatitis and neuritic pains. Used in nausea of pregnancy and radiation sickness, muscular dystrophy, pellagra, etc.

pyrimethamine (pi-ri-meth'-a-min). A powerful antimalarial widely used in prophylaxis. Suitable for administration to children.

pyrogen (pī'-rō-jen) [G. *pyr*, fire]. A substance capable of producing a pyrexia—pyrogenic, adj.

Pyroscan (pī'-rō-skan). An apparatus for thermography (q.v.). Used as a screening procedure for breast cancer.

pyrosis (pī-rō'-sis) [G. firing]. Heartburn; water-brash. Eructation of acid gastric contents into the mouth, accompanied by a burning sensation felt behind the sternum.

pyrotherapy (pī-rō-ther'-a-pi). Production of fever by artificial means. See MALARIAL THERAPY.

pyuria (pī-ūr'-i-á) [G. *pyon*, pus; *ouron*, urine]. Pus in the urine (more than 3 leucocytes per high-power field)—pyuric, adj.

Q

Quellada (qwel'-ad-á). Gammabenzene hexachloride (q.v.). Less irritant, devoid of odour and requiring only one application.

Q-fever. Febrile disease caused by *Coxiella burnetti*. Human infection transmitted from sheep and cattle in which the organism does not produce symptoms. Pasteurization of milk kills the *C. burnetti*.

quadriceps (kwod'-ri-seps) [L. *quattuor*, four; *caput*, head]. The q. extensor femoris muscle of the thigh which possesses four heads.

quadriplegia (kwod-ri-plē-ji-á) [L. *quattuor*, four; *plege*, stroke]. Paralysis of all four limbs.

quadruple vaccine (kwod-rū'-pl). A vaccine for immunization against diphtheria, pertussis, poliomyelitis and tetanus.

qualitative (kwol'-i-tat-ēv). Pertaining to quality.

quantitative (kwon'-ti-tat-ēv). Pertaining to quantity.

quarantine (kwawr'-an-tēn). Period of isolation of infected or suspected people with the objective of preventing spread to others. For contacts it is usually the same period as the longest incubation period for the specific disease.

quartan (kwawr'-tan) [L. *quartus*, fourth]. The term applied to intermittent fever with paroxysms occurring every 72 hours.

Queckenstedt's test (kvek'-en-stets). Performed during lumbar puncture. Compression on internal jugular vein produces a rise in CSF pressure, if there is no obstruction to circulation of fluid in the spinal region. [Hans Queckenstedt, German physician, d. 1918.]

Questran (kwes'-tran). Lemon-flavoured cholestyramine (q.v.).

'quickening.' The first perceptible fetal movements felt by the mother, usually at 16 to 18 weeks gestation.

quicklime. Calcium oxide.

quicksilver. Mercury.

quiescent (kwī-es'-ent) [L. *quiescere*, to become still]. Becoming quiet. Used especially of a skin disease, which is settling under treatment.

quinalbarbitone (kwin-al-bár'-bit-ōn). A short-acting barbiturate with the general properties of the group, used in mild insomnia and anxiety conditions. Useful as 'night cap' for those with ischaemic limbs as it produces vasodilation.

quinethazone (qwin-eth'-az-ōn). Thiazide diuretic. See CHLOROTHIAZIDE.

quinestrol (kwin-es'-trol). Suppresses lactation.

quinidine (kwin-i-din). An alkaloid similar to quinine, but with a specific effect on the atrial muscle of the heart. Used in early atrial fibrillation, but only about 50 per cent of patients respond. Therapy should not be continued for more than 10 days unless adequate response has been obtained.

quinine (kwin-ēn). The chief alkaloid of cinchona, once the standard treatment for malaria. For routine use and prophylaxis, synthetic antimalarials such as mepacrine, proguanil and pyrimethamine are now preferred. The drug also has some oxytocic action and has been employed as a uterine stimulant in labour. **quinine urethane,** sclerosing agent used for injection treatment of varicose veins. The main use is in management, of 'night cramps' where it is given as 300–600 mg of bisulphate.

quininism (kwin'-in-izm). Headache, noises in the ears and partial deafness, disturbed vision and nausea arising from an idiosyncrasy to, or long-continued use of quinine.

quinsy (kwin'-zi). Acute inflammation of the tonsil and surrounding loose tissue, with abcess formation. Peritonsillar abscess.

quotient (kwō'-shent). A number obtained by division. **intelligence q., IQ**, see INTELLIGENCE. **respiratory q.**, the ratio between inspired oxygen and expired carbon dioxide during a specified time.

R

rabid (rā'-bid) Infected with rabies (q.v.).

rabies (rā'-bēz) [L. madness]. Hydrophobia (q.v.) Fatal infection in man caused by a virus; infection follows the bite of a rabid animal, e.g. dog, cat, fox, vampire bat. Worldwide distribution; vaccines available—rabid, adj.

racemose (ras'-i-mōs) [L. *racemus*, clusters]. Resembling a bunch of grapes.

radical (rad'-ik-al) [L. *radix*, root]. Pertaining to the root of a thing. **radical operation**, usually extensive so that it is curative, not palliative.

radioactive (rā-di-ō-ak'-tiv). Giving off penetrating rays due to spontaneous breaking up of atoms. **radioactive gold**, used for investigation of liver disease. **radioactive iodine**, see IODINE. **radioactive mercury**, used for investigation of brain lesions. **radioactive technetium**, used for investigation of visceral lesions.

radiobiology (rā-di-ō-bī-ol'-oj-i) [L. *radius*, ray; G. *bios*, life; *logos*, discourse]. The study of the effects of radiation on living tissue—radiobiological, adj.; radiobiologically, adv.

radiocaesium (rā-di-ō-kē'-zi-um). A radioactive form of the element caesium used in radiation treatment of disease.

radiocarbon (rā-di-ō-kár'-bon). A radioactive form of the element carbon used for research into metabolism, etc.

radiograph (rā'-di-ō-graf)[L.*radius*,ray; G. *graphein*, to write]. The finished X-ray picture—radiographic, adj.

radiographer (rā-di-og'-ra-fèr). X-ray technician.

radiography (rā-di-og'-ra-fi) [L. *radius*, ray; G. *graphein*, to write]. The making of radiographs.

radioiodinated human serum albumin. Used for detection and localization of brain lesions, determination of blood and plasma volumes, circulation time and cardiac output.

radioisotope (rā-di-ō-ī'-sō-tōp) [L. *radius*, ray; G. *isos*, equal; *topos*, place]. An element which has the same atomic number as another but a different atomic weight, exhibiting the property of spontaneous decomposition. When fed or injected can be traced by a Geiger-Müller counter. **radioisotope scan**, pictorial representation of the distribution and amount of radioactive isotope present.

radiokymogram (rā-di-ō-kī'-mō-gram) [L. *radius*, ray; G. *kyma*, wave; *gramma*, letter]. A graphic record of movement of the silhouette of a part of the body.

radiologist (rā-di-ol'-oj-ist). Specialist in X-ray diagnosis.

radiology (rā-di-ol'-o-ji) [L. *radius*, ray; G. *logos*, discourse]. The study of the diagnosis of disease by the use of X-rays—radiological, adj.; radiologically, adv.

radiomimetic (rā-di-ō-mim-et'-ik) [L. *radius*, ray; G. *mimetikos*, imitative]. Produces effects similar to those of radiotherapy. See CYTOTOXIC.

radiosensitive (rā-di-ō-sen'-sit-iv). Affected by X-rays. Applied to tumours, curable by X-rays.

Radiostoleum (rā-di-ō-stō'-le-um). A solution of vitamins A and D (calciferol).

radiotherapist (rā-di-ō-ther'-ap-ist). Specialist in the treatment of disease by X-rays.

radiotherapy (rā-di-ō-ther'-a-pi) [L. *radius*, ray; G. *therapeia*, treatment]. The treatment of disease by X-rays and other forms of radiation. **endolymphatic r.**, adaptation of diagnostic lymphography, a method of introducing a radioactive substance into lymphatic channels and nodes in order to irradiate and thereby destroy malignant cells.

radium (rā'-di-um). A radioactive element occurring in nature, and used in radiotherapy.

radon seeds (rā'-don-sēds). Capsules containing radon—a radioactive gas produced by the breaking up of radium atoms. Used in radiotherapy.

râle (rál)[F.]. Abnormal sound heard on

auscultation of lungs when fluid is present in bronchi.

Ramstedt's operation. An operation to relieve pyloric stenosis in infants by dividing the pyloric muscle, leaving the mucous lining intact. [Conrad Ramstedt, Emeritus Chief Surgeon, Rafael Clinic, Münster, 1867– .]

ranula (ran'-ū-lá) [L. frog]. A cystic swelling beneath the tongue—ranular, adj.

raphe (raf'-ē) [G. *rhaphe*, seam]. A seam, suture, ridge or crease; the median furrow on the dorsal surface of the tongue.

Rapitard (rap'-i-tard) (Crystal II) Bovine insulin 3 parts in Actrapid (q.v.) 1 part at pH 7.

rarefaction (rā-ri-fak'-shun) [L. *rarefacere*, to make thin]. Becoming less dense, as applied to diseased bone.

rash. Skin eruption. **nettle r.**, urticaria, formation of weals on the skin.

Rashkind's septostomy. When the pulmonary and systemic circulations do not communicate, an artificial atrial septal communication is produced by passing an inflatable balloon-ended catheter through the foramen ovale, filling the balloon with contrast media and pulling it back into the right atrium.

Rastinon (ras'-tin-on). Tolbutamide (q.v.).

rat-bite fever. A relapsing fever caused by *a Spirillum minus* or by *Streptobacillus moniliformis*. The blood Wassermann test is positive in the spirillary infection.

rationalization (rash-on-al-ī-zā'-shun) [L. *rationalis*, reasonable]. A mental process whereby a person explains his behaviour by substituting an unconscious excuse that is more acceptable than the truth, both to himself and to others. The excuse must be acceptable enough for self-deception and he feels completely justified.

rauwolfia (rau-wol'-fi-á). The root of an Indian plant. It is used in hypertension and as a central depressant, but the action of the drug is slow, and time is required before full response is achieved. Used mainly as the alkaloid reserpine (q.v.). Has tranquillizing property but in susceptible subjects can cause profound depression.

Raynaud's disease (rā'-nō). Idiopathic trophoneurosis. Paroxysmal spasm of the digital arteries producing pallor or cyanosis of fingers or toes, and occa-

sionally resulting in gangrene. Disease of young women. [Maurice Raynaud, French physician, 1834–81.]

RDS. Respiratory distress syndrome (q.v.).

reaction (rē-ak'-shun). 1. Response to a stimulus. 2. A chemical change, e.g. acid or alkaline reaction to litmus paper. **allergic r.** (see SENSITIZATION) is a hypersensitivity disorder to certain proteins to which the patient is brought into contact through the medium of his skin, his digestive or respiratory tract, resulting in eczema, urticaria, hay fever, etc. Inheritance and emotion contribute to the allergic tendency. The basis of the condition is probably a local antigen-antibody reaction.

reagent (rē-ā'-jent). An agent capable of producing a chemical reaction.

reagin (rē'-ag-in). An antibody associated with allergic reactions. Present in the serum of naturally hypersensitive people.

rebore. Disobliteration (q.v.).

recalcitrant (rē-kal'-si-trant) [L. *re*, again; *calcitrare*, to kick against the prick]. Refractory. Describes medical conditions which are resistant to treatment.

recall (rē-kawl'). Part of the process of memory. Memory consists of memorizing retention and recall.

recannulation (rē-kan-ū-lā'-shun). Re-establishment of patency of a vessel.

receptaculum (rē-sep-tak'-ū-lum) [L. receptacle]. Receptacle, often acting as a reservoir. **receptaculum chyli,** the pear-shaped commencement of the thoracic duct in front of the first lumbar vertebra. It receives digested fat from the intestine.

receptor (rē-sep'-tor) [L. *recipere*, to receive]. Sensory afferent nerve endings capable of receiving and transmitting stimuli.

recessive (rē-ses'-iv) [L. *ecessio*, withdrawn]. Receding; having a tendency to disappear. **recessive trait,** an inherited characteristic which remains latent when paired with a dominant trait in selective mating. See MENDEL'S LAW.

recipient. See BLOOD GROUPS.

Recklinghausen's disease (rek'-ling-howz-en). Name given to two conditions: (1) osteitis fibrosa cystica—the result of overactivity of the parathyroid glands (hyperparathyroidism) resulting in decalcification of bones and formation of cysts; (2) multiple neurofibromatosis—a skin disease in which tumours of all sizes appear on the skin all over the body. [Friedrich Daniel von Recklinghausen, German pathologist, 1839–1910.]

recliners reflux syndrome. This is due to severe disturbance of the antireflux mechanism which allows stomach contents to leak at any time whatever position the patient is in, although it is most likely to happen when the patient lies down or slumps in a low chair.

recrudescence (rē-kroo-des′-ens) [L. *recrudescere*, to become raw again]. The return of symptoms.

rectocele (rek′-tō-sēl) [L. *rectus*, straight; G. *kele*, hernia]. Prolapse (q.v.) of the rectum, so that it lies outside the anus. Cf. procidentia. Usually reserved for herniation of anterior rectal wall into posterior vaginal wall caused by injury to the levator muscles at childbirth. Repaired by a posterior colporrhaphy.

rectoscope (rek′-tō-skōp) [L. *rectus*, straight; G. *skopein*, to examine]. An instrument for examining the rectum. See ENDOSCOPE—rectoscopic, adj.

rectosigmoid (rek-tō-sig′-moid) [L. *rectus*, straight; *sigmoeides*, E shaped]. Pertaining to the rectum and sigmoid portion of colon.

rectosigmoidectomy (rek-tō-sig-moid-ek′-to-mi) [L. *rectus*, straight; G. *sigmoides*, E shaped; *ektome*, excision]. Surgical removal of the rectum and sigmoid colon.

rectouterine (rek-tō-ū′-ter-īn) [L. *rectus*, straight; *uterus*, womb]. Pertaining to the rectum and uterus.

rectovaginal (rek-tō-va-jī′-nal) [L. *rectus*, straight; *vagina*, sheath]. Pertaining to the rectum and vagina.

rectovesical (rek-tō-ve-sīk′-al) [L. *rectus*, straight; *vesica*, bladder]. Pertaining to the rectum and bladder.

rectum (rek′-tum) [L. *rectus*, straight]. The lower part of the large intestine between the sigmoid flexure and anal canal—rectal, adj.; rectally, adv.

recumbent (rē-kum′-bent) [L. *recumbere*, to recline]. Lying or reclining—recumbency, n.

red lotion. Contains zinc sulphate which acts as an astringent and assists granulation.

Redoxon (re-doks′-on). Ascorbic acid (q.v.).

Redul (red′-ul). One of the sulphonamidopyrimidines (q.v.).

referred pain. Pain occurring at a distance from its source, e.g. pain felt in the upper limbs from angina pectoris; that from the gall bladder felt in the scapular region.

reflex (rē′-fleks) [L. *reflexus*, bent back]. Reflected or thrown back. **accommodation r.**, constriction of the pupils and convergence of the eyes for near vision. **reflex action**, an involuntary motor or secretory response by tissue to a sensory stimulus, e.g. sneezing, blinking, coughing. The testing of various reflexes provides valuable information in the localization and diagnosis of diseases involving the nervous system. **conditioned r.**, a reaction acquired by repetition or practice. **corneal r.**, a reaction of blinking when the cornea is touched (often absent in hysterical conditions).

reflux (rē′-fluks) [L. *re*, back; a flow]. Backward flow.

refraction (rē-frak′-shun). The bending of light rays as they pass through media of different densities. In normal vision, the light rays are so bent that they meet on the retina—refractive, adj.

refractory (rē-frak′-tor-i). Resistent to treatment; stubborn, unmanageable; rebellious.

regeneration (rē-jen-er-ā′-shun) [L. *regenerare*, to beget again]. Renewal of tissue.

regression (rē-gre′-shun) [L. *regressio*, turn back]. In psychiatry, reversion to an earlier stage of development, becoming more childish. Occurs in dementia, especially senile dementia.

regurgitation (rē-gur-ji-tā′-shun) [L. *re*, back; *gurgitare*, to flood]. Backward flow, e.g. of stomach contents into, or through, the mouth.

rehabilitation. A planned programme in which the convalescent or disabled person progresses towards, or maintains, the maximum degree of physical and psychological independence of which he is capable.

Reiter's syndrome. A condition in which arthritis occurs together with conjunctivitis and urethritis (or cervicitis in women). It is commonly, but not always, a venereal infection and should be considered as a cause of knee effusion in young men when trauma has not occurred. [Hans Reiter, German physician, 1881–1969.]

relapsing fever. Louse-borne or tick-borne infection caused by spirochaetes of genus Borrelia. Prevalent in many parts of the world. Characterized by a febrile period of a week or so, with apparent recovery, followed by a further bout of fever.

relaxant (rē-laks'-ant) [L. *re*, again; *laxo*, to loosen]. That which reduces tension. See MUSCLE.

relaxin (rē-laks'-in). Polypeptides secreted by the ovaries to soften the cervix and loosen the ligaments in preparation for birth.

remission (rē-mi'-shun) [L. *remissio*, a sending back]. The period of abatement of a fever or other disease.

remittent (rē-mit'-ent) [L. *remittere*, to send back]. Increasing and decreasing at periodic intervals.

renal (rē'-nal) [L. *renalis*, of the kidney]. Pertaining to the kidney. **renal asthma**, hyperventilation of lungs occurring in uraemia as a result of acidosis. **renal calculus** (q.v.), stone in the kidney. **renal glycosuria** occurs in patients with a normal blood sugar and a lowered r. threshold for sugar. **renal rickets**, see RICKETS. **renal uraemia** is uraemia (q.v.) following kidney disease itself, in contrast to uraemia from failure of the circulation of the blood (extrarenal uraemia).

renin (rē'-nin). An enzyme, released into the blood from the kidney cortex and stimulated by sodium loss. A cause of hypertension in man. See ANGIOTENSIN, ALDOSTERONE.

Sodium loss
↓
Renin
↓
Angiotensin
↓
Aldosterone from adrenal cortex
↓
Prevents sodium loss

rennin (ren'-in). Milk curdling enzyme of gastric juice, converting soluble caseinogen into insoluble casein.

renogram (rē'-nō-gram) [L. *rena*, kidney; G. *gramma*, letter]. X-ray of renal shadow following injection of opaque medium, demonstrated in aortograph series. **isotope r.**, see TEST: RADIOISOTOPE RENOGRAM—renographical, adj.; renographically, adv.

reovirus (rē'-ō-virus). Respiratory enteric orphan virus (q.v.).

replogle tube. A double lumen aspiration catheter, attached to low pressure suction apparatus. It is kept patent by half hourly instillation of ½ ml of saline into the lumen not attached to suction.

repression (rē-presh'-un) [L. *repressum*, press back]. The refusal to recognize the existence of urges and feelings which are painful, or are in conflict with the individual's accepted moral principles. Freud called this refusal 'repression,' because the painful idea was repressed into the unconscious mind.

resection (rē-sek'-shun) [L. *resecare*, to cut off]. Surgical excision. **submucous r.**, incision of nasal mucosa, removal of deflected nasal septum, replacement of mucosa.

resectoscope (rē-sek'-tō-skōp) [L. *resecare*, to cut off; G. *skopein*, to examine]. An instrument passed along the urethra; it permits resection of tissue from the base of the bladder and prostate under direct vision. See PROSTATECTOMY.

resectotome (rē-sek'-to-tōm) [L. *resecare*, to cut off]. Instrument used for resection.

reserpine (rē-ser'-pin). The chief alkaloid of rauwolfia (q.v.). Used mainly in hypertension, sometimes with other drugs. Severe depression has occurred after full and prolonged therapy. Interferes with transmission in sympathetic adrenergic nerves, especially sympathetically mediated vascular reflexes and thus can lead to postural and exercise hypotension.

residual (rē-zid'-ū-al) [L. *residuus*, that is left behind]. Remaining. **residual air**, the air remaining in the lung after forced expiration. **residual urine**, urine remaining in the bladder after micturition.

resin (res'-in). A mixture of complex organic substances which can occur naturally or be manufactured synthetically. **ion exchange r.**, administered orally, acts on the gut to effect a change in plasma ions.

resistance (rē-zis'-tens) [L. *resistere*, to withstand]. Power of resisting. In psychology the name given to the force which prevents repressed thoughts from re-entering the conscious mind from the unconscious. **resistance to infection**, the power of the body to withstand infection. See IMMUNITY. **peripheral r.**, that offered by the capillaries to the blood passing through them.

Resochin (res'-ō-chin). Chloroquine (q.v.).

resolution (rez-ō-loo'-shun) [L. *resolvere*, to loosen]. The subsidence of inflammation; describes the earliest indications of a return to normal, as when, in lobar pneumonia, the consolidation begins to liquefy.

resonance (rez'-ō-nans) [L. *resonare*, to resound]. The musical quality elicited on percussing a cavity which contains air. **vocal r.** is the reverberating note heard through the stethoscope when the patient is asked to say 'one, one, one' or 'ninety-nine.'

Resonium (re-sō'-ni-um). A synthetic resin that can absorb potassium. Given in hyperkalaemic states, anuria, shock and other conditions of high potassium blood level.

resorcinol (re-zor'-sin-ol). A mild antiseptic derived from phenol. Used in hair lotions and antipruritic ointments. It should not be used for long periods on open surfaces.

resorption (rē-sorp'-shun) [L. *resorbere*, to drink in]. To absorb again, e.g. absorption of (1) callus following bone fracture, (2) roots of the deciduous teeth, (3) blood from a haematoma.

respiration (res-pi-rā'-shun) [L. *respirare*, to breathe]. The act or function of breathing. **abdominal r.**, the use of the diaphragm and abdominal muscles in breathing. **anaerobic r. result**, if the availability of oxygen to the fetus is limited, with the production of lactic and pyruvic acids, and a fall in the pH value of fetal blood; this can be measured in labour once the cervix has dilated, by taking a microsample of blood from the fetal scalp. **paradoxical r.**, during inspiration air drawn into unaffected lung via normal route and from lung on affected side, during expiration air forced from lung on unaffected side, some of which enters lung on affected side, resulting in inadequate oxygenation of blood; occurs when ribs are fractured in two places. **periodic r., (Cheyne Stokes r.)**, cyclical waxing and waning of respiration, characterized at the extremes by deep, fast breathing and by apnoea; it generally has an ominous prognosis. **tissue r.**, oxygen used by living cells to release the chemical energy that is stored in foodstuffs—respiratory, adj.

respirator (res'-pi-rā-tor)[L. *respirare*, to breathe again]. 1. An apparatus worn over the nose and mouth and designed to purify the air breathed through it. 2. An apparatus which artificially and rhythmically inflates and deflates the lungs as in normal breathing, when for any reason the natural nervous or muscular control of respiration is impaired. The apparatus may work on either positive or negative pressure or on electrical stimulation. **pump r.**, heart–lung machine by which the blood can be removed from a vein for oxygenation, after which it is returned to the vein.

respiratory distress syndrome. Dyspnoea in the newly born. Due to failure of secretion of protein–lipid complex (pulmonary surfactant) by type II pneumocytes in the tiny air spaces of the lung on first entry of air. Causes atelectasis. Formerly called hyaline membrane disease. Environmental temperature of 32–34º C (90–94 F), oxygen and infusion of sodium bicarbonate are used in treatment. Clinical features include severe retraction of chest wall with every breath, cyanosis, an increased respiratory rate and an expiratory grunt.

respiratory failure. A term used to den-

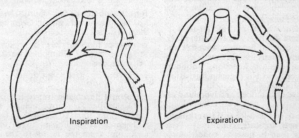

Paradoxical breathing

Inspiration   Expiration

ote failure of the lungs to oxygenate the blood adequately. **acute r.f.** denotes respiratory insufficiency secondary to an acute insult to the lung; hypoxaemia develops, frequently terminating in bronchopneumonia. **acute-on-chronic r.f.**, hypoxaemia resulting from chronic obstructive airways disease such as chronic bronchitis and emphysema.

respiratory syncytial virus. Causes severe respiratory infection with occasional fatalities in very young children. Infections are less severe in older children.

responaut. Person with permanent severe respiratory paralysis needing a mechanical device.

resuscitation (rē-sus′-i-tā-shun) [L. *resuscitare*, to revive]. Restoration to life of one who is apparently dead (collapsed or shocked). See CARDIAC. **expired air r.**, see KISS OF LIFE—resuscitation, n.; resuscitative, adj.

retching. Straining at vomiting.

retention (rē-ten′-shun) [L. *retinere*, to hold back]. 1. Retaining of facts in the mind. 2. Accumulation of that which is normally excreted. **retention of urine**, accumulation of urine within the bladder due to interference of nerve supply, obstruction or psychological factors.

reticular (re-tik′-ū-lar) [L. *reticulum*, little net]. Resembling a net.

reticulocyte (ret-ik′-ū-lō-sīt) [L. *reticulum*, little net; G. *kytos*, cell]. A young circulating red blood cell which still contains traces of the nucleus which was present in the cell when developing in the bone marrow.

reticulocytoma. See EWING'S TUMOUR.

reticulocytosis (ret-ik-ū-lō-sī-tō′-sis) [L. *reticulum*, little net; G. *kytos*, cell; -*osis*, condition]. An increase in the number of reticulocytes in the blood indicating active red blood cell formation in the marrow.

reticuloendothelial system (ret-ik′-ū-lō-end-oth-ē′-li-al). A widely scattered system of cells, of common ancestry and fulfilling many vital functions, e.g. defence against infection, antibody, blood cell and bile pigment formation, etc. Main sites of r.e. cells are bone marrow, spleen, liver and lymphoid tissue.

reticulosis (ret-ik-ū-lō′-sis) [L. *reticulum*, little net; G. -*osis*, condition]. Term loosely used to describe conditions in which there is a reaction of reticuloendothelial cells. **malignant r.**, neoplastic disorder affecting the reticuloendothelial system; now called malignant lymphoma—reticuloses, pl.

retina (ret′-i-na) [L. *rete*, net]. The light-sensitive internal coat of the eyeball, consisting of eight superimposed layers, seven of which are nervous and one pigmented. It is soft in consistency, translucent and of a pinkish colour—retinal, adj.

retinitis (ret-in-ī′-tis) [L. *rete*, net; G. -*itis* inflammation]. Inflammation of the retina. **retinitis pigmentosa**, a familial, degenerative condition which progresses to blindness.

retinoblastoma (ret-in-ō-blas-tō′-má) [L. *rete*, net; G. *blastos*, shoot; -*oma*, tumour]. A malignant tumour of the neuroglial element of the retina, occurring exclusively in children.

retinopathy (ret-in-op′-ath-i) [L. *rete*, net; G. *pathos*, disease]. Any non-inflammatory disease of the retina.

retinoscope (ret′-in-ō-skōp) [L. *rete*, ret; G. *skopein*, to examine]. Instrument for detection of refractive errors by illumination of retina using a mirror.

retinotoxic (ret-in-ō-toks′-ik). Usually applied to drugs which may damage the retina in some instances.

retractile (rē-trak′-tīl). Capable of being drawn back, i.e. retracted.

retractor (rē-trak′-tor). A surgical instrument for holding apart the edges of a wound to reveal underlying structures.

retrobulbar (ret-rō-bul′-bar) [L. *retro*, behind; *bulbus*, bulb]. Pertaining to the back of the eyeball. **retrobulbar neuritis**, inflammation of that portion of the optic nerve behind the eyeball.

retrocaecal (re-trō-sēk′-al) [L. *retro*, behind; *coecus*, blind]. Behind the caecum, e.g. a retrocaecal appendix.

retroflexion (ret-rō-flek′-shun). The state of being bent backwards. Opp., anteflexion.

retrograde (ret′-rō-grād) [L. *retrogradi*, to go backward]. Going backward. **retrograde pyelography** (q.v.).

retrogression (ret-rō-gresh′-un). See REGRESSION.

retrolental fibroplasia (ret-rō-len′-tal fi-brō-plāz′-i-á) [L. *retro*, behind; *lens*, lentil; *fibra*, fibre; G. *plassein*, to form]. The presence of fibrous tissue in the vitreous, from the retina to the lens, causing blindness. Noticed shortly after birth, more commonly in premature babies who have had continuous oxygen therapy.

retro-ocular (ret-rō-ok'-ū-lar) [L. *retro*, behind; *oculus*, eye]. Behind the eye.

retroperitoneal (re-trō-pe-ri-ton-ē'-al) [L. *retro*, behind; G. *peri*, around; *teinein*, to stretch]. Behind the peritoneum.

retropharyngeal (re-trō-far-in-jē'-al) [L. *retro*, behind; G. *pharygx*, pharynx]. Behind the pharynx.

retroplacental (re-trō-pla-sen'-tal) [L. *retro*, behind; *placenta*, a cake]. Behind the placenta.

retropleural (re-trō-plū'-ral) [L. *retro*, behind; G. *pleuro*, rib]. Behind the pleura.

retropubic (ret-rō-pū'-bik) [L. *retro*, behind; *pubes*, the private parts]. Behind the pubis.

retrospection (ret-rō-spek'-shun). Morbid dwelling on the past.

retrosternal (ret-rō-stėr'-nal) [L. *retro*, behind; G. *sternon*, breast]. Behind the breast bone.

retrotracheal (ret-rō-trak-ē'-al) [L. *retro*, behind; G. *trachus*, rough]. Behind the trachea.

retroversion (ret-rō-vėr'-shun) [L. *retro*, behind; G. *vertere*, to turn]. Turning backward. **retroversion of the uterus**, tilting of the whole of the uterus backward with the cervix pointing forward—retroverted, adj.

revascularization (rē-vas-kūl-ar-īz-ā'-shun) [L. *re*, again; *vasculum*, small vessel]. The regrowth of blood vessel into a tissue or organ after deprivation of its normal blood supply.

Reverin (rev'-er-in). Broad spectrum antibiotic of the tetracycline series. Of good local and general tolerance.

reverse barrier nursing. Every attempt is made to prevent carrying infection to the patient. Used for agranulocytosis and immunosuppressive treatment.

Rh. Rhesus factor. See BLOOD GROUPS.

rhagades (rag'-a-dēz) [G. *rhagas*, fissure]. Superficial elongated scars radiating from the nostrils or angles of the mouth and which are pathognomonic of congenital syphilis. See STIGMATA.

rhei (rē'-ī). Genitive of Rheum, i.e. rhubarb (q.v.).

Rheomacrodex (rē-ō-mak'-rō-deks). A low molecular weight dextran (q.v.). Antithrombotic. Used to prevent clots in grafted vein.

rhesus factor. See BLOOD GROUPS.

rheumatic (roo-mat'-ik) [G. *rheumatikos*, subject to a flux]. Pertaining to rheumatism. See CHOREA.

rheumatism (roo'-mat-izm) [G. *rheumatismos*, that which flows]. A non-specific term embracing a diverse group of diseases and syndromes which have in common, disorder or diseases of connective tissue and hence usually present with pain, or stiffness, or swelling of muscles and joints. The main groups are rheumatic fever, rheumatoid arthritis, ankylosing spondylitis, non-articular rheumatism, osteoarthritis and gout. **acute r.** (rheumatic fever), a disorder, tending to recur but initially commonest in childhood, classically presenting as fleeting polyarthritis of the larger joints, pyrexia and carditis within 3 weeks following a streptococcal throat infection. Atypically, but not infrequently, the symptoms are trivial and ignored, but carditis may be severe and result in permanent cardiac damage. **non-articular r.**, involves the soft tissues and includes fibrositis, lumbago, etc.

rheumatoid (roo'-mat-oid) [G. *rheuma*, stream; *eidos*, form]. Resembling rheumatism. **rheumatoid arthritis**, a disease of unknown aetiology, characterized by a chronic polyarthritis mainly affecting the smaller peripheral joints, accompanied by general ill health and resulting eventually in varying degrees of crippling joint deformities and associated muscle wasting. It is not just a disease of joints. Every system may be involved in some way. Many rheumatologists therefore prefer the term 'rheumatoid disease.' There is some question of it being an autoimmune process. **rheumatoid factors**. macro gamma-globulins found in most people with severe r. arthritis. They affect not only joints but lung and nerve tissues and small arteries. It is not yet known whether they are the cause of, or the result of, arthritis. See PNEUMOCONIOSIS and STILL'S DISEASE.

rheumatology (roo-mat-ol'-o-ji) [G. *theumatikos*, subject to a flux; *logos*, discourse]. The science or the study of rheumatic disease.

rhinitis (rī-nī'-tis) [G. *rhis*, nose; *-itis*, inflammation]. Inflammation of the nasal mucous membrane.

rhinology (rīn-ol'-o-ji) [G. *rhis*, nose; *logos*, discourse]. The study of diseases affecting the nose—rhinologist, n.

rhinophyma (rī-nō-fī'-må) [G. *rhis*, nose; *phyma*, tumour]. Nodular enlargement of skin of nose.

rhinoplasty (rī-nō-plas'-ti) [G. *rhis*, nose; *plassein*, to form]. Plastic surgery of the nose.

rhinorrhoea (rīn-or-ē'-å) [G. *rhis*, nose; *rheein*, to flow]. Nasal discharge.

rhinoscopy (rīn-os'-kop-i). Inspection of the nose using an instrument, a nasal speculum or a rhinoscope.

rhinosporidosis (rī-nō-spor-i-dō'-sis). A fungal condition affecting the mucosa of the nose, eyes, ears, larynx and occasionally the genitalia; characterized by persistent polypi.

Rhinosporidium (rī-nō-spor-id'-i-um) [G. *rhis*, nose; *spora*, seed]. A genus of fungi, parasitic to man.

rhinovirus (rī-nō-vī'-rus). There are about 100 different varieties which can cause the common cold.

rhizotomy (rī-zot'-o-mi) [G. *rhiza*, root; *tome*, a cutting]. Surgical division of a root; usually the posterior root of a spinal nerve. **chemical r.**, accomplished by injection of a chemical, often phenol.

rhodopsin (rō-dop'-sin) [G. *rhodon*, rose; *opsis*, vision]. The visual purple contained in the retinal rods. Its colour is preserved in darkness; bleached by daylight. Its formation is dependent on vitamin A.

rhomboid (rom'-boid) [G. *rhombos*, magic wheel; *eidos*, form]. Diamond shaped.

rhonchus (rong'-kus) [G. *rhogchos*, wheezing]. An adventitious sound heard on auscultation of the lung. Passage of air through bronchi obstructed by oedema or exudate produces a musical note. See SIBILUS.

rhubarb (roo'-barb). The dried root of Chinese Rheum officinale. It is purgative in large doses, astringent in small doses. Used in mist gent c rhei, etc.

riboflavine (rī-bō-flā'-vēn). A constituent of the vitamin B group. Given in Ménière's disease, angular stomatitis and a variety of other conditions.

ribonuclease (rī-bō-nū'-klē-āz). Enzyme that breaks down ribonucleic acid. Has been made synthetically.

ribonucleic acid. RNA. See DEOXYRIB-ONUCLEIC ACID.

ribosomes (rī'-bō-sōms). Submicroscopic protein-making agents inside all cells.

ribs. The twelve pairs of bones which articulate with the twelve dorsal vertebrae posteriorly and form the walls of the thorax. The upper seven pairs are **true r.** and are attached to the sternum anteriorly by costal cartilage. The remaining five pairs are the **false r.** The first three pairs of these do not have an attachment to the sternum but are bound to each other by costal cartilage. The lower two pairs are the **floating r.** which have no anterior articulation. **cervical r.** are formed by an extension of the transverse process of the seventh cervical vertebra in the form of bone or a fibrous tissue band; this causes an upward displacement of the subclavian artery. A congenital abnormality.

rice-water stool. The stool of cholera. The 'rice grains' are small pieces of desquamated epithelium from the intestine.

rickets (ri'-kets). A disorder of calcium and phosphorus metabolism associated with a deficiency of vitamin D, and beginning most often in infancy and early childhood between the ages of 6 months and 2 years. There is proliferation and deficient ossification of the growing epiphyses of bones, producing 'bossing,' softening and bending of the long weight-bearing bones, muscular hypotonia, head sweating and, if the blood calcium falls sufficiently, tetany. **fetal r.**, see ACHONDROPLASIA. **renal r.**, a condition of decalcification (osteoporosis) of bones associated with chronic kidney disease and clinically simulating rickets, occurs in later age groups and is characterized by excessive urinary calcium loss. **vitamin D resistant r.**, due to disease of the lower extremities producing short legs. Genetic illness. No deficiency of vitamin D. Serum levels of phosphorus low. No associated renal disease. Thought to be due to a defect in the tubular reabsorption of phosphorus and a lowered calcium absorption from the gut causing secondary hyperthyroidism and a vitamin D abnormality.

Rickettsia (ri-ket'-si-aå). Small pleomorphic parasitic micro-organisms which have their natural habitat in the cells of the gut of arthropods. Some are pathogenic to mammals and man, in whom they cause the typhus group of fevers. They are smaller in size than bacteria and larger than the viruses. Many of their physiological characters resemble the bacteria, but like the viruses they are obligate intracellular parasites. [Howard Taylor Ricketts, American pathologist, 1871–1910.]

rickety rosary. Series of protuberances (bossing) at junction of ribs and costal cartilages in children suffering from rickets.

rider's bone. A bony mass in the adductor muscles of the thigh, from repeated minor trauma in horse-riding.

Rifadin (rī-fa'-din). Rifampicin (q.v.).

Rifaldazine (rīf-al'-daz-ēn). Main indication is as a secondary drug in treating drug resistant tuberculosis.

rifampicin (ri-fam'-pi-sin). Antibiotic. Main indication is as a secondary drug in treating drug-resistant tuberculosis. Bacteriostatic. Active against a wide range of bacteria and Gram-positive cocci, *Mycobacterium tuberculosis*, but with limited action against Gram-negative bacteria. Useful for leprosy.

rifamycin (rī-fa-mī'-sin). Antibiotic. From Streptomyces group of organisms. Useful in resistant tuberculosis; also effective in staphylococcal infections. Some of the drug is excreted in tears and it has some antiviral properties.

rigor (rī'-gor) [L. stiffness]. A sudden chill, accompanied by severe shivering. The body temperature rises rapidly and remains high until perspiration ensues and causes a gradual fall in temperature. **rigor mortis** the stiffening of the body after death.

RIHSA. Radio-iodinated human serum albumin (q.v.).

Rimactane (rī-mak'-tān). Rifampicin (q.v.).

Rimifon (ri'-mi-fon). Isoniazid (q.v.).

ringworm. Generic term used to describe contagious infection of the skin by a fungus, because the common manifestations are circular (circinate) scaly patches. See also TINEA and MYCOSIS.

risus sardonicus (rī'-sus sár-don'-ik-us). The spastic grin of tetanus (q.v.).

Ritalin. Methyl phenidate (q.v.).

river blindness. A form of onchocerciasis (q.v.).

RNA. Ribonucleic acid (q.v.).

Robert Jones's abduction frame. A metal frame with a leather saddle used to treat hip disease. [Sir Robert Jones, English orthopaedic surgeon, 1858–1933.]

Rondomycin (ron-dō-mī'-sin). Methacycline (q.v.).

Roentgen or **Röntgen** (ront'-gen) rays. X-rays. [Wilhelm Konrad von Röntgen, German physicist, 1845–1923.]

Rogitine (roj'-i-tēn). Phentolamine (q.v.).

Romberg's sign. A sign of ataxia (q.v.). Inability to stand erect (without swaying) when the eyes are closed and the feet together. Also called 'Rombergism.' [Moritz Romberg, German neurologist, 1795–1873.]

Rondomycine (ron-do-mī'-sēn). Methacycline (q.v.).

Ronicol (ron'-i-kol). Nicotynyl alcohol (q.v.).

rosacea (rō-zā'-sē-à). A skin disease which shows on flush areas of the face, especially in women at menopause. In areas affected there is chronic dilation of superficial capillaries and hypertrophy of sebaceous follicles, often complicated by an acneiform eruption.

rose bengal (rōz ben'-gàl). A straining agent used to detect threads of mucus in the eye afflicted with keratoconjunctivitis.

roseola (rō-zē-ō'-là). The earliest manifestation of secondary syphilis (q.v.). This syphilide is a faint, pink spot, widespread in distribution except for the skin over the hands and face.

rotaviruses. Viruses associated with gastroenteritis in children and infants. Related to, but easily distinguished from reoviruses.

rotator (rō-tā'-tor) [L. *rotare*, to turn round.] A muscle having the action of turning a part.

Roth spots Round white spots in the retina in some cases of bacterial endocarditis; thought to be of embolic origin. [Moritz Roth, Swiss physician and pathologist, 1839–1915.]

roughage (ruf'-āj). Coarse food containing much indigestible vegetable fibre, composed of cellulose. It provides bulk in the diet and by this means helps to stimulate peristalsis and eliminate waste products. Lack of r. may cause atonic constipation. Too much r. may cause spastic constipation.

rouleaux (roo'-lō) [F.]. A row of red blood cells, resembling a roll of coins.

roundworm *(Ascaris lumbricoides)*. Look like earth worms. Worldwide distribution. Parasitic to man. Eggs passed in stools; ingested; hatch in bowel, migrate through tissues, lungs and bronchi before returning to the bowel as mature worms. During migration worms can be coughed up—which is unpleasant and frightening. Heavy infections can produce pneumonia. A tangled mass can cause intestinal obstruction or appendicitis. The best drug for treatment is piperazine. Roundworm of the cat and dog is called Toxocara.

Rous sarcoma virus (RSV). A virus of chickens which can cause tumours (sarcomas). A typical member of the RNA tumour virus group; despite much research no viruses belonging to this group have as yet been isolated from human tumours.

Roux-en-Y operation. Originally the distal end of divided jejunum was anastomosed to the stomach, and the proximal jejunum containing the duodenal and pancreatic juices was anastomosed to the jejunum about 76.2 mm below the first anastomosis. The term is now used to include joining of the distal jejunum to a divided bile duct, oesophagus or pancreas, in major surgery of these structures. [César Roux, Swiss surgeon, 1857–1926.]

Rovsing's sign. Pressure in the left iliac fossa causes pain in the right iliac fossa in appendicitis. [Niels Thorkild Rovsing, Danish surgeon 1862–1927.]

RPCF. Reiter protein complement fixation.

RSV. 1. Respiratory syncytial virus (q.v.). **2.** Rous sarcoma virus (q.v.).

rubefacients (roo-bi-fā'-shènts) [L. *rubefacere*, to make red]. Substances which, when applied to the skin, cause redness (hyperaemia).

rubella (roo-bel'-á) [L. *rubellus*, reddish]. Syn., German measles. An acute, infectious, eruptive fever (exanthema) caused by a virus and spread by droplet infection. There is pyrexia, coryza, conjunctivitis, a pink rash, enlarged occipital and posterior cervical glands. Complications are rare, except when contracted in the first three months of pregnancy it may produce fetal deformities. See HPV-77.

rubidomycin (roo-bid-ō-mī'-sin). Daunorubicin (q.v.).

rugae (roo'-jē) [L.]. Wrinkles, corrugations, folds, often of an impermanent nature and allowing for distension.

rupia (roo'-pē-á) [G. *rhypos*, filth]. Stuck-on crusts which look like limpets. Rupial syphilide, a late manifestation of secondary syphilis.

rupture (rup'-tūr) [L. *ruptura*, a break].. Tearing, splitting, bursting of a part. A popular name for hernia (q.v.).

Russell traction. Weighted skin traction using slings and pulleys. [William Russell, Edinburgh physician, 1852–1940.]

Ryan virus. Identified as an amoeba of the genus Hartmannella.

Ryle's tube (rīlz). A small-bore gastric tube, weighted at the tip. [John A. Ryle, British physician, 1889–   .]

S

Sabin vaccine. Living attenuated poliovirus which can be given orally. Produces active immunity against poliomyelitis. [Albert Bruce Sabin, American bacteriologist, 1906–   .]

sac [L. *saccus*, sack]. A small pouch or cyst-like cavity—saccular, sacculated, adj.

saccharides (sak'-a-rīdz). The carbohydrate grouping contained in each of the three main classes of carbohydrates.

saccharin (sak'-a-rin). A well-known sugar substitute. The soluble form is sometimes given intravenously as a test for circulation time, the end-point being the perception of a sweet taste in the mouth.

saccharolytic (sak-ar-ō-lit'-ik) [G. *sakcharon*, sugar; *lysis*, a loosening]. Having the capacity to ferment or disintegrate carbohydrates—saccharolysis, n.

Saccharomyces (sak-á-rō-mi'-sēz). A genus of yeasts which includes baker's and brewer's yeast.

saccharose (sak'-ar-ōs). Cane sugar; sucrose.

sacculation (sak-ū-lā'-shun) [L. *sacculus*, little sac]. Appearance of several saccules.

saccule (sak'-ūl) [L. *sacculus*, little sac]. A minute sac—saccular, sacculated, adj.

sacral (sā'-kral), Pertaining to the sacrum (q.v.).

sacroanterior (sā'-krō an-tē'-ri-èr) [L. *sacer*, sacred; *anterior*, foremost]. Used to describe a breech presentation in midwifery. The fetal sacrum is directed to one or other acetabulum of the mother—sacroanteriorly, adv.

sacrococcygeal (sā-krō-koks-ij'-ē-al) [L. *sacer*, sacred; G. *kokkyx*, cuckoo]. Pertaining to the sacrum and the coccyx.

sacroiliac (sā-krō-il'-i-ak) [L. *sacer*,

sacred; *ilium,* flank]. Pertaining to the sacrum and the ilium.

sacrolumbar (sā-krō-lum'-bar) [L. *sacer,* sacred; *lumbus,* loin]. Pertaining to the sacrum and the loins.

sacroposterior (sā'-krō pos-tē'-ri-ĕr) [L. *sacer,* sacred; *post,* behind]. Used to describe a breech presentation in midwifery. The fetal sacrum is directed to one of other sacroiliac joint of the mother—sacroposteriorly, adv.

sacrum (sā'-krum) [L. *sacer,* sacred]. The triangular bone lying between the fifth lumbar vertebra and the coccyx. It consists of five vertebrae fused together, and it articulates on each side with the innominate bones of the pelvis, forming the sacroiliac joints—sacral, adj.

saddlenose. One with a flattened bridge; often a sign of congenital syphilis.

sadism (sā'-dizm). The obtaining of pleasure from inflicting pain, violence or degradation on another person, or on the sexual partner. Opp. masochism.

Safapryn (sā'-fa-prin). 'Safe' aspirin. It is claimed that it does not cause gastric bleeding.

sagittal (saj'-it-al) [L. *sagitta,* arrow]. Resembling an arrow. In the anteroposterior plane of the body. **sagittal suture,** the immovable joint formed by the union of the two parietal bones.

Salazopyrin (sal-as-ō-pī'-rin). Salicylazosulphapyridine (q.v.).

salbutamol (sal-būt'-a-mol). Bronchodilator derived from isoprenaline. Does not produce cardiovascular side effects when inhaled in the recommended dose.

salicylamide (sal-is-il'-a-mīd). Mild analgesic similar in action to the salicylates, but less likely to cause gastric disturbance.

salicylazosulphapyridine (sal-is-il-ā-zō-sul-fa-pi'-ri-dēn). A sulphonamide compound which, after ingestion, is said to be distributed largely in connective tissue. It is used in the treatment of ulcerative colitis.

salicylic acid (sal-i-sil'-ik as'-id). Has fungicidal and bacteriostatic properties, and is used in a variety of skin conditions. It is a constituent of Whitfield's ointment. The plaster is used to remove corns and warts.

saline (sā'-līn) [L. *sal,* salt]. A solution of salt and water. Normal or physiological s. is a 0.9 per cent solution with the same osmotic pressure as that of blood. See HYPERTONIC, HYPOTONIC, ISOTONIC.

saliva (sal-ī'-vá) [L.]. The secretion of the salivary glands; spittle. It contains water, mucus and ptyalin (q.v.)—salivary, adj.

salivary (sal'-iv-a-ri). Pertaining to saliva. **salivary calculus,** a stone formed in the salivary ducts. **salivary glands,** the glands which secrete saliva, viz., parotid, submaxillary and sublingual.

salivation (sal-iv-ā'-shun) [L. *salivare,* to spit out]. An increased secretion of saliva. Ptyalism.

Salk vaccine (solk vak'-sēn). A preparation of killed poliomyelitis virus used as an antigen to produce active artificial immunity to poliomyelitis. By injection. [Jonas Edward Salk, American bacteriologist, 1914–   ]

Salmonella (sal-mon-el'-á). A genus of bacteria. Gram-negative rods. Parasitic in many animals and man in whom they are often pathogenic. Some species, such as *Salmonella typhi,* are host-specific, infecting only man, in whom they cause typhoid fever. Others, such as *S. typhimurium,* may infect a wide range of host species, usually through contaminated foods.

salpingectomy (sal-pin-jek'-to-mi) [G. *salpigx,* trumpet; *ektome,* excision]. Excision of a Fallopian tube.

salpingitis (sal-pin-jī'-tis) [G. *salpigx,* trumpet; *-itis,* inflammation]. Acute or chronic inflammation of the Fallopian tubes. See HYDROSALPINX, PYOSALPINX.

salpingogram (sal-ping'-ō-gram) [G. *salpigx,* trumpet; *gramma,* letter]. Radiological examination of tubal patency by injecting an opaque substance into the uterus and along the tubes—salpingography, n.; salpingographic, adj.; salpingographically, adv.

salpingo-oophorectomy (sal-ping-gō-ō-ō-for-ek'-to-mi) [G. *salpigx,* trumpet; *oon,* egg; *pherein,* to bear; *ektome,* excision]. Excision of a Fallopian tube and ovary.

salpingostomy (sal-ping-gos'-to-mi) [G. *salpigx,* trumpet; *stoma,* mouth]. The operation performed to restore tubal patency.

salpinx (sal'-pingks) [G. *salpigx,* trumpet]. A tube, especially the Fallopian tube or the Eustachian tube.

Sulupres. Hypotensive. Combination of reserpine and hydrochlorothiazide.

Saluric (sal-ū'-rik). Chlorothiazide (q.v.).

salve (sáv). An ointment.

sal volatile (sal vol-at'-i-li). Aromatic solution of ammonia. A household analeptic.

Salyrgan (sal-ir'-gan). Mersalyl (q.v.).

Sanamycin (san-a-mī'-sin). See ACTINOMYCIN C.

sandfly (*Phlebotomus*). Responsible for short, sharp, pyrexial fever called 'sandfly fever' of the tropics. Likewise transmits leishmaniasis (q.v.).

sanguineous (sang-gwin'-i-us) [L. *sanguis*, blood]. Pertaining to or containing blood.

santonin (san'-ton-in). An anthelmintic once used for round worm, but less toxic and more reliable drugs such as piperazine (q.v.) are now preferred.

saphenous (saf-ē'-nus). Apparent; manifest. The name given to the two main veins in the leg, the internal and the external, and to the nerves accompanying them.

saponification (sa-pon-i-fik-ā'-shun) [L. *sapo*, soap; *facere*, to make]. Conversion into a soapy substance.

sapraemia (sap-rē'-mj-á) [G. *sapros*, putrid; *haima*, blood]. A general bodily reaction to circulating toxins and breakdown products of saprophytic (non-pathogenic) organisms, derived from one or more foci in the body.

saprophyte (sap'-rō-fīt). Free-living micro-organisms obtaining food from dead and decaying animal or plant tissue—saprophytic, adj.

sarcoid (sár'-koid) [G. *sarkoeides*, flesh-like]. A term applied to a group of lesions in skin, lungs or other organs, which resemble tuberculous foci in structure, but the true nature of which is still uncertain.

sarcoidosis (sár-koid-ō'-sis) [G. *sarkoeides*, flesh-like; *-osis*, condition]. A granulomatous disease of unknown aetiology in which histological appearances resemble tuberculosis. May affect any organ of the body, but most commonly presents as a condition of the skin, lymphatic glands or the bones of the hand. See LUPUS.

sarcoma (sár-kō'-má) [G. *sarkoma*, fleshy overgrowth]. Malignant growth of mesodermal tissue (e.g. connective tissue, muscle, bone—sarcomatous, adj.; sarcomata, pl.

sarcomatosis (sár-kō-má-tō-sis). A condition in which sarcomata are widely spread throughout the body.

Sarcoptes (sár-kop'-tēz). Genus of Acerina. *Sarcoptes scabiei* is the itch mite which causes scabies (q.v.).

Saroten. Amitriptyline (q.v.). See ANTIDEPRESSANT.

sartorius (sár-tōr'-i-us) [L. *sartor*, patcher]. The tailor's muscle of the thigh, since it flexes one leg over the other.

SAT. Sodium antimony tartrate (q.v.).

Saventrine. Long-acting isoprenaline. A sustained release preparation active for 8 hours. Given to raise the heart rate to more than 40 by increasing the rate of the idioventricular rhythm. Toleration may avoid artificial pacing.

Savlon (sav'-lon). Chlorhexidine 1.5 per cent and centrimide 15 per cent.

scab. A dried crust forming over an open wound.

scabies (skā'-bi-ēz) [L. the itch.]. A parasitic skin disease caused by the itch mite. Highly contagious. See QUELLADA.

scald (skawld). An injury caused by moist heat.

scalenus syndrome (skal-ē'-nus sin'-drōm). Pain in arm and fingers, often with wasting, because of compression of the lower trunk of the brachial plexus behind scalenus anterior muscle at the thoracic outlet.

scalp (skalp). The hair-bearing skin which covers the cranium.

scalpel (skal-pel). A surgeon's knife which may or may not have detachable blades.

scan. See SCINTISCANNING.

scanning speech. A form of dysarthria occurring in disseminated sclerosis. The speech is jumpy or staccato or slow.

scaphoid (skāf'-oid) [G. *skaphe*, boat; *eidos*, form]. Boat-shaped as a bone of the tarsus and carpus.

scapula (skap'-ū-lá) [L.]. The shoulder-blade—a large, flat, triangular bone—scapular, adj.

scar. The dense, avascular white fibrous tissue, formed as the end-result of healing, especially in the skin. Cicatrix.

scarification (skar-i-fik-ā'-shun) [L. *scarificare*, to scratch open]. The making of a series of small, superficial incisions or punctures in the skin.

scarlatina (skar-la-tē'-ná). Scarlet fever.

Infection by haemolytic streptococcus producing a rash. Occurs mainly in children. Begins commonly with a throat infection, leading to pyrexia and the outbreak of a punctate erythematous eruption of the skin. Characteristically the area around the mouth escapes (circumoral pallor)—scarlatinal, adj.

scarlet red. A dye used as a stimulating ointment (2 to 5 per cent) for clean but slow-healing ulcers, wounds and pressure sores.

Scheuermann's disease. Osteochondritis of spine affecting the ring epiphyses of the vertebral bodies. Occurs in adolescents. [Holger Werfel Scheuermann, radiologist and orthopaedic surgeon of Copenhagen, 1877-1960.]

Schilder's disease. Genetically determined degenerative disease associated with mental subnormality. [Paul Schilder, German-American psychiatrist, 1886-1940.]

Schiötz tonometer. See TONOMETER. [Hjalmar Schiötz, Norwegian physician, 1850-1927.]

Schistosoma (skis-tō-sō'-má) [G. *schistos,* cleft; *soma,* body]. A genus of trematode worms or flukes which infest man. *Schistosoma mansoni* occurs in Africa, the West Indies and Brazil. *Schistosoma japonicum* occurs in the Far East.

schistosomiasis (skis-to-sō-mī'-a-sis) [G. *schistos,* cleft; *soma,* body; N.L. *-iasis,* condition]. Infestation of the human body by Schistosoma ('blood flukes') from drinking, or bathing in infected water. *Schistosoma haematobium* results in vesical schistosomiasis with haematuria as a characteristic symptom. *Schistosoma mansoni* and *Schistosoma japonicum* produce intestinal schistosomiasis characterized at first by diarrhoea and later by hepatosplenic disease.

schistosomicides (skis-to-sō'-mi-sīd) [G. *schistes,* cleft; *soma,* body; L. *coedere,* to kill]. Lethal to Schistosoma—schistosomicidal, adj.

schizophrenia (skiz'-ō-frē'-ni-á) [G. *schizein,* to cleave; *phren,* mind]. A mental disease first described by Kraepelin in 1896 as dementia praecox, Bleuler coined the name s. in 1911. A group of mental illnesses characterized by disorganization of the patient's personality, often resulting in chronic life long ill-health and hospitalization. The onset, commonly in youth or early adult life, is

either sudden or insidious. Bleuler described four main types, (1) **s. simplex,** (2) **catatonic s,** (3) **paranoid s,** (4) **hebephrenic s,** but the terms have disappeared from common usage. There are three elements common to all cases: a shallowness of emotional life; an inappropriateness of emotion; unrealistic thinking.

schizophrenic (skiz-ō-fren'-ik). Pertaining to schizophrenia. **schizophrenic syndrome in childhood** considered to be the best diagnostic label, rather than autism or psychosis in childhood. A working party (1961) formulated nine diagnostic points for this condition.

Schlatter's disease. Also Osgood-Schlatter's disease. Osteochondritis of the tibial tubercle. [Carl Schlatter, Swiss surgeon, 1864-1934. Robert Bayley Osgood, American orthopaedic surgeon, 1873-1934.]

Schlemm's canal. A lymphaticovenous canal in the inner part of the sclera, close to its junction with the cornea, which it encircles. [Friedrich Schlemm, German anatomist, 1795-1858.]

Scholz's disease. Genetically determined degenerative disease associated with mental subnormality. [Willibald Scholz, German neurologist, 1899 .]

Schönlein's disease. A form of anaphylactoid purpura occurring in young adults, associated with damage to the capillary walls and accompanied by swollen, tender joints and mild fever. See PURPURA. [Johann Lukas Schönlein, German physician. 1793-1864.]

Schwartze's operation. Opening of the mastoid process for the excision of infected bone and drainage of cellular suppuration. [Hermann H. R. Schwartze, German otologist. 1837-1910.]

sciatica (sī-at'-ik-á) [G. *ischion,* hip joint]. Pain in the line of distribution of the sciatic nerve (buttock, back of thigh, calf and foot).

scintillography: scintiscanning (sin-til-og'-ra-fi:sin-ti-skan'-ning) [L. *scintilla,* spark]. Visual recording of radioactivity over selected areas after administration of suitable radioisotope.

scirrhous (skir'-us [G. *skiros,* hard]. Hard; resembling a scirrhus.

scirrhus (skir'-us) [G. *skiros,* hard]. A carcinoma which provokes a considerable growth of hard, connective tissue; a hard carcinoma of the breast.

scissor leg deformity. The legs are crossed in walking—following double hip-joint disease, or as a manifestation of Little's disease (spastic cerebral diplegia).

sclera (sklēr'-à) [G. *skleros,* hard]. The 'white' of the eye; the opaque bluish-white fibrous outer coat of the eyeball covering the posterior five-sixths; it merges into the cornea at the front—scleral, adj.; sclerae, pl.

sclerema (sklēr-ē'-mà), **scleroderma** (sklēr-ō-der'-mà), **scleroedema** (sklēr-ē-dē'-mà) [G. *skleros,* hard]. Progressive atrophy of the skin in localized or diffuse patches. Localized s. is called 'morphea.' The diffuse form leads to severe limitation of movement over joints and in the face.

scleritis (sklēr-ī'-tis) [G. *skleros,* hard; *-itis,* inflammation]. Inflammation of the sclera.

sclerocorneal (sklēr-ō-kor'-ni-al) [G. *skleros,* hard; L. *corneus,* horny]. Pertaining to the sclera and the cornea, as the circular junction of these two structures.

scleroderma (sklē-rō-der'-mà) [G. *skleros,* hard; *derma,* skin]. A disease in which localized oedema of the skin is followed by hardening, atrophy, deformity and ulceration. Occasionally it becomes generalized, producing immobility of the face, contraction of the fingers; diffuse fibrosis of the myocardium, kidneys, digestive tract and lungs. See COLLAGEN and DERMATO-MYOSITIS.

scleroma (sklēr-ō'-mà) [G. *skleros,* hard; *-oma,* tumour]. Hardening of a tissue.

sclerosis (skler-ō'-sis) [G. *sklerosis,* hardening]. Term used in pathology to describe abnormal hardening or fibrosis of a tissue. **disseminated s.** (syn. **multiple s.**), a variably progressive disease of the nervous system, most commonly first affecting young adults, in which patchy, degenerative changes occur in nerve sheaths in the brain, spinal cord and optic nerves, followed by sclerosis (glial scar). The presenting symptoms can be diverse, ranging from diplopia to weakness or unsteadiness of a limb; disturbances of micturition are common. See TEST: platelet stickiness. **tuberose s.,** see EPILOIA—sclerotic, adj.

sclerotherapy (sklēr-ō-ther'-à-pi) [G. *skleros,* hard; *therapeia,* treatment]. Injection of sclerosing agent for treatment of varicose veins. **compression s.,** rubber pads are bandaged into position over the injection sites to increase localized compression in these areas.

sclerotic (skler-ōt'-ik). Pertaining to sclerosis.

sclerotomy (sklēr-ot'-o-mi) [G. *skleros,* hard; *tome,* a cutting]. Incision of sclera for relief of acute glaucoma, prior to doing a decompression operation.

scolex (skō'-leks) [L.]. The head of the tapeworm by which it embeds into the intestinal wall, and from which the segments (proglottides) develop.

Scoline (skō'-lēn). Suxamethonium (q.v.).

scoliosis (skō'-li-ō-sis) [G.]. Lateral curvature of the spine.

scopolamine (sko-pol'-a-min). Hyoscine (q.v.).

scorbutic (skor-bū'-tik). Pertaining to scorbutus, the old name for scurvy.

scotoma (sko-tō'-mà) [G. *skotos,* darkness]. Blind spot in field of vision. May be normal or abnormal—scotomata, pl.

scotopic vision. The ability to see well in poor light.

Scott's dressing. Ung. hydrarg. co. An ointment containing camphor, olive oil, mercury and beeswax is spread on strips of lint and applied to swollen joints. [John Scott, English surgeon, 1799–1846.]

'screening.' See FLUOROSCOPY.

scrapie (skrā-pē). Virus disease of sheep and goats.

scrofula (skrof'-ū-là). Tuberculosis of bone or lymph gland—scrofulous, adj.

scrofuloderma (skrof-ū-lō-der'-ma). An exudative and crusted skin lesion, often with sinuses, resulting from a tuberculous lesion underneath, as in bone or lymph glands.

scrotum (skrō'-tum) [L.]. The pouch in the male which contains the testicles—scrotal, adj.

scurf. A popular term for dandruff.

scurvy (skur'-vi). A deficiency disease caused by lack of vitamin C (ascorbic acid). Clinical features include fatigue and haemorrhage. Latter may take the form of oozing at the gums or large ecchymoses. Tiny bleeding spots on the skin around hair follicles are characteristic. In children painful subperiosteal haemorrhage (rather than other types of bleeding) is pathognomonic.

scybala (sib'-a-là) [G. *skybalon,* dung].

Rounded, hard, faecal lumps—scybalum, sing.

Sea Legs. Meclozine. See ANTIHISTAMINES.

sebaceous (sē-bā'-shus) [L. *sebaceus*, a tallow candle]. Pertaining to fat or suet. **sebaceous glands**, the cutaneous glands which secrete an oily substance called 'sebum.' The ducts of these glands are short and straight and open into the hair follicles.

seborrhoea (seb-o-rē'-á) [L. *sebum*, tallow; G. *rheein*, to flow]. Greasy condition of the scalp, face, sternal region and elsewhere due to overactivity of sebaceous glands. The seborrhoeic type of skin is especially liable to conditions such as alopecia, seborrhoeic dermatitis, acne, etc.

sebum (sē'-bum) [L.]. The normal secretion of the sebaceous glands; it contains fatty acids, cholesterol and dead cells.

Seclomycin (sek-lō-mī'-sin). Mixture of streptomycin and penicillin, broad spectrum antibiotic.

Seconal (sek'-on-al). Quinalbarbitone (q.v.).

secretin (sē-krē'-tin) [L. *secernere*, to separate]. A hormone produced in the duodenal mucosa, which causes a copious secretion of pancreatic juice. Available as snuff.

secretion (sē-krē'-shun) [L. *secretio*, separation]. A fluid or substance, formed or concentrated in a gland, and passed into the alimentary tract, the blood or to the exterior.

secretory (sē-krēt'-o-ri) [L. *secernere*, to separate]. The process of secretion: describes a gland which secretes.

sedation (sē-dā'-shun) [L. *sedare*, to soothe]. The production of a state of lessened functional activity.

sedative (sed'-at-iv) [L. *sedare*, to soothe]. An agent which lessens functional activity.

Sedormid (sed'-or-mid). A mild sedative and hypnotic. A useful alternative to barbiturates, but it may cause purpura in sensitive patients.

segment (seg'-ment) [L. *segmentum*, piece]. A small section; a part -segmental, adj.; segmentation, n.

segregation (seg-rē-gā'-shun) [L. *segregare*, to separate]. A setting apart, usually for a particular purpose, e.g. those suffering from the same or similar disease.

Seidlitz powder (sed'-litz). A popular aperient. It is dispensed as two powders, one containing sodium potassium tartrate and sodium bicarbonate, the other containing tartaric acid. Both powders are dissolved in water, and taken as an effervescent draught. [Named from a mineral spring in Bohemia.]

Seldinger intra-arterial catheter. See diagram.

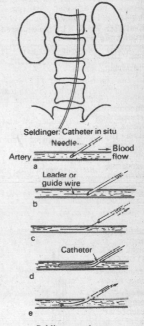

Seldinger: Catheter in situ

a

b

c

d

e

Seldinger catheter

Selenomethionine (sel-en-ō'-meth-ī'-o-nēn). An injection in which the sulphur atom present in the amino acid methionine is replaced by radioactive selenium. Taken up selectively by the pancreas; valuable in diagnosis of pancreatic disease.

sella turcica (sel'-á tur'-sik-á) [L. *sella*, saddle; *turcicus*, Turkish]. Now called 'pituitary fossa.'

semen (sē'-men) [L. seed]. The secretion from the testicles and accessory male organs, e.g. prostate. It contains the spermatozoa.

semicircular canals (se-mi-sir'-kū-lar ka-nalz'). Three membranous semicircular tubes contained within the bony labyrinth of the internal ear. They are concerned with appreciation of the body's position in space.

semicomatose (se-mi-kō'-ma-tōz). Condition bordering on the unconscious.

semilunar (sem-i-loon'-ar) [L. *semi*, half; *luna*, moon]. Shaped like a crescent or half moon. **semilunar cartilages**, the crescentic interarticular cartilages of the knee joint (menisci).

seminal (sem'-in-al) [L. *semen*, seed]. Pertaining to semen.

seminiferous (sem-in-if'-er-us) [L. *semen*, seed; *ferre*, to carry]. Carrying or producing semen.

seminoma (sem-in-ō'-má) [L. *semen*, seed; G. *-oma*, tumour]. A malignant tumour of the testis—seminomata, pl.; seminomatous, adj.

semipermeable (se-mi-pēr'-mē-ab-l). Used to describe a membrane which is permeable to some substances in solutions, but not to others.

senescence (sē-nes'-ens) [L. *senescere*, to grow old]. Normal changes of mind and body in increasing age—senescent, adj.

Sengstaken tube. For compression of bleeding oesophageal varices.

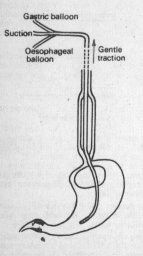

Gastric balloon

Suction

Oesophageal balloon

Gentle traction

Sengstaken tube

senile (sēn'-īl) [L. *senilis*, aged]. Senescence complicated by morbid processes—senility, n.

senna (sen'-na). Leaves and pods of a purgative plant from Egypt and India. Once used extensively as Black Draught or compound senna mixture.

Senokot. Standardized senna (q.v.).

sensible (sen'-sib-l). 1. Endowed with the sense of feeling. 2. Detectable by the senses.

sensitization (sen-si-tī-zā'-shun). Rendering sensitive. Persons may become sensitive to a variety of substances which may be food (e.g. shellfish), bacteria, plants, chemical substances, drugs, sera, etc. Liability is much greater in some persons than others. Sensitizing agent acts as an antigen leading to development of antibodies in the blood. See ALLERGY, ANAPHYLAXIS.

sensorineural (sen-sor-i-nūr'-al) [L. *sensus*, sense; G. *neuron*, nerve]. Pertaining to sensory neurones. **sensorineural deafness**, a discriminating term for nerve deafness.

sensory (sen'-sor-i) [L. *sensus*, sense]. Pertaining to sensation. **sensory nerves**, those which convey impulses to the brain and spinal cord.

sentiment (sen'-ti-ment) [L. *sentire*, to feel]. A group of emotionally charged tendencies centred on some person or object. Sentiments increase with experience of the environment.

sepsis (sep'-sis) [G. putrefaction]. The state of being infected with pus-producing organisms—septic, adj.

septicaemia (sep-ti-sēm'-i-á) [G. *sepsis*, putrefaction; *haima*, blood]. The persistence and multiplication of living bacteria in the blood stream—septicaemic, adj.

Septrin (sep'-trin). Tablets containing 80 mg trimethoprim and 400 mg sulphamethoxazole.

septum (sep'-tum). A partition between two cavities, e.g. between the nasal cavities—septa, pl.; septal, septate, adj.

sequela (sē-kwē'-lá) [L. *sequi*, to follow]. Pathological consequences of a disease, e.g. pock-marks of smallpox—sequelae, pl

sequestrectomy (sē-kwes-trek'-to-mi) [L. *sequester*, standing apart; G. *ektome*, excision]. Excision of a sequestrum (q.v.).

sequestrum (sē-kwes'-trum) [L. *seques-*

ter, standing apart]. A piece of dead bone which separates from the healthy bone but remains within the tissues—sequestra, pl.

Serenace. Haloperidol (q.v.).

Serenid-D (ser′-e-nid). Oxazepam (q.v.).

serology (sē-rol′-oj-i) [L. *serum,* whey; G. *logos,* discourse]. The branch of science dealing with the study of sera—serological, adj; serologically, adv.

seropurulent (sē-rō-pūr′-ū-lent) [L. *serum,* whey; *purulentus,* purulent]. Containing serum and pus.

serosa (sē-rōz′-ä) [L. *serum,* whey]. A serous membrane, e.g. the peritoneal covering of the abdominal viscera—serosal, adj.

serositis (sē-rō-sī′-tis) [L. *serum,* whey; G. *itis,* inflammation]. Inflammation of a serous membrane.

serotonin (sē-rō-tōn′-in). A product of cell metabolism. Liberated by blood platelets after injury. Together with histamine may be concerned in allergic reactions.

serous (sē′-rus) [L. *serum,* whey]. Pertaining to serum. **serous membrane,** one lining a cavity which has no communication with the external air.

Serpasil (sėr′-pa-sil). See RESERPINE.

serpiginous (sėr-pij′-in-us) [L. *serpere,* to creep]. Snakelike, coiled, irregular and used to describe the margins of skin lesions, especially ulcers and ringworm.

serration (ser-ā′-shun) [L. *serra,* saw]. A saw-like notch—serrated, adj.

serum (sē′-rum) [L. whey]. Supernatant fluid which forms when blood clots. **antitoxic s.,** prepared from the blood of an animal which has been immunized by the requisite toxin; it contains a high concentration of antitoxin. **serum sickness,** the symptoms arising as a reaction about ten days after the administration of serum: urticarial rash, pyrexia and joint pains—seta, pl.

serum gonadotrophin (sē′-rum gŏn-ad-ō-trō′-fin). An ovarian-stimulating hormone obtained from the blood serum of pregnant mares. It is used in amenorrhoea, often in association with oestrogens.

sesamoid (ses′-a-moid). Resembling a seed. **sesamoid bones,** small bony masses formed in the tendons, e.g. the patella and the pisiform (wrist) bone.

sessile (ses′-īl) [L. *sedere,* to sit]. Non-pedunculated; having a broad base.

sex-linked, Refers to genes which are located on the sex chromosomes.

SGOT. Serum glutamic oxalacetic transaminase. See TEST, ENZYME.

SGPT. Serum glutamic pyruvic transaminase. See TEST, ENZYME.

SH 420. Norethisterone (q.v.).

shelf operation. An open reduction of a congenital dislocation of hip joint, involving the use of a bone graft. Performed at 7 to 8 years, after failure of conservative treatment.

Shigella (shē-gel′-ä). A genus of bacteria containing some of the organisms causing dysentery, *Shigella sonnei, S. flexneri, S. shigae.*

shin bone. The tibia, the medial bone of the foreleg.

shingles. See HERPES.

Shirodkar's operation. Placing of a purse-string suture around an incompetent cervix, during pregnancy. It is removed when labour starts.

shock. The circulatory disturbance produced by severe injury or illness and due in large part to reduction in blood volume. There is discrepancy between the circulating blood volume and the capacity of the vascular bed. Initial cause is reduction in circulating blood volume; perpetuation is due to vasoconstriction, therefore vasoconstrictor drugs are not given. Its features include a fall in blood pressure, rapid pulse, pallor, restlessness, thirst and a cold clammy skin.

short-circuit operation. An anastomosis designed to bypass an obstruction in a conducting channel, e.g. gastrojejunostomy

short-sightedness. Myopia (q.v.).

shoulder girdle. Formed by the clavicle and scapula on either side.

shoulder lift. See AUSTRALIAN LIFT.

'show.' A popular term for the blood-stained vaginal discharge at the commencement of labour.

shunt. A term applied to the passage of blood through other than the usual channel.

sialagogue (sī-al′-a-gog) [G. *sialon,* saliva; *agogos,* leading]. An agent which increases the flow of saliva.

sialogram (sī-al-ō-gram) [G. *sialon,* saliva; *gramma,* letter]. Radiographic picture of the salivary glands and ducts, usually after injection of radio-opaque medium—sialography, n.; sialographic, adj.; sialographically, adv.

sialolith (sī-al'-ō-lith) [G. *sialon,* saliva; *lithos,* stone]. A stone in a salivary gland or duct.

sibling (sib'-ling). One of a family of children having the same parents.

sickle-cell anaemia. Familial, hereditary haemolytic anaemia peculiar to Negroes. The red cells are crescent-shaped.

side effect. Any physiological change other than the desired one from drug administration, e.g. the antispasmodic drug propantheline causes the s.e. of dry mouth in some patients. The term also covers undesirable drug reactions. Some are predictable being the result of a known metabolic action of the drug, e.g. yellowing of skin and eyes with mepacrine; thinning of skin and bone and formation of striae with corticosteroid; loss of hair with cyclophosphamide. Unpredictable reactions can be: (1) Immediate: anaphylactic shock, angioneurotic oedema. (2) Erythematous: all forms of erythema, including nodosum and multiforme and purpuric rashes. (3) Cellular reactions: eczematous rashes and contact dermatitis. (4) Specific reactions: e.g. light-sensitive eruptions with Ledermycin and griseofulvin.

siderosis (sid-er-ō'-sis) [G. *sideros,* iron;-*osis,* condition]. Excess of iron in the blood or tissues. Inhalation of iron oxide into the lungs can produce a s. as one form of pneumoconiosis (q.v.).

Sigmamycin (sig-ma-mī'-sin). Capsules of tetracycline (q.v.) and oleandomycin (q.v.). The mixture is claimed to have a wider range of activity than either antibiotic alone.

sigmoid (sig'-moid) [G. letter sigma]. Shaped like the letter S. **sigmoid flexure,** an S-shaped curve joining the descending colon above to the rectum below.

sigmoidoscope (sig-moid'-o-skōp) [G. letter sigma; *skopein,* to examine]. An instrument for visualizing the rectum and sigmoid flexure of the colon. See ENDOSCOPE—sigmoidoscopic, adj.; sigmoidoscopy, n.

sigmoidostomy (sig-moid-os'-to-mi) [G. letter sigma; *stoma,* mouth]. The formation of a colostomy in the sigmoid (pelvic) colon.

sign (sīn) [L. *signum*]. Any objective evidence of disease.

Silbephylline (sil-bef'-i-lin). Diprophylline (q.v.).

silicones (si'-li-kōns). Organic compounds which are water-repellant.

silicosis (si-li-kō'-sis) [L. *silex,* flint; G. *-osis,* condition]. Fibrosis of the lung from the inhalation of uncombined silica. A form of pneumoconiosis or 'industrial dust disease', found in metal grinders, stone-workers, etc.

silver nitrate (sil'-ver nī'-trāt). In the form of small sticks, is used as a caustic for warts. Occasionally used as antiseptic eye drops (1 per cent), and as an application to ulcers. Now being used in ½ per cent solution for burns to control bacterial infection in postburn period. Causes sodium and chloride loss from wound surface. Sodium chloride given orally or intravenously. Urine tested for chlorides.

silver sulphadiazine (sil'-ver sul-fa-dī'-a-zēn). Silver derivative of sulphadiazine (q.v.). Topical bacteriostatic agent.

Silverman score. A method of rating respiratory distress by assessing movement of accessory muscles and degree of expiratory grunt.

Simmonds' disease. Patient becomes emaciated, suffers from early senility: face unduly wrinkled, hair grey and sparse, blood pressure low, pulse slow, bones become frail. Previously incorrectly called hypopituitary cachexia. [Morris Simmonds, physician in Germany, 1855–1925.]

Sinemet (sin'-i-met). Levodopa (q.v.). combined with carbidopa (q.v.). in 10:1 ratio.

sinequan (sin'-e-qwan). Doxepin (q.v.).

sinew (sin'-ū)A ligament or tendon.

sinoatrial node (sī-nō-āt'-ri-al). See NODE.

sinogram (sī'-nō-gram) [L. *sinus,* cavity; G. *gramma,* letter]. Radiographic picture of a sinus after injection of radio-opaque medium.

Sintisone (sin'-ti-sōn). Oral preparation of prednisolone that does not produce 'mooning' of face.

sinus (sī'-nus) [L.]. 1. A hollow or cavity, especially the nasal sinuses. 2. A channel containing blood, especially venous blood, e.g. the sinuses of the brain. 3. A recess or cavity within a bone. 4. Any suppurating tract or channel. **coronary s.,** the dilated terminal part of the great cardiac vein. It is about 25.4 mm in length and opens into the right atrium. **frontal s.,** two cavities in the frontal bone, one on each side of the medial line, which open into the upper part of the nasal cavity—See PILONIDAL, CAVERNOUS.

sinusitis (sĭ-nŭ-sī'-tis) [L. *sinus,* hollow; G. *-itis,* inflammation]. Inflammation of a sinus, used exclusively for the paranasal sinuses.

sinusoid (sī'-nŭ-soid) [L. *sinus,* hollow; G. *eidos,* form]. A dilated channel into which arterioles open in some organs and which take the place of the usual capillaries.

sitz-bath (sits-bath) [G. *sitzen,* to sit]. Hip bath.

Sjögren-Larsson syndrome. Genetically determined congenital ectodermosis. Associated with mental subnormality.

Sjögren's syndrome (swä'-grens). Deficient secretion from lacrimal, salivary and other glands, mostly in postmenopausal women. There is keratoconjunctivitis, dry tongue and hoarse voice. Thought to be due to an autoimmune process. Also called **keratoconjunctivitis sicca.** [Henrik Samuel Conrad Sjögren, Swedish ophthalmologist, 1899- .]

skeleton (skel'-ē-ton). The bony framework of the body, supporting and protecting the soft tissues and organs. **appendicular s.,** the bones forming the upper and lower extremities. **axial s.,** the bones forming the head and trunk— **skeletal,** adj.

Skene's glands. Two small glands at the entrance to the female urethra; the paraurethral glands. [Alexander Johnston Chalmers Skene, American gynaecologist, 1838-1900.]

skin. The tissue which forms the outer covering of the body; it consists of two main layers: (1) the epidermis, or cuticle, forming the outer coat; (2) the dermis, or cutis vera, the inner or true skin, lying beneath the epidermis.

Skopyl (skop'-il). Methylscopolamine (q.v.).

skull. The bony framework of the head. See CRANIUM.

sleeping sickness. A disease endemic in Africa, characterized by increasing somnolence caused by infection of the brain by trypanosomes. See TRYPANOSOMIASIS.

sleep-walking. See SOMNAMBULISM.

slough (sluf). Septic tissue which becomes necrosed and separates from the healthy tissue.

Slow K. Slow-release potassium chloride.

smallpox. Variola. Caused by a virus eradicated from most parts of the world following WHO campaign. Headache, vomiting, and high fever precede the eruption of a widespread rash which is papular, vesicular and finally pustular. The eruption follows a set pattern of dissemination, commencing on the head and face. When the final stage of desiccation is passed scars (pockmarks) are left to disfigure the skin. Prophylaxis against the disease is by vaccination. See VACCINIA.

smear. A film of material spread out on a glass slide for microscopic examination. **cervical s.,** microscopic examination of cells scraped from the cervix to detect carcinoma-in-situ. See CARCINOMA.

smegma (smeg'-ma) [G. *unguent*]. The sebaceous secretion which accumulates beneath the prepuce and clitoris.

smelling salts. A mixture of compounds usually containing some form of ammonia, which acts as a stimulant, when inhaled.

Smith-Petersen nail. A trifid, cannulated metal nail used to provide internal fixation for intracapsular fractures of the femoral neck. [Marius Nygaard Smith-Petersen, American surgeon, 1886-1953.]

Smith-Petersen nail.

snare (snār). A surgical instrument with a wire loop at the end; used for removal of polypi.

Snellen's test types. A chart for testing visual acuity. [Hermann Snellen, Dutch ophthalmologist, 1834-1908.]

snow. Solid carbon dioxide. Used for local freezing of the tissues in minor surgery.

snuffles (snuf-lz). A snorting inspiration

due to congestion of nasal mucous membrane. It is a sign of early congenital (prenatal) syphilis when the nasal discharge may be purulent or bloodstained.

sociocultural (sō-si-ō-kul'-tur-al). Pertaining to culture in its sociological setting.

sociology (sō-si-ol'-o-ji) [L. *socius,* companion; G. *logos* discourse]. The scientific study of interpersonal and intergroup social relationships—sociological adj.

sociomedical (sō-si-ō-med'-ik-al). Pertaining to the problems of medicine as affected by sociology (q.v.).

sodium acetrizoate (sō'-di-um á-sĕt-tri-zō'-āt). An organic iodine compound used as a contrast agent in intravenous pyelography.

sodium acid phosphate (sō'-di-um as'-id fos'-fāt). Saline purgative and diuretic. It increases the acidity of the urine, and is given with hexamine as a urinary antiseptic.

sodium and meglumine diatrizoates (sō'-di-um meg'-lū-mīn dī-á-trī-zō'-ātz). Water soluble, radio-opaque form of iodine given before an X-ray using a fluorescent screen.

sodium amytal. Amylobarbitone (q.v.).

sodium antimonylgluconate (sō'-di-um an-tim'-on-il-gloo'-kon-āt). Used intravenously in schistosomiasis.

sodium antimony tartrate (sō'-di-um an-tim'-on-i tar'-trāt). SAT. Used intravenously in schistosomiasis.

sodium benzoate (sō'-di-um ben'-zō-āt). An acidifying diuretic, given when a lowering of the urinary pH is desired.

sodium bicarbonate (sō'-di-um bī-kár'-bon-āt). A domestic antacid, given for heartburn, etc. For prolonged therapy alkalis that cause less rebound acidity are preferred.

sodium chloride (sō'-di-um klōr'-īd). Salt, present in body tissues. Used extensively in shock and dehydration as intravenous normal saline, or as dextrosesaline in patients unable to take fluids by mouth. Used orally as replacement therapy in Addison's disease, in which salt loss is high. When salt is lost from the body, there is compensating production of renin (q.v.).

sodium citrate (sō'-di-um sit'-rāt). An alkaline diuretic very similar to potassium citrate. Used also as an anticoagulant for stored blood, and as an addition to milk feeds to reduce curdling.

sodium fusidate (sō'-di-um fū'- si-dāt). Expensive drug for the treatment of staphylococcal infections.

sodium gentisate (sō'-di-um jen-tis'-āt). A salicylate-like compound, used in rheumatic conditions when salicylates are not tolerated.

sodium iodide (sō'-di-um ī'-ō-dīd). Used occasionally as an expectorant, and as a contrast agent in retrograde pyelography.

sodium morrhuate (sō'-di-um mor'-rū-āt). A sclerosing agent sometimes used in the obliterative treatment of varicose veins.

sodium perborate (sō'-di-um per-bor'-āt). Aqueous solutions have antiseptic properties similar to those of hydrogen peroxide, and are used as mouthwashes, etc.

sodium propionate (sō'-di-um prō'-pi-on-āt). Used as an antimycotic in fungal infections as gel, ointment, lotion and pessaries.

sodium salicylate (sō'-di-um sal-is'-il-āt). Has the analgesic action of salicylates in general, but of particular value in rheumatic fever. Large doses are essential. Chronic rheumatoid conditions do not respond so well.

sodium stibogluconate (sō'-di-um stib-ō-gloo'-kon-āt). Used in treatment of leishmaniasis.

sodium sulphate (sō'-di-um sul'-fāt). A popular domestic purgative. A 25 per cent solution is used as a wound dressing. Given intravenously as a 4.3 per cent solution in anuria.

Soframycin (sof-rá-mī'-sin). Framycetin (q.v.).

soft sore. The primary ulcer of the genitalia occurring in the venereal disease chancroid (q.v.).

Solacen (sol'-ā-sen). Tybamate (q.v.).

solapsone (sol-ap'-sōn). Chemically related to dapsone (q.v.).

solar plexus (sō'-lar pleks'-us). A large network · of sympathetic (autonomic) nerve ganglia and fibres, extending from one adrenal gland to the other. It supplied the abdominal organs.

Solpadeine (sol'-pa-dēn). Soluble tablets of paracetamol with codeine and caffeine.

solute (sol-ūt'). That which is dissolved in a fluid.

solution (sol-ū'-shun). A fluid which contains a dissolved substance. **saturated s.**, one in which as much of the solid is dissolved as will be held in solution without depositing or floating.

solvent (sol'-vent). An agent which is capable of dissolving other substances.

somatic (sō-mat'-ik) [G. *somatikos*, of the body]. Pertaining to the body. **somatic nerves**, nerves controlling the activity of striated, skeletal muscle.

somatostatin (sō-ma-tō-stat'-in). Growth hormone release-inhibiting hormone (GH-RIH). Remarkable hypothalamic tetradecapeptide.

somatotrophin (sō-ma-tō-trō'-fin) [G. *soma*, body; *trophe*, nourishment]. The growth factor secreted by anterior pituitary gland.

somnambulism (som-nam'-bū-lizm) [L. *somnus*, sleep; *ambulare*, to walk]. Sleepwalking; a state of dissociated consciousness in which sleeping and waking states are combined. Considered normal in children but as an illness having a hysterical basis in adults.

Sonalgin. (son-al'-jin). Butobarbitone (q.v.), codeine (q.v.) and phenacetin (q.v.).

Soneryl Son'-er-il). Butobarbitone (q.v.).

Sonicaid (son'-i-kad). Diagnostic ultrasound machine used to detect movement inside body.

Sonne dysentery (son'-nē dis'-en-tèr-i). Bacillary dysentery caused by infection with *Shigella sonnei* (Sonne bacillus), the commonest form of dysentery in the United Kingdom. The organism is excreted by cases and carriers in their faeces, and contaminates hands, food and water, from which new hosts are infected. [Carl Sonne, Danish bacteriologist, 1882–1948.]

sonograph (sō'-nō-graf). Graphic record of sound waves.

soporific (sop-or-if'-ik) [L. *sopor*, sleep; *facere*, to make]. An agent which induces profound sleep.

sorbide nitrate (sor'-bīd nīt'-rāt). Improves effort tolerance in angina.

Sorbitol (sor'-bit-al). Liquid for parenteral feeding.

sordes (sor'-dēz) [L.]. Dried, brown crusts which form in the mouth, especially on the lips and teeth, in illness.

souffle (soo-fl) [F.]. Puffing or blowing sound. **funic s.**, auscultatory murmur of pregnancy. Synchronizes with the fetal heart-beat and is caused by pressure on the umbilical cord. **uterine s.**, soft, blowing murmur which can be auscultated over the uterus after the fourth month of pregnancy.

sound. An instrument to be introduced into a hollow organ or duct so as to detect a stone, or to dilate a stricture.

Sourdille's operation. Multiple-stage operation for the relief of deafness. See FENESTRATION. [Maurice Sourdille, French otologist, 1885–1961.]

soya bean (soi'-á bēn). A highly nutritious legume used in Asiatic countries in place of meat. It contains high-quality protein and little starch. Is useful in diabetic preparations.

spansules. A chemical means of preparing drugs so that there is controlled release via oral route.

Sparine. Promazine (q.v.).

spasm. Convulsive, involuntary muscular contraction.

spasmolytic (spas-mō-lit'-ik). Current term for antispasmodic drugs—spasmolysis, n.

spastic (spas'-tik) [G. *spastikos*, drawing in]. In a condition of muscular rigidity or spasm, e.g. spastic diplegia (Little's disease (q.v.)).

spasticity (spas-tis'-it-i) [G. *spastikos*, drawing in]. Condition of rigidity or spasm.

spatula (spat'-ū-lá). A flat flexible knife with blunt edges for making poultices and spreading ointment. **tongue s.**, a rigid, blade-shaped instrument for depressing the tongue.

species (spē'-shēz) [L. kind]. A subdivision of genus. A group of individuals having common characteristics and differing only in minor details.

specific (spe-sif'-ik) [L. *species*, kind; *facere*, to make]. Special; characteristic; peculiar to **specific disease**, one that is always caused by a specified organism. **specific gravity**, the weight of a substance, as compared with that of an equal volume of water, the latter being represented by 1000.

spectrophotometer (spek-trō-fō-tom'-et-ēr). A spectroscope combined with a photometer for quantitatively measuring the relative intensity of different parts of a light spectrum.

spectroscope (spek'-trō-skōp). An

instrument for observing spectra of light.

speculum (spek'-ū-lum) [L. mirror]. An instrument used to hold the walls of a cavity apart, so that the interior of the cavity can be examined—specula, pl.

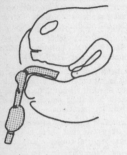

Auvard's vaginal speculum

sperm [G. *sperma*, seed]. Abbreviation for spermatozoon.

spermatic (spér-mat'-ik) [G. *sperma*, seed]. Pertaining to or conveying semen. **spermatic cord**, suspends the testicle in the scrotum and contains the s. artery and vein and the vas deferens.

spermaticidal (sper-mat-i-sī'-dal) [G. *sperma*, seed; L. *coedere*, to kill]. Lethal to spermatozoa.

spermatogenesis (sper-mat-ō-jen'-e-sis) [G. *sperma*, seed; *genesis*, descent]. The formation and development of sperms—spermatogenetic, adj.

spermatorrhoea (spér-mat-o-rē'-á) [G. *sperma*, seed; *rheein*, to flow]. Involuntary discharge of semen without orgasm.

spermatozoon (spér-mat-ō-zō'-on) [G. *sperma*, seed; *zoion*, living being]. A mature, male reproductive cell—spermatozoa, pl.

spermicide (spér'-mi-sīd) [G. *sperma*, seed; L. *coedere*, to kill]. An agent that kills spermatozoa. Also **spermatocide**—spermicidal, adj.

Spersin (sper'-sin). An insufflation of Polymyxin and Neomycin.

sphenoid (sfē'-noid) [G. *sphen*, wedge; *eidos*, form]. A wedge-shaped bone at the base of the skull—sphenoidal, adj.

spherocyte (sfer'-ō-sīt) [G. *sphaira*, sphere; *kytos*, cell]. Round red blood cell, as opposed to biconcave—spherocytic, adj.

spherocytosis (sfer-ō-sī-tō'-sis) [G. *sphaira*, sphere; *kytos*, cell; *-osis*, condition]. Syn. for acholuric jaundice. A heredofamilial genetic disorder transmitted as a dominant gene, i.e. with a one in two chance of transmission. It exists from birth but can remain in obeyance throughout life; sometimes discovered by 'accidental' examination of the blood. See JAUNDICE.

sphincter (sfink'-tér) [G. *sphinggein*, to bind tight]. A circular muscle, contraction of which serves to close an orifice.

sphincterotomy (sfink-ter-ot'-omi) [G. *sphigkter*, that which binds tight; *tome*, a cutting]. Surgical division of a muscular sphincter.

sphygmocardiograph (sfig-mō-kár'-di-ō-graf) [G. *sphygmos*, pulse; *kardia*, heart; *graphein*, to write]. An apparatus for simultaneous graphic recording of the radial pulse and heart-beats—sphygmocardiographic, adj.; sphygmocardiographically, adv.

sphygmograph (sfig'-mō-graf) [G. *sphygmos*, pulse; *graphein*, to write]. An apparatus attached to the wrist, over the radial artery, which records the movements of the pulse-beat—sphygmographic, adj.

sphygmomanometer (sfig-mō-man-om'-et-ér) [G. *sphygmos*, pulse; *manos*, rare; *metron*, a measure]. An instrument used for measuring the blood pressure.

spica (spī'-ká) [L.]. A bandage applied in a figure-of-eight pattern.

spicule (spī'-kūl) [L. *spica*, spike]. A small, spike-like fragment, especially of bone.

spigot (spig'-ot). Glass, wooden or plastic peg used to close a tube.

spina bifida (spī'-ná bif'-id-á). A congenital defect in which the vertebral neural arches fail to close, so exposing the contents of the spinal canal posteriorly. The fissure usually occurs in the lumbosacral region. The contents of the canal may or may not protrude through the opening: this latter condition is called 'spina bifida occulta'.

spinal (spī'-nal) [L. *spina*, thorn]. Pertaining to the spine. **spinal anaesthetic**, a local anaesthetic solution is injected into the subarachnoid space, so that it renders the area supplied by the selected s. nerves insensitive. **spinal canal**, the central hollow throughout the s. column. **spinal caries**, disease of the vertebral bones. **spinal column**, a bony structure formed from 33 separate bones; the lower ones fuse together; the rest are separated by pads of cartilage.

spinal cord, the continuation of nervous tissue of the brain down the s. canal to the level of the first or second lumbar vertebra. **spinal nerves,** 31 pairs leave the s. cord and pass out of the s. canal to supply the periphery.

spine (spīn) [L. *spina,* thorn]. A popular term for the bony spinal or vertebral column. A sharp process of bone—spinous, spinal, adj.

spiramycin (spī-ra-mī'-sin) [L.]. An orally active antibiotic with a range of activity similar to that of penicillin and erythromycin.

Spirillum (spī-ril'-um) [L. *spira,* a spiral]. A bacterial genus. Cells are rigid screws or portions of a turn. Common in water and organic matter. *Spirillum minus* is found in rodents and may infect man, in whom it causes one form of rat-bite fever—spirilla, pl.; spirillary, adj.

spirochaete (spī'-rō-kēt). A bacterium having a spiral shape—spirochaetal, adj.

spirochaetaemia (spī-rō-kēt-ē'-mi-á) [G. *speira,* coil; *chaite,* a bristle; *haima,* blood]. Spirochaetes in the blood stream. This kind of bacteraemia occurs in the secondary stage of syphilis and in the syphilitic fetus—spirochaetaemic, adj.

spirograph (spī'-rō-graf) [L. *spirare,* to breathe; G. *graphein,* to write]. An apparatus which records the movement of the lungs—spirographic, adj.; spirographically, adv.; spirography, n.

spirometer (spī-rom'-et-ér) [L. *spirare,* to breathe; G. *metron,* a measure]. An instrument for measuring the capacity of the lungs. See BRONCHOSPIRO-METER—spirometric, adj.; spirometry, n.

spironolactone. Aldactone-A. Antialdosterone preparation. Acts on the complex biochemical processes involved in oedematous accumulation and causes renal excretion of sodium and water.

spittle (spit'-l). Sputum; that which is expectorated.

Spitz-Holter valve. Used to drain hydrocephalus (q.v.).

splanchnic (splangk'-nik) [G. *splagchna,* inward parts]. Pertaining to or supplying the viscera.

splanchnicectomy (splang-knik-ek'-to-mi) [G. *splagchna,* inward parts; *ektome,* excision]. Surgical removal of the splanchnic nerves, whereby the viscera are deprived of sympathetic impulses; occasionally performed in the treatment of hypertension or for the relief of certain kinds of visceral pain.

splanchnology (splangk-nol'-o-ji) [G. *splagchna,* inward parts; *logos,* discourse]. The study of the structure and function of the viscera.

spleen (splēn) [G. *splen*]. A lymphoid, vascular organ immediately below the diaphragm, at the tail of the pancreas, behind the stomach. It can be enlarged in reactive and neoplastic conditions affecting the reticuloendothelial system (q.v.).

splenectomy (splen-ek'-to-mi) [G. *splen,* spleen; *ektome,* excision]. Surgical removal of the spleen.

splenic anaemic, See BANTI'S DISEASE.

splenitis (splen-ī'-tis) [G. *splen,* spleen; *-itis,* inflammation]. Inflammation of the spleen.

splenocaval (splen-ō-ka'-val) [G. *splen,* spleen; L. *Cavum,* hollow]. Pertaining to the spleen and inferior vena cava, usually referring to anastomosis of the splenic vein to the IVC.

splenogram (splen'-ō-gram) [G. *splen,* Spleen; *gramma,* letter]. Radiographic picture of the spleen after injection of radio-opaque medium—splenograph, splenography, n.; splenographical, sdj.; splenographically, adv.

splenomegaly (splen-ō-meg'-al-i) [G. *splen,* spleen; *megas,* large]. Enlargement of the spleen.

splenoportal (splen-ō-por'-tal) [G. *splen,* spleen; L. *porta,* gate]. Pertaining to the spleen and portal vein.

splenoportogram (splen-ō-port'-ō-gram) [G. *splen,* spleen; L. *porta,* gate; G. *gramma,* letter]. Radiographic picture of the spleen and portal vein after injection of radio-opaque medium—splenoportograph, splenoportography, n.; splenoportographical, adj.; splenoportographically, adv.

splenorenal (splen-ō-rē'-nal) [G. *splen,* spleen; L. *ren,* kidney]. Pertaining to the spleen and kidney, as anastomosis of the splenic vein to the renal vein; a procedure carried out in some cases of portal hypertension.

splenovenography (splen-ō-ven-og'-ra-fi). See SPLENOGRAM.

spondyl(e) (spon'-dil) [G. *spondylos*, vertebra]. A vertebra.

spondylitis (spon-dil-ī'-tis) [G. *spondylos*, vertebra; *-itis*, inflammation]. Inflammation of one or more vertebrae—spondylitic, adj. **ankylosing s.**, a condition characterized by ossification of the spinal ligaments and ankylosis of sacroiliac joints. It occurs chiefly in young men.

spondylolisthesis (spon-dil-ō-lis-thē'-sis) [G. *spondylos*; vertebra; *olisthesis*, a slipping and falling]. Forward displacement of lumbar vertebra(e)—spondylolisthetic, adj.

spondylosis deformans (spon-dil-ō'-sis dē-form'-ans) [G. *spondylos*, vertebra; *-osis*, condition; L. misshapen]. Degeneration of the whole intervertebral disc, with new bone formation at the periphery of the disc. Commonly called 'osteoarthritis of spine'.

spongioblastoma multiforme (spon-ji-ō-blas-tō'-má mul'-ti-form). A highly malignant rapidly growing brain tumour.

sporadic (spor-ad'-ik) [G. *sporadikos*, scattered]. Scattered; occurring in isolated cases; not epidemic—sporadically, adv.

spore (spōr) [G. *sporos*, seed]. A phase in the life-cycle of a limited number of bacterial genera where the vegetative cell becomes encapsulated and metabolism almost ceases. These spores are highly resistant to environmental conditions such as heat and desiccation. The spores of important species such as *Clostridium tetani* and *C. botulinum* are ubiquitous so that sterilization procedures must ensure their removal or death.

sporicidal (spor-i-sī'-dal) [G. *sporos*, seed; L. *coedere*, to kill]. Lethal to spores—sporicide, n.

sporotrichosis (spor-ō-trī-kō'-sis) [G. *sporos*, seed; *thrixtrichos*, hair; *-osis*, condition]. Infection of a wound by a fungus (*Sporotrix schenkic*). There results a primary sore with lymphangitis and subcutaneous painless granulomata. Occurs amongst those working with soil.

sporulation (spor-ū-lā'-shun) [G. *spora*, seed]. The formation of spores by bacteria.

spotted fever. 1. Cerebrospinal fever. Organism responsible is the meningococcus transferred by droplet infection. Occurs in epidemics. **2.** Rocky Mountain spotted fever is a tick-borne typhus fever.

sprain (sprān). Injury to the soft tissues surrounding a joint, resulting in discoloration, swelling and pain.

Sprengel's shoulder deformity. Congenital high scapula, a permanent elevation of the shoulder, often associated with other congenital deformities, e.g. the presence of a cervical rib or the absence of vertebrae [Otto G. K. Sprengel, German surgeon, 1852-1915.]

sprue (sproo). A chronic malabsorption disorder associated with glossitis, indigestion, weakness, anaemia and steatorrhoea.

sputum (spū'-tum) [L. spittle]. Matter which is expectorated from the lungs.

squamous (skwā'-mous) [L. *squamosus*, scaly]. Scaly. **squamous epithelium,** the non-glandular epithelial covering of the external body surfaces. **squamous carcinoma,** carcinoma arising in squamous epithelium; epithelioma.

squills (skwillz). Dried bulbs of Mediterranean plant, used in Gee's linctus and other cough preparations as an expectorant.

squint (skwint). Syn., strabismus. Incoordinated action of the muscles of the eyeball, such that the visual axes of the two eyes fail to meet at the objective point. **convergent s.,** when the eyes turn towards the medial line. **divergent s.,** when the eyes turn outwards.

staccato speech (stak-ā'-tō). With interruptions between words or syllables. The scanning speech of disseminated sclerosis and cerebellar disease.

Stacke's operation. Plastic operation on posterior membranous wall of the aural canal. [Ludwig Stacke, German otologist, 1859-1918.]

stagnant loop syndrome. Stagnation of contents of any surgically created 'loop' of intestine with consequent increase in bacterial population and interference with absorption of food.

St Anthony's fire. Erysipelas (q.v.); and sometimes used for gangrene resulting from ergotism.

stapedectomy (stā-ped-ek'-to-mi). Surgical removal of stapes for otosclerosis and insertion of 1. Teflon piston (Schuknecht's operation). 2. Vein graft. 3. Plug of fat. After s., stapes can be replaced by a prosthesis. Normal hearing is restored in 90 per cent of patients.

stapedial mobilization (stā-pēd'-i-al). Release of a stapes, rendered immobile by otosclerosis.

stapediolysis (stā-pēd-i-ol'-i-sis). See STAPEDIAL MOBILIZATION.

stapes (stā'-pēz). The stirrup-shaped medial bone of the middle ear. **mobilization of s.**, forcible pressure on s. to restore its mobility. Gain in hearing not permanent, but a stapedectomy can be done later —stapedial, adj.

Staphylococcus (staf-i-lō-kok'-us) [Gr. *staphyle*, bunch of grapes]. A genus of bacteria. Gram-positive cocci occurring in clusters. May be saprophytes or parasites. Common commensals of man, in whom they are responsible for much minor pyogenic infection, and a lesser amount of more serious infection. Produce several exotoxins. These include leucocidins which kill WBC and hâemolysins which destroy RBC. A common cause of hospital cross-infection—staphylococcal, adj.

staphyloma (staf-il-ō'-má) [G.]. A protrusion of the cornea or sclera of the eye—staphylomata, pl.

starch. The carbohydrate present in potatoes, rice, maize, etc. Widely used as an absorbent dusting powder.

stasis (stā'-sis) [G.]. Stagnation; cessation of motion. **Intestinal s.**, sluggish bowel contractions resulting in constipation.

status (stā'-tus) [L.]. State. Condition. **status asthmaticus** is a prolonged and refractory attack of asthma. **status epilepticus** describes epileptic attacks following each other almost continuously. **status lymphaticus** is a condition found postmortem in patients who have died without apparent cause. The thymus may be found hypertrophied with increase in lymphatic tissue elsewhere.

steapsin (stē-ap'-sin). The lipase of the pancreatic juice which splits fat into fatty acids and glycerine.

steatorrhaea (stē-at-or-ē'-á) [G. *stear*, fat; *rheein*, to flow] A syndrome of varied aetiology associated with multiple defects of absorbtion from the gut and characterized by the passage of pale, bulky, greasy stools.

stegomyia (steg-ō-mī'-i-á) [G. *stegos*, roof; *myia*, fly]. A genus of mosquitoes, some of which transmit the malaria parasite. Found in most tropical and subtropical countries.

Stein-Leventhal syndrome. Secondary amenorrhoea, sterility, bilateral polycystic ovaries and hirsutism occurring in the second or third decades of life. Treated by wedge resection of ovary.

Steinmann's pin. An alternative means to the use of a Kirschner wire (q.v.) of applying skeletal traction to a limb. It has its own introducer and stirrup. [Fritz Steinmann, Swiss surgeon, 1872-1932.]

Stelazine. Trifluoperazine (q.v.).

stellate (stel'-āt) [L. *stella*, star]. Starshaped **stellate ganglion**, a large collection of nerve cells (ganglion) on the sympathetic chain in the root of the neck.

Stellwag's sign. Occurs in exophthalmic goitre (Graves' disease). Patient does not blink so often as usual, and the eyelids close only imperfectly when he does so. [Carl Stellwag von Carion, Austrian ophthalmologist, 1823-1904.]

Stemetil (stem'-et-il). Prochlorperazine (q.v.).

stenosis (sten-ō'-sis) [G.]. A narrowing—stenoses, pl.; stenotic, adj.

sterkobilin (ster-kō-bī'-lin). The brown pigment of faeces; it is derived from the bile pigments.

stercobilinogen. Urobilinogen (q.v.).

stercoraceous (ster-kor-ā'-shus) [L. *stercus*, dung]. Pertaining to or resembling faeces—stercoral, adj.

stereotactic surgery (stē-rē-ō-tak'-tik). Electrodes and cannulae are passed to a predetermined point in the brain for physiological observation or destruction of tissue in diseases such as paralysis agitans, multiple sclerosis and epilepsy. Intractable pain can be relieved by this method. Also stereotaxic.

sterile (ste'-rīl). Free from micro-organisms —sterility, n.

sterilization (ster-il-ī-zā'-shun). 1. The process of ridding material or tissue of living microbes. 2. Rendering incapable of reproduction.

sternoclavicular (ster-nō-klav-ik'-ū-lar) [G. *sternon*, breast; L. *clavicula*, small key]. Pertaining to the sternum and the clavicle.

sternocleidomastoid muscle (ster-nō-klī-dō-mas'-toid) [G. *sternon*, breast; *kleis*, hook; *mastos*, breast]. A strap-like neck muscle arising from the sternum and clavicle, and inserting into the mastoid process of temporal bone. See TORTICOLLIS.

sternocostal (stèr-nō-kos'-tal) [G. *sternon,* breast; L. *costa,* rib]. Pertaining to the sternum and ribs.

sternotomy (stèr-not'-om-i) [G. *sternon,* breast; *tome,* a cutting]. Surgical division of the sternum.

sternum (stèr'-num) [G. *sternon,* breast]. The breast bone—sternal, adj.

Sterogyl 15. Calciferol forte (NF—National Formulary).

steroids (ster'-oidz) [G. *stereos,* solid; *eidos,* form]. A term embracing a naturally occurring group of chemicals allied to cholesterol and including sex-hormones, adrenal cortical hormones, bile acids, etc. By custom if often now implies the natural adrenal glucocorticoids, viz., hydrocortisone and cortisone, or synthetic analogues such as prednisolone and prednisone.

sterol (ster'-ol) [G. *steros,* solid; *-ol,* alcohol]. A solid alcohol. Cholesterol and many hormones secreted by the adrenal cortex and the gonads are examples. They all contain the same basic ring structure.

stertor (ster'-tor) [L. *stertere,* to snore]. Loud snoring; sonorous breathing—stertorous, adj.

stethoscope (steth'-o-skōp) [G. *stethos,* breast; *skopein,* to examine]. An instrument used for listening to the various body sounds, especially those of the heart and chest. See MEDETRON—stethoscopic, adj.; stethoscopically, adv.

Stevens-Johnson syndrome. Severe variant of the allergic response—erythema multiforme. It is an acute hypersensitivity state and can follow a viral or bacterial infection, drugs—such as long-acting sulphonamides, some anticonvulsants and some antibiotics. In some cases no cause can be found. Lung complications during the acute phase can be fatal. Mostly it is a benign condition, and there is complete recovery. [Albert Mason Stevens, American paediatrician, 1884–1945. Frank Chambliss Johnson, American paediatrician, 1894–1934.]

stibocaptate (stib-ō-kap'-tāt) Trivalent antimonial, effective in the treatment of intestinal schistosomiasis. Given intramuscularly. Admission to hospital essential and patient should be kept lying down for a few hours after each injection. BAL should be available to reverse any severe toxic effects.

stibophen (stib'-ō-fen). A complex antimony compound used in the treatment of schistosomiasis.

stigmata (stig'-ma-tá) [G. *stigma,* mark or brand]. Marks of disease, or congenital abnormalities, e.g. facies of congenital syphilis—stigma, sing.

stilboestrol (stil-bēs'-trol). An orally active synthetic oestrogen, indicated in all conditions calling for oestrogen therapy. Large doses are given in prostatic carcinoma.

stilette (stil-et'). A wire or metal rod for maintaining patency of hollow instruments.

stillborn. Born dead.

Still's disease. A form of rheumatoid polyarthritis, involving enlargement of the spleen, lymphatic nodes and glands, occurring in infants and young children. Sufferers are often retarded. Also called 'arthritis deformans Juvenilis'. [George Fredric Still, English physician, 1868–1941.]

stimulant (stim'-ū-land)]L. *stimulare,* to goad]. Stimulating. An agent which excites or increases function.

stimulus (stim'-ū-lus) [L. *stimulare,* to goad]. Anything which excites functional activity in an organ or part.

stitch. 1. A sudden, sharp, darting pain. 2. A suture.

Stockholm technique. A method of treating carcinoma of the cervix by radium on three successive occasions at weekly intervals.

Stokes-Adams syndrome. A fainting (syncopal) attack, commonly transient, which occurs in patients with heart block. If severe, may take the form of a convulsion, or patient may become unconscious. [William Stokes, Irish physician, 1804–78. Robert Adams, Irish physician, 1791–1875]

stoma (stō'-má) [G.]. The mouth; any opening—stomal, adj.; stomata, pl.

stomach (stum'-ak) [G. *stomachos,* gullet]. The most dilated part of the digestive tube, situated between the oesophagus (cardiac orifice) and the beginning of the small intestine (pyloric orifice); it lies in the epigastric, umbilical and left hypochondriac regions of the abdomen. The wall is composed of four coats: serous, muscular, submucous and mucous. **hour glass s.,** one partially divided into two halves by an equatorial constriction following scar formation.

stomachics (stom-ak'-iks) Agents which

increase the appetite, especially bitters.

stomatitis (stō-mat-ī'-tis) [G. *stoma*, mouth; *-itis*, inflammation]. Inflammation of the mouth. **angular s.**, fissuring in the corners of the mouth consequent upon riboflavine deficiency. Sometimes misapplied to: (1) the superficial maceration and fissuring at the labial commisures in perlèche (q.v.) and (2) the chronic fissuring at the site in elderly persons with sagging lower lip or malapposition of artificial dentures. **aphthous s.**, recurring crops of small ulcers in the mouth. Relationship to herpes simplex suspected, but not proven. See APHTHAE. **gangrenous s.**, see CANCRUM ORIS.

stone (stōn). Calculus; a hardened mass of mineral matter.

stool. The faeces. An evacuation of the bowels.

Stovarsol (stov-ár'-sol). Acetarsol (q.v.).

stove-in chest. There may be multiple anterior or posterior fractures of the ribs (causing paradoxical breathing) and fractures of sternum, or a mixture of such fractures.

STP. Psychedelic drug that engenders hallucinations comparable to those experienced in schizophrenic states.

strabismus (strab-iz'-mus) [G. *strabismos*, squinting]. See SQUINT.

stramonium (stra-mō'-ni-um). A plant resembling belladonna in its properties, and used as an antispasmodic in bronchitis and Parkinsonism.

strangulation (strang'-gū-lā-shun) [G. *straggale*, halter]. Constricted so as to impede the circulation—strangulated, adj.

strangury (strang'-gū-ri) [G. *stragx*, drop; *ouron*, urine]. Slow and painful micturition.

Strassman operation. A plastic operation to make a bicornuate uterus a near normal shape. [Paul F. Strassman, German gynaecologist, 1866–1938.]

stratified (strat'-i-fīd) [L. *stratum*, a covering; *facere*, to make]. Arranged in layers.

stratum Strā'-tum) [L.]. A layer or lamina, e.g. the various layers of the epithelium of the skin, viz., s. granulosum, s. lucidum.

Streptobacillus (strep-tō-bas-il'-us). Gram-positive, rod-shaped bacteria.

Streptococcus (strep-tō-kok'-us) [G. *streptos*, curved; *coccus*, berry]. A genus of bacteria. Gram-positive cocci, often occurring in chains of varying length. Require enriched media for growth and the colonies are small. Saprophytic and parasitic species. Pathogenic species produce powerful exotoxins. These include leucocidins which kill WBC and haemolysins which kill RBC. In man they are responsible for numerous infections such as scarlatina, tonsillitis, erysipelas, endocarditis, rheumatic fever, glomerulonephritis, and wound infections in hospital—streptococcal, adj.

streptodornase (streptō-dor'-nās). An enzyme used with streptokinase (q.v.) in liquefying pus and blood clots.

streptoduocin (strep-tō-dū'-ō-sin). A mixture of streptomycin and dihydrostreptomycin, said to have a lower toxicity.

streptokinase (strep-tō-kī'-nāz). An enzyme derived from cultures of certain haemolytic streptococci. Plasminogen activator. Used with streptodornase (q.v.). Its fibrinolytic effect has been used with thrombolytic therapy to speed removal of intravascular fibrin.

streptolysins (strep-tō-lī'-sinz) [G. *streptos*, curved; *lysis*, a loosening]. Haemolytic toxins produced by streptococci. Antibody produced in the tissues against streptolysin may be measured and taken as an indicator of recent streptococcal infection.

streptomycin (strep-tō-mī'-sin). An antibiotic effective against many organisms, but used mainly in tuberculosis. Treatment is usually combined with other drugs to reduce drug resistance. It is not absorbed when given orally, hence used in some intestinal infections.

Streptothrix (strep'-tō-thriks) [G. *streptos*, curved; *thrix*, thread]. A filamentous bacterium which shows true branching.

Striatran. Emylcamate (q.v.).

striae (strī'-ē) [L. furrows]. Streaks; stripes; narrow bands. **striae gravidarum**, lines which appear, especially on the abdomen, as a result of stretching of the skin in pregnancy; due to rupture of the lower layers of the dermis. They are red at first and then become silvery-white—stria, sing.; striated, adj.

stricture (strik'-tūr) [L. *strictura*, compression]. A narrowing, especially of a tube or canal, due to scar tissue or tumour.

stridor (strī'-dor) [L. harsh sound]. A harsh sound in breathing, caused by air passing through constricted air passages—stridulous, adj.

stroke (strōk). Popular term for apoplexy resulting from a vascular accident in the brain, usually resulting in hemiplegia. Heat-stroke is hyperpyrexia due to inhibition of heat-regulating mechanism in conditions of high temperature or high humidity, or because sweating is interfered with.

stroma (strō'-mà) [G. bed]. The interstitial or foundation substance of a structure.

Strongyloides (strong'-i-loids). Intestinal worms that can infest man.

strongyloidiasis (strong-i-loid-ī'-a-sis). Infestation with *Strongyloides stercoralis*, usually acquired through skin from contaminated soil, but can be through mucous membrane. At site of larval penetration there may be an itchy rash. As the larvae migrate through the lungs there may be pulmonary symptoms with larvae in sputum. There may be varying abdominal symptoms. Because of autoinfective life cycle, treatment aims at complete elimination of the parasite. Thiabendazole 25 mg per kg twice daily for 2 days; given either as a suspension or tablets which should be chewed. Driving a car is inadvisable during therapy.

strontium 90. Radioactive isotope with a relatively long half-life (28 years). It is incorporated into bone tissue where turnover is slow.

strophanthus (strō-fan'-thus). African plant with cardiac properties similar to digitalis, but of more rapid action. The active principle, strophanthin, is sometimes given by intravenous injection.

strophulus (strof'-ūl-us). Prickly heat; miliaria (q.v.).

strychnine (strik'-nēn). A bitter alkaloid obtained from nux vomica. Used as a tonic in association with other bitter drugs.

stupe (stūp). A medical fomentation (q.v.). Opium may be added to relieve pain. Turpentine may be added to produce counterirritation.

stupor (stū'-por) [L]. A state of marked impairment of, but not complete loss of consciousness. The victim shows gross lack of responsiveness, usually reacting only to noxious stimuli. In psychiatry there are three main varieties of s.: depressive, schizophrenic and hysterical—stuporous, adj.

Sturge-Weber syndrome. A genetically determined congenital ectodermosis, i.e. a capillary haemangioma above eye may be accompanied by similar changes in vessels inside skull giving rise to epilepsy and other cerebral manifestations. Naevoid amentia. [William A. Sturge, English physician, 1850–1919. Frederick Parkes Weber, English physician, 1863–   ].

St Vitus' dance. See CHOREA.

stye (stī). An abscess in the follicle of an eyelash. Syn., hordeolum.

styloid (stī'-loid) [G. *stylos* pillar; *eidos,* form]. Long and pointed; resembling a pen or stylus.

styptic (stip'-tik). An astringent applied to stop bleeding. Haemostatic.

Stypven (stip'-ven). A preparation of viper venom, used by local application as a haemostatic.

Styrion (sti'-ri-on). A synthetic resin capable of absorbing acids. It is sometimes useful in peptic ulcer.

Suavitil (sū-āv'-it-il). Benactyzine (q.v.).

subacute (sub-ak-ūt') [L. *sub,* under; *acutus,* pointed]. Moderately severe. Often the stage between the acute and chronic phases of disease. **subacute bacterial endocarditis,** septicaemia superimposed on previous valvular heart lesion. Petechiae of the skin and embolic phenomena are characteristic. **subacute combined degeneration of the spinal cord** is a complication of pernicious anaemia (PA) and affects the posterior and lateral columns.

subarachnoid space (sub-a-rak'-noid)[L. *sub,* under; G. *arachne,* spider; *eidos,* form]. The space beneath the arachnoid membrane, between it and the pia mater. It contains cerebrospinal fluid.

subcarinal (sub-kar-ī'-nal) [L. *sub,* under; *carina,* keel]. Below a carina, usually referring to the carina tracheae.

subclavian (sub-klā'-vi-an) [L. *sub,* under; *clavis,* key]. Beneath the clavicle.

subclinical (sub-klin'-ik-al) [L. *sub,* under; G. *klinikos,* of a bed]. Insufficient to cause the classical identifiable disease.

subconjunctival (sub-con-jungk-ti'-val) [L. *sub,* under; *conjunctivus,* serving to connect]. Below the conjunctiva—subconjunctivally, adv.

subconscious. That portion of the mind

outside the range of clear consciousness, but capable of affecting conscious mental or physical reactions.

subcostal (sub-kos'-tal) [L. *sub*, under; *costa*, rib]. Beneath the rib.

subcutaneous (sub-kū-tā'-ni-us) [L. *sub*, under; *cutis*, skin]. Beneath the skin—subcutaneously, adv.

subcuticular (sub-kū-tik'-ū-lar) [L. *sub*, under; *cuticula*, cuticle]. Beneath the cuticle, as a s. abscess.

subdural (sub-dū'-ral) [L. *sub*, under; *durus*, hard]. Beneath the dura mater; between the dura and arachnoid membranes.

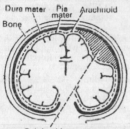

Dura mater   Pia   Arachnoid
            mater
Bone

Subdural haematoma

subendocardial (sub-end-ō-kár'-di-al) [L. *sub*, below; G. *endon*, within; *kardia*, heart]. Immediately beneath the endocardium.

subhepatic (sub-hep-at'-ik) [L. *sub*, under; G. *hepar*, liver]. Beneath the liver.

subinvolution (sub-in-vol-ū'-shun) [L. *sub*, under; *involvere*, to roll up]. Failure of the gravid uterus to return to its normal size within a normal time after childbirth. See INVOLUTION.

subjective (sub-jek'-tiv) [L. *subjectivus*]. Internal; personal; arising from the senses and not perceptible to others. Opp., objective.

sublimate (sub'-lim-āt) [L. *sublimare*, to elevate]. A solid deposit resulting from the condensation of a vapour. In psychiatry, to redirect a primitive desire into some more socially acceptable channel, e.g. a strong tendency to agressiveness subliminated into sporting activity—sublimation, n.

subliminal (sub-lim'-in-al) [L. *sub*, under; *limen*, threshold]. Inadequate for perceptible response. Below the threshold of consciousness. See LIMINAL.

sublingual (sub-ling'-gwal) [L. *sub*, under; *lingua*, tongue]. Beneath the tongue.

subluxation (sub-luks-ā'-shun) [L. *sub*, under; *luxatio*, dislocation]. Incomplete dislocation of a joint. Term usually implies that joint can return to normal position without formal reduction.

submandibular (sub-man-dib'-ū-lar) [L. *sub*, under; *mandibula*, jaw]. Below the mandible.

submaxillary (sub-maks-ilL-lar-i) [L. *sub*, under; *maxilla*, jaw]. Beneath the lower jaw.

submucosa (sub-mū-kō'-sā) [L. *sub*, under; *mucosus*, mucous]. The layer of connective tissue beneath a mucous membrane—submucous, submucosal, adj.

submucous (sub-mū'-kus). Below mucous membrane. **submucous resection**, straightening of a deflected nasal septum.

subnormality. A state of arrested or incomplete development of mind (not amounting to severe s.) which includes subnormality of intelligence and is of a nature or degree which requires or is susceptible to medical treatment or other special care or training of the patient. **severe s.**, a state of arrested or incomplete development of mind which includes subnormality of intelligence and is of such a nature or degree that the patient is incapable of living an independent life or of guarding himself against serious exploitation, or will be so incapable when of an age to do so.

suboccipital (sub-oks-ip'-it-al) [L. *sub*, under; *occiput*, back of head]. Beneath the occiput; in the nape of the neck.

subperiosteal (sub-per-i-os'-ti-al) [L. *sub*, under; G. *periosteos*, around the bones]. Beneath the periosteum of bone.

subphrenic (sub-fren'-ik) [L. *sub*. under; G. *phren*, midriff]. Beneath the diaphragm.

subsultus (sub-sul'-tus) [L. *subsultare*, to leap]. Muscular tremor. **Subsultus tendinum**, twitching of tendons and muscles particularly around the wrist in severe fever, such as typhoid.

succinylcholine (sucks-in-il-kō'-lēn). Short-acting muscle relaxant.

succinylsulphathiazole (suk-sin-il-sul-fa-thī'-a-zol). A sulphonamide used in gastrointestinal infections and in bowel surgery. It is poorly absorbed and is not effective against systemic infections.

succus (suk'-us) [L. juice]. A juice, especially that secreted by the intestinal glands and called 's. entericus'.

succussion (suk-ush'-on) [L. *succutere,* to fling from below]. Splashing sound produced by fluid in a hollow cavity on shaking the patient, e.g. liquid content of dilated stomach in pyloric stenosis. **hippocratic s.,** the splashing sound, on shaking, when fluid accompanies a pneumothorax.

sucrose (sū'-krōs). Cane, beet or maple sugar. A disaccharide. It is normally converted into dextrose and levulose in the body.

sucrosuria (sū-krō-sū'-ri-á). The presence of sucrose in the urine.

sudamina (sū-dam'-in-á) [L. *sudare,* to sweat]. Sweat rash.

Sudan blindness. A form of onchocerciasis.

sudor (sū'-dor) [L.]. Sweat—sudoriferous, adj.

sudorific (sū-dor-if'-ik) [L. *sudor,* sweat; *facere,* to make]. An agent which induces sweating. Diaphoretic.

suggestibility (suj-jest'-ib-il'-it-i) [L. *suggerere,* to suggest]. Amenable to suggestion (q.v.); is heightened in hospital patients, in the dependence on others that illness brings, in children, in the mentally subnormal and those with a tendency to hysteria.

suggestion (suj-jest'-chun) [L. *suggestio,* suggest]. The implanting in a person's mind of an idea which he accepts fully without logical reason. Suggestion is utilized when the idea of recovery is given to, and accepted by, a patient. In psychiatric practice s. is used as a therapeutic measure sometimes under hypnosis or narcoanalysis (q.v.).

sulcus (sul'-kus) [L.]. A furrow or groove, particularly those separating the gyri or convolutions of the cortex of the brain—sulci, pl.

sulfametopyrazine (sul-fa-met-o-pī-ra-zēn). Particularly useful for urinary infections.

Sulfamylon (sul-fa-mī'-lon). Mefenide acetate (q.v.).

Sulfasuxidine (sul-fa-suks'-i-dēn). Succinylsulphathiazole (q.v.).

sulphacetamide (sul-fa-set'-a-mīd). A sulphonamide used mainly as eye drops, and systemically for urinary tract infections.

sulphadiazine (sul-fa-dī'-a-zēn). Powerful sulphonamide compound for systemic use in many infections. Often drug of choice in meningococcal infections as penetration into CSF is greater. It is less effective against staphylococcal infections.

sulphadimidine (sul-fa-di'-mi-dēn). One of the most effective and least toxic of the sulphonamides, and reduced incidence of side effects increases its value in paediatrics. The sodium salt may be given by injection.

sulphaemoglobinaemia (sulf-hēm-ō-glōb-in-ē'-mi-á). A condition of circulating sulphmethaemoglobin in the blood.

sulphafurazole (sul-fa-fūr'-a-zol). A sulphonamide of wide application, but used mainly in urinary infections owing to its high solubility.

sulphaguanidine (sul-fa-gwan'-i-dēn). Once used in gastrointestinal infections but now largely replaced by less soluble compounds such as phthalylsulphathiazole.

sulphamerazine (sul-fa-mer'-a-zēn). A longer acting sulphonamide, effective in 8-hourly doses, but the slow elimination may cause toxic side effects.

Sulphamethazine (sul-fa-meth'-a-zēn). Sulphadimidine (q.v.).

sulphamethoxazole (sul-fa-meth-oks'-a-zol). Sulphonamide that has a pattern of absorption and excretion very similar to trimethoprim.

sulphamethoxydiazine (sul-fa-meth-oks'-i-dī'-a-zēn). A variant of the sulphonamides (q.v.).

sulphamethoxypryridazine (sul-fa-meth-ok'-si-pi-ri-dā-zēn). A long-acting, small-dosage sulphonamide.

sulphapyridine (sul-fa-pi'-ri-dēn). One of the early sulphonamides, now replaced by less toxic drugs. Occasionally used in low dose in dermatitis herpetiformis.

sulphathiazole (sul-fa-thī'-a-zol). A powerful but rapidly excreted sulphonamide. Toxic effects are common with this drug, and it is now used less frequently, except in association with other sulphonamides.

Sulphatriad (sul-fa-trī'-ad). Contains sulphadiazine, sulphamerazine and sulphathiazole. Sulphonamide mixtures reduce the risk of toxic side effects.

sulphinpyrazone (sul-fin-pir'-á-zōn). Uricosuric agent.

sulphmethaemoglobin (sulf-met-hēm-ō-glōb'-in). Syn., sulphaemoglobin. A sulphide oxidation product of haemoglobin, produced in vivo by certain drugs. This compound cannot transport oxygen or carbon dioxide and, not being reversible in the body, is an indirect poison.

sulphonamides. A group of bacteriostatic agents, effective orally, but must be maintained in a definite concentration in the blood. Antimetabolites. Inhibit formation of folic acid, which for many organisms is an essential metabolite.

sulphonamidopyrimidines (sul-fon-a-mid'-ō-pi-ri-mid'-ēnz). Oral blood-sugar lowering agents.

sulphones (sul'-fōns). A group of synthetic drugs useful for leprosy.

sulphonylureas (sul-fon-il-ū'-rē-as). Sulphonamide derivatives that are oral hypoglycaemic agents. They increase insulin output from the pancreas.

sulphur (sul'-fur). An insoluble yellow powder once used extensively as sulphur ointment for scabies. Still used in lotions for acne and other skin disorders, and internally as a laxative.

sulphuric acid (sul-fū'-rik as'-id). The concentrated acid is widely employed in industry, and is very corrosive. The dilute acid (10 per cent) has been given for its astringent action, but is now rarely used.

sulthiame (sul-thī'-am). For temporal lobe and Jacksonian epilepsy.

sunstroke. Syn., heat-stroke. See STROKE.

supercilium (sū-per-sil'-i-um) [L. eyebrow]. The eyebrow—superciliary, adj.

superior (sū-pē'-ri-or) [L. higher]. In anatomy, the upper of two parts.

supernumerary (sū-per-nū'-mėr-ár-i). In excess of the normal number; additional.

supinate (sū'-pin-āt) [L. supinare, to bend backward]. Turn face or palm upward. Opp., pronate—supination, n.

supinator (sū-pin-ā'-tor). That which supinates, usually applied to a muscle. Opp., pronator.

supine (sū'-pīn) [L. supinus, thrown backward]. Lying on the back with face upwards, palm upwards. Opp., prone.

suppository (sup-os'-i-tri). Medicament in a base that melts at body temperature. Inserted rectally.

suppression (sup-resh'-un) [L. supprimere, to press down]. Cessation of a secretion (e.g. urine) or a normal process (e.g. menstruation). In psychology, the voluntary forcing out of the mind of painful thoughts. This often results in the precipitation of a neurosis (q.v.).

suppuration (sup-ūr-ā'-shun) [L. suppurare, to suppurate]. The formation of pus—suppurative, adj.; suppurate, v.i.

supraclavicular (soop-ra-klav-ik'-ū-lar) [L. supra, above; clavicula, little key]. Above the collar bone (clavicle).

supracondylar (soop-ra-kond'-il-ar) [L. supra, above, G. kondylos, knob]. Above a condyle.

supraorbital (soop-ra-or'-bit-al) [L. supra, above; orbis, circle]. Above the orbits. **supraorbital ridge,** the ridge covered by the eyebrows.

suprapubic (soop-ra-pū'-bik) [L. supra, above; pubes, private parts]. Above the pubis.

suprarenal (soop-ra-rēn'-al) [L. supra, above; renes, kidneys]. Above the kidney. See ADRENAL.

suprasternal (soop-ra-stèr'-nal) [L. supra, above; G. sternon, breast]. Above the breast bone (sternum).

suramin (sū'-ra-min). Drug used i.v. in the early stages of trypanosomiasis, filariasis and onchocerciasis. Contraindications: renal disease or adrenal insufficiency.

surgery (sur'-je-ri). That branch of medicine which treats diseases, deformities and injuries, wholly or in part, by manual or operative procedures.

Surmontil (sur-mon'-til). Trimipramine (q.v.).

susceptibility (sus-sep-tib-il'-it-i) [L. suscipere, to take up]. The opposite of resistance. Usually refers to a disposition to infection.

Sustac (sus'-tak). Sustained action glyceryl trinitrate (q.v.).

suture (sū'-tūr). The junction of cranial bones; in surgery, a stitch. See LIGATURE.

suxamethonium (suks-a-meth-ō'-ni-um). A muscle relaxant used in minor operative work. The action is very brief, lasting 2 to 5 min, but a longer effect can be achieved by continuous intravenous drip infusion. Usually preceded by an intravenous barbiturate to reduce initial muscular fibrillation. Normally hydrolysed by the serum enzyme pseudocholinesterase. An abnormal pseudocholinesterase affects a person's reaction to s. and can give rise to s. **apnoea.**

SVC. Vaginal tablets containing acetarsol (q.v.).

swab (swob). 1. A small piece of cotton wool or gauze. 2. A small piece of sterile cotton wool, or similar material, on the end of a shaft of wire or wood, enclosed in a protecting tube. It is used to collect material for bacteriological examination.

sweat (swet). The secretion from the sudoriferous glands.

Swenson's operation. For congenital intestinal aganglionosis (Hirschsprung's disease).

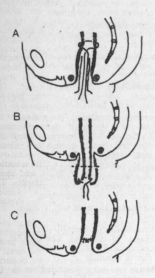

Swenson's operation

sycosis (sī-kō'-sis) [G. *sykosis,* fig-like ulcer]. Barber's itch. **sycosis barbai** is a pustular folliculitis of the beard area in men. **sycosis nuchae** is a similar folliculitis at the nape of the neck which leads to keloid thickening (acne keloid).

symbiosis (sim-bī-ō'-sis) [G. living together]. A relationship between two or more organisms in which the partici-

pants are of mutual aid and benefit to one another—symbiotic, adj.

symblepharon (sim-blef'-a-ron) [G. *syn,* with; *blepharon,* eyelid]. Adhesion of the lid to the eyeball.

Syme's amputation. Amputation just above ankle joint. Provides an end-bearing stump. Especially useful in primitive conditions where elaborate artificial limbs are not available. [James Syme, Scottish surgeon, 1799–1870.]

Symmetril (sim'-et-ril). Amantadine (q.v.).

sympathectomy (sim-path-ek'-to-mi) [G. *sympathein,* to feel for; *ektome,* excision]. Surgical excision of part of the sympathetic nervous system.

sympathetic (sim-path-et'-ik) [G. *sympathein,* to feel for]. A portion of the autonomic nervous system. It is composed of a chain of ganglia on either side of the vertebral column in the thoracolumbar region, and sends fibres to all plain muscle tissue.

sympathomimetic (sim-path-ō-mim-et'-ik) [G. *sympathein,* to feel for; *mimokos,* imitating]. Capable of producing changes similar to those produced by stimulation of the sympathetic nerves.

symphysis (sim'-fis-is) [G. *symphysis,* growing together]. A fibrocartilaginous union of bones—symphyseal, adj.

symptom (simp'-tom) [G. *symptoma,* anything that happens]. A subjective phenomenon or manifestation of disease. **symptom complex,** a group of symptoms which, occurring together, typify a particular disease or syndrome—symptomatic, adj.

symptomatology (simp-tom-at-ol'-o-ji) [G. *symptoma,* anything that happens; *logos,* discourse]. The branch of medicine concerned with symptoms. The combined symptoms typical of a particular disease.

Synacthen (sin-ak'-then). Tetrocosactrin (q.v.).

Synalar (sin'-à-lar). Fluocinolone (q.v.).

synapse (sī'-naps) [G. *synapsis,* contact]. The point of communication between two adjacent neurones. Syn., synapsis.

synchysis (sing'-ki-sis). Degenerative condition of vitreous humor of the eye, rendering it fluid. **synchysis scintillans,** fine opacities in vitreous.

syncope (sing'-ko-pi) [G. *syngkope,* sudden loss of strength]. A faint. Caused by reduced cerebral circulation often following a fright, when vasodilation is responsible. May be symptomatic of cardiac arrhythmia, e.g. heart block—syndactylous, adj.

syndactyly (sin-dak'-ti-li) [G. *syn*, with; *daktylos*, finger]. Webbed fingers or toes. Also **syndactylism, syndactylia**—syndactylous, adj.

syndrome (sin'-drōm) [G. *syndromos*, a running together]. A group of symptoms and/or signs which, occurring together, produce a pattern or symptom complex, typical of a particular disease.

synechia (sin-ek'-i-á) [G. *synecheia*, continuity]. Abnormal union of parts, especially adhesion of the iris to the cornea in front, or the lens capsule behind—synechiae, pl.

synergism (sin'-ér-jizm) [G. *synergos*, co-operator]. The harmonious working together of two agents, such as drugs, micro-organisms, muscles, etc. Also **synergy**—synergic, adj.

synergist (sin'-ér-jist). An agent co-operating with another. One partner in a synergic action.

Synkavit (sin'-kav-it). A water-soluble compound possessing high vitamin K activity.

synovectomy (sī-nov-ek'-to-mi) [N.L. *synovia*; G. *ektome*, excision]. Excision of synovial membrane. Current early treatment for rheumatoid arthritis especially of the hands.

synovia (sī-nō'-vi-á) [N.L.]. The fluid secreted by the membrane lining a joint cavity—synovial adj.

synovial membrane (sī-nō'-vi-al mem'-brān). That lining a joint capsule; it does not cover the articular surfaces. See BURSA.

synovioma (sī-nō-vi-ō'-má) [N.L. *synovia*; G. *-oma*, tumour]. A tumour of synovial membrane—benign or malignant.

synovitis (si-nov-ī'-tis) [N.L. *synovia*; G. *-itis*, inflammation]. Inflammation of a synovial membrane.

synthesis (sin'-the-sis) [G. a putting together]. The chemical building up of complex substances from simpler substances—synthetic, adj.

Syntocinon. Synthetic oxytocin (q.v.).

Syntometrine (sin-tō-met'-rin). Ergometrine maleate 0.5 mg and synthetic oxy-

tocin 5 units in one ampoule. Combines the rapid action of oxytocin with the more sustained action of ergometrine on the uterus.

syphilide (sif'-il-īd) [N.L. syphilis]. A syphilitic skin lesion.

syphilis (sif'-il-is). [Syphilus, syphilitic shepherd in poem by Fracastorius (1530), in which the term first appears.] The most severe venereal disease, caused by *Treponema pallidum*. Infection is acquired (may be accidentally) or congenital—when it is prenatal. Acquired syphilis manifests in: (1) The primary stage, appears 4 to 5 weeks (or later) after infection when a primary chancre associated with swelling of local lymph glands appears. (2) The secondary stage in which the skin eruption (syphilide) appears. (3) The third stage occurs 15 to 30 years after initial infection. Gummata appear, or neurosyphilis and cardiovascular syphilis supervene. The commonest types of nervous system involvement are general paralysis of the insane and tabes dorsalis (locomotor ataxia). Cardiovascular involvement produces cerebrovascular disasters, aortic aneurysm and impairment or destruction of the aortic valve—syphilitic, adj.

syringomyelia (si-ring-gō-mī-ē'-li-á) [G. *syrigx*, pipe; *myelos*, marrow]. An uncommon, progressive disease of the nervous system of unknown cause, beginning mainly in early adult life. Cavitation and surrounding fibrous tissue reaction, in the upper spinal cord and brain stem, interfere with sensation of pain and temperature, and sometimes with the motor pathways. The characteristic symptom is painless injury, particularly of the exposed hands. Touch sensation is intact.

syringomyelocele (si-ring-gō-mī'-el-ō-sēl) [G. *syrigx*, pipe; *myelos*, marrow]. Most severe form of meningeal hernia (spina bifida). The central canal is dilated and the thinned-out posterior part of the spinal cord is in the hernia.

systole (sis'-to-li) [G. a drawing together]. The contraction phase of the cardiac cycle—systolic, adj.

systolic murmur. Abnormal quality of first heart sound usually related to the area of one of the heart valves, e.g. systolic mitral murmur.

Sytron (sit'-ron) Elixir. Sodium iron edetate. For iron deficiency anaemia.

TAB 290

T

TAB. A vaccine containing killed *Salmonella typhi*, *S. paratyphi A* and *S. paratyphi B*; and used to produce active artificial immunity in man, against typhoid and paratyphoid fever. Sometimes used therapeutically to produce pyrexia.

tabes (tā'-bēz) [L.]. Wasting away. **tabes dorsalis** (locomotor ataxia) is a variety of neurosyphilis in which the posterior (sensory) columns of the spinal cord and the sensory nerve roots are diseased. **tabes mesenterica** is tuberculous enlargement of peritoneal glands found in children—tabetic, adj.

taboparesis (tā-bō-par-ē'-sis) [L. *tabes*, a wasting; G. *paresis*, paralysis]. A condition of general paralysis of the insane in which the spinal cord shows the same lesions as in tabes dorsalis (q.v.).

Tace (tās). Chlorotrianisene (q.v.).

tachistoscope (tak-is'-to-skōp) [G. *tachys*, swift; *skopein*, to examine]. Enables words and patterns to be presented for predetermined periods in the R. or L. visual field. Used in centres for training 'word blind' people.

tachycardia (tak-i-kár'-di-á) [G. *tachys*, swift; *kardia*, heart]. Excessively rapid action of the heart. **paroxysmal t.**, a temporary but sudden marked increase in frequency of heart-beats, because the conducting stimulus is originating in an abnormal focus.

tachyphasia (tak-i-fā'-zi-á) [G. *tachys*, swift; *phasis*, speech]. Extreme rapidity of flow of speech occurring in some mental disorders.

tachypnoea (tak-ip'-nē-á) [G. *tachys*, swift; *pnein*, to breathe]. Abnormal frequency of respiration—tachypnoeic, adj.

tactile (tak'-tīl) [L. *tactilis*, that may be touched]. Pertaining to the sense of touch.

Taenia (tē'-ni-á) [G. *tainia*, band]. A genus of flat, parasitic worms; cestodes or tapeworms. *Taenia echinococcus*, the adult worm lives in the dog's intestine (the definitive host) and man (the intermediate host) is infested by swallowing eggs from the dog's excrement. These become embryos in the human small intestine, pass via the blood stream to organs, particularly the liver, and develop into hydatid cysts. *Taenia saginata*, larvae present in infested, undercooked beef. Commonest species in Britain. In man's (the definitive host) intestinal lumen they develop into the adult tapeworm, which by its four suckers attaches itself to the gut wall. Treated with two 500 mg tablets of Yomesan—chewed and swallowed with water before breakfast. This drug partially digests the worms, hence it must never be used in *T. solium* infections. *Taenia solium*, resembles *T. saginata*, but has hooklets as well as suckers. Commonest species in Eastern Europe. The larvae are ingested in infested, undercooked pork; man can also be the intermediate host for this worm by ingesting eggs which, developing into larvae in his stomach, pass via the bowel wall to reach organs, and there develop into cysts. In the brain these may give rise to epilepsy. Treatment in hospital with 1 g mepacrine hydrochloride via duodenal tube followed in 30 min by saline purge.

taenia (tēn'-i-á) [G. *tainia*, band]. A flat band. **taenia coli**, three flat bands running the length of the large intestine and consisting of the longitudinal muscle fibres.

taeniacide (tēn'-i-a-sīd) [G. *tainia*, band; L. *caedere*, to kill]. An agent that destroys tapeworms—taeniacidal, adj.

taeniafuge (tēn'-i-á-fūj) [G. *tainia*, band; L. *fugere*, to flee]. An agent that expels tapeworms.

Tagamet (tag'-a-met). Cimetidine (q.v.).

Talampicillin (tal-am-pi-sil'-lin). Hydrolysed in mucous membrane to release free ampicillin (q.v.).

talc. A naturally occurring soft white powder, consisting of magnesium silicate. Used extensively as a dusting powder, prior to the donning of surgical gloves. K285 (q.v.) now preferred.

talipes (tal'-i-pēz) [L. *talus*, ankle; *pes*,

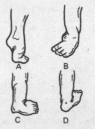

A Talipes equinus   C Talipes valgus
B Talipes varus   D Talipes calcaneus

foot]. Congenital deformity of foot—
'club-foot'. Club-foot includes t. equinovarus and t. calcaneovalgus.

talus (tāl'-us) [L.]. The astragalus; situated between the tibia proximally and
the calcaneus distally, thus directly
bearing the weight of the body. It is the
second largest bone of the ankle.

tamponade. Insertion of a tampon. See
CARDIAC.

Tanderil (tan'-der-il). Oxyphenbutazone
(q.v.).

Tannafax (tan'-a-faks). A proprietary
preparation containing tannic acid in
jelly form. Useful for superficial burns
and scalds

tannic acid (tan'-nik as'-id). A brown
powder obtained from oak galls. It has
astringent properties, and is used as a
rectal irrigation in colitis, as suppositories for haemorrhoids and as a jelly for
mild burns.

tantalum (tant'-a-lum). A rare metal
sometimes used in the form of wire or
gauze to reinforce weak areas in the
body, as in the repair of a large hernia

tapeworm. Taenia (q.v.).

tapping. Aspiration. Paracentesis (q.v.).

tar. Usually refers to wood tar, which,
like coal tar, is used in a variety of skin
disorders **coal t.,** a black viscid substance obtained as a by-product from
coal distillation. Liq. picis carb. is an
alcoholic solution of coal t., used in
dermatological conditions.

Taractan. Chlorprothixene (q.v.)

tarsalgia (tár-sal'-ji-á) [G. *tarsos,* flat
surface; *algos,* pain]. Pain in the foot.

tarsometatarsal (tár-sō-met'-a-tár-sal)
[G. *tarsos,* flat surface; *meta* between,
tarsos]. Pertaining to the tarsal and
metatarsal region.

tarsoplasty (tár'-sō-plás-ti). [G. *tarsos,*
flat surface; *plassein,* to form]. Any
plastic operation to the eyelid.

tarsorrhaphy (tár-sor-raf-i) [G. *tarsos,*
flat surface; *rhaphe,* suture]. Suturing
of the lids together in order to protect
cornea when it is anaesthetic, or to
allow healing.

tarsus (tár'-sus) [G. *tarsos,* flat surface].
1. The seven small bones of the foot. 2.
The thin elongated plates of dense connective tissue found in each eyelid,
contributing to its form and support—
tarsal, adj.

tartar (tár'-tèr). The deposit which forms
on the teeth. **cream of t.,** potassium

bitartrate. **tartar emetic,** antimony and
potassium tartrate.

Tay-Sachs' disease. Primary defect
appears to be a deficiency of the enzyme
β-D-N-acetylhexosaminidase which
leads to a massive accumulation on a
specific lipid substance called GM_2, or
Tay-Sachs ganglioside—hence the alternative name, gangliosidosis. [Warren
Tay, English physician, 1843-1927.
Bernard Sachs, New York neurologist,
1858-1944.]

tears (tērz). The secretion formed by the
lacrimal gland. It contains the enzyme
lysozyme which acts as an antiseptic.

tease (tēz). To draw or pull out into fine
threads, as in separating the fibres of a
particle of muscle tissue.

teat (tēt). A nipple.

teclothiazide (tek-lo-thī'-a-zīd). Oral diuretic. See CHLOROTHIAZIDE.

teeth (tēth). The structures used for mastication. The deciduous, milk or temporary set, 20 in number, is shed by the
age of 7. The permanent set, 32 in
number, is usually complete in the late
teens. **canine** or **eye t.** have sharp fanglike edge for tearing food. **Hutchinson's
t.** have a notched edge and are characteristic of congenital syphilis. **incisor t.**
have knife-like edge for biting food
premolar and **molar t.** have a squarish
termination for chewing and grinding
food. **wisdom t.** are the last molar teeth,
one at either side of each jaw.

Tegretol (teg'-ret-ol). Carbamazepine
(q.v.).

tegument (teg'-ū-ment) [L. *tegumentum,*
covering]. The skin or covering of the
animal body.

telangiectasis (tel-an-ji-ek'-ta-sis) [G.
telos, end; *aggeion,* vessel; *ektasis,*
extension]. Dilatation of the capillaries
on a body surface.

Telepaque (tel-ē'-pak). Iopanoic acid
(q.v.).

teleradium (te-lē-rā'-di-um) [G. *tele,* far
off]. Radium whose radiation is
directed into the body from an external
source; radium beam.

teletherapy (te-lē-ther'-a-pi) [G. *tele,* far
off; *therapeia,* treatment]. By custom
refers to treatment with teleradium.
Now includes cobalt or caesium
beams—teletherapeutic, adj.; teletHerapeutically, adv

TEM. Tretamine (q.v.).

temperament (tem'-pèr-a-ment) [L. *tem-*

peramentum, mixing in proportion]. The habitual mental attitude of the individual. Four classicial types described originally—sanguine, phlegmatic, bilious, melancholic.

temple (tem'-pl) [L. *tempora*]. That part of the head lying between the outer angle of the eye and the top of the ear-flap.

temporal (tem'-por-al). Relating to the temple. **temporal bones,** one on each side of the head below the parietal bone, containing the middle ear.

temporomandibular (tem'-por-ō-mandib'-ū-lar) [L. *tempora,* temples; *mandibula,* jaw]. Pertaining to the temporal region or bone, and the lower jaw.

Temposil (tem'-pō-sil). Analogue of disulphiram (q.v.).

TEN. Toxic epidermal necrolysis (q.v.).

tendon (ten'-don) [G. *tenon*]. A firm, white, fibrous inelastic cord which attaches muscle to bone—tendinous, adj.

tenesmus (ten-ez'-mus) [G. *telnein,* to stretch]. Painful, ineffectual straining to empty the bowel or bladder.

tenoplasty (tēn'-ō-plas-ti) [G. *tenon,* tendon; *plassein,* to form]. A plastic operation on a tendon—tenoplastic, adj.

Tenormal (ten-orm'-al). Pempidine (q.v.).

tenorrhaphy (tēn-or'-raf-i) [G. *tenon,* tendon; *rhaphe.* suture]. The suturing of a tendon.

tenosynovitis (tē-nō-sī-no-vī'-tis) [G. *tenon,* tendon; N.L. *synovia,* synovia; G. *-itis,* inflammation]. Inflammation of the thin synovial lining of a tendon sheath, as distinct from its outer fibrous sheath. It may be caused by mechanical irritation or by bacterial infection.

tenotomy (ten-ot'-om-i) [G. *tenon,* tendon; *tome,* cutting]. Division of a tendon.

TEPP. Ethyl pyrophosphate (q.v.).

teratogen (ter'-at-o-jen) [G. *teras,* monster]. Anything capable of disrupting fetal growth and producing malformation. Classified as drugs, poisons, radiations physical agents such as ECT, infections—e.g. rubella, and rhesus and thyroid antibodies. See DYSMORPHOGENIC—teratogenic, teratogenetic, adj.; teratogenicity, teratogenesis, n.

teratology (ter-at-ol'-o-ji) [G. *teras,* monster; *logos,* discourse]. The scientific study of teratogens and their mode of action—teratologist, n.; teratological adj.; teratologically, adv.

teratoma (te-ra-tō'-má) [G. *teras,* monster; *-oma,* tumour]. A tumour of embryonic origin and composed of various structures, including both epithelial and connective tissues; most commonly found in the ovaries and testes, the majority being malignant—teratomata, pl.; teratomatous, adj.

Terra-Cortril (ter-ra-kor'-tril). Terramycin, hydrocortisone and polymyxin B. Mainly used as eye, ear and nose drops and for topical application.

Terramycin (ter-ra-mī'-sin). Oxytetracycline (q.v.).

Tersavid (ter'-sa-vid). Pivhydrazine (q.v.).

tertiary (ter'-shi-a-ri). Third in order.

Tertroxin (ter-troks'-in). A preparation of liothyronine (q.v.) that has a standardized activity.

TEST

adrenal function tests. Abnormal adrenal-cortical function can be detected by measuring the 24-hour urinary output of 17 oxosteroids and 17 hydroxycorticoids or by estimating the 11-hydroxycorticosteroids in plasma. In doubtful cases the estimations can be repeated following the administration of ACTH. See METAPYRONE TEST. Increased adrenal medullary function may be detected by measuring urinary vanyl mandelic acid (VMA) excretion.

Astrup test. Estimates degree of acidosis by measuring gas (O_2 and CO_2) pressures in arterial blood.

augmented histamine test. See HISTAMINE TEST.

basophil test. Distinguishes between immediate and delayed hypersensitivity states. There is a basophil reaction in all of the immediate allergic states.

Bence-Jones' protein test. See BENCE-JONES' PROTEIN.

breath-H_2(hydrogen) test. For disaccharide intolerance. Indirect method for detecting lactase deficiency.

bromosulphthalein test. A test used to assess hepatic function; 5 mg per kg body weight of bromosulphthalein (BSP) are injected intravenously. The dye is usually excreted in the bile; if more than 5 per cent of the dye is circulating in the blood 45 min after injection there is impaired hepatic function.

calcium test. In a normal person sudden increase of calcium by i.v. infusion causes raised phosphate level in blood and urine. In hyperparathyroidism this does not occur.

caloric test (ka-lor'-ik). The assessment of vestibular function by means of heat. Investigation of vestibular disease.

Casoni test. Intradermal injection of 0.2 ml of fresh, sterile hydatid fluid. A white papule indicates a hydatid cyst.

colloidal gold test. One of the laboratory tests of cerebrospinal fluid (CSF) with special application in the diagnosis of syphilis of brain or spinal cord. Different dilutions of a colloidal gold solution show precipitation of the metal when added to an abnormal CSF. The degree of precipitation is shown by corresponding colour changes and the colours are reported as numbers from 1 to 5. Ten dilutions are commonly tested. Tabes dorsalis gives a pattern of numbers such as 0012344321; general paralysis of the insane (GPI), demyelination diseases —e.g. multiple sclerosis, carcinomatous meningitis and subacute inclusion-body encephalitis gives a pattern of numbers such as 5554433210.

complement fixation test. See COMPLEMENT.

Coombs' test. A highly sensitive test designed to detect immune antibodies, attached to red blood cells or present in serum: the 'direct' method detects the former; the 'indirect' method detects the latter. Especially useful in the diagnosis of haemolytic syndromes. [R. R. A. Coombs, contemporary British scientist.]

cortisone suppression test. Differentiates primary from secondary hypercalcaemia. Sarcoidosis causes secondary hypercalcaemia. Primary hyperparathyroidism causes primary hypercalcaemia.

creatine test. See CREATINE.

Demco test. Done on centrifuged blood for glandular fever.

dextroxylase test. See XYLOSE TEST.

diagnex blue test. A means of showing production of acid by the stomach without passing a stomach tube; tablets and granules taken orally.

The findings are revealed by testing the urine.

Duke's test. See BLEEDING TIME. Skin pricked, blood continuously removed with absorbent paper until it ceases to flow. Normal 3 to 5 min.

echo encephalogram. A new test for detecting intracerebral space-occupying lesions causing midline shift.

edrophonium test. For myasthenia gravis. A small i.m. dose of edrophonium. A chloride will immediately relieve symptoms, albeit temporarily, while quinine sulphate will increase the muscular weakness.

enzyme tests. The presence of abnormally high concentrations of serum enzymes may indicate underlying disease. Those enzyme tests in common use and the diseases which cause high levels include:

Acid phosphatase—carcinoma of prostate.
Aldolase—muscle disease.
Alkaline phosphatase—obstructive jaundice and various forms of bone disease.
Amylase—acute pancreatitis; see DIASTASE.
Creatinephosphokinase (CPK)—raised only in acute myocardial infarction and not in other cardiopathics.
Dopamine-β-hydroxylase (DBH)—for high blood pressure.
Glutamic oxalacetic transaminase (GOT)—myocardial infarction.
Glutamic-pyruvic transaminase (GPT)—liver disease.
Hydroxybutyrate dehydrogenase—myocardial infarction.
Lactate dehydrogenase (LDH)—when tissue of high metabolic activity dies tissue necrosis is quickly reflected by increased LDH.

flocculation test. Serum set up against various salts—gold, thymol, cephalin, cholesterol. Presence of abnormal serum proteins results in cloudiness. Abnormal forms of albumin and globulin made by diseased liver cells.

fluorescein string test. A test used to detect the site of obscure upper gastrointestinal haemorrhage. The patient swallows a radio-opaque knotted string. Fluorescein is injected intravenously and after a few minutes the string is withdrawn. If staining has occurred the site of bleeding can be determined.

galactose test. Forty g galactose in 500 ml water taken after fasting. Five hours later urine collected. If it contains 2 g or more g it indicates liver damage.

glucose tolerance test. Useful in the diagnosis of diabetes mellitus and other causes of glycosuria. Serial collections of blood are estimated for blood glucose following the oral or intravenous administration of 50g glucose, and urine samples are simultaneously tested for glucose.

gonococcal complement fixation test. A specific serological test for the diagnosis of gonorrhoea.

growth hormone (GH) test. The effect of growth hormone that is used clinically in measurement is its reciprocal relationship with blood glucose. Blood is therefore taken for estimation of GH during a standard 50 g oral glucose tolerance test. In acromegaly, not only is the resting level of GH higher, but it does not show normal suppression with glucose.

Guthrie test. Assay of phenylalanine from a drop of blood dried on special filter paper. Done on the sixth day of life. It is necessary to confirm the diagnosis in those infants with a positive test.

haemagglutination tests for pregnancy. All based on the same principle, are almost as accurate as the Hogben test and can be performed more rapidly. The addition of urine from a pregnant person will prevent haemagglutination occurring between red cells pretreated with human chlorionic gonadotrophin (HCG) in the presence of specific antisera.

haematoporphyrin test. One to 3 h after injection haematoporphyrin localizes in rapidly multiplying cells and fluoresces under ultraviolet light. In many instances investigators can detect the exact extent of malignant or precancerous tissue.

Heaf test. Multiple puncture of epidermis with special 'gun' through a layer of filter paper soaked in tuberculin strength 1 in 1000 or 1 in 100. Inflammatory reaction is positive.

Hess test. Sphygmomanometer cuff applied and inflated. Petechial eruption in surrounding area after 5 min denotes a positive reaction, i.e. weakness of the capillary walls. [Walter Rudolf Hess, Swiss physiologist. 1881– .]

Hickey-Hare test. Intravenous infusion of hypertonic saline causes increase in urinary output. Administration of 0.2 to 0.3 ml of ADH decreases output.

histamine test. Designed to determine the maximal gastric secretion of hydrochloric acid. A Levin's tube is positioned in the most dependent part of the stomach of a fasting, weighted patient. Following the collection of a control specimen and the injection of an appropriate dose of an antihistamine (100 mg mepyramine maleate) 0.04 mg per kg body weight histamine acid phosphate is injected subcutaneously and gastric secretions are collected for a further hour. By titrating the collections against a standard alkaline solution the acidity of the gastric secretions can be determined.

Hogben test. A female Xenopus toad is injected with a preparation obtained from the early morning urine of a woman suspected of pregnancy. In the case of pregnancy the toad lays eggs after 8 to 24 h. The test is over 99 per cent accurate [Lancelot Hogben, British scientist. 1895– .]

human chorionic gonadotrophin (HCG) test. Presence of HCG in urine detectable in early morning specimen of urine from 6th week of pregnancy. Result can be given in 2 min and confirmed in 2 h.

insulin test. For determining the completeness or otherwise of surgical vagotomy. Hyoglycaemia is the response to i.v. insulin when the vagus nerve is intact. Complete vagotomy gives a negative response.

jelly test. Old tuberculin in a jelly is applied to skin, usually between shoulder blades in babies. If positive, inflammation appears at site of application.

Kahn test. A serological test for the diagnosis of syphilis. The patient's serum reacts with an heterologous antigen prepared from mammalian tissue, and flocculation is produced if syphilitic antibodies are present, [Reuben Leon Kahn, American bacteriologist. 1887– .]

Kay's augmented histamine test. See HISTAMINE TEST.

kidney function tests. Various tests are available for measuring renal function. All require careful collection of urine specimens. Those in common use are: paraaminohippuric acid clearance test for measuring renal blood flow; creatinine clearance test for measuring glomerular filtration rate; ammonium chloride test for measuring tubular ability to excrete hydrogen ion; urinary concentration and dilution tests for measuring tubular function; radioisotope renogram (q.v.). See INDIGOCARMINE.

Kveim test. An intradermal test for sarcoidosis using tissue prepared from person known to be suffering from the condition. [Morten Ansgar Kveim, Oslo physician, 1892–1966.]

levulose test. See LAEVULOSE.

leptospiral agglutination tests. Serological tests used in the diagnosis of specific leptospiral infections, e.g. Weil's disease.

Makari intradermal test for cancer. The detection of antigen–antibody complexes in response to interaction of antigen (TPS, tumour polysaccharide substances) and serum antibodies by use of a skin test.

Mantoux test. Intradermal injection of old tuberculin or PPD (purified protein derivative—a purified type of tuberculin) into anterior aspect of forearm. Inspection after 48 to 72 h. If positive there will be an area of induration and inflammation greater than 5 mm in diameter.

match test. A rough test of respiratory function. If a person is unable to blow out a lighted match held 4 inches from a fully open mouth there is significant reduction of respiratory function.

metapyrone test. A test of pituitary and adrenal function. The urinary excretion of 17 hydroxycorticosteroids is estimated before and after the oral administration of metapyrone. Disease of the pituitary or adrenal cortex causes an abnormal result.

pancreatic function test. Levin's tubes are positioned in the stomach and second part of duodenum. The response of the pancreatic gland to various hormonal stimuli can be measured by analysing the duodenal aspirate. See SELENOMETHIONINE.

Pandy test. For excess globulin in CSF. Only significant if total protein is normal, when it suggests a diagnosis of demyelinating disease (e.g. multiple sclerosis) or syphilis.

patch test. Old tuberculin incorporated in a strapping dressing. Usually applied to skin between shoulder blades in babies. If positive, there is inflammation at site of application.

Paul-Bunnell test. A serological test used in the diagnosis of infective mononucleosis. Antibodies which occur in patients with this disease agglutinate sheep's erythrocytes. [J. R. Paul, American physician, 1893– . W. W. Bunnell, American physician, 1902– .]

pentagastrin test. When injected, p. causes parietal cells to secrete acid to their utmost capacity, expressed as mEq H^+ in 1 h, for the peak 30 min after injection—PAO (peak acid output).

protein-bound iodine (PBI) test. Blood taken for serum protein-bound iodine which corresponds to circulating thyroid hormone levels. In preparation for test—no iodine-containing medicines and a fish-free diet.

platelet stickiness test. Increased in multiple sclerosis and rapidly growing tumours. May be consequent on degradation of neural tissue, as it is rich in phospholipid, fractions of which have been shown to be potent aggregators of platelets in suspension.

prognosticon test. For pregnancy.

prothrombin test. Indirectly reveals amount of p. in the blood. To a sample of oxalated blood are added all the factors needed to bring about clotting, except prothrombin time taken for clot to form is therefore dependent on amount of p. present. Normal time, 10 to 12 seconds.

radioiodine uptake test. The person is given a small dose of radioactive iodine, and the radioactivity of the thyroid gland is subsequently measured. If the gland is overactive more than 45 per cent of the iodine will be taken up by the gland within 4 h. If the gland is underactive less than 20 per cent will be taken up after 48 h.

radioisotope renogram. A kidney function test in which renal blood flow, tubular function and renal excretion can be roughly estimated following the intravenous injection of a radioactive labelled substance which is rapidly accumulated and excreted by the kidneys. Simultaneous counting of the radioactivity over the kidneys allows comparison of the function of the two kidneys. Counters placed over renal tract can detect obstruction such as a stone in the ureter.

rheumatoid arthritis (RA) latex test. Discerns the presence in the blood of rheumatoid factor.

respiratory function tests. Numerous tests are available for assessing respiratory function. These include measurements of the vital capacity (VC), forced vital capacity (FVC), forced expiratory volume (FEV) (which is the volume of air that can be expired in 1 second) and the maximal breathing capacity (MBC) which is that quantity of air that can be shifted in 1 min.

Rinne's test. Testing of air conduction and bone conduction hearing, by tuning fork. [Friedrich Heinrich Rinne, German otologist, 1819–68.]

Rogitine test. If hypertension is permanent, an adrenalytic substance, Rogitine (phentolamine) 5 mg, is injected intravenously. A fall in excess of 35 mmHg in the systolic, and 25 mmHg in the diastolic pressure, occurring within 2 min of injection, is highly suggestive of phaeochromocytoma.

Saxona test. Radioreceptor assay test for pregnancy yielding results in 1 h. Can identify those with a tendency to abort.

SCAT (Sheep cell agglutination test). Presence in the blood of rheumatoid factor detected by the sheep cell agglutination titre.

Schick test. A test used to determine a person's susceptibility or immunity to diphtheria. It consists in the injection of 2 or 3 minims of freshly prepared toxin beneath the skin of the left arm. A similar test is made into the right arm, but in this the serum is heated to 75°C for 10 min, in order to destroy the toxin but not the protein. A positive reaction is recognized by the appearance of a round red area on the left arm within 24 to 48 h, reaching its maximum intensity on the fourth day, then gradually fading with slight pigmentation and desquamation. This reaction indicates susceptibility or absence of immunity. No reaction indicates that the subject is immune to diphtheria. Occasionally a pseudoreaction occurs, caused by the protein of the toxin; in this case the redness appears on both arms, hence the value of the control. [Bela Schick, Austrian paediatrician, 1877–1967.]

Schilling test. Estimation of absorption of radioactive vitamin B_{12} for confirmation of pernicious anaemia.

Schultz-Charlton test. A blanching produced in the skin of a patient showing scarlatinal rash, around an injection of serum from a convalescent case, indicating neutralization of toxin by antitoxin. [Werner Schultz, German physician, 1878–1947.]

Scriver test. Remarkably efficient in detecting, by a single procedure, 22 aminoacidopathies.

secretin test. A quantitative and qualitative test to estimate secretion of pancreatic juice in response to the enzyme secretin.

sweat test. Petri dish prepared with agar, silver nitrate and potassium chromate. With palm of hand pressed to this, excessive chorides in sweat gives distinctive white print, as mucoviscidosis.

synacthen test. Synacthen is a proprietary preparation of tetrosactrin which is synthetic ACTH. Intramuscular infusion of s. normally produces pituitary stimulation for increased secretion of steroid hormones by adrenal cortex, measured by estimation of plasma cortisol. Lack of response denotes inactivity of adrenal cortex as in Addison's disease.

Thyopac test. A resin uptake test to measure circulating thyroid hormone levels.

thyroid antibody test. Thyroid antibody levels indicate the presence and severity of autoimmune thyroid disease.

thyroid stimulating hormone (TSH) test. Radio-immunoassay of level of serum thyroid stimulating hormone. Useful in diagnosing mild hypothyroidism.

tolbutamide test. Fasting blood sugar taken. Intravenous infusion of tolbutamide. Blood taken for glucose level 20 and 30 min later. Normal response—rapid fall of blood sugar due to increased manufacture of insulin. Mature type diabetic response—delayed fall. Prematurity type diabetic response—none.

triple test. A Dreiling tube is passed through the mouth into the duodenum and pancreatic function tests are carried out. In these, the enzymes secretin and pancreozymin are given to stimulate the pancreas and the juice is aspirated as it flows into the duodenum. It is possible to recognize a tumour in the pancreas from analysis of the volume and chemistry of this juice. Some of the juice is then examined by the pathologist using Papanicolaou's method to show cancer cells, and thirdly, the radiologist performs a hypotonic duodenogram which, unlike the conventional barium meal, frequently demonstrates tumours of the pancreas or ampulla. The test takes 2 hours to complete.

urea clearance test, urea concentration test. Procedures for measuring the efficiency of kidney function and both require urine collection under specified conditions.

van den Bergh's test. Estimation of serum bilirubin. Direct positive reaction (conjugated) in obstructive and hepatic jaundice. Indirect positive reaction (unconjugated) in haemolytic jaundice. See BILIRUBIN.

vitamin K test. After injection of vitamin K, serum prothrombin rises in obstructive jaundice, remains depressed in toxic jaundice.

Volmer test. Tuberculin jelly applied to skin and covered with adhesive. Inflammation indicates positive reaction.

von Pirquet's test. Old tuberculin applied to cleansed skin followed by scarification. If positive, inflammation appears at site of scarification.

TPI test. *Treponema pallidum* immobilization test. A modern, highly specific test for syphilis in which syphilitic serum immobilizes and kills spirochaetes grown in pure culture.

Wassermann test. Carried out in the diagnosis of syphilis. It is a complement-fixation test and is not entirely specific. See also under TPI test. [August von Wassermann, German bacteriologist, 1866–1925.]

Weber's test. Tuning fork test for the diagnosis of conduction deafness.

[Friedrich Eugen Weber, German otologist. 1832–91]

Weil-Felix test. An agglutination reaction used in the diagnosis of the typhus group of fevers. Patient's serum is titrated against an heterologous antigen. [Edmund Weil, German physician in Prague, 1880–1922. Arthur Felix, Prague bacteriologist, 1887–1956.]

wool test. A test for detecting colour blindness. The person is asked to select skeins of wool of matching colours.

Widal test (vē'-dal). An agglutination reaction for typhoid fever. The patient's serum is put in contact with *Salmonella typhi.* The result is positive it agglutination occurs, proving the presence of antibodies in the serum. [Georges F.I. Widal, French physician, 1862–1929.]

xylose test. More convenient than fat balance and equally as accurate. Xylose given orally and its urinary excretion measured. Normally 25 per cent of loading dose is excreted. Less than this indicates malabsorption syndrome.

testicle (tes'-tik-l) [L. *testiculus,* dim. of testis]. Testis—testicular, adj.

testis (tes'-tis). One of the two glandular bodies contained in the scrotum of the male; they form sperms and also the male sex-hormones. **undescended t.,** the organ remains in the pelvis or inguinal canal. Cryptorchism (q.v.)—testes, pl.

testosterone (tes-tos'-ter-ōn). The hormone derived from the testes and responsible for the development of the secondary male characteristics. Used in carcinoma of the breast, to control uterine bleeding and in male underdevelopment.

tetanus (tet'-an-us) [G. *tetanos*]. Lockjaw. Disease caused by *Clostridium tetani,* an anaerobe which may be present in road dust and manure. Patient develops spasm and rigidity of muscles. Tetanus toxoid injection produces active immunity. ATS injection produces passive immunity—tetanic, adj.

tetany (tet'-en-i) [G. *tetanos,* convulsive spasm]. Condition of muscular hyperexcitability in which mild stimuli produce cramps and spasms (cf. carpopedal spasm). Found in parathyroid deficiency and alkalosis. Associated in infants with gastrointestinal upset and rickets.

Tetmosol (tet′-mo-sol). Monosulfiram (q.v.).

tetrabenazine. Nitoman. Tranquillizer.

tetrachlor(o)ethylene (tet-ra-klor-eth′-i-lēn). An anthelmintic given in hookworm. A single dose is used.

tetracoccus (tet-ra-kok′-us). Coccal bacteria arranged in cubical packets of four.

tetracycline (tet-ra-sī′-klin). A broad spectrum antibiotic related to both aureomycin and terramycin and used for similar purposes. As a rule it causes less gastrointestinal disturbances. There is less absorption of oral t. when the stomach is full, or contains aluminium, calcium and magnesium. Causes fluroescence in body cells. This disappears rapidly from normal cells when the drug is discontinued and is retained by cancerous cells for 24–30 h after dosage ceases. Can be used for tuberculosis.

Tetracyn (tet′-ra-sin). Tetracycline (q.v.).

tetradactylous (tet-ra-dak′a-til-us) [G. *tetra,* four; *daktylos,* finger]. Having four digits on each limb.

tetradecapeptide (tet-ra-dek-a-pep′-tīd) [G. *tetra,* four; *deka,* ten; *peptikos,* to cook]. A sophisticated peptide (q.v.).

tetrahydroaminacrine (tet-ra-hī′-drō-a-mēn′-ō-krēn). Counteracts the narcotic and respiratory depressant effect of other drugs, e.g. morphine.

tetralogy of Fallot. A form of congenital heart defect which includes narrowing of the pulmonary artery, a septal defect between the ventricles, hypertrophy of the right ventircle, and displacement of the aorta to the right. [Etienne Louis Arthur Fallot, French physician, 1850–1911.]

Tetralysal (tet-ra-lī-sal). A tetracycline derivative which maintains higher blood serum levels with fewer doses, resulting in greater efficiency in combating infections of the respiratory system.

tetraplegia (tet-ra-plē′-ji-à) [G. *tetra,* four; *plege,* stroke]. Paralysis of all four limbs. Also QUADRIPLEGIA.

tetrocosactrin (tet-ro-kō′-sak-trin). Synthetic ACTH. As it does not cause allergic reactions, it should replace ACTH in treatment of asthma, etc.

THA. Tetrahydroaminacrine (a.v.).

thalamotomy (thal-am-ot′-o-mi) [G. *thalamos,* chambers; *tome,* cutting].

Usually operative (stereotaxic) destruction of a portion of thalamus. Can be done for intractable pain.

thalamus (thal′-a-mus) [G. *thalamos,* chamber]. A collection of grey matter at the base of the cerebrum. Sensory impulses from the whole body pass through on their way to the cerebral cortex—thalami, pl.; thalamic, adj.

thalassaemia (thal-as-ēm′-i-à) [G. *thalassa,* the sea; *haima,* blood]. Cooley's anaemia (q.v.). Genetically transmitted haemoglobin abnormality.

Thalazole (thal′-a-zol). Phthalylsulpha-thiazole (q.v.).

THAM. Tris hydroxylmethyl amino methane. (q.v.).

thanatology (than-at-ol′-o-ji) [G. *thanatos,* death; *logos,* discourse]. The study of death to discover a trustworthy way of deciding that death beyond resuscitation has taken place.

theca (thē′-kà) [G. *theke;* case]. An enveloping sheath, especially of a tendon. **theca vertebralis,** the membranes enclosing the spinal cord—thecal, adj.

theine (thē′-in). An alkaloid found in tea.

thenar (thē′nàr) [G. palm]. The palm of the hand and the sole of the foot. **thenar eminence,** the palmar eminence below the thumb.

theobromine (thē-ō-brō′-mēn). A drug allied to caffeine, but with a less stimulating and more powerful diuretic action. Sometimes given with phenobarbitone to reduce frequency and severity of anginal attacks.

Theo-nar (thē′-ō-nar). Theophylline and noscapine capsules that give immediate release of part of dose, and delayed release of remaining dose for control of bronchospasm.

Theophorin (thē-of′-or-in). Phenindamine (q.v.).

theophylline (thē-of′-il-lin). A diuretic related to caffeine but more powerful. It is used mainly as its derivative amniophylline in the treatment of congestive heart failure, dyspnoea and asthma. Present in mersalyl and Neptal injections.

therapeutics (ther-à-pū′-tiks) [G. *therapeutikos,* wait on; cure]. The branch of medical science dealing with the treatment of disease—therapeutic, adj; therapeutically, adv.

therapy (ther′-à-pi) [G. *therapeia*]. Treatment.

thermal (thĕr'-mal) [G. *therme*, heat]. Pertaining to heat.

thermogenesis (thĕr-mo-jen'-e-sis) [G. *therme*, heat; *genesis*, production]. The production of heat—thermogenetic, adj.

thermography (ther-mog'-ra-fi) [G. *therme*, heat; *graphein*, to write]. Temperature differences throughout the body are recorded on photographic film for diagnostic purposes—thermographic, adj.; thermographically, adv.; thermograph, n.

thermolabile (thĕr-mō-lā'-bil) [G. *therme*, heat; L. *labilis*, slipping]. Capable of being altered by heat.

thermolysis (ther-mol'-i-sis) [G. *therme*, heat; *lysis*, a loosening]. Loss of heat—thermolytic, adj.

thermometer (thĕr-mom'-et-ĕr) [G. *therme*, heat; *metron*, a measure]. An instrument containing a substance, the volume of which is altered by temperature—thermometric, adj. The low reading clinical thermometer is marked either

$$\left(\begin{array}{c|c} 85° & \\ 29° & \end{array} \middle| \begin{array}{c} 05° \text{ F} \\ 41° \text{ C} \end{array}\right)$$

or

$$\left(\begin{array}{c|c} 70° & \\ 21° & \end{array} \middle| \begin{array}{c} 102° \text{ F} \\ 39° \text{ C} \end{array}\right)$$

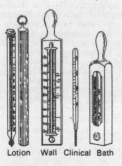

Lotion   Wall   Clinical   Bath

Thermometers

thermophil (thĕr'-mō-fil) [G. *therme*, heat; *philein*, to love]. A micro-organism accustomed to growing at a high temperature—thermophilic, adj.

Thermoscan (ther'-mō-skan). Apparatus capable of scanning the distribution of heat over an area. Sufficiently sensitive to record temperature differentials

down to 0.2° C. Among the many conditions which can be studied are blood flow disorders, viability of skin grafts, onset of malignant breast tumours and the extent of varicose veins.

thermostable (thĕr-mō-stā'-bl) [G. *therme*, heat; L. *stabilis*, stable]. Remaining unaltered at a high temperature, which is usually specified—thermostability, n.

thermotherapy (thĕr-mō-ther'-a-pi) [G. *therme*, heat; *therapeia*, treatment]. Heat treatment.

thesaurosis (thĕs-awr-ō'-sis) [G. *thesauros*, store; *-osis*, condition]. Term currently concerned with hair sprays. Macromolecules taken up by cells of the reticuloendothelial system with a consequent inflammatory reaction. Similar to sarcoidosis.

thiabendazole (thī-a-bend'-az-ol). Can be used as single dose treatment for threadworms. Effective orally for larva migrans caused by some species of Ancylostoma. Best available treatment for strongyloides infestation. No starvation or purgation necessary. Stated to clear the infection in about 50 per cent of patients with trichuriasis.

thiacetazone (thī-a-set'-a-zōn). Synthetic antitubercular compound. As effective as PAS and cheaper. Can be used in a regimen of one dose per day with isoniazid.

thialbarbitone (thī-al-bár'-bit-ōn). A barbiturate used as an intravenous anaesthetic in a similar way to thiopentone. It is said to cause less laryngeal spasm of respiratory depression.

thiambutosine (thī-am-būt'-ō-sēn). Antileprotic drug.

thiamine (thī'-a-mēn). See ANEURINE.

Thiersch skin graft (teersh). Films of epidermis with a portion of dermis applied to a raw area shaved smooth from granulations. [Karl Thiersch, German surgeon, 1822–95.]

thiethylperazine (thī-eth-il-per'-a-zēn). For nausea, vomiting and vertigo.

Thiomerin (thi-ōm'-er-in). A mercury-containing diuretic, similar in action to mersalyl, but suitable for subcutaneous injection.

thiomersalate (thī-ō-mér'-sal-āt). An organic mercurial antiseptic and fungicide. Used for skin sterilization and as a lotion.

thiopentone (thī-ō-pen'-tōn). A barbiturate given by intravenous injection as a short-acting basal anaesthetic. The effect can be extended by additional doses, and in combination with curare compounds adequate relaxation for major surgery can be achieved.

thiopropazate (thī-ō-prō'-paz-āt). Sedative and antiemetic used widely for psychoneurotic states.

thioquanine (thī-o-qwan'-ēn). Antimetabolite. Interferes with synthesis of nucleoprotein, thus useful in acute luekaemia.

thioridazine (thī-ō-rid'-a-zēn). Sedative, tranquillizer. Closely resembles chlorpromazine.

Thiotepa (thī-o'-tē'-pa). Triethylene thiophosphoramide (q.v.).

thiothixene (thī-ō-thiks'-ēn). Antipsychotic, used in schizophrenia.

thoracentesis (thor-a-sen-tē'-sis) [G. *thorax*, chest; *kentesis*, puncture]. Paracentesis (q.v.) of the pleural cavity.

thoracic (thor-as'-ik). Pertaining to the thorax. **thoracic duct**, a channel conveying lymph (chyle) from the receptaculum chyli in the abdomen to the left subclavian vein. **thoracic inlet syndrome**, see CERVICAL RIB.

thoracoplasty (thor'-ak-ō-plas-ti) [G. *thorax*; *plassein*, to form]. An operation on the thorax in which the ribs are resected to allow the chest wall to collapse and the lung to rest; used in the treatment of pulmonary tuberculosis.

thoracoscope (thor'-ak-ō-skōp) [G. *thorax*, thorax; *skopein*, to examine]. An instrument which can be inserted into the pleural cavity through a small incision in the chest wall, to permit inspection of the pleural surfaces and division of adhesions by electric diathermy—thoracoscopic, adj.; thoracoscopy, n.

thoracotomy (thor-a-ko'-to-mi) [G. *thorax*, thorax; *tome*, a cutting]. Surgical exposure of the thoracic cavity.

thorax (thō'-raks) [G.]. The chest cavity—thoracic, adj.

thorium X (thō'-ri-um). A substance allied to radium, but with only a brief radioactive life. It is used as a varnish or ointment in the treatment of various skin conditions.

threadworm (thred). *Enterobius (Oxyuris) vermicularis*. Tiny threadlike worms that infest man's intestine. Females migrate to anus to lay eggs, thus spread of, and reinfestation easy. The whole family should be treated simultaneously using piperazine over a week, together with hygiene measures to prevent reinfestation. A further course after 10 days interval is advisable to deal with worms that have since hatched, as the eggs are not affected by the drug.

threonine (thrē'-ō-nin). An essential amino acid (q.v.).

thrill. Vibration as perceived by the sense of touch.

thrombectomy (throm-bek'-to-mi) [G. *thrombus*, clot; *ektome* excision]. Surgical removal of a thrombus from within a blood vessel.

thrombin (throm'-bin) [G. *thrombos*, clot]. Not normally present in circulating blood; generated from prothrombin (Factor II). See BLOOD CLOTTING. The extrinsic and intrinsic pathways lead to production of thrombin. The extrinsic pathway is tested by the prothrombin time (PT). The intrinsic pathway involves principally Factors IX and VIII among others. The partial thromboplastin time (PTT) or a modification called the partial thromboplastin time with kaolin (PTTK) detects abnormalities in this pathway. See CHRISTMAS DISEASE and HAEMOPHILIA.

thromboangiitis (throm-bō-an-ji-ī'-tis) [G. *thrombos*, clot; *aggeion*, vessel; *-itis*, inflammation]. Clot formation within an inflamed vessel. **thromboangiitis obliterans** (syn., Buerger's disease), an uncommon disorder of unknown cause, occurring mainly in young adult Jewish males, characterized by patchy, inflammatory, obliterative, vascular disease, principally in the limbs (sometimes in the cardiac or cerebral vessels), and presenting usually as calf pains, or more severely as early gangrene of the toes and following a chronic progressive course.

thromboarteritis (throm-bō-ar-te-rī'-tis) [G. *thrombos*, clot; *arteria*, artery; *-itis*, inflammation]. Inflammation of an artery with clot formation.

thrombocyte (throm'-bō-sīt) [G. *thrombos*, clot; *kytos*, cell]. Syn., blood platelet. Plays a part in the clotting of blood.

thrombocythaemia. Syn., thrombocytosis (q.v.).

thrombocytopenia (throm-bō-sī-tō-pēn'-i-á) [G. *thrombos*, clot; *kytos*, cell; *penia*, want]. A reduction in the number of platelets in the blood—thrombocytopenic, adj.

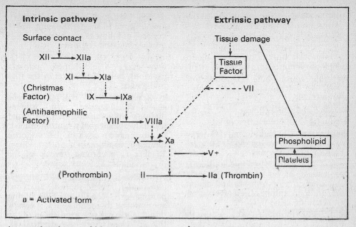

Intrinsic pathway

Surface contact

XII ---→ XIIa

XI ---→ XIa

(Christmas
Factor)   IX ---→ IXa

(Antihaemophilic
Factor)   VIII ---→ VIIIa

X ---→ Xa

(Prothrombin)   II ---→ IIa (Thrombin)

a = Activated form

Extrinsic pathway

Tissue damage

Tissue
Factor

----- VII

Phospholipid

Platelets

→V+

A cascade scheme of blood coagulation reactions leading to thrombin formation

thrombocytopenic purpura (thrombō-sī-tō-pē′-nik pur′-pū-rá). A syndrome characterized by a low blood platelet count, intermittent mucosal bleeding and purpura (q.v.). It can be symptomatic, i.e. secondary to known disease or to certain drugs; or idiopathic, a rare condition of unknown cause (syn., purpura haemorrhagica) occurring principally in children and young adults. In both forms the bleeding time is prolonged.

thrombocytosis (throm-bō-sīt-ō′-sis) [G. *thrombos*, clot; *kytos*, cell; *-osis*, condition]. An increase in the number of platelets in the blood.

thromboembolic (throm-bō-em-bol′-ik) [G. *thrombos*, clot; *embolos*, plug]. Used to describe the phenomenon whereby a thrombus or clot detaches itself and is carried to another part of the body in the bloodstream to block a blood vessel there.

thromboendarterectomy (throm-bō-end-art-er-ek′-to-mi) [G. *thrombos*, clot; *endon*, within; *arteria*, artery; *ektome*, excision]. Removal of a thrombus from an artery following reboring.

thromboendarteritis (throm-bō-end-art-e-rī′-tis) [G. *thrombos*, clot; *endon*, within; *arteria*, artery *-itis*, inflammation]. Inflammation of the inner lining of an artery with clot formation.

thrombogen (throm′-bō-jen). Precursor of thrombin (q.v.).

thrombogenic (throm-bō-jen′-ik) [G. *thrombos*, clot; *genesis*, descent]. Capable of clotting blood—thrombogenesis, thrombogenicity, n.; thrombogenetic, adj.; thrombogenetically, adv.

thrombokinase (throm-bō-kīn′-āz) [G. *thrombos*, clot] Syn., thromboplastin (q.v.).

thrombolytic (throm-bō-lit′-ik) [G. *thrombos*, clot; *lysis*, a loosening]. Pertaining to disintegration of a blood clot. **thrombolytic therapy**, the attempted removal of preformed intravascular fibrin occlusions using fibrinolytic agents—thrombolysis, n.

thrombophlebitis (throm-bō-flē-bī′-tis) [G. *thrombos*, clot; *phleps*, vein; *-itis*, inflammation]. Inflammation of the wall of a vein with secondary thrombosis within the involved segment. **thrombophlebitis migrans**, recurrent episodes of t. affecting short lengths of superficial veins. Deep vein t. uncommon and pulmonary embolism rare—thrombophlebitic, adj.

thromboplastin (throm-bō-plas′-tin) [G. *thrombos*, clot; *plassein*, to form]. An enzyme which converts prothrombin into thrombin. **intrinsic t.**, produced by the interaction of several factors during the clotting of blood. Much more active than tissue thromboplastin. **tissue t.**, thromboplastic enzymes are present in many tissues, and tissue extracts are used in clotting experiments and in the estimation of prothrombin time.

thrombosis (throm-bō′-sis) [G. *thrombos*, clot; *-osis*, condition]. The intravascular formation of a blood clot—thrombotic, adj.; thromboses, pl.

thrombus (throm′-bus) [G. *thrombos*, clot]. An intravascular blood clot—thrombi, pl.

thrush. Candidiasis (q.v.).

Thylin (thī-lin). Nifenazone (q.v.).

thymectomy (thī-mek′-to-mi) [G. *thymos*, soul; *ektome*, excision]. Surgical excision of the thymus.

thymol (thī′-mol). The chief antiseptic constituent of oil of thyme. Widely employed in mouthwashes and dental preparations, and has been given as an anthelmintic in hookworm.

thymoleptic (thī-mō-lep′-tik). A current term for drugs primarily exerting their effect on the brain, thus influencing 'feeling' and behaviour.

thymoma (thī-mō′-mà) [G. *thymos*, soul; *-oma*, tumour]. A tumour arising in the thymus—thymomata, pl.

thymosin (thī′-mo-sin). Hormone secreted by the epithelial cells of the thymus gland. Provides the stimulus for lymphocyte production within the thymus; confers on lymphocytes elsewhere in the body the capacity to respond to antigenic stimulation.

thymoxamine (thī-moks′-a-mēn). Vasodilator drug. Blocks alpha receptors of sympathetic nervous system. Useful in Ménière's disease.

thymus (thī′-mus). A gland lying behind the breast bone and extending upward as far as the thyroid gland. It is well developed in infancy and attains its greatest size towards puberty; and then the lymphatic tissue is replaced by fatty tissue. It has an immunological role. Autoimmunity is thought to result from pathological activity of this gland—thymic, adj.

thyroglossal (thī′-rō-glos′-al). Pertaining to the thyroid gland and the tongue. **thyroglossal** duct, the fetal passage from the thyroid gland to the back of the tongue where its vestigial end remains as the foramen caecum. Thyroglossal cyst or fistula can occur.

thyroid (thī′-roid). The ductless gland found on both sides of the trachea. It secretes thyroxine, which controls the rate of metabolism. The commercial material is the t. gland of the ox, sheep

or pig, dried and reduced to powder, and adjusted in strength to contain 0.1 per cent of iodine as thyroxine. Used in myxoedema and cretinism.

thyroidectomy (thī-roid-ek′-to-mi) [G. *thureoeides*, shield-shaped; *ektome*, excision]. Surgical removal of the thyroid gland.

thyroiditis (thī-roid-ī′-tis) [G. *thureoeides*, shield-shaped; *-itis*, inflammation]. Inflammation of the thyroid gland. **lymphadenoid t.** (autoimmune t. or Hashimoto's disease), a firm goitre ultimately resulting in hypothyroidism. **Riedel's t.**, a chronic fibrosis of the thyroid gland; ligneous goitre.

thyrotoxicosis (thī-rō-toks-i-kō′-sis) [G. *thureoeides*, shield-shaped; *toxikon*, poison; *-osis*, condition]. One of the autoimmune thyroid diseases. A condition due to excessive production of the thyroid gland hormone (thyroxine), probably in response to stimulation by an excessive production of pituitary thyrotrophic hormone, and resulting classically in anxiety, tachycardia, sweating, increased appetite with weight loss, and a fine tremor of the outstretched hands, and prominence of the eyes. It is much commoner in women than in men. In older patients cardiac irregularities may be a prominent feature—thyrotoxic, adj.

thyrotrophic (thīr′-ō-trof-ik). A substance which stimulates the thyroid gland, e.g. the t. hormone secreted by the anterior pituitary gland.

thyroxine (thī-roks′-in). The principal hormone of the thyroid gland. It raises the basal metabolic rate.

tibia (tib′-i-à) [L.]. The shin-bone; the larger of the two bones in the lower part of the leg; it articulates with the femur, fibula and talus—tibial, adj.

tibiofibular (ti-bi-ō-fib′-ū-lar) [L. *tibia*, shin-bone; *fibula*, clasp]. Pertaining to the tibia and the fibula.

tic (tik). Purposeless involuntary, spasmodic muscular movements and twitchings, due partly to habit, but often associated with a psychological factor.

tic douloureux (doo-lêr-oo′). Trigeminal neuralgia. Spasms of excruciating pain in distribution of trigeminal nerve.

tick (tik). A blood-sucking parasite, larger than a mite. Some of them are concerned in the transmission of relapsing fever, typhus, etc.

timolol maleate (tim'-ō-lol mal'-ē-āt) Hypotensive beta-blocking agent.

tincture (tink-tūr). Solution of a drug in alcohol.

tinea (tin'-ē-á) [L. gnawing worm]. See RINGWORM. **tinea barbae** (barber's itch), ringworm of the beard. **tinea capitis**, ringworm of the head. **tinea corporis** (also circinata), ringworm of the body. **tinea cruris** ('Dhobie itch'), ringworm of the crutch area. **tinea pedis** (dermatophytosis), ringworm of the foot.

tinnitus (ti-nī'-tus) [L.]. A buzzing, thumping or ringing sound in the ears.

tissue (tis'-ū). A collection of cells or fibres of similar function, forming a structure.

titration (ti-trā'-shun). Volumetric analysis by aid of standard solutions.

titre (tē'-tér). A standard of strength per volume.

tobramycin (tob-ra-mī'-sin) Antibiotic particularly effective against *Pseudomonas aeruginosa* and *Staphylococcus aureus*. Such infections can be lethal to those afflicted with cystic fibrosis.

tocography (tok-og'-raf-i) [G. *tokos,* birth; *graphein,* to write]. Process of recording uterine contractions using a tocograph or a parturiometer.

tocopherol (tok-of'-er-ol). Synthetic vitamin E, similar to that found in wheat-germ oil. It has been used in habitual abortion, and empirically in many other conditions with varying success.

Tofranil. Imipramine (q.v.). See ANTIDEPRESSANT.

Tolanase (tol'-an-āz). Tolazamide (q.v.).

tolazamide (tol-az'-a-mīd). Oral antidiuretic agent. One of the sulphonylureas.

tolazoline (tol-az'-o-lēn). A peripheral vasodilator, of value in circulatory disorders such as Raynaud's disease and related conditions. Has also been used in ophthalmic conditions such as keratitis.

tolbutamide (tol-bū'-ta-mīd). A sulphonamide derivative which stimulates the islets of Langerhans to pour out more insulin. Has been used with success in the oral treatment of diabetes, so that insulin injections may be reduced or withdrawn. Not suitable for juvenile or severe diabetes.

tolerance. Ability to tolerate the application or administration of a substance,

usually a drug. One may have to increase the dose of the drug as t. develops, e.g. nitrites. **exercise t.,** exercise accomplished without pain or marked breathlessness. American Heart Association's classification of functional capacity: Class I—no symptoms on ordinary effort; Class II—slight disability on ordinary effort (in Britain it is usual to subdivide this class into Class IIa—able to carry on with normal housework under difficulty—and Class IIb—cannot manage shopping or bed-making except very slowly); Class III—marked disability on ordinary effort which prevents any attempt at housework; Class IV—symptoms at rest or heart failure.

tolnaflate (tol'-naf-lāt). Antifungal agent, useful for athlete's foot.

Tolnate, Prothipendyl (q.v.).

tomograph (tō'-mō-graf) [G. *tomos,* cutting; *graphein,* to write]. Differential radiograph demonstrating a selected layer in a specified region of the body. A series of such films with the 'in focus' layer set at various depths allows a three dimensional impression to be built up. Shows extent of cysts, tubercular foci, cancer, calculi, etc.—tomography, n.; tomographic, adj.; tomographically, adv.

tone (tōn); **tonus** (ton'-us). The normal, healthy state of tension.

tongue (tung). The mobile muscular organ contained in the mouth; it is concerned with speech, mastication, swallowing and taste. **strawberry t.,** thickly furred with projecting red papillae. As the fur disappears the t. is vividly red, like an overripe strawberry. Characteristic of scarlet fever.

tonic (ton'-ik) [G. *tonos,* tension]. Used to describe a state of continuous muscular contraction, as opposed to intermittent contraction. Cf. clonus.

tonography (ton-og'-ra-fi) [G. *tonos,* tone; *graphein,* to write]. Continuous measurement of blood, or intraocular, pressure. **carotid compression t.,** normally occlusion of one common carotid artery causes an ipsilateral fall of intraocular pressure. Screening test for carotid insufficiency.

tonometer (ton-om'-et-ér) [G. *tonos,* tension; *metron,* a measure]. An instrument for measuring intraocular pressure.

tonsillectomy (ton-sil-ek'-to-mi) [L. *ton-*

sillae, tonsils; G. *ektome,* excision]. Removal of the tonsils.

tonsillitis (ton-sil-ī'-tis) [L. *tonsillae,* tonsils; G. *-itis,* inflammation]. Inflammation of the tonsils.

tonsilloliths (ton'-sil-o-liths) [L. *tonsillae,* tonsils; G. *lithos,* stone]. Concretions arising in the body of the tonsil.

tonsillopharyngeal (ton-sil-ō-far-in-jē'-ăl) [L. *tonsillae,* tonsils; G. *pharynx,* pharynx]. Pertaining to the tonsil and pharynx.

tonsillotome (ton'-sil-ō-tōm) [L. *tonsillae,* tonsils; G. *tome,* a cutting]. Instrument for excision of tonsils.

tonsils (ton'-silz) [L. *tonsillae*]. The small bodies, one on each side, covered by mucous membrane, embedded in the fauces between the palatine arch; composed of about 10 to 18 lymph follicles—tonsillar, adj.

topectomy (top-ek'-to-mi). Modified frontal lobotomy. Small incisions made in thalamofrontal tracts.

tophus (tō'-fus) [L.]. A small, hard concretion forming on the ear-lobe, on the joints of the phalanges, etc. in gout—tophi, pl.

topical (top'-ik-al) [G. *topos,* place]. Local—topically, adv.

topography (top-og'-ra-fi) [G. *topos,* place; *graphein,* to write]. A description of the regions of the body—topographical, adj.; topographically, adv.

Torecan (tor'-ē-kan). Thiethylperazine (q.v.).

torsion (tor'-shun). Twisting.

torticollis (tor-ti-kol'-is) [L. *torquere,* to twist; *collum,* neck]. Wryneck; a painless contraction of one sternomastoid muscle. The head is slightly flexed and drawn towards the contracted side, with the face rotated over the other shoulder.

Tosmilen (tos-mil'-en). Anticholinesterase eyedrops, useful in glaucoma. Miotic.

Toti's operation. See DACRYOCYSTOR-HINOSTOMY. [Addeo Toti, Italian ophthalmologist and laryngologist, 1861-1946.]

tourniquet (toor'-nē-kā) [F.]. An apparatus for the compression of the blood vessels of a limb. Designed for compression of a main artery to control bleeding. Is also often used to obstruct the venous return from a limb and so facilitate the withdrawal of blood from a

vein. Tourniquets vary from a simple rubber band to a pneumatic cuff.

tow (tō). Coarse flax.

toxaemia (toks-ē'-mi-ă) [G. *toxikon,* poison; *haima,* blood]. A generalized poisoning of the body by the products of bacteria or damaged tissue—toxaemic, adj.

toxic (toks'-ik). Poisonous.

toxic epidermal necrolysis (toks'-ik ep-i-dér'-mal ne -krol'-is-is) [G. *toxikon,* poison; *epi,* on; *derma,* skin; *nekros,* corpse; *lysis,* a loosening]. A syndrome in which the appearance is of scalded skin. It can occur in response to drug reaction, staphylococcal infection, systemic illness, and it can be idiopathic.

toxicity (toks-is'-it-i) [G. *toxikon,* poison]. The quality or degree of being poisonous.

toxicology (toks-i-kol'-o-ji) [G. *toxikon,* poison; *logos,* discourse]. The science dealing with poisons—toxicological, adj.; toxicologically, adv.

toxicomania (toks-ik-ō-mā'-ni-ă). WHO definition: Periodic or chronic state of intoxication produced by repeated consumption of a drug harmful to the individual or society. Characteristics are: (1) Uncontrollable desire or necessity to continue consuming the drug and to try to get it by all means. (2) Tendency to increase the dose. (3) Psychic and physical dependency as a result.

toxin (toks'-in). A product of bacteria poisonous to other cells which, on injection into animal or man, stimulates the production of an antibody (i.e. antitoxin) to it. **non-bacterial t.,** a poisonous nitrogenous compound such as that liberated from diseased or injured tissue.

Toxocara (toks-ō-car'-ă). Genus of roundworm of the cat and dog. Man can be infested (toxocariasis) by eating with hands soiled from these pets. The worms cannot become adult in man (incorrect host) so the larval worms wander through the body, attacking mainly the liver and the eye. Treatment is unsatisfactory, but the condition usually clears after several months.

toxoid (toks'-oid) [G. *toxikon,* poison: *eidos,* form]. A toxin altered in such a way that it has lost its poisonous properties but retained its antigenic properties. Vaccines are prepared from toxins by accelerating the change to toxoid with oxidizing agents.

toxoid-antitoxin (toks-oid-an-ti-toks'-in). A mixture of toxoid and homologous antitoxin in floccule form, used as a vaccine, e.g. in immunization against diphtheria.

Toxoplasma (toks-ō-plas'-má). A genus of parasite which causes toxoplasmosis.

toxoplasmosis (toks-ō-plas-mō'-sis) [G. *toxikon* poison; *plasma,* anything formed; *-osis,* condition]. Infection by Toxoplasma parasites which, commonly occurring in mammals and birds, may infect man. Intrauterine fetal and infant infections are often severe, producing encephalitis, convulsions hydrocephalus and eye diseases, resulting in death or, in those who recover, mental retardation and impaired sight. Infection in older children and adults may result in pneumonia, nephritis or skin rashes. Skull X-ray reveals flecks of cerebral calcification. Skin and antibody tests confirm the diagnosis.

trabeculae (tra-bek'-ū-lē)[L. little beam]. The fibrous bands or septa projecting into the interior of an organ, e.g. the spleen; they are extensions from the capsule surrounding the organ—trabecula, sing.; trabecular, adj.

trabeculotomy (trab-ek-ū-lot'-o-mi). Operation for glaucoma. It aims at creating a channel through the trabecular meshwork from the canal of Schlemm to the angle of the anterior chamber.

trace elements. Metals and other elements that are regularly present in very small amounts in the tissues and known to be essential for normal metabolism (e.g. copper, cobalt, manganese, fluorine, etc.).

tracer (trā'-ser). A substance or instrument used to gain information. Radioactive tracers have extended knowledge in physiology; some are used in diagnosis.

trachea (trak-ē'-á) [G. *trachus,* rough]. The windpipe; the fibrocartilaginous tube lined with mucous membrane passing from the larynx to the bronchi. It is about 11.43 cm long and about 25.4 mm wide—tracheal, adj.

tracheitis (trak-ē-ī'-tis) [G. *trachus,* rough; *-itis,* inflammation]. Inflammation of the trachea.

trachelorrhaphy (trak-el-or'-raf-i) [G. *trachelos,* neck; *rhaphe,* suture]. Operative repair of a uterine cervical laceration.

tracheobronchial (trak-ē-ō-brong'-ki-al) [G. *trachus,* rough; *brongchos,* bronchial tube]. Pertaining to the trachea and the bronchi.

tracheobronchitis (trak-ē-ō-brong-kī'-tis). Inflammation of the trachea and bronchi.

tracheo-oesophageal (trak-ē-ō-ē-sof-aj-ē-'al) [G. *trachus,* rough; *oisophagos,* gullet]. Pertaining to the trachea and the oesophagus.

tracheostomy (tr-kē-os'-to-mi) [G. *trachus,* rough; *stoma,* mouth]. Fenestration in the anterior wall of the trachea by removal of circular piece of cartilage from third and fourth rings, for establishment of a safe airway and reduction of 'dead space'—tracheostome, n.

tracheotomy (tr-kē-ot'-o-mi) [G. *trachus,* rough; *tome,* cutting]. Vertical slit in the anterior wall of the trachea at the level of the third and fourth cartilaginous rings. Usually performed in young children.

trachoma (tra-kō'-má) [G.]. Contagious inflammation affecting conjunctiva, cornea and eyelids. Due to Bedsonia, which resembles a virus. It behaves like a bacterium, though it multiplies intracellularly. Sensitive to sulphonamides and antibiotics. If untreated it leads to blindness. Medical Research Council's Trachoma Research Unit is trying out a vaccine—trachomatous, adj.

traction (trak'-shun). A drawing or pulling on the patient's body to overcome muscle spasm, and to reduce or prevent deformity. A steady pulling exerted on some part (limb or head) by means of weights and pulleys. See BALKAM BEAM, BRAUN'S FRAME, BRYANT'S TRACTION, RUSSELL TRACTION.

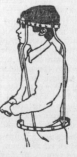

Halo-pelvic traction

tractotomy (trak-tot'-o-mi). Incision of a nerve tract. Surgical relief of intractable pain. Using stereotactic measures this operation is now being done for some forms of mental illness.

tragus (trā'-gus) [G. *tragos*, a goat]. The projection in front of the external auditory meatus—tregi, pl.

trait (trā). An individual characteristic forming part of the whole personality.

trance (trāns) [L. *transire*, to pass over]. A term used for hypnotic sleep and for certain self-induced hysterical stuporous states.

tranquillizers (tran'-kwi-lī-zers) [L. *tranquillus*, calm]. These drugs do not affect a basic disease, but reduce symptoms so that patient feels more comfortable and is more accessible to help from psychotherapy. Greatly exaggerate the effects of alcohol. Chlordiazepoxide (Librium), meprobamate (Equanil, Miltown), hydroxyzine (Atarax) and methylpentynol (Oblivon). Syn., ataractic, neuroleptic, anxiolytic, thymoleptic.

transabdominal (trans-ab-dom'-in-al) [L. *trans*, through; *abdomen*, belly]. Through the abdomen as the t. approach for nephrectomy—transabdominally, adv.

transamniotic (trans-am-ni-ot'-ik) [L. *trans*, through; G. *amnion*, membrane round fetus]. Through the amniotic membrane and fluid as a t. transfusion of the fetus for haemolytic disease.

transection (tran-sek'-shun) [L. *trans*. through; *sectio*, a cutting]. The cutting across or mechanical severance of a structure.

transfrontal (trans-front'-al) [L. *trans*, through; *frons*, forehead]. Through the frontal bone; an approach used for hypophysectomy.

transfusion (trans-fū'-zhun) [L. *transfundere*, to transfuse]. The introduction of fluid into the tissue or into a blood vessel. **blood t.**, the transfer of blood into a vein. **intrauterine t.** of the fetus endangered by rhesus incompatibility. Red cells are transfused directly into the abdominal cavity of the fetus, on one or more occasions. This enables the induction of labour to be postponed until a time more favourable to fetal welfare. Also called **intraabdominal prenatal t.**

transillumination (trans-il-ū-min-ā'-shun). The transmission of light through the sinuses for diagnostic purposes.

transirrigation (trans-ir-ri-gā'-shun) [L. *trans*, through; *irrigare*, to irrigate]. Diagnostic puncture and lavage, as performed in maxillary sinusitis.

Transithal (trans'-i-thal). Buthalitone (q.v.).

translocation (trans-lo-kā'-shun). Transfer of a segment of a chromosone to a different site on the same chromosome or to a different one. Can be the cause of congenital abnormality.

translucent (trans-lū'-sent) [L. *trans*, through; *lucere*, to shine]. Intermediate between opaque and transparent.

translumbar (trans-lum'-bar) [L. *trans*, through; *lumbus*, loin]. Through the lumbar region. Route used for injecting aorta prior to aortography.

transmigration (trans-mī-grā'-shun) [L. *trans*, through; *migrare*, to migrate]. The transit of a cell through a membrane.

transmural (trans-mū'-ral) [L. *trans*, through; *murus*, wall]. Through the wall, e.g. of a cyst, organ or vessel—transmurally, adv.

transonic (tran-son'-ik). Allowing the passage of ultrasound. See ULTRASONIC.

transperitoneal (trans-per-it-on-ē'-al) [L. *trans*, through; G. *peri*, around; *teinein*, to stretch]. Across or through the peritoneal cavity. See DIALYSIS.

transnasal (trans-na'-zal) [L. *trans*, through; *nasus*, nose]. Through the nose—transnasally, adv.

transplacental (trans-pla-sen'-tal) [L. *trans*, through; *placenta*, cake]. Through the placenta—transplacentally, adv.

transplantation (trans-plan-tā'-shun) [L. *transplantare*, to transplant]. Grafting on to one part, tissue or an organ taken from another part or another body.

transrectal (trans-rek'-tal) [L. *trans*, through; *rectus*, straight]. Through the rectum as a t. injection into a tumour—transrectally, adv.

transsphenoidal (trans-sfen-oid'-al) [L. *trans*, through; *sphenoeides*, wedgeshaped]. Through the sphenoid bone; an approach used for hypophysectomy.

transthoracic (trans-thor-as'-ik) [L. *trans*, through; G. *thorax*, thorax]. Across or through the chest.

transudate (trans'-ū-dāt) [L. *trans*, through; *sudare*, to sweat]. A fluid that has passed out of the cells either into a body cavity (e.g. ascitic fluid in the peritoneal cavity) or to the exterior (e.g. serum from the surface of a burn)—transudation, n.

transurethral (trans-ū-rēth'-ral) [L. *trans*, through; G. *ourethra*, urethra]. By way of the urethra.

transvaginal (trans-va-jīn'-al) [L. *trans*, through; *vagina*, sheath]. Through the vagina as an incision to drain the utero-rectal pouch, t. injection into a tumour, pudendal block or culdoscopy—transvaginally, adv.

transventricular (trans-ven-trik'-ū-lar) [L. *trans*, through; *ventriculum*, ventricle]. Through a ventricle. Term used mainly in cardiac surgery—transventricularly, adv.

transvesical (trans-ves-ik-al) [L. *trans*, through; *vesica*, bladder]. Through the bladder, by custom referring to the urinary bladder—transvesically, adv.

tranylcypromine (tran-il-si-pro'-min). Monamine oxidase inhibitor (q.v.).

Trasylol (trā'-sil-ol). Aprotinin (q.v.).

trauma (traw'-ma) [G.]. Bodily injury; emotional shock—traumatic, adj.

traumatology (traw-mat-ol'-o-ji). The branch of surgery dealing with injury from accident.

Trematoda (trem-a-tō'-da). A class of parasitic worms which include many pathogens of man such as the Schistosoma of bilharziasis.

tremor (trem'-or) [L. *tremere*, to tremble]. Involuntary trembling. **coarse t.**, violent trembling. **fine t.**, slight trembling as seen in the outstretched hands or tongue of a patient suffering from thyrotoxicosis. **intention t.**, only occurs on voluntary movement; characteristic of disseminated sclerosis.

Trendelenburg's operation. Ligation of the long saphenous vein in the groin at its junction with the femoral vein. Used in cases of varicose veins. [Friedrich Trendelenburg, German surgeon, 1844–1924.]

Trendelenburg's sign. A test of the stability of the hip, and particularly of the ability of the hip abductors (gluteus medius and minimus) to steady the pelvis upon the femur. Principle: normally, when one leg is raised from the ground the pelvis tilts upwards on that side, through the hip abductors of the standing limb. If the abductors are inefficient (e.g. in poliomyelitis, severe coxa vara, and congenital dislocation of the hip), they are unable to sustain the pelvis against the body weight, and it tilts downwards instead of rising. [Friedrich Trendelenburg, German surgeon, 1844–1924.]

trephine (trē-fin') [G. *trypaein*, to bore]. An instrument with sawlike edges for removing a circular piece of tissue, such as the cornea or skull.

Treponema [G. *trepein*, to turn; *nema*, thread]. A slender spiral-shaped bacterium which is actively motile. Best visualized with dark-ground illumination. Cultivated in the laboratory with great difficulty. *Treponema pallidum* is the causative organism of syphilis; *T. pertenue* the spirochaete that causes yaws (q.v.); *T. carateum* the spirochaete that causes pinta (q.v.).

treponematosis. See YAWS.

treponemicide (trep-on-em'-i-sīd) [G. *trepein*, to turn; L. *coedere*, to kill]. Lethal to Treponema—treponemicidal, adj.

Trescatyl (tres'-kat-il). Ethionamide (q.v.).

tretamine (tret'-a-mēn). A cytostatic drug with an action similar to that of mustine, but active orally. Used in leukaemia and Hodgkin's disease.

Trevintex (trev'-in-teks). Prothionamide (q.v.).

triamcinolone. Steroid with good anti-inflammatory effect and very little electrolyte retaining activity. Due to stimulation of protein breakdown it can cause muscle wasting.

triamterene (trī-am'-ter-ēn). Diuretic that increases excretion of sodium chloride but lessens potassium loss at distal kidney tubule.

TRIC agent. Trachoma inclusion conjunctivitis. Responsible for infections of eye, genital tract and urethritis. See CONJUNCTIVITIS.

triceps (trī'-seps) [L. having three heads]. The three-headed muscle on the back of the upper arm.

trichiasis (trik-ī'-a-sis) [G.]. Abnormal eyelashes causing irritation from friction on the eyeball.

trichinosis (trik-in-ō'-sis) [G. *trichinos*, hair-like; *-osis*, condition]. A disease caused by eating undercooked pig meat infected with *Trichinella spiralis* (the trichina worm). The female worms living in the small bowel produce larvae which invade the body and, in particular, form cysts in skeletal muscles; the usual symptoms are diarrhoea, nausea, colic, fever, facial oedema, muscular pains and stiffness.

trichloracetic acid (trī-klor-as-et'-ik). Powerful caustic and astringent. Used as a crystal for application to warts and ulcers.

trichlorethylene (trī-klor-eth'-i-lēn). Liquid similar to chloroform, and also used as an inhalation anaesthetic. Inhaled in small doses, it is useful in relieving the pain of trigeminal neuralgia.

trichomonacide (trī-kō-mō'-na-sīd). Lethal to the protozoa belonging to the genus Trichomonas.

Trichomonas (trī-kō-mō'-nas). A protozoan parasite of man. *Trichomonas vaginalis* produces infection of the urethra and vagina often associated with profuse discharge (leucorrhoea). The organism is best recognized by microscopic examination of the discharge. See PROTOZOA, AMOEBA.

trichomoniasis (trī-kō-mon-ī-'a-sis). Inflammation of the vagina (urethra in males) caused by *Trichomonas vaginalis*.

Trichomycin. An antibiotic trichomonacide. Vaginal and oral tablets. Ointment relieves pruritis.

trichophytosis (trī-kō-fī-tō'-sis). Infection with a species of the fungus Trichophyton, e.g. ringworm of the hair or skin.

Trichuris (tri-kū'-ris) [G. *thrixtrichos,* hair; *oura,* tail]. A genus of nematodes. *Trichuris trichiura,* the whipworm (q.v.).

trichuriasis (trik-ū-rī'-a-sis) [G. *thrixtrichos,* hair, *oura,* tail]. Infestation with whipworm (*Trichuris trichiura*).

triclofos (tri'-klō-fos). Derivative of chloral hydrate causing less gastric irritation.

Tricloryl (trī-klor'-il). Triclofos (q.v.).

tricuspid (trī-kus'-pid) [L. *tri-,* three; *cuspis,* point]. Having three cusps. **tricuspid valve,** that between the right atrium and ventricle of the heart.

Tridione (trī'-di-ōn). Troxidone (q.v.).

triethylene thiophosphoramide. Alkalylating cytotoxic agent.

trifluoperazine (trī-floo-ō-pėr'-zēn). Tranquillizer and antiemetic. More potent and less sedative than chlorpromazine.

trigeminal (trī-jem'-in-al) [L. *trigeminus,* triplet]. Triple; separating into three

sections, e.g. the t. nerve, the fifth cranial nerve, which has three branches, supplying the skin of the face, the tongue and teeth. **trigeminal neuralgia,** see TIC DOULOUREUX.

trigger finger. A condition in which the finger can be actively bent but cannot be straightened without help; usually due to a thickening on the tendon which prevents free gliding.

trigone (trī'-gōn) [G. *trigonos,* three-cornered]. A triangular area, especially applied to the bladder base bounded by the ureteral openings at the back, and the urethral opening at the front—trigonal, adj.

tri-iodothyronine (trī-i-ō-dō-thī'-rō-nēn). A thyroid hormone that plays a part in maintaining the body's metabolic process.

Trilene (trī'-lēn). Trichlorethylene (q.v.).

trimeprazine (trī-mep'-ra-zēn). Antihistamine with sedative action. Phenotriazine derivative. Used in treatment of pruritis, urticaria and pre-operatively for children.

trimester (trī-mes'-tėr) [L. *trimestris,* of 3 months]. A period of 3 months.

trimetaphan (trī-met'-a-fan). Brief-acting blocking agent used by i.v. injection to produce a fall in blood pressure during bloodless field surgery.

trimethadione (trī-meth-à-dī'-ōn). An anticonvulsant with a specific action in petit mal. May produce toxic effects such as agranulocytosis and drug rash, and some patients experience visual disturbances.

trimethoprim (trī-meth'-ō-prim). Antibacterial agent. Has selective inhibiting action on the enzyme that converts folic acid into folinic acid, needed by many bacteria. When used with sulphonamides the ensuing action is bactericidal. The sulphonamide must have a similar pattern of absorption and excretion.

trimipramine (trīm-īp'-ra-mēn). Antidepressant similar to imipramine (.v.).

trinitrine caffeine (trī-nīt'-rēn kaf'-ēn). Glyceryl trinitrate (q.v.).

Triostam (trī-os-tam). Sodium antimony gluconate (q.v.).

tripelennamine (trī-pel-en'-a-mēn). Antihistamine, useful in treatment of allergy.

triple antigen. Contains diphtheria, whooping-cough and tetanus antigens.

Triplopen (trip'-lo-pen). Benethamine

penicillin G, procaine penicillin G and sodium penicillin G. Used for acute localized infections.

Triptafen (trip'-ta-fen). Amitriptyline (q.v.).

tris-hydroxylmethyl aminomethane (tris hī-droks'-il-meth'-il am-in-ō-mē'-thān). An alkali used to treat acidosis.

trismus (triz'-mus) [G. a grinding]. Spasm in the muscles of mastication.

trisomy (trī'-so-mi). Division into three giving an extra chromosome, i.e. 47 in man.

trocar (trō'-kár). A pointed rod which fits inside a cannula.

trochanters (trō-kan'-tèrz). Two processes, the larger one (t. major) on the outer, the other (t. minor) on the inner side of the femur between the shaft and neck; they serve for the attachment of muscles—trochanteric, adj.

trochlea (trok'-lē-á) [G. *trochilia*, pulley]. Any part which is like a pulley in structure or function—trochlear, adj.

Tromexan (trō-meks'-an). Ethyl biscoumacetate (q.v.).

trophic (trō'-fik) [G. *trophe*, nourishment]. Pertaining to nutrition.

trophoblastic tissue (trō-fō-blas'-tik tis'-ū) [G. *trophe*, nourishment; *blastos*, germ]. Cells covering the embedding ovum and concerning with the nutrition of the ovum.

trophoneurosis (trō-fō-nū-rō'-sis). See RAYNAUD'S DISEASE.

Trousseau's sign. See CARPOPEDAL SPASM. [Armand Trousseau, French physician, 1801–67.]

Troxidone (troks'-i-dōn). Trimethadione (q.v.).

Trypanosoma (tri-pan-ō-sō'-má). A genus of parasitic protozoa. Their life cycle alternates between blood-sucking arthropods and vertebrate hosts, and in the latter they appear frequently in the blood stream as fusiform, actively motile structures some 12 to 40 μm in length. A limited number of species are pathogenic to man.

trypanosomiasis (tri-pan-o-som-ī'-a-sis). Disease produced by infestation with Trypanosoma. In man this may be with *Trypanosoma rhodesiense* in East Africa or *T. gambiense* in West Africa, both transmitted by the tsetse fly, and with *T. cruzii*, transmitted by bugs in South America. In West Africa infection of the brain commonly produces the symptomatology of 'sleeping sickness'.

tryparsamide (trī-pár'-sa-mīd). An organic arsenic compound of value in the treatment of trypanosomiasis. It is usually given by intravenous injection, as it is more irritant and less effective orally.

trypsin (trip'-sin). A proteolytic enzyme present in pancreatic juice. Given in digestive disorders. Specially purified forms are used to liquefy clotted blood and other secretions, and in ophthalmology to facilitate removal of cataracts.

Tryptizol. Armitriptyline (q.v.). See ANTIDEPRESSANT. In small doses can be used to prevent bed-wetting in adults. Not suitable for the elderly. Makes one aware of full bladder even though one is sleeping soundly.

tryptophane (trip'-tō-fān). One of the essential amino acids necessary for growth.

tsetse fly (tset'-sē) A fly of the genus Glossina. A common vector of Trypanosoma in Africa. The Trypanosoma live part of their life cycle in the flies and are transferred to new hosts, including man, in the salivary juices when the fly bites for a blood meal.

tubal (tū'-bal). Pertaining to a tube. **tubal pregnancy** see ECTOPIC PREGNANCY.

Tubarine (tū'-bar-ēn). Tubocurarine (q.v.).

Tubegauz (tūb'-gawz). A special type of woven circular bandage, applied with a special applicator.

tubercle (tūb'-èr-kl) [L. *tuberculum*, small lump]. 1. A small rounded prominence usually on bone. 2. The specific lesion produced by *Mycobacterium tuberculosis*.

tuberculide (tū-ber'-kūl-īd) [L. *tuberculum*, small lump]. Also **tuberculid.** Metastatic manifestation of tuberculosis producing a skin lesion, e.g. papulonecrotic t., rosacealike t. (Cf. syphilide.)

tuberculin. A sterile extract of either the crude (old t.) or refined (PPD) complex protein constituents of the tubercle bacillus. Its commonest use is in determining whether a person has or has not previously been infected with the tubercle bacillus, by injecting a small amount into the skin and reading the reaction, if any, in 48 to 72 hours; negative reactors have escaped previous infection. See MANTOUX.

tuberculoid (tū-ber'-kū-loid). Resembling tuberculosis. Describes one of the two types of leprosy.

tuberculoma (tū-ber-kū-lō'-má). A caseous tubercle, usually large, its size suggesting a tumour.

tuberculosis (tū-ber-kū-lō'-sis) [L. *tuberculum,* small swelling; G. *-osis,* condition]. A specific, infective disease caused by *Mycobacterium tuberculosis* (Koch's tubercle bacillus). **avian t.,** endemic in birds and rarely seen in man. **bovine t.,** endemic in cattle and transmitted to man via infected cow's milk, causing disease of the glands and rarely of the lungs and joints. **human t.,** endemic in man and the usual cause of pulmonary and other forms of tuberculosis. **miliary t.,** a generalized acute form in which, as a result of bloodstream dissemination, minute, multiple tuberculous foci are scattered throughout many organs of the body—tubercular, tuberculous, adj.

tuberculostatic (tū-ber-kū-lō-stat'-ik). Inhibiting the growth of the tubercle bacillus (*Mycobacterium tuberculosis*).

tuberose (tuberous) sclerosis. See EPILOIA.

tuberosity (tū-ber-os'-it-i) [L. *tuber,* swelling]. A bony prominence.

Tubigrip (tū'-bi-grip). Supporting hose. Can be worn during a operation and early postoperative period to prevent deep vein thrombosis.

tubocurarine (tū-bō-kū-rár'-ēn). The muscle-relaxing drug obtained from the South American arrow poison curare. Action reversed by neostigmine given intravenously together with atropine which depresses vagus nerve and so quickens the heart beat.

tubo-ovarian (tū-bō-ov-ār'-i-an) [L. *tubus,* tube; *ovum,* egg]. Pertaining to or involving both tube and ovary, e.g. tubo-ovarian abscess.

tubular necrosis (tū'-būl-ar ne-krō'-sis). Degenerative change resulting from renal ischaemia. May terminate fatally with uraemia. Syndrome occurs in shock such as the crush syndrome (q.v.), severe burns, hypotension, intrauterine haemorrhage and dehydration. Represents a type of acute renal failure.

tubule (tū'-būl) [L. *tubulus,* small tube]. A small tube. **collecting t.,** straight tube in the kidney medulla conveying urine to the kidney pelvis. **convoluted t.,** coiled tube in the kidney cortex. **seminiferous t.,** coiled tube in the testis. **uriniferous t.,** syn. nephron (q.v.).

Tuinal (tū'-in-al). Hypnotic. A mixture of quinalbarbitone (q.v.) and amylobarbitone (q.v.).

tularaemia (tū-lar-ē'-mi-á). Syn., deer-fly fever; tick fever; rabbit fever, etc. An endemic disease of rodents, caused by *Pasteurella tularensis*; transmitted by biting insects and acquired by man either in handling infected animal carcases or by the bite of an infected insect. Suppuration at the inoculation site is followed by inflammation of the draining lymph glands and by severe constitutional upset—tularaemic, adj.

tulle gras (tūl'-grá'). Non-adhesive dressing for wounds. Gauze impregnated with soft paraffin, and sterilized.

tumescence (tū-mes'-ens) [L. *tumescere,* to swell]. A state of swelling; turgidity.

tumour (tū'-mor) [L.]. A swelling. A mass of abnormal tissue which resembles the normal tissues in structure, but which fulfils no useful function and which grows at the expense of the body. Benign, simple or innocent tumours are encapsulated, do not infiltrate adjacent tissue or cause metastases and are unlikely to recur if removed. **malignant t.,** not encapsulated, infiltrate adjacent tissue and cause metastases. See CANCER—tumorous, adj.

tunica (tūn'-ik-á) [L. a tunic]. A lining membrane; a coat. **tunica adventitia,** the outer coat of an artery. **tunica intima,** the lining of an artery. **tunica media,** the middle muscular coat of an artery.

tunnel reimplantation operation. See LEADBETTER-POLITANO OPERATION.

turbinate (tur'-bin-āt) [L. *turbinatus*]. Shaped like a top or inverted cone. **tubinate bone,** one on either side forming the lateral nasal walls.

turbinated (tur'-bin-ā-ted) [L. *turbinatus,* cone-shaped]. Scroll-shaped, as the three ethmoidal t. processes which project from the lateral nasal walls.

turbinectomy (tur-bin-ek'-to-mi) [L. *turbo,* whirled; *ektome,* excision]. Removal of turbinate bones.

turgid (tur'-jid) [L. *turgescere,* to swell]. Swollen; firmly distended, as with blood by congestion—turgescence, n.; turgidity, n.

Turner's syndrome. Gonadal dysgenesis. Can be identified at birth: 45 chromosomes instead of 46; one sex chromosome missing. Brought up as girl though genetic male. Such an individual has small female genitalia, scanty pubic hair. atrophic ovaries, webbed neck and valgus of the elbows. [Henry H. Turner, American endocrinologist, 1892- .]

tussis (tus´-sis) [L]. A cough.

tybamate (tī´-bam-āt). Analogue of meprobamate (q.v.).

tympanic (tim-pan´-ik) [G. *tympanon,* drum]. Pertaining to the tympanum. **tympanic membrane** (membrane tympani), the eardrum.

tympanites (tim-pan-īt´-ēz) [G. *tympanon,* drum]. Abdominal distension due to accumulation of gas in the intestine. Also called 'tympanism'.

tympanitis (tim-pan-ī´-tis) [G. *tympanon,* drum; *-itis,* inflammation]. Inflammation of the tympanum.

tympanoplasty (tim´-pan-ō-plas´-ti). Any reconstructive operation on the middle ear designed to improve hearing. Normally carried out in ears damaged by chronic suppurative otitis media with associated conductive deafness—tympanoplastic, adj.

tympanum (tim´-pan-um) [G. *tympanon,* drum]. The cavity of the middle ear.

typhoid fever (tī-foid). An infectious fever usually spread by contamination of food, milk or water supplies with *Salmonella typhi,* either directly by sewage, indirectly by flies, or by faulty personal hygiene. Symptomless carriers harbouring the germ in the gall-bladder and excreting it in their stools are the main source of outbreaks of disease in this country. The average incubation period is 10 to 14 days. A progressive febrile illness marks the onset of the disease, which develops as the germ invades lymphoid tissue, including that of the small intestine (Peyer's patches) to profuse diarrhoeal (pea soup) stools which may become frankly haemorrhagic; ultimately recovery usually begins at the end of the third week. A rose-coloured rash may appear on the upper abdomen and back at the end of the first week. See TAB.

typhus (tī´-fus) [G. *typhos,* delusion]. An acute infectious disease characterized by high fever, a skin eruption, and severe headache. It is a disease of war, famine or catastrophe, being spread by lice, ticks or fleas. It is only sporadic in Britain. Infecting organism is *Rickettsia prowazekii,* sensitive to sulphonamides and antibiotics.

tyramine (tī´-rá-mēn). An enzyme present in several foodstuffs. See MONOAMINE OXIDASE.

tyrosine(e) (ti´-rō-sin). An amino acid associated with growth. Combines with iodine to form thyroxine.

tyrosinosis (tī-rō-sin-ō´-sis). Due to abnormal metabolism of tyrosin, *p*-hydroxyphenylpyruvic acid is excreted in the urine.

tyrothricin (ti-rō-thrī´-sin). A mixture of gramicidin and other antibiotics. It is too toxic for systemic therapy, but is valuable in a number of infected skin conditions.

U

UCB 1549. Drug for Parkinsonism.

Ulbreval (ul-brē´-val). Buthalitone (q.v.).

ulcer (ul´-sėr). An open sore in a body surface. Curling's u., a peptic u., associated with extensive burns and scalds. [Thomas Blizard Curling, English surgeon, 1811-88.] decubitis u., pressure sore (q.v.). dendritic u. (q.v.). penetrating u., one which is locally invasive and may erode a blood vessel, causing haematemesis or melaena in the case of gastric or duodenal ulcer. peptic u. occurs in the stomach (gastric ulcer), in the duodenum (duodenal ulcer). perforating u., one which erodes through the wall of an organ. rodent u., a slowly growing, locally invasive tumour of the skin commonly found on the face. varicose u., indolent type which occurs in the lower third of a leg afflicted with varicose veins. Syn., gravitational ulcer.

ulcerative (ul´-sėr-āt-iv). Pertaining to, or of the nature of an ulcer. see COLITIS.

ulcerogenic (ul-ser-ō-jen´-ik) [L. *ulcus,* a sore; G. *genesis,* descent]. Capable of producing an ulcer.

Ultralanum (ul-tral-an´-um). Fluocortolone (q.v.).

ultramicroscopic (ul-tra-mī-krō-skop´-ik). Too small to be seen by means of the microscope, usually referring to the light microscope.

ultrasonic. Relating to mechanical vibrations of very high frequency (above 30000 Hz). In diagnostic ultrasound information is derived from echoes which occur when a controlled beam of this energy crosses the boundary between adjacent tissues of differing physical properties. **Power** ultrasound has a destructive effect and has been used in the treatment of frostbite, Ménière's disease and in brain surgery. See ECHOENCEPHALOGRAPHY.

Ultrapen (ul'-tra-pen). Propicillin (q.v.).

ultrasonography (ul-tra-son-og'-ra-fi) [L. *ultra*, beyond; *sonus*, sound; G. *graphein*, to write]. Production of visual image from application of ultrasound, sound waves with a frequency of over 20000 Hz (cycles per second) and inaudible to the human ear—ultrasonographically, adv.; ultrasonograph, n.

ultrasound (ul-tra-sownd'). Can be used for cleansing and nebulizing.

umbilicated (um-bil'-i-kā-ted) [L. *umbilicus*, middle]. Having a central depression, e.g. a smallpox vesicle.

umbilicus (um-bil-ī'-kus) [L. middle]. The abdominal scar left by the separation of the umbilical cord (q.v.) after birth; the naval—umbilical, adj.

uncinate (un'-sin-āt) [L. *uncinus*, hook]. Hook-shaped. Unciform.

unconsciousness (un-kon'-shus-nes) [A.S. *un*, not; *conscire*, to know, be aware]. State of being unconscious; insensible.

undine (un'-dēn) [L. *unda*, a wave]. A small, thin glass flask used for irrigating the eyes.

undulant fever (un'-dū-lant) [L. *unda*, a wave]. The condition is also called (abortus f.', 'Malta f.' and 'Mediterranean f'. See BRUCELLA, BRUCELLOSIS.

unguentum (ung-gwen'-tum) [L.]. Ointment.

unicellular (ū-ni-sel'-ū-lar) [L. *unus*, one; *cellula*, cell]. Consisting of only one cell.

unilateral (ū-ni-lat'-e-ral) [L. *unus*, one; *latus*, side]. Relating to or on one side only—unilaterally, adv.

uniocular (ū-ni-ok'-ū-lar) [L. *unus*, one; *oculus*, eye]. Pertaining to, or affecting, one eye.

uniovular (ū-ni-ov'-ū-lar) [L. *unus*, one; *ovum*, egg]. Pertaining to one ovum, as u. twins (identical). (Cf. binovular.)

unipara (ū-nip'-a-rá) [L. *unus*, one; *parere*, to bring forth]. A woman who has borne only one child—uniparous, adj.

Unna's paste (un'-nas). A glycogelatin

and zinc oxide preparation, used in the treatment of varicose veins in association with supportive bandaging. [Paul Gerson Unna, German dermatologist, 1850–1929.]

urachus (ū'-rak-us) [G. *ouron*, urine; *echein*, to hold]. The stemlike structure connecting the bladder with the umbilicus in the fetus; in postnatal life it is represented by a fibrous cord situated between the apex of the bladder and the umbilicus, known as the median umbilical ligament—urachal, adj.

uracil mustard (ū'-rá-sil mus'-tard). Uramustine (q.v.).

uraemia (ū-rē'-mi-á). A clinical syndrome due to renal failure resulting from either disease of the kidneys themselves, or from disorder or disease elsewhere in the body which induces kidney dysfunction, and which results in gross biochemical disturbance in the body, including retention of urea and other nitrogenous substances in the blood. Depending on the cause it may or may not be reversible. The fully developed syndrome is characterized by nausea, vomiting, headache, hiccough, weakness, dimness of vision, convulsions and coma—uraemic, adj.

uramustine (ū-rá-mus'-tēn). Antimitotic agent occasionally used in cancer.

uraemic snow. See URIDROSIS.

urate (ū'-rāt). A salt of uric acid; such compounds are present in the blood and urine.

uraturia (ū-rat-ūr'-ē-á) [G. *ouron*, urine]. Excess of urates in the urine—uraturic, adj.

urea (ū-rē'-á). The end waste product of protein metabolism; it is excreted in the urine of which it is the main chemical constituent. Can be given orally as a diuretic.

Ureaphil (ū-rē'-á-fil). Urea compound used to produce dehydration in cerebral oedema, raised intraocular pressure, and as a diuretic in resistant cases. Has a low potential for sodium retention, thus increases urinary output.

ureter (ū'-rē-ter) [G. *oureter*]. The tube passing from each kidney to the bladder for the conveyance of urine; its average length is from 25.00 to 30.48 cm—ureteric, ureteral, adj.

ureterectomy (ūr-ēt-er-ek'-to-mi) [G. *oureter*, ureter; *ektome*, excision]. Excision of a ureter.

ureteritis (ū-rēt-er-ī'-tis) [G. *oureter*, ureter; -itis, inflammation]. Inflammation of a ureter.

ureterocolic (ūr-ēt-er-o-kol'-ik) [G. oureter, ureter; kolon, colon]. Pertaining to the ureter and colon.

ureterocolostomy (ūr-ēt-er-ō-kol-os'-to-mi) [G. oureter, ureter; kolon, colon; stoma, mouth]. Surgical transplantation of the ureters from the bladder to the colon so that urine is passed by the bowel; sometimes carried out to relieve strangury in tuberculosis of the bladder, or prior to cystectomy for bladder tumours.

ureteroileal (ūr-ēt-er-ō-il'-ē-al) [G. oureter, ureter; L. ilia, flanks]. Pertaining to the ureters and ileum as the anastomosis necessary in ureteroileostomy.

ureteroileostomy (ūr-ēt-er-ō-īl-ē-os'-to-mi) [G. oureter, ureter; L. ilia, flanks; G. stoma, mouth]. More usually 'ileoureterostomy' (q.v.).

ureterolith (ū-rēt'-er-ō-lith) [G. oureter, ureter; lithos, stone]. A calculus in the ureter.

ureterolithotomy (ūr-ēt-er-ō-lith-ot'-o-mi) [G. oureter, ureter; lithos, stone; tome, a cutting]. Surgical removal of a stone from a ureter.

ureterosigmoidostomy (ūr-ēt'-er-ō-sig-moid-os'-to-mi). See URETEROCOLOSTOMY.

ureterostomy (ū-rēt-er-os'-tō-mi) [G. oureter, ureter; stoma, mouth]. The formation of a permanent fistula, through which the ureter discharges urine. cutaneous u., transplantation of the ureter to the skin. See BLADDER.

ureterovaginal (ū-rēt-er-ō-vaj-ī'-nal) [G. oureter, ureter; L. vagina, sheath]. Pertaining to the ureter and vagina.

ureterovesical (ū-rēt-er-ō-ves'-ik-al) [G. oureter, ureter; L. vesica, bladder]. Pertaining to the ureter and bladder.

urethane (ūr'-ēth-ān). This compound has diuretic, hypnotic and cytostatic properties.

urethra (ū-rē'-thrà) [G. ourethra]. The passage from the bladder through which urine is excreted; in the female it measures 25.4 to 38.1 mm; in the male 25.00 cm—urethral, adj.

urethral syndrome. Symptoms of urinary infection although the urine is sterile when withdrawn by catheter. Suggests that infection is confined to the urethra and adjoining glands.

urethritis (ū-rē-thrī'-tis) [G. ourethron,

urethra; -itis, inflammation]. Inflammation of the urethra. non-specific u. (NGU), now listed by the DHSS as a venereal disease.

urethrocele (ūr-ēth'-rō-sēl) [G. ourethron, urethra; kele, hernia]. Prolapse of the urethra, usually into the anterior vaginal wall.

urethrogram (ūr-ēth'-rō-gram). X-ray of urethra. Can be part of cystography (q.v.) or the dye may be inserted into bladder by catheter. X-ray taken on voiding bladder.

urethrography (ūr ēth rog' rà-fi). X-ray examination of the urethra. See UROGRAPHY.

urethrometry (ūr-ēth-rom'-et-ri) [G. ourethron. urethra; metron, a measure]. Measurement of the urethral lumen using a urethrometer—urethrometric, adj.; urethrometrically, adv.

urethroplasty (ūr-ēth-rō-plas'-ti) [G. ourethra, urethra; plassein, to form]. Any plastic operation on the urethra urethroplastic, adj.

urethroscope (ūr-eth'-rō-skōp) [G. ourethra, urethra; skopein, to examine]. An instrument designed to allow visualization of the interior of the urethra—urethroscopic, adj.; urethroscopically, adv.; urethroscopy, n.

urethrostenosis (ūr-ēth-rō-sten-ō'-sis) [G. ourethra, urethra; a narrowing]. Urethral stricture.

urethrotomy (ur-eth-rot'-o-mi) [G. ourethra, urethra; tome, a cutting]. Incision into the urethra; usually part of an operation for stricture.

urethrotrigonitis (ūr-ēth-rō-trī-gon-ī'-tis) [G. ourethra, urethra, trigonos, three-cornered; -itis, inflammation]. Inflammation of the bladder. See TRIGONE.

uric acid (ūr'-ik as'-id). An acid formed in the breakdown of nucleoproteins in the tissues, and excreted in the urine. It is relatively insoluble and liable to give rise to stones. Present in excess in the blood in gout and a gout-like syndrome occurring in male infants, manifesting as early as 4 months with self-destructive behaviour, cerebral palsy and mental retardation.

uricosuric (ū-ril-ō-sū'-rik). Enhances renal excretion of uric acid due to impairment of tubular reabsorption. Such substances used in chronic gout.

uridrosis (ū-ri-drō'-sis) [G. ouron, urine; hidrosis, sweating]. Excess of urea in the sweat; it may be deposited on the skin as fine white crystals. 'Uraemic snow.'

urinalysis (ū-rin-al'-i-sis)[L. *urina*, urine; G. *lysis*, a loosening]. Examination of the urine.

urinary (ūr-in'-ar-i). Pertaining to urine. **urinary diversion**, see BLADDER.

urination (ū-rin-ā'-shun) [L. *urina*, urine]. Micturition (q.v.).

urine (ū'-rin) [L. *urina*]. The amber-coloured fluid which is excreted from the kidneys at the rate of about 1500 ml every 24 hours in the adult; it is slightly acid and has a specific gravity of 1005 to 1030.

uriniferous (ū-rin-if'-er-us) [L. *urina*, urine; *ferre*, to carry]. Conveying urine.

urinogenital (ū-rin-ō-jen'-it-al). See UROGENITAL.

urinometer (ū-rin-om'-e-tèr) [L. *urina*, urine; G. *metron*, a measure]. An instrument for estimating the specific gravity of urine.

Urispas (ūr'-is-pas). Flavoxate (q.v.).

urobilin (ū-rō-bīl'-in). [G. *ouron*, urine; L. *bilus*, bile]. A pigment formed by the oxidation of urobilinogen and excreted in the urine and faeces.

urobilinogen (ū-rō-bīl-in'-ō-jen). A pigment formed from bilirubin in the intestine by the action of bacteria. It may be reabsorbed into the circulation and converted back to bilirubin in the liver or excreted in the urine.

urobilinuria (ū-rō-bīl-in-ūr'-i-á). The presence of increased amounts of urobilin in the urine. Evidence of increased production of bilirubin in the liver, e.g. after haemolysis.

urochrome (ū'-rō-chrōm). The pigment which gives urine its normal colour. Its chemical composition and origin are unknown.

urogenital (ū-rō-jen'-it-al) [G. *ouron*, urine; L. *genitalis*, genital]. Pertaining to the urinary and the genital organs.

urogram (ū'-rō-gram) [G. *ouron*, urine; *gramma*, letter]. Radiograph of urinary tract after injection of contrast media.

urografin (ūr-ō-gräf'-in). Sodium and meglumine diatrizoates (q.v.).

urography (ūr-og'-ra-fi) [G. *ouron*, urine; *graphein*, to write]. X-ray examination of urinary tract by means of contrast media, e.g. pyelography, cystography, cystourethrograpy, urethrography.

urokinase (ū-rō-kīn'-ās). An enzyme which dissolves fibrin clot. Used for traumatic and postoperative hyphaema. It has been tried in hyaline membrane disease.

urologist (ū-rol'-o-jist) [G. *ouron*, urine; *logos*, discourse]. A person who specializes in disorders of the female urinary tract, and the male genitourinary tract.

urology (ū-rol'-o-ji) [G. *ouron*, urine; *logos*, discourse]. That branch of science which deals with disorders of the female urinary tract and the male genitourinary tract—urological, adj., urologically, adv.

Urolucosil (ūr-ō-luk'-o-sil). A sulphonamide highly effective in urinary infections. The low dose (0.1 g) markedly reduces the risk of renal complications.

Uropac (ūr'-ō-pak). Iodoxyl (q.v.).

Uroselectan (ūr-rō-sē-lek'-tan). Iodoxyl (q.v.).

urticaria (ur-ti-kā'-ri-á). Syn., nettle-rash or hives. An allergic skin eruption characterized by multiple, circumscribed, smooth, raised, pinkish, itchy weals, developing very suddenly, usually lasting a few days, and leaving no visible trace. Common provocative agents in susceptible subjects are ingested foods such as shellfish, injected sera, and contact with, or injection of, antibiotics such as penicillin and streptomycin. See ANGIOHEUROTIC OEDEMA.

uteroplacental (ū-ter-ō-plas-en'-tal). Pertaining to the uterus and placenta.

uterorectal (ū-ter-ō-rek'-tal) [G. *uterus*, womb; L. *rectus*, straight]. Pertaining to the uterus and the rectum.

uterosacral (ū-ter-ō-sā'-kral) [L. *uterus*, womb; *sacer*, sacred]. Pertaining to the uterus and sacrum.

uterosalpingography (ū-ter-ō-sal-ping-og'-raf-i) [L. *uterus*, womb; G. *salpigx*, trumpet; *graphein*, to write]. X-ray by means of injection of contrast media (for patency of Fallopian tubes).

uterovaginal (ū-ter-ō-vaj-īn'-al) [L. *uterus*, womb; *vagina*, sheath]. Pertaining to the uterus and the vagina.

uterovesical (ū-ter-ō-ves'-ik-al) [L. *uterus*, womb; *vesica*, bladder]. Pertaining to the uterus and the bladder.

uterus (ū'-tèr-us) [L.]. The womb; a hollow muscular organ into which the ovum is received through the uterine tubes, and where it is retained during development, and from which the fetus is expelled through the vagina. **bicornu-**

ate u., a uterus with two horns. **gravid u.**, a pregnant uterus—uterine, adj.; uteri, pl.

utricle (ū'-trik-l) [L. *utriculus*, small bag]. A little sac or pocket.

uvea (ū'-vi-à) [L. *uva*, grape]. The pigmented part of the eye, including the iris, ciliary body and choroid—uveal, adj.

uveitis (ū-vē-ī'-tis) [L. *uva*, grape; G. *-itis*, inflammation]. Inflammation of the uvea.

uvula (ū'-vū-là) [L. *uva*, grape]. The central, tag-like structure hanging down from the free edge of the soft palate.

uvulectomy (ū-vūl-ek'-to-mi) [L. *uva*, grape; G. *ektome*, excision]. Excision of the uvula.

uvulitis (ū'-vūl-ī'-tis) [L. *uva*, grape; G. *-itis*, inflammation]. Inflammation of the uvula.

V

vaccination (vak-sin-ā'-shun) [L. *vacca*, cow]. Originally described the process of inoculating persons with discharge from cowpox to protect them from smallpox. Now applied to the inoculation of any antigenic material for the purpose of producing active artificial immunity.

vaccines (vak'-sēnz). Suspensions or extracts of dead or attenuated bacterial cells, used chiefly in the prophylactic treatment of certain infections by production of active immunity. Triple vaccine protects against diphtheria, tetanus and whooping-cough. In addition to these, quadruple vaccine protects against poliomyelitis. See SABIN, SALK, TAB, BCG.

vaccinia (vak-sin'-i-à) [L. *vaccinus*, of cows]. Virus used to confer immunity against smallpox. Its origins are obscure but it is probably a cowpox-smallpox hybrid—vaccinial, adj.

vaccinotherapy (vak-sin-ō-ther'-à-pi). The use of a vaccine for the treatment of disease. Most often this is non-specific, as in the use of TAB vaccine for producing artificial pyrexia.

vagal (vā'-gal). Pertaining to the vagus (q.v.).

vagina (va-jīn'-à) [L.]. A sheath; the musculomembranous passage extending from the cervix uteri to the vulva; it measures 76.2 mm along the anterior wall and 88.9 mm along the posterior—vaginal, adj.

vaginismus (vaj-in-iz'-mus) [L. *vagina*]. Painful muscular spasm of the vaginal walls resulting in dyspareunia or painful coitus.

vaginitis (vaj-in-ī'-tis) [L. *vagina*, sheath; G. *-itis*, inflammation]. Inflammation of the vagina. **senile v.**, can cause adhesions which may obliterate the vaginal canal. **trichomonas v.**, characterized by an intensely irritating discharge; due to a ciliated protozoon which normally inhabits the bowel. See TRICHOMONAS.

vagolytic (vā-gō-lit'-ik). [L. *vagus*, wandering; G. *lysis*, a loosening]. That which neutralizes the effect of a stimulated vagus nerve.

vagotomy (vā-got'-o-mi) [L. *vagus*, wandering; G. *tome*, a cutting]. Surgical division of the vagus nerves; done in conjunction with gastroenterostomy in the treatment of peptic ulcer or pyloroplasty.

vagus (vā'-gus) [L. wandering]. The parasympathetic pneumogastric nerve; the tenth cranial nerve, composed of both motor and sensory fibres, with a wide distribution in the neck, thorax and abdomen, sending important branches to the heart, lungs stomach, etc.—vagal, adj.; vagi, pl.

valgus (val'-gus) [L.]. Displacement or angulation away from the midline of the body, e.g. hallux valgus.

valine (vā'-lēn). One of the essential amino acids (q.v.).

Valium (val'-i-um). Diazepam (q.v.).

Vallergan. Trimeprazine (q.v.).

Valoid (val'-oid). Cyclizine (q.v.).

valve (valv) [L. *valva*, fold]. A fold of membrane in a passage or tube permitting the flow of contents in one direction only. **valvular replacement,**

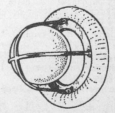

Prosthetic heart valve

operation for insertion of prosthetic mitral or aortic valve—valvular, adj.

valvoplasty (val-vō-plas'-ti) [L. *valva,* fold; *plassein,* to form]. A plastic operation on a valve, usually reserved for the heart; includes valve replacement and valvulotomy—valvoplastic, adj.

valvotomy (val-vot'-om-i). See VALVU-LOTOMY.

valvulitis (val-vū-lī'-tis) [L. *valva,* fold; G. *-itis,* inflammation]. Inflammation of a valve, particularly in the heart.

valvulotomy (val-vūl-ot'-om-i) [L. *valva,* fold; G. *tome,* cutting]. Incision of a valve, by custom referring to the heart.

Vamin Scientifically prepared solution for parenteral feeding.

vancomycin (van-ko-mī'-sin). Antibiotic for overwhelming staphylococcal infections. Natural resistance to v. rare. Has to be given intravenously Ototoxic.

Vandid (van'-did). Vanillic acid diethylamide (q.v.).

vanillic acid diethylamide. Chemoreceptor stimulant, especially useful in promoting respiration.

Vanquin (van'-qwin). Viprynium embonate (q.v.).

Vaquez's disease. Polycythaemia vera (q.v.). [Louis Henri Vaquez, French physician, 1860–1936.]

varicella (va-ri-sel'-lá). Chickenpox (q.v.)—varicelliform, adj.

varices (vār'-i-sēz) [L.]. Dilated, tortuous (or varicose) veins—varix, sing.

varicocele (va'-ri-kō-sēl) [L. *varicosus,* full of dilated veins; G. *kele,* tumour]. Varicosity of the veins of the spermatic cord.

varicose (va'-ri-kōs) [L. *varicosus,* full of dilated veins]. Dilated varicosity, n. varicose veins, dilated veins, the valves of which become incompetent so that blood flow may be reversed. Most commonly found in the lower limbs, rectum (haemorrhoids) or lower oesophagus (oesophageal varices).

varicotomy (va-ri-kot'-o-mi) [L. *varicosus,* full of dilated veins; G. *tome,* cutting]. Excision of a varicose vein.

Varidase. Streptokinase (q.v.) and streptodornase (q.v.).

variola (va-ri'-ō-lá) [L.]. Smallpox (q.v.).

varioloid (va'-ri-ō-loid) [L. *variola,* smallpox]. Attack of smallpox modified by previous vaccination.

Varistab (va-ri-stab'). Ethyloleamine (q.v.).

varix (vā'-iks) [L.]. A dilated and tortuous vein—varices, pl.

varus (vār'-us) [L.]. Displacement or angulation towards the midline of the body, e.g. coxa vara.

vas [L.]. A vessel—vasa, pl.

vas deferens (vas def'-er-enz). The excretory duct of the testis.

vasa vasorum (va'-zá vaz-or'-um). The minute nutrient vessels of the artery and vein walls.

vascular (vas'-kū-lar) [L. *vasculum,* small vessel]. Supplied with vessels, especially referring to blood vessels.

vascularization (vas-kū-lar-ī-zā'-shun) [L. *vasculum,* small vessel]. The acquisition of a blood supply. The process of becoming vascular.

vasculitis (vas-kūl-ī'-tis) [L. *vasculum,* small vessel; G. *-itis,* inflammation]. Inflammation of a blood vessel. Also angiitis.

vasectomy (vas-ek'-to-mi) [L. *vas,* vessel; G. *ektome,* excision]. Surgical excision of part of the vas deferens.

vasoconstrictor (vā-sō-kon-strik'-tor) [L. *vas,* vessel; *constringere,* to draw tight]. Any agent which causes a narrowing of the lumen of blood vessels.

vasodilator (vā-sō-dī'-la-tor) [L. *vas,* vessel; *dilatare,* to dilate]. Any agent which causes a widening of the lumen of blood vessels.

vasoepididymostomy (va'-sō-ep-i-did-i-mos'-to-mi) [L. *vas,* vessel; G. *epi,* on; *didumoi,* twins; *stoma,* mouth]. Anastomosis of the vas deferens to the epididymis.

vasomotor nerves (vā-sō-mō'-tėr) [L. *vas,* vessel; *movere,* to move]. Nerves which cause changes in the calibre of the blood vessels.

vasopressin (vaz-ō-pres'-in). Formed in the hypothalamus. Passes down the nerves in the pituitary stalk to be stored in the posterior lobe of the pituitary gland. It is the antidiuretic hormone (ADH). Can be given by injection or as snuff in diabetes insipidus. Synthetic preparation available–Pitressin.

vasospasm (vā'-sō-spazm) [L. *vas,* vessel; G. *spasmos,* spasm]. Constricting spasm of vessel walls—vasospastic, adj.

vasovagal attack. Faintness, pallor, sweating, feeling of fullness in epigastrium. When part of the post-gastrectomy syndrome it occurs a few minutes after a meal.

Vasoxine (vaz-oks'-ēn). Methoxamine (q.v.).

Vatensol (vat'-en-sol). Guanoclor (q.v.).

VBI. Vertebrobasilar insufficiency (q.v.).

vector (vek'-tor) [L. *vehere,* to carry]. Carrier of disease.

Veganin (vej'-a-nin). A preparation similar to tab. codeine co. (BNF), containing aspirin, phenacetin and codeine.

vegetations (vej-e-tā'-shuns) [L. *vegetare,* enliven]. Growths or accretions composed of fibrin and platelets occurring on the edge of the cardiac valves in endocarditis.

vegetative (vej-e-tā'-tiv) [L. *vegetare,* enliven]. Pertaining to the non-sporing stage of a bacterium.

Vegolysen (vej-ō-lī'-sen). Hexamethonium (q.v.).

vehicle (vē'-i-kl) [L. *vehiculum,* conveyance]. An inert substance in which a drug is administered, e.g. water in mixtures.

vein (vān) [L. *vena,* vein]. A vessel conveying blood from the capillaries back to the heart. It has the same three coats as an artery, the inner one being fitted with valves—**venous,** adj.

Velactin (vel-ak'-tin). A substitution for milk in milk-free diets.

Velbe (vel'-bē). Vinblastine (q.v.).

venepuncture (vē-ni-pungk'-tūr) [L. *vena,* vein; *punctura,* a puncture]. Insertion of a needle into a vein.

venereal (ven-ē'-rē-al) [L. *venereus,* from Venus, goddess of love]. Pertaining to or caused by sexual intercourse. **venereal disease,** gonorrhoea, non-specific urethritis, syphilis and soft sore.

venereology (ven-ē-rē-ol'-o-ji). The study and treatment of venereal disease.

venesection (vē-ni-sek'-shun) [L. *vena,* vein; *sectio,* cutting]. A clinical procedure, formerly by opening cubital vein with scalpel (now usually by venepuncture), whereby blood volume is reduced in congestive heart failure.

venoclysis (vē-nō-klī'-sis) [L. *vena,* vein; G. *klysis,* a drenching]. The introduction of nutrient or medicinal fluids into a vein. See CLYSIS.

venogram (vē'-nō-gram) [L. *vena,* vein; G. *gramma,* letter]. A radiograph of venous system after opaque media injection.

venography (vēn-og'-ra-fi) [L. *vena,* vein; G. *graphein,* to write] X-ray examination of venous system by injection of opaque media—venographic, adj.; venographically, adv.

venous (vē'-nus) [L. *vena,* vein]. Pertaining to the veins.

Ventolin (ven'-tol-in). Salbutamol (q.v.).

Ventouse extraction. Use of the vacuum extractor in obstetrics.

ventral (ven'-tral) [L. *venter,* belly]. Pertaining to the abdomen or the anterior surface of the body—ventrally, adv.

ventricle (ven'-trik l) [L. *ventriculum*]. A small belly-like cavity. **ventricle of the brain,** four cavities filled with cerebrospinal fluid within the brain. **ventricle of the heart,** the two lower muscular chambers of the heart—ventricular, adj.

ventriculocysternostomy (ven-trik'-ū-lō-sis-tern-os'-to-mi) [L. *ventriculum,* ventricle; *cisterna,* cistern; G. *stoma,* mouth]. Artificial communication between cerebral ventricles and subarachnoid space. One of the drainage operations for hydrocephalus.

ventriculography (ven-trik-ū-log'-ra-fi) [L. *ventriculum,* ventricle; G. *graphein,* to write]. X-ray examination of ventricles after injection of an opaque medium—ventriculographic, adj.

ventriculoscope (ven-trik'-ūl-ō-skōp). An instrument via which the cerebral ventricles can be examined.

ventriculostomy (ven-trik-ūl-os'-to-mi) [L. *ventriculum,* ventricle; G. *stoma,* mouth]. An artificial opening into a ventricle. Usually refers to a drainage operation for hydrocephalus.

ventrosuspension (ven-tro-sus-pen'-shun). Fixation of displaced uterus to anterior abdominal wall.

venule (ven'-ūl) [L. *venula*]. A small vein. A syringe-like apparatus for collecting blood from a vein.

Veramon (ve'-ra-mon). See AMIDOPYRINE.

verapamil (ver-a-pam'-il). Synthetic drug which appears to have a quinidine-like action on the myocardium. Useful for angina of effort.

Verecolate (ver-ē-kō'-lāt). Cholagogue (q.v.).

Veriloid (ve'-ri-loid). Preparations of green hellebore. Useful in hypertension, particularly in association with similar drugs.

vermicide (vėr'-mi-sīd) [L. *vermis,* worm; *coedere,* to kill]. An agent which kills intestinal worms—vermicidal, adj.

vermiform (vėr'-mi-form) [L. *vermis,* worm; *forma,* form]. Wormlike. **vermiform appendix,** the vestigial, hollow, wormlike structure attached to the caecum.

vermifuge (vėr'-mi-fūj) [L. *vermis,* worm; *fugere,* to flee]. An agent that expels intestinal worms.

vernix caseosa (ver'-niks kā-zi-ō'-zà). The fatty substance which covers the skin of the fetus at birth and keeps it from becoming sodden by the liquor amnii.

Veronal (ve'-ron-al). Barbitone (q.v.), one of the first compounds of this type to be used therapeutically.

verruca (ve-roo'-kà) [L.]. Wart. Non-venereal warts of the genitals are called 'condylomata acuminata' (q.v.). **verruca necrogenica,** postmortem wart, develops as result of accidental inoculation with tuberculosis. **verruca plana juvenilis,** the common multiple, flat, tiny warts often seen on children's hands and knees. **verruca plantaris,** a flat wart on the sole of the foot. Highly contagious. **verruca seborrhoeica,** the brown, greasy wart seen in seborrhoeic subjects commonly on chest or back. **verruca vulgaris,** the common wart of the hands, of brown colour and rough pitted surface—verrucous, verrucose, adj.; verrucae, pl.

Versapen (vėr'-sa-pen). Hetacillin (q.v.).

Versene EDTA. A chelating agent, the calcium and sodium salts of which have been used to remove harmful substances from the body, e.g. lead, radioactive heavy metals. The newly formed stable chelate compounds are excreted in the urine.

version (vėr'-shun) [L. *vertere,* to turn]. Turning—applied to the manoeuvre to alter the position of the fetus *in utero.* **cephalic v.,** turning the child so that the head presents. **external v.** is turning the child by manipulation through the abdominal wall. **internal v.** is turning the child by one hand in the uterus, and the other on the patient's abdomen. **podalic v.,** turning the child to a breech presentation. This v. may be external or internal.

vertebrobasilar insufficiency. Syndrome caused by lack of blood to the hindbrain. May be progressive, episodic, or both. Clinical manifestations include giddiness and vertigo, nausea, ataxia, drop attacks and signs of cerebellar disorder such as nystagmus.

vertex (vėr'-teks) [L. top]. The top of the head.

vertigo (vėr-tī'-gō) [L.]. Giddiness, dizziness—vertiginous, adj.

vesical (ves'-i-kal) [L. *vesica,* bladder]. Pertaining to the bladder.

vesicant (ves'-i-kant) [L. *vesica,* bladder]. A blistering substance.

vesicle (ves'-ik-l) [L. *vesicula*]. A small bladder, cell or hollow structure. A skin blister—vesicular, adj.; vesiculation, n.

vesicostomy (ve-si-kos'-to-mi) [L. *vesica,* bladder; G. *stoma,* mouth]. Syn., cystostomy. **cutaneous v.,** the bladder is drained on to the anterior abdominal wall to which an ileostomy bag is attached. A tube of bladder muscle conducts urine from bladder to surface.

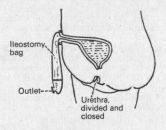

Ileostomy bag

Outlet

Urethra, divided and closed

Vesicostomy

vesicoureteric (ve-si-kō-ū-rēt-er'-ik) [L. *vesica,* bladder; G. *oureter,* ureter]. Pertaining to the urinary bladder and ureter. Vesicouretic reflux can cause pyelonephritis.

vesicovaginal (ve-si-kō-vaj-īn'-al) [L. *vesica,* bladder; *vagina,* sheath]. Pertaining to the urinary bladder and the vagina.

vesiculitis (ves-ik-ū-lī'-tis) [L. *vesicula,* vesicle; G. *-itis,* inflammation]. Inflammation of a vesicle, particularly the seminal vesicles.

vesiculopapular (ves-ik-ū-lō-pa'-pū-lar) [L. *vesicula,* vesicle; *papula,* pimple]. Pertaining to or exhibiting both vesicles and papules.

vessel (ves'-el) [L. *vascellum*]. A tube, duct or canal, holding or conveying fluid, especially blood and lymph.

vestibule (ves'-ti-būl) [L. *vestibulum,* passage]. 1. The middle part of the internal ear, lying between the semicircular canals and the cochlea. 2. The triangular area between the labia minora—vestibular, adj.

vestigial (ves-tij'-i-al) [L. *vestigium*, trace]. Rudimentary; indicating a remnant of something formerly present.

viable (vī'-a-bl). Capable of living a separate existence—viability, n.

Viacutan (vī-a-kūt'-an). Available as tulle dressing and emulsion. Promotes healing under an aseptic cover. Active against Gram-positive and Gram-negative bacteria, including Pseudomonas and Proteus. Activity enhanced rather than diminished in presence of serum, pus and tissue debris. Bacterial resistance does not occur and local sensitivity reactions are uncommon.

Vibramycin (vib-ra-mī'-sin). Doxycycline (q.v.).

vibration syndrome. Impotency and paralysis of the arm and hands in workers using vibrating machines. Syn., Raynaud's phenomenon.

Vibrio (vib'-ri-ō) [L. *vibrare*, to vibrate]. A genus of curved, motile, microorganisms. *Vibrio cholerae* or *comma* causes cholera.

vicarious (vī-kār'-i-us) [L. *vicarius*, substituted]. Substituting the function of one organ for another. **vicarious menstruation**, bleeding from the nose or other part of the body when menstruation is abnormally suppressed.

villus (vil'-us) [L. shaggy hair]. A microscopic fingerlike projection, such as found in the mucous membrane of the small intestine, or on the outside of the chorion of the embryonic sac—villi, pl.; villous, adj.

vinblastine (vin-blas'-tēn). Alkaloid from periwinkle. Antimitotic used mainly in Hodgkin's disease and choriocarcinoma resistant to other therapy. Given intravenously.

vincristine (vin-kris'-tēn). Antileukaemic drug. Derived from an extract of the periwinkle plant. Given intravenously.

Vineberg operation. For angina pectoris. Internal mammary artery dissected from chest wall and implanted with bleeding side holes into the wall of the left ventricle. Established vascular connections with the coronary circulation. First performed by Vineberg in 1950.

Vinesthene (vīn'-es-thēn). Vinyl ether (q.v.).

vinyl ether (vī'-nīl ēth'-er). An inhalation anaesthetic similar to ether, but more rapid and less sustained in effect.

Viocin (vī'-ō-sin). Viomycin (q.v.).

viomycin (vī-ō-mī'-sin). An antibiotic used in the treatment of tuberculosis when the disease is resistant to other drugs.

Vionactone (vī-on-ak'-tōn). Viomycin (q.v.).

viprynium (vip-rin'-i-um). Anthelmintic effective against threadworms. Stools become red.

viraemia (vīr-ēm'-i-ā) [L. *virus*, poison; G. *haima*, bleed]. The presence of virus in the blood. **maternal v.** can cause fetal damage—viraemic, adj.

viricidal (vī-ri-sī'-dal) [L. *virus*, poison; *caedere*, to kill]. Lethal to a virus—viricide, n.

virilism (vir'-il-izm) [L. *virilis*, manly]. The appearance of secondary male characteristics in the female.

virology (vī-rol'-o-ji) [L. *virus*, poison; G. *logos*, discourse]. The study of viruses and the diseases caused by them—virological, adj.

Virugon (vīr-ū'-gon). Antiviral drug effective in influenzal type illness.

virulence (vir'-ū-lens) [L. *virulentus*, poisonous]. Infectiousness; the disease-producing power of a micro-organism; the power of a micro-organism to overcome host resistance—virulent, adj.

virus (vī'-rus) [L.]. Very small micro-organisms parasitic within living cells. Differ from bacteria in having only one kind of nucleic acid, either DNA or RNA, in lacking the apparatus necessary for energy production and protein synthesis, and by not reproducing by binary fission but by independent synthesis of their component parts which are then assembled. Cause many kinds of acute and chronic diseases in man, can cause tumours in animals. Some of the more important groups are: (1) **poxviruses**, e.g. smallpox, molluscum contagiosum. (2) **herpesviruses**, e.g. herpes simplex v., cytomegalovirus, varicella zoster v., EB virus. (3) **adenoviruses**. (4) **papovaviruses**, e.g. polyoma virus, which can cause tumours in laboratory animals. (5) **reoviruses**, e.g. rotaviruses. (6) **togaviruses**, e.g. yellow fever v. (7) **picornaviruses**. (8) **myxoviruses**. (9) **paramyxoviruses**. (10) **rhabdoviruses**, e.g. rabies v. (11) **coronaviruses**, e.g. some common cold viruses. (12) **arenaviruses**, e.g. Lassa fever v. Groups 1–4 are DNA viruses, groups 5–12 are RNA viruses. Viruses spread by arthropods—insects and ticks—are known as arboviruses, these include reoviruses, togaviruses and rhabdoviruses.

viscera (vis'-ĕr-ȧ) [L. inner organs]. The internal organs—viscus, sing.; visceral, adj.

visceroptosis (vis-e-rop-tō'-sis) [L. *viscero*, inner organs; G. *ptosis*, a falling]. Downward displacement or falling of the abdominal organs.

viscid (vis'-kid). Sticky, glutinous.

Viscopaste (vis'-ko-pāst). A medicated bandage impregnated with Unna's paste (q.v.).

visual (viz'-ū-al) [L. *visus*, sight]. Pertaining to vision. **visual field**, the area within which objects can be seen. **visual purple**, the purple pigment in the retina of the eye. Rhodopsin.

vital capacity. The amount of air expelled from the lungs after a deep inspiration.

vitallium (vī-tal'-li-um). An alloy which can be left in the tissues in the form of nails, plates, tubes, etc.

vitamins (vī'-ta-mins) [L. *vita*, life; and 'amine']. Essential food factors, chemical in nature, present in certain foodstuffs. Some can now be synthesized commercially. Their absence causes deficiency diseases. See page 374.

vitamin E deficiency syndrome. Occurs in small infants, less than 2 kg and under 35 weeks gestation. At diagnosis between 6 and 11 weeks, low haemoglobin; there is good response to vitamin E including a rise in haemoglobin and loss of oedema.

vitiligo (vit-il-ī'-gō) [L.]. Leucoderma (q.v.).

vitreous (vit'-ri-us) [L. *vitreus*, of glass]. Resembling jelly. **vitreous chamber**, the cavity inside the eyeball. **vitreous humor**, the jelly-like substance contained in the vitreous chamber.

vocal cords. Membranous folds stretched anteroposteriorly across the larynx. Sound is produced by their vibration as air from the lungs passes between them.

volatile (vol'-a-tīl) [L. *volatilis*, flying]. Evaporating rapidly.

volition (vō-lish'-un) [L. *velle*, wish]. The will to act—volitional, adj.

Volkmann's ischaemic contracture (is-

kē'-mik). A flexion deformity of wrist and fingers from fixed contracture of the flexor muscles in the forearm. The cause is ischaemia of the muscles by injury or obstruction to the brachial artery, near the elbow. [Richard von Volkmann, German surgeon, 1830–89.]

voluntary (vol'-un-ta-ri) [L. *voluntarious*]. Under the control of the will; free and unrestricted; as opposed to reflex or involuntary.

volvulus (vol'-vū-lus) [L. *volvere*, to roll]. A twisting of a section of bowel, so as to occlude the lumen.

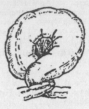

Volvulus

vomit (vom'-it) [L. *vomere*, to vomit]. Ejection of the stomach contents through the mouth; sickness.

vomiting of pregnancy. See HYPEREMESIS.

vomitus (vom'-i-tus) [L.]. Vomited matter.

von Recklinghausen's disease. Multiple neurofibromatosis of the skin. The picture is one of multiple soft tumours in the skin, their origin being the connective tissue of cutaneous nerves. Molluscum fibrosum. [Freidrich Daniel von Recklinghausen, German pathologist, 1833–1910.]

von Willebrand's disease. Bleeding disease with capillary defect, with or without AHG deficiency. [E. A. von Willebrand, Finnish physician, 19th century.]

Voss operation. Described in 1956 for relief of pain in early degenerative disease of the hip joint. Division of surrounding main muscles allows healing of articulating surfaces and increases the joint space.

vulva (vul'-vȧ) [L.]. The external genitalia of the female—vulval, adj.

vulvectomy (vul-vek'-to-mi) [L. *vulva*, covering; G. *ektome*, excision]. Excision of the vulva.

vulvitis (vul-vī'-tis) [L. *vulva*, covering; G. *-itis*, inflammation]. Inflammation of the vulva.

vulvovaginal (vul-vō-vaj-īn'-nal) [L. *vulva*, covering; *vagina*, sheath]. Pertaining to the vulva and the vagina.

vulvovaginitis (vul-vō-vaj-in-ī'-tis) [L. *vulva*, covering; *vagina*, sheath; G. *-itis*, inflammation]. Inflammation of the vulva and vagina.

vulvovaginoplasty (vul'-vō-vag'-in-ō-plas'-ti.) [L. *vulva*, covering; *vagina*, sheath; G. *plassein*, to form]. Recently devised operation for congenital absence of the vagina, or acquired disabling stenosis—vulvovaginoplastic, adj.

W

Waldeyer's ring. A lymphatic circle surrounding the pharynx. [Wihelm von Waldeyer-Hartz, German anatomist, 1836–1921.]

Wängensteen tube. Has radio-opaque tip. Used for gastrointestinal aspiration. [Owen H. Wängensteen, American surgeon, 1898–   .]

warfarin (wawr'-far-in). Oral anticoagulant. Coumarin derivative. See DICOUMAROL.

wart (wawrt) [A.S. *wearte*]. See VERRUCA.

washing soda. Sodium carbonate.

water-brash. See PYROSIS.

Waterhouse-Friderichsen syndrome. Shock with widespread skin haemorrhages occurring in meningitis, especially meningococcal. There is bleeding in the adrenal glands. [Rupert Waterhouse, British physician, 1893–1958. Carl Friderichsen, Danish physician, 1886–   ]

Waterston's operation. Anastomosis of the right pulmonary artery to the ascending aorta. Used as a palliative measure in the treatment of Fallot's tetralogy in the young child.

weal (wēl). Superficial blister, characteristic of urticaria, nettle-stings, etc.

Weil's disease (vīlz). Spirochaetosis icterohaemorrhagica. A type of jaundice with fever caused by a small spirochaete voided in the urine of rats. A disease of miners, sewer workers, etc. who work in dirty water. [Adolph Weil, German physician, 1848–1916.]

Welldorm. Dichloralphenazone (q.v.).

wen. A sebaceous cyst (q.v.).

Wertheim's hysterectomy. An extensive operation for removal of carcinoma of the cervix, where the uterus, cervix, upper vagina, tubes, ovaries and regional lymph glands are removed. [Ernst Wertheim, Austrian gynaecologist. 1864–1920.]

Wharton's jelly. A jelly-like substance contained in the umbilical cord. [Thomas Wharton, English physician, 1616–73.]

Wheelhouse's operation. External urethrotomy for impassable stricture. [Claudius Galen Wheelhouse, English surgeon, 1826–1909.]

whipworm (*Trichuris trichiura*). A roundworm which infests the intestine of man in humid tropics. Eggs are excreted in the stools. The worms do not normally produce symptoms, but heavy infestations of over 1000 worms cause bloody diarrhoea, anaemia and prolapse of the rectum. Treatment unsatisfactory but recently thiabendazole has cleared the infestation in about 50 per cent of patients treated.

Whitehead's varnish. A solution of iodoform, benzoin, storax and tolu in ether, used as an antiseptic and protective application to wounds. [Walter Whitehead, English surgeon, 1840–1913.]

white fluids. Emulsions of taracids and phenols in water, widely used for general disinfectant purposes.

white leg. See THROMBOPHLEBITIS.

'whites.' A popular term for leucorrhoea (q.v.).

White's tar paste. Zinc paste with the addition of about 6 per cent coal tar. Valuable in infantile eczema. [James C. White, American dermatologist, 1833–1916.]

Whitfield's ointment. An antifungal preparation containing salicylic and benzoic acids. [Arthur Whitfield, English dermatologist, 1867–1947.]

whitlow (wit'-low). Paronychia (q.v.).

whooping-cough. Pertussis (q.v.).

widow's itch. Pruritus (q.v.) and secondary skin eruptions occurring shortly after bereavement.

Wilms' tumour. A congenital, highly malignant, kidney tumour. [Max Wilms, German surgeon, 1867–1918.]

Wilson's disease. Hepaticolenticular degeneration with choreic movements. Due to disturbance of copper metabolism. No urinary catecholamine excretion. Associated with mental subnormality. Can be treated with BAL and penicillamine. Asymptomatic relatives can be given prophylactic penicillamine. [Sir William J. E. Wilson, English dermatologist, 1809–84.]

windpipe. The trachea (q.v.).

wintergreen, oil of. Methyl salicylate (q.v.).

winter vomiting disease. Caused by a ubiquitous, yet still unidentified virus. Syndrome simulates food poisoning.

witch-hazel. See HAMAMELIDIS.

womb (woom). The uterus (q.v.).

Wood's glass (or light). Special glass (or light) used for the detection of ringworm. Hailed as 'God's gift to dermatologists'. [Robert W. Wood, American physicist, 1868–1955.]

woolsorter's disease. Anthrax (q.v.).

worms. See ASCARIDES, TAENIA and TRICHURIS.

Woulfe's bottle. A special bottle for washing gases. [Peter Woulfe, British chemist, 1727–1803.]

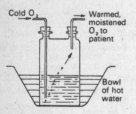

Woulfe's bottle

wrist (rist) [A.S. *writham*, to twist]. The carpus (q.v.).

wryneck (rī′-nek). See TORTICOLLIS.

Wyovin (wī′-ō-vin). Dicyclomine (q.v.).

X

xanthelasma (zan-thel-az′-ma) [G. *xanthos*, yellow; *elasma*, metal plate]. A variety of xanthoma. **xanthelasma palpebrarum**, small yellowish plaques appear on the eyelids.

xanthine (zan′-thin). Dioxypurine found in liver, muscle, pancreas and urine. Some derivatives are diuretic. Present in some renal calculi.

xanthoma (zan-thō′-má). A collection of cholesterol under the skin producing a

yellow discolouration—xanthomata, pl.

xenon (zē′-non). A rare gas that is chemically inert, but which can induce general anaesthesia.

Xenopsylla (zen-op-sil′-á). A genus of fleas. *Xenopsylla cheopis* is the rat flea that transmits bubonic plague.

xeroderma (zē-rō-děr′-má). [G. *xeros*, dry; *derma*, skin]. Also **xerodermia**. Dryness of the skin. See ICHTHYOSIS. **xerodermia pigmentosum**, Kaposi's disease, is a familial dermatosis probably caused by photosensitization. Pathological freckle formation (ephelides) may give rise to keratosis, neoplastic growth and a fatal termination.[Moritz Kaposi, Hungarian dermatologist, 1837–1902.]

xerophthalmia (zē-rof-thal′-mi-á). Dryness and ulceration of the cornea which may lead to blindness. Associated with lack of vitamin A.

xerosis (zē-rō′-sis) [G. *xeros*, dry; *-osis*, condition]. Dryness. **xerosis conjunctivae**, see BITOT'S SPOTS.

Xerostomia (zē-ros-tō′-mi-á) [G. *xeros*, dry; *stoma*, mouth]. Dry mouth.

X-rays. Short rays of electromagnetic spectrum.

xylene (zī-lēn). A clear inflammable liquid resembling benzene. Has been used as an ointment in pediculosis.

xylocaine (zī′-lō-kān). Lignocaine (q.v.).

xylol (zī′-lol). Xylene (q.v.).

xylotox (zī′-lō-toks). Lignocaine (q.v.).

XYY syndrome. Syn., Klinefelter's syndrome (q.v.).

Y

yaws. A tropical disease which resembles syphilis so closely that they may be one and the same disease but modified by differences of climate, social habit and hygiene. Pinta (S. America) and bejel (Transjordan) may be similar variants. All these diseases are caused by an identical spirochaete and produce a positive Wassermann test in the blood. Syphilis, alone, is a venereal disease. The general term for the group is 'treponematosis'.

yeast (yēst) Saccharomyces. A unicellular fungus which will cause fermentation and which reproduces by budding only. Said to be rich in vitamin B complex.

yellow fever. Acute febrile illness of tropical areas, caused by a group B arbovirus and spread by a mosquito (*Aedes aegypti*). Characteristic features are jaundice, black vomit and anuria. An attenuated virus variant known as 17D is prepared as vaccine for immunization.

Yersinia (yer-sin′-i-á). Current name for Pasteurella.

Yomesan (yom′-ē-san). Niclosamide (q.v.).

yttrium 90 (^{90}Y). A substance emitting beta particles with a half-life of 64 hours. Implantations of this in bone wax are left in the pituitary fossa after hypophysectomy for breast cancer.

Z

Zactirin. Ethoheptazine (q.v.).

Zarontin (zar′-on-tin). Ethosuximide (q.v.).

Zinamide (zin′-á-mīd). Pyrazinamide (q.v.).

zinc oxide (zingk oks′-īd). A widely used mild astringent, present in calamine lotion and cream, Lassar's paste, Unna's paste and many other dermatological applications.

zinc peroxide (zingk per-oks′-īd). A white powder with an antiseptic action similar to that of hydrogen peroxide, but much slower and prolonged in action. Used as ointment, lotion and mouthwash.

zinc stearate (zingk stē′-ar-āt). A mild astringent used as a dusting powder in eczematous conditions.

zinc sulphate (zingk sul′-fāt). A constituent of red lotion (q.v.) and other stimulating lotions for the treatment of ulcers. Occasionally used as an emetic.

zingiber (zin′-jib-er). Ginger.

Zollinger-Ellison syndrome. Ulcerogenic tumour of the pancreatic islets of Langerhans, hypersecretion of gastric acid, fulminating ulceration of oesophagus, stomach, duodenum and jejunum. Frequently accompanied by diarrhoea. Diagnosed by peroral biopsy. [Robert M. Sollinger, American surgeon, 1903– . E. H. Ellison, American physician.]

zona (zo′-ná) [G. *zone*, belt]. A zone; a girdle; herpes zoster. **zone pellucida**, the vitelline membrane surrounding the ovum.

zonula ciliaris (zōn′-ū-lá si-li-ar′-is). Suspensory ligament attaching periphery of lens of eye to ciliary body (q.v.).

zonule (zon′-ūl). Small zone, belt or girdle. Zonula.

zonulolysis (zōn-ūl′-ol-is-is) [L. *zone*, belt; G. *lysis*, a loosening]. Breaking down the zonula ciliaris—sometimes necessary before intracapsular extraction of the lens—zonulolytic, adj.

zoonosis (zō-on-ō′-sis) [G. *zoon*, animal; -*osis*, condition]. Disease in man transmitted from animal. Abbattoir and farm workers at risk—zoonoses, pl.

zygoma (zi-gō′-má) The cheekbone—zygomatic, adj.

zygote (zī′-gōt) [G. *zygon*, yoke]. The fertilized ovum.

Zyloric (zī-lor′-ik). Allopurinal (q.v.).

zymogen (zī′-mō-jen). The granular precursor, within the secretory cell, of enzymes.

Appendix

Prefixes which can be used as combining forms in compounded words

Prefix	Meaning	Prefix	Meaning
a-	without, not	cephal-	head
ab-	away from	cerebro-	brain
abdo-	} abdominal	cervico-	cervix
abdomino-		cheil-	lip
acro-	extremity	cervico-	cervix
ad-	towards	cheil-	lip
adeno-	glandular	cheir-	hand
amb-	} both, on both sides	chemo-	chemical
ambi-		chol-	bile
amido-	NH$_2$ group united to an acid radical	cholecysto-	gall bladder
		choledocho-	common bile duct
amino-	NH$_2$ group united to a radical other than an acid radical	chondro-	cartilage
		chrom-	colour
		cine-	film
amphi-	on both sides, around	circum-	around
amyl-	starch	co-	} together
an-	not, without	con-	
andro-	male	coli-	bowel
angi-	vessel (blood)	colpo-	vagina
aniso-	unequal	contra-	against
ant-	} against, counteracting	costo-	rib
anti-		crani-	} skull
ante-	} before	cranio-	
antero-		crypt-	hidden
antro-	antrum	cysto-	bladder
aorto-	aorta	cyto-	cell
arthro-	joint		
auto-	self	dacryo-	tear
		dactyl-	finger
bi-	twice, two	de-	away, from, reversing
bili-	bile	deca-	ten
bio-	life	deci-	tenth
blenno-	mucus	demi-	half
bleph-	eyelid	dent-	tooth
brachio-	arm	derma-	} skin
brady-	slow	dermat-	
broncho-	bronchi	dextro-	to the right
		dip-	double
cardio-	heart	dis-	separation, against
carpo-	wrist	dorso-	dorsal
cata-	down	dys-	difficult, painful, abnormal
centi-	a hundredth		

Prefix	Meaning	Prefix	Meaning
ecto-	outside, without, external	iatro-	physician
		idio-	peculiar to the individual
electro-	electricity	ileo-	ileum
em-	in	ilio-	ilium
en-		immuno-	immunity
end-	in, into, within	in-	not, in, into, within
endo-		infra-	below
ent-	within	inter-	between
entero-	intestine	intra-	within
epi-	on, above, upon	intro-	inward
ery-	red	ischio-	ischium
eu-	well, normal	iso-	equal
ex-	away from, out, out of	karyo-	nucleus
exo-		kerato-	horn, skin, cornea
extra-	outside	kypho-	rounded, humped
ferri-	iron	lact-	milk
ferro-		laparo-	flank
fibro-	fibre, fibrous tissue	laryngo-	larynx
flav-	yellow	lepto-	thin, soft
feto-	fetus	leuco-	white
fore-	before, in front of	leuko-	
		lympho-	lymphatic
gala-	milk		
gastro-	stomach	macro-	large
genito-	genitals, reproductive	mal-	abnormal, poor
glosso-	tongue	medi-	middle
glyco-	sugar	mega-	large
gnatho-	jaw	melano-	pigment, dark
		meso-	middle
haema-	blood	meta-	between
haemo-		metro-	uterus
hemi-	half	micro-	small
hepa-		milli-	a thousandth
hepatico-	liver	mio-	smaller
hepato-		mono-	one, single
hetero-	unlikeness, dissimilarity	muco-	mucus
hexa-	six	multi-	many
histo-	tissue	myc-	fungus
homeo-	like	myelo-	spinal cord, bone marrow
homo-	same	myo-	muscle
hydro-	water		
hygro-	moisture	narco-	stupor
hyper-	above	neo-	new
hypo-	below	nephro-	kidney
hystero-	uterus	neuro-	nerve

Prefix	Meaning	Prefix	Meaning
noct-	night	proto-	first
normo-	normal	pseudo-	false
nucleo-	nucleus	psycho-	mind
nyc-	night	pyelo-	pelvis of the kidney
		pyo-	pus
oculo-	eye	pyr-	fever
odonto-	tooth		
oligo-	deficiency, diminution	quadri-	four
onycho-	nail		
oo-	egg, ovum	radio-	radiation
oophor-	ovary	re-	again, back
ophthalmo-	eye	ren-	kidney
opisth-	backward	retro-	backward
orchido-	testis	rhin-	nose
oro-	mouth		
ortho-	straight	sacchar-	sugar
os-	bone, mouth	sacro-	sacrum
osteo-	bone	salpingo-	Fallopian tube
oto-	ear	sapro-	dead, decaying
ovari-	ovary	sarco-	flesh
		sclero-	hard
pachy-	thick	scota	darkness
pan-	all	semi-	half
para-	beside	sero-	serum
patho-	disease	socio-	sociology
ped-	child, foot	spleno-	spleen
penta- ⎫	five	steato-	fat
pento- ⎭		sterno-	sternum
per-	by, through	sub-	below
peri-	around	supra-	above
perineo-	perineum	syn-	together, union, with
pharyngo-	pharynx		
phlebo-	vein	tabo-	tabes
phono-	voice	tachy-	fast
photo-	light	tarso-	foot, edge of eyelid
phren-	diaphragm, mind	teno-	tendon
pleuro-	pleura	tetra-	four
pluri-	many	thermo-	heat
pneumo-	lung	thoraco-	thorax
podo-	foot	thrombo-	blood clot
polio-	grey	thyro-	thyroid gland
poly-	many, much	tibio-	tibia
post-	after	tox-	poison
pre- ⎫	before	tracheo-	trachea
pro- ⎭		trans-	across, through
proct-	anus	tri-	three

Prefix	Meaning	Prefix	Meaning
trich-	hair	vaso-	vessel
tropho-	nourishment	veno-	vein
		vesico-	bladder
ultra-	beyond		
uni-	one		
uretero-	ureter	xanth-	yellow
urethro-	urethra	xero-	dry
uro-	urine, urinary organs	xiphi-	} ensiform cartilage of
utero-	uterus	xipho-	sternum

Suffixes which can be used as combining forms in compounded words

Suffix	Meaning	Suffix	Meaning
-able	able to, capable of	-iatric	practice of healing
-aemia	blood	-itis	inflammation of
-aesthesia	sensibility, sense-percept		
-agra	attack, severe pain	-kinesis	motion
-al	characterized by, pertaining to	-lith	calculus, stone
-algia	pain	-lithiasis	presence of stones
-an	belonging to, pertaining to	-logy	science of, study of
		-lysis (lytic)	breaking down, disintegration
-ase	catalyst, enzyme, ferment		
		-malacia	softening
-blast	cell	-megaly	enlargement
		-meter	measure
-caval	pertaining to venae cavae		
-cele	tumour, swelling	-ogen	precursor
-centesis	to puncture	-oid	likeness, resemblance
-cide	destructive, killing	-ol	alcohol
-clysis	infusion, injection	-ology	the study of
-coccus	spherical cell	-oma	tumour
-cule	little	-opia	eye
-cyte	cell	-ose	sugar
		-osis	condition, disease, excess
-derm	skin	-ostomy	to form an opening or outlet
-desis	to bind together		
-dynia	pain	-otomy	incision of
		-ous	like, having the nature of
-ectasis	dilation, extension		
-ectomy	removal of	-pathy	disease
		-penia	lack of
-form	having the form of	-pexy	fixation
-fuge	expelling	-phage	ingesting
		-phagia	swallowing
-genesis	formation, origin	-phasia	speech
-genetic		-philia	affinity for, loving
-genic	capable of causing	-phobia	fear
-gogue	increasing flow	-phylaxis	protection
-gram	a tracing	-plasty	reconstructive surgery
-graph	description, treatise, writing	-plegia	paralysis
		-pnoea	breathing
		-poiesis	making
-iasis	condition of, state	-ptosis	falling

Suffix	Meaning	Suffix	Meaning
-rhage	to burst forth	-stasis	stagnation, cessation of movement
-rhaphy	suturing		
-rhoea	excessive discharge	-sthenia	strength
-rhythmia	rhythm	-stomy	to form an opening or outlet
-saccharide	basic carbohydrate molecule	-taxia	arrangement, co-ordination, order
-scope	instrument for visual examination	-taxis	
		-taxy	
-scopy	to examine visually	-tome	cutting instrument
-somatic	pertaining to the body	-tomy	incision of
-somy	pertaining to chromosomes	-trophy	nourishment
-sonic	sound	-uria	urine

Poisoning: some common causes, symptoms and treatment

In all cases of poisoning, certain general principles should be followed. It is a common misconception that for each poison there is a specific antidote. In practice, a true pharmacological antagonist is available in only 2.0 per cent of poisonings. In the great majority of instances, therefore, the treatment consists primarily in the application of basic principles of supportive treatment. If the poison is a gas, or the vapour of a volatile liquid, the patient must be removed at once to fresh air and given oxygen and artificial respiration if needed. Subsequent treatment is supportive to maintain vital functions. If the poison has been ingested in most cases it is necessary to remove as much as possible of the unabsorbed substance from the stomach. Outside hospital this is best achieved by pharyngeal irritation using the finger or a blunt spoon handle. In hospital, gastric aspiration and lavage should be given provided the patient retains an adequate cough and gag reflex, or is sufficiently unconscious to allow the introduction of a cuffed endotracheal tube to protect the airway. These procedures should only be performed with the patient lying on his side with the head dependent. An adequate size of tube must be used, e.g. in an adult 30 English gauge, and 300 ml quantities of lukewarm water should be used for lavage until the recovered fluid runs clear. As a general rule nothing should be left in the stomach after lavage for fear of subsequent vomiting and pulmonary aspiration. Emetic drugs have been enthusiastically recommended to avoid the use of gastric aspiration and lavage. Apomorphine may cause prolonged vomiting which may result in shock and should not be used. Copper salts have been advised as an emetic in children but are uncertain in their effects, slow in action, and as significant absorption may result in toxicity are best avoided. Syrup of ipecacuanha is quite widely used in a dose of 15 ml followed by 200 ml of water, and provided its limitations are recognized is the treatment of choice in children. The onset of its emetic effect is usually delayed for about 18 min and occasionally it may produce undesirable toxic effects after absorption.

Common errors in treatment

1. *Analeptic Therapy.* Bemegride is not a specific barbiturate antagonist and its use in poisonings due to hypnotic drugs is associated with frequent serious side effects including cardiac arrhythmias, convulsions and even irreversible brain damage. The use of analeptics cannot be justified.

2. *Bladder Catheterization.* This highly dangerous procedure is seldom necessary even in deeply unconscious patients. With adequate nursing care, there should be no undue risk of skin breakdown due to incontinence of urine. Bladder catheterization is justified in prolonged bladder distension and occasionally when forced diuresis therapy is being given.

3. *Prophylactic Antibiotics.* With good nursing care, including frequent turning of the patient and careful attention to mouth hygiene prophylactic administration of antibiotics is unnecessary. These drugs should be given only when there is clear clinical or X-ray evidence of infection.

334

Substance	Clinical Features	Treatment
Acids Strong hydrochloric acid. Spirits of salts. Strong sulphuric acid (oil of vitriol). Strong nitric acid. (See separate heading for oxalic acid) **Alkalis** Caustic soda (sodium hydroxide). Caustic potash (potassium hydroxide). Strong ammonia	Severe burning of mouth and throat, causing dyspnoea due to oedema of glottis. Severe abdominal pains, thirst, shock, dark and bloodstained vomit, gastroenteritis	Plenty of water to dilute the poison. *Acids:* Neutralize with cream of magnesia or calcium hydroxide (56 g to ½ litre of warm water). Carbonates, as chalk, sodium bicarbonate and washing soda also effective, but cause liberation of carbon dioxide. Soap can be used if no other alkali available. *Alkalis:* Neutralize with acetic acid (56 g to ½ litre), or vinegar (112 g to ½ litre); lemon juice also effective, if available in sufficient quantity. General measures include morphine for pain, and arachis or olive oil as demulcent.
Amphetamine and related substances	Alertness, tremor, confusion, delirium, hallucinations, panic attacks, lethargy, exhaustion, headache, sweating, cardiac arrhythmias, hypertension or hypotension, dryness of mouth, diarrhoea and abdominal colic, ulcers of the lips in addicts, convulsions and deep unconsciousness	Gastric aspiration and lavage. If markedly excited chlorpromazine i.m. is the most effective treatment. Intensive supportive therapy. Forced acid diuresis

Anticoagulants Phenindione Warfarin Rodenticides	Haematuria, haemoptysis, bruising and haematemesis; occasionally bleeding elsewhere. Orange yellow urine. Prolonged prothrombin time	Gastric aspiration and lavage. Vit. K, 25 mg i.v. Blood transfusion if necessary
Antidepressants Amitriptyline Imipramine Nortriptyline Desipramine Trimipramine Doxepin Protriptyline	Dryness of the mouth, dilated pupils, tachycardia leading to bizarre cardiac arrhythrias, hypotension, cardiac failure or arrest, urinary retention, varying degrees of unconsciousness, pressure of speech, increased limb reflexes, convulsions, torticollis and ataxia. Respiratory failure. Cardiac complications are common and particularly dangerous in children	Gastric aspiration and lavage. Intensive supportive therapy. In the majority of patients these measures are all that are necessary. The central nervous system effects and some of the cardiac abnormalities can be abolished by the slow i.v. injection of physostigmine salicylate 1–3 mg, which may be repeated once after 10 min. If ineffective, convulsions may be controlled by diazepam 10 mg i.v. or sodium phenobarbitone 300 mg i.m. β-Adrenergic blocking drugs may correct difficult cardiac arrhythmias
Antihistamines	In adults, toxic doses cause deep central depression. In children and infants, the effect is often stimulatory, and confusion and convulsions may result. Hypotension, tachycardia and occasionally cardiac arrhythmias. Respiratory depression. Dryness of the mouth, nausea and constipation. Hyperpyrexia. Agranulocytosis and aplastic anaemia may develop	Intensive supportive therapy. Gastric aspiration and lavage. Sedation may be required in the form of diazepam or sodium phenobarbitone i.m. Antibiotics, steroid drugs and blood tranfusion may be necessary in severe blood dyscrasia

336

Substance	Clinical Features	Treatment
Atropine Belladonna Scopolamine Homatropine Propantheline Deadly Nightshade	Blurring of vision, ataxia, mental confusion, hallucinations. Tachycardia, hypertension, cardiac arrhythmias. Dryness and burning of the mouth with marked thirst, nausea and vomiting. Urinary urgency and possible acute retention. Hyperpyrexia. Death usually results from respiratory failure	Intensive supportive therapy. Gastric aspiration and lavage. Peripheral effects may be relieved by subcutaneous injection of neostigmine 0.25 mg. When central nervous stimulation is marked, sedation with a short-acting barbiturate or diazepam may be necessary. Physostigmine salicylate (1–4 mg) i.m. or i.v. will rapidly antagonize the central nervous complications, but repeat doses may be required every 1 to 2 hours.
Barbiturates *Long-acting:* Barbitone Phenobarbitone *Medium-acting:* Allobarbitone Butobarbitone Amylobarbitone *Short-acting:* Pentobarbitone Cyclobarbitone Quinalbarbitone *Ultra-short-acting:* Hexobarbitone Thiopentone	Impaired level of consciousness. Limb reflexes very variable. Withdrawal fits and delirium during the phase of recovery occur in patients habituated to the drug. Cardiovascular depression with hypotension and 'shock'. Respiratory depression. Hypothermia. Renal failure. Bullous lesions occur in 6 per cent of patients with this condition	Intensive supportive therapy. Gastric aspiration and lavage. Forced osmotic alkaline diuresis and/or haemodialysis are of value in patients severely poisoned with long-acting barbiturates but are less effective with the other types

Benzodiazepins	Physical dependence may occur when the drug has been taken for some time. Also an additive effect occurs when taken in combination with alcohol, barbiturate, phenothiazine, monoamine oxidase inhibitors and imipramine. Loss of consciousness, bradycardia and hypotension. Respiratory depression	Intensive supportive therapy. Gastric aspiration and lavage
Bleaches (a) Containing sodium hypochlorite	If inhaled: Cough and pulmonary oedema. If ingested: Irritation of the mouth and pharynx; oedema of pharynx and larynx. Nausea and vomiting	Gastric aspiration and lavage using 2.5 per cent sodium thiosulphate (if not available milk or milk of magnesia). If severely ill sodium thiosulphate (1 per cent) 250 ml i.v.
(b) Containing oxalic acid	Irritation of the mouth and throat. Nausea and vomiting. Muscular twitchings and convulsions. Shock and cardiac arrest. Acute renal failure the onset of which may be delayed	Intensive supportive therapy. Gastric aspiration and lavage adding 10 g calcium lactate to the lavage fluid. Calcium gluconate 10 per cent 10 ml i.v. and repeat as necessary. Provided the renal output is adequate at least 5 litres of fluid should be given for three days
Carbamates Meprobamate Ethinamate Methylpentynol	Impairment of consciousness, muscle weakness and incoordination, nystagmus. Respiratory depression. Hypotension. Hypothermia. Withdrawal fits may occur	Intensive supportive therapy. Gastric aspiration and lavage. Forced osmotic alkaline diuresis in severely poisoned patients and, if ineffective, haemodialysis

Substance	Clinical Features	Treatment
Carbon monoxide and coal gas	Vertigo and ataxia: acute agitation and confusion; deep coma may develop. Papilloedema, increased limb reflexes and possibly extensor plantar responses. Acute myocardial infarction, tachycardia, arrhythmias and hypotension. Respiratory stimulation, which may progress to respiratory failure. Nausea, vomiting, haematemesis and faecal incontinence are common. Bullous lesions may occur. Sequelae include Parkinsonism, hemiparesis and impairment of higher intellectual function	Urgent. Remove from exposure. Intensive supportive therapy. Give a mixture of 95 per cent O_2 and 5 per cent CO_2. In the presence of cerebral oedema 500 ml of 20 per cent mannitol i.v. over 15 min followed by 500 ml 5 per cent dextrose over the next 4 hours
Chlorate salts	Nausea, vomiting, colic and diarrhoea. Jaundice and hepatic failure. Methaemoglobinaemia. Oliguria or anuria. Initial confusion followed by convulsions and coma	Intensive supportive therapy. Gastric aspiration and lavage. If cyanosis severe, methylene blue 25 ml of 1 per cent solution, slowly intravenously. Forced diuresis and/or haemodialysis in severe poisoning. Conventional treatment for hepatic or renal failure.
Contraceptive pills	Mild nausea or vomiting. Withdrawal bleeding in girls may occur	Intensive supportive therapy. Gastric aspiration and lavage

Cresol Phenol Lysol	Strong smell of carbolic acid in patient's breath or vomit. Corrosion of lips and buccal mucosa but little pain. Marked abdominal pain, nausea and vomiting. Haematemesis or gastric perforation. After absorption, initial excitement then impaired consciousness. Hypotension. Dark urine, oliguria and renal failure. Liver failure may occur. Respiratory failure is a common cause of death	Intensive supportive therapy. Gastric aspiration and lavage with care. Wash ulcers with copious water or 50 per cent alcohol. Medical measures for hepatic and renal failure. Haemodialysis may be required
Cyanide	Very toxic. *Mild poisoning:* Headache, dyspnoea, vomiting, ataxia and loss of consciousness occur gradually. *Severe poisoning:* The above features develop very rapidly and the patient becomes deeply unconscious. The smell of bitter almonds is not necessarily present. The skin remains pink unless breathing has ceased. Rapid, thready pulse	Speed is essential. As long as the heart sounds are audible, recovery may be anticipated with appropriate treatment. Four forms of treatment are available: (1) If the poisoning is due to inhalation, remove from contaminated atmosphere. (2) Break an ampoule of amyl nitrite under the patient's nose whilst applying artificial respiration where this is necessary. Also inject 10 ml 3 per cent sodium nitrite intravenously. (3) Very slow infusion of 25 ml 50 per cent sodium thiosulphate. (4) If the poison has been ingested, gastric aspiration and lavage should also be done and 300 ml 25 per cent *(contd. overleaf)*

Substance	Clinical Features	Treatment
Cyanide (contd.)	Hypotension. Limb reflexes are often absent and the pupils are dilated	sodium thiosulphate should be left in the stomach. An emergency kit containing the above solution is commercially available and should be part of the equipment of all Casualty Departments. An alternative to nitrite treatment is the use of Kelocyanor (cobalt edetate). Many consider this to be the treatment of choice. Initially 40 ml (600 mg) is given i.v. over 1 min. Hypotension and nausea may be produced but recovery usually is very rapid. If this does not occur within 1 to 2 min a further 20 ml (300 mg) is given i.v. immediately followed by 50 ml 5 per cent dextrose i.v.
Detergents	Nausea, vomiting and diarrhoea. Most are not very toxic	Supportive therapy
Digitalis	Nausea and vomiting, diarrhoea. Bradycardia. Cardiac arrhythmias. Mental confusion	Intensive supportive therapy. Gastric aspiration and lavage. Potassium chloride 1.0 g orally every 20 min; if vomiting occurs 1 g in 200 ml 5 per cent dextrose infused over 30 min. Lignocaine 500 mg in 500 ml saline/dextrose i.v. administered at a rate depending on the clinical

		response is the best treatment for ventricular ectopics. Atropine sulphate 0.6 mg i.m. repeated as necessary for bradycardia. Cardiac pacing may occasionally be required
Glutethimide	Similar to barbiturate poisoning, but depth of coma may vary considerably. Sudden apnoea may occur, probably due to sudden raised intracranial pressure. Pupils dilated and unresponsive to light. Hypotension may be severe. Myocardial infarction may occur	Intensive supportive therapy. Gastric aspiration and lavage. If there is any suspicion of raised intracranial pressure give 500 ml 20 per cent mannitol i.v. over 20 min followed by 500 ml 5 per cent dextrose over next 4 hours
Iron salts	*Stage 1.* Epigastric pain, nausea and vomiting. Haematemesis. Tachypnoea and tachycardia. *Stage 2.* An interval of hours or even several days may elapse during which there are no further signs and symptoms. Then severe headache, confusion, delirium, convulsions and loss of consciousness. Respiratory and circulatory failure. *Stage 3.* If patient survives, liver failure and renal failure may occur	Intensive supportive therapy. Gastric aspiration and lavage with cesferrioxamine 2 g in 1 litre of water. Afterwards 10 g desferrioxamine should be left in the stomach. Immediately inject desferrioxamine 15 mg/kg per hour to a maximum dose of 80 mg/kg per 24 hours Medical measures for hepatic and renal failure may be necessary

Substance	Clinical Features	Treatment
Laburnum	Burning in mouth, nausea, intractable vomiting, diarrhoea, exhaustion and collapse. Delirium, convulsions and coma	Intensive supportive therapy. Gastric aspiration and lavage
Lead	Severe abdominal pain, vomiting, diarrhoea, oliguria, collapse, coma. 'Shock' and hepatic failure may occur. Acute haemolytic anaemia	Intensive supportive therapy. Gastric aspiration and lavage. When colic is severe calcium gluconate (10 per cent) 10 ml i.v. Calcium disodium versenate (Versene) 75 mg per kg body weight i.v. in 24 hours plus BAL 24 mg per kg in 24 hours. This regimen should be continued for 3 to 5 days. Peritoneal or haemodialysis in severe poisoning
Methyl alcohol Methanol Wood alcohol	Headache, blurring of vision which may lead to blindness, dilatation of pupils and papilloedema, loss of consciousness. Nausea and vomiting Hyperventilation	Intensive supportive therapy. Gastric aspiration and lavage. Ethylalcohol 50 per cent 1 ml per kg stat. then 0.5 ml per kg every 2 hours. If impaired vision, peritoneal dialysis or haemodialysis is essential
Methaqualone	Hypertonia, myoclonia, extensor plantar responses, papilloedema and impairment of level of consciousness. Tachycardia, acute myocardial infarction. Respiratory depression. Bleeding tendencies may occur	Intensive supportive therapy. Gastric aspiration and lavage. Haemodialysis in severe poisoning

Opium alkaloids Diamorphine Morphine Pethidine Codeine Dipipanone Pentazocine Propoxyphene	Impaired level of consciousness; pinpoint pupils. Convulsions may occur particularly in young children. Respiratory and circulatory depression. Methaemoglobinaemia may occur	A true antidote is available. Intensive supportive therapy. Gastric aspiration and lavage. Naloxone 0.4 mg i.v. and 0.8 mg repeated i.v. 3 min later is usually sufficient to re-establish normal respiration and conscious level
Organophosphorous compounds	These insecticides are very toxic. Headache, restlessness, ataxia, muscle weakness, convulsions. Salivation, nausea, vomiting, colic and diarrhoea. Bradycardia, hypotension, peripheral circulatory failure. Bronchospasm, cyanosis, acute pulmonary oedema. Respiratory failure is the usual cause of death	Intensive supportive therapy. Gastric aspiration and lavage if ingested. As soon as cyanosis is corrected, atropine sulphate 2 mg i.v. and repeated at 15-min intervals until fully atropinized. Pralidoxime 30 mg per kg i.v. slowly and repeat half-hourly as necessary. If sedation or control of convulsions is required, short-acting barbiturates may be used but with the greatest caution
Paracetamol	Pallor, nausea and sweating. Hypotension, tachycardia and other cardiac arrhythmias Excitement and delirium progressing to CNS depression and stupor. Hypothermia, hypoglycaemia and metabolic acidosis. Tachypnoea. Haemolysis. Renal failure. Jaundice and hepatic failure, which is the commonest mode of death. Severity of poisoning best assessed	Intensive supportive therapy. If the plasma paracetamol half-life is greater than 4 hours cysteamine hydrochloride 2.0 g i.v. over 10 min followed by three 400 mg doses in 500 ml of 5 per cent dextrose i.v. over 4, 6 and 8 hours has been shown to reduce and even prevent liver damage. Intravenous infusions of sodium bicarbonate to correct acidaemia, i.v. glucose for (*contd. overleaf*)

Substance	Clinical Features	Treatment
Paracetamol (*contd.*)	on blood levels. If the plasma paracetamol level is above 2000 mmol per litre and especially if the plasma half-life is greater than 4 hours hepatic damage is likely	hypoglycaemia, and if haemolysis is severe corticosteroids and blood transfusion may be necessary. Haemodialysis may be required for renal failure
Paraquat	Burning sensation in mouth at time of ingestion. After a few hours painful buccal ulceration develops. Several days after ingestion a progressive alveolitis and bronchiolitis is probable and is the usual cause of death. Severe renal and hepatic impairment may occur	Careful gastric aspiration and lavage. If paraquat ingested within 2 hours leave 500 ml of 7 per cent bentonite suspension in stomach. Intensive supportive therapy. Immediate forced diuresis is safe before renal damage occurs
Petroleum distillates	Nausea, vomiting and diarrhoea. If inhaled or aspirated, intense pulmonary congestion and chemical pneumonitis. Depression of consciousness and respiration with occasionally convulsions	*No* gastric aspiration or lavage. 250 ml liquid paraffin orally If pneumonitis, hydrocortisone 100 mg i.m. 6-hourly for 48 hours with antibiotics as indicated. Mechanical ventilation may be necessary
Phenothiazines	Impaired level of consciousness, Parkinsonism, torticollis, oculogyric crises, restlessness and convulsions. Hypotension, tachycardia, cardiac arrhythmias. Hypothermia. Respiratory depression in severe poisoning	Intensive supportive therapy. Gastric aspiration and lavage. Convulsions should be treated with diazepam and if this fails, with barbiturates. Cogentin (benztropine mesylate) 2 mg i.v. is effective for Parkinsonism

Phenytoin	Stimulation and possibly euphoria, vertigo, headache, cerebellar ataxia, nystagmus, tremor, loss of consciousness. Nausea, and vomiting. Respiratory depression	Intensive supportive therapy. Gastric aspiration and lavage
Primidone	Similar to phenytoin but loss of consciousness tends to be more marked	Intensive supportive therapy. Gastric aspiration and lavage. Forced alkaline osmotic diuresis or haemodialysis may be necessary in severe poisoning.
Quinine and quinidine	Tinnitus; blurred vision; headache and dizziness. Impaired consciousness; rapid, shallow breathing. Tachycardia, hypotension, cardiac arrhythmias and arrest may occur. Acute haemolysis and renal failure	Intensive supportive therapy. Gastric aspiration and lavage. ECG monitoring is required and cardiac arrhythmias treated with appropriate drugs. In marked visual impairment stellate ganglion block may produce dramatic improvement. Forced acid diuresis may be of value in severe poisoning
Salicylate Acetyl salicylate Methyl salicylate Sodium salicylate	Alertness and restlessness, tinnitus, deafness. Hyperventilation. Hyperpyrexia and sweating. Nausea and vomiting. Dehydration and oliguria. Unconsciousness may occur in severe poisoning; hypoprothrombinaemia occurs in some patients. Hypokalaemia may be severe.	Gastric aspiration and lavage in all patients. Forced alkaline diuresis if the plasma salicylate is above 3.6 mmol per litre. In very severe poisoning haemodialysis. Intensive supportive therapy

346

Substance	Clinical Features	Treatment
Salicylate (*contd.*)	Metabolic acidaemia and hypoglycaemia are often marked in children	
Snake bite Adder bite (Viper berus)	Local features: Swelling, pain and redness. General features: Agitation, restlessness, abdominal colic, vomiting and diarrhoea. Collapse and respiratory failure may result	Specific antivenom should *not* be used as serious anaphylactic shock may result, unless in the severely ill patient when only the Zagreb antivenom should be given by i.v. infusion. Cleanse the site and immobilize the bitten part. Hydrocortisone 100 mg i.m. Antibiotics and tetanus antitoxin should be given. Intensive supportive therapy
Thiazides	Polyuria, dehydration, hypokalaemia, hyponatraemia, hypochloraemia and alkalaemia. Acute renal failure may occur. Also acute hepatic failure is occasionally found and in susceptible patients an acute attack of gout may result	Intensive supportive therapy. Gastric aspiration and lavage. Potassium chloride 2 g 3-hourly depending on the degree of hypokalaemia. Intravenous fluids may be necessary to correct dehydration

Further information may be obtained from various Poisons Information Centres.

Telephone numbers

Belfast 0232-30503
Cardiff 0222-33101
Dublin Dublin 45588
Edinburgh 031-229 2477
London 01-407 7600

Side-room Testing

Tests that are carried out in ward side-rooms, surgeries and other places without full laboratory facilities are mainly concerned with urine, but some quick tests are available for use on blood, serum, plasma and faeces. This section, therefore, starts with urine analysis, and has two shorter sections at the end dealing respectively with tests for glucose, ketones and urea in blood, serum or plasma, and for blood and sugars in faeces.

A. Urine testing

COLLECTION OF URINE SPECIMEN

Fresh specimens of urine should be used for all tests, because changes in the composition occur when the urine is allowed to stand, especially if it is infected. The complete specimen should be well mixed, but not centrifuged or filtered, before taking out a portion for testing.

The specimen container should be absolutely clean and free from contaminants, e.g., antiseptics or detergents, and nothing should be added to the specimen before analysis.

PHYSICAL EXAMINATION

Physical examination of the urine should include noting its quantity, colour, odour, sediment after a portion has been left to settle, and specific gravity.

Quantity. The output of urine of a normal adult over 24 hours averages between 1200 and 1500 ml, and depends on fluid intake and the amount of fluid lost from the body by routes other than the kidney, such as perspiration. The amount excreted can vary also in nervous and hysterical states, in various diseases and according to climatic conditions. Some drugs can increase or decrease the volume of urine.

Colour. The colour of normal urine is usually amber but can vary from pale straw to brown. It is caused by various pigments, primarily urochrome which is always present in normal urine. The colour may be affected by various factors in the following ways:

Greenish-orange, caused by bile
Smoky or pale reddish, caused by blood
Whitish opalescent, caused probably by pus
Very pale amber, caused by dilution as a result of polyuria
Various shades resulting from ingestion of drugs.

Odour. In certain diseases the characteristic smell of normal urine may be altered. For examples, in diabetic ketoacidosis the urine smells of acetone and in cystitis it has a fishy odour.

Sediment. A pinkish curdy deposit is caused by an excess of urates, and a white sediment usually indicates phosphates.

Specific gravity. The specific gravity (sp. gr.) of normal urine varies between 1.015 and 1.025. As a general rule, the greater the volume of urine passed the lower is its sp. gr., and where there is diminished volume of urine, as in febrile states, the sp. gr. will be higher. Occasionally, as in diabetes mellitus, there is increased volume of urine with a high sp. gr.

The sp. gr. is taken with a urinometer (hydrometer) as shown in the diagram. This is floated in the urine, care being taken to prevent it touching the side of the test glass used. The urine must be allowed to reach room temperature before its sp. gr. is read. The reading taken is the level of the bottom of the meniscus of the urine on the scale up the stem of the urinometer; it is important that this is done with at eye level with the liquid surface.

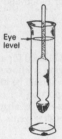

Eye level

If there is insufficient urine to float the urinometer, either use a narrower urinometer or, *after the chemical testing has been done*, dilute the urine with an equal amount of water, measure the sp. gr. of this and correct it by doubling the last two figures of the reading.

The osmolality of urine may sometimes be more informative than its sp. gr., but is less easily measured.

CHEMICAL ANALYSIS

Routine chemical analysis of urine generally includes testing for pH (acidity), protein, reducing sugars, glucose, ketones, blood, bilirubin, urobilinogen and nitrite (as an indication of infection). In some instances other tests may be required as well, and these are mentioned at the end of the section, e.g. tests for phenylketones, chlorides.

Usually it is sufficient to obtain semiquantitative or even qualitative estimates of urinary components. The older 'side-room' tests are described, and the Ames strip or tablet tests. Ames strip tests for pH, proteins, glucose, ketones, blood, bilirubin, urobilinogen and nitrite are available, singly (in most cases) or in various combinations on multiple-test strips up to N-Multistix strips, which carry all the above eight; for simplicity, the single tests will be described under the heading for each substance to be investigated. When using any Ames test it is important to follow exactly the instructions for use and for preservation of the product in good condition, and to check that the product is within its expiration date shown on the label. Instructions for the Ames tablet tests are given individually in the sections which follow; those for the strip tests are similar for all of them and can be summarized thus:

(a) Completely immerse all reagent areas of the strip in fresh, well-mixed, uncentrifuged urine and remove immediately.

(b) Tap edge of strip against the side of urine container to remove excess urine. Hold the strip in a horizontal position to prevent possible soiling of hands with urine or mixing of chemicals from adjacent reagent areas, making sure that the test areas face upwards.

(c) Compare test areas closely with corresponding colour charts on the bottle label at the times specified. Hold strip close to colour blocks and match carefully.

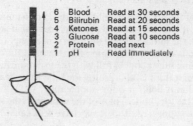

6	Blood	Read at 30 seconds
5	Bilirubin	Read at 20 seconds
4	Ketones	Read at 15 seconds
3	Glucose	Read at 10 seconds
2	Protein	Read next
1	pH	Read immediately

Regular quality control checks are now standard practice in the analysis of clinical specimens. For Ames tests this is easily done with Tek-Chek controls for routine urinalysis (also from Ames). These synthetic solutions provide positive and negative checks, and their use is recommended when a new bottle of reagents is opened and also each day, hidden among the batch of urines to be tested. The negative control gives confidence that no false positives are obtained and provides an appropriate negative reaction to make sure that comparison to the 'negative' colour blocks is being made properly. The appropriate positive control gives confidence that the reagents are reacting properly with positive specimens.

pH

Ames pH test (on Hema-Combistix, Labstix, Bili-Labstix, N-Labstix, Multistix and N-Multistix strips, but not available singly).

The Ames pH test covers the range 5–9 units and can be read to one unit. It should be read immediately after dipping the strip.

It is not affected by variations in the urinary buffer concentration, but care should be taken, by tapping the strip to remove excess urine and by holding it level while reading it, to avoid contamination from reagents from the adjacent protein test portion, which would tend to cause an underestimate of an alkaline or neutral pH.

Protein

The excess protein excreted as a result of most of the common causes of proteinuria is mainly albumin, but globulins also may be present.

1. Albustix strips (and all Ames multiple-test strips except Keto-Diastix)

This test is based on the 'protein error of indicators' principle using buffered tetrabromophenol blue, and may be read immediately. It has colour blocks marked negative, trace, 30 mg/dl (+), 100 mg/dl (++), 300 mg/dl (+++), 1000 or more mg/dl (++++), the figures referring to albumin. Its sensitivity is 5–20 mg/dl albumin. It is more sensitive to albumin than to globulin, haemoglobin, Bence-Jones protein and mucoprotein. Clinical judgement must determine the significance of 'trace' results; particularly in urines of high specific gravity, the test area may most closely match 'trace' despite only physiological concentrations of protein. Falsely positive results can be obtained from alkaline and/or highly buffered urines, or from contamination with quaternary ammonium salts.

2. Boiling test (heat plus acetic acid test)

(a) Check that the urine pH is mildly acidic (5 or 6 units) or just acidic to litmus paper; if it is not so, add 10 per cent acetic acid solution until it is. Failure to check the initial pH and adjust it if necessary can invalidate this test. If the urine is cloudy, filter some for this procedure.

(b) Fill a boiling tube about ¾ full with the urine and heat the top inch of liquid gently over a spirit lamp, turning the tube while heating to prevent it from cracking. Let it boil for a few moments.

(c) Compare the top, boiled, part of the urine with the lower part to see if any cloudiness has appeared. If so, it may have been caused by either protein or phosphates.

(d) Add 3 drops of 10 per cent acetic acid and reboil the top portion. If cloudiness persists, proteins are indicated. If cloudiness disappears, phosphates are indicated.

3. Salicylsulphonic acid test

(a) If the urine is cloudy, filter some for this test.

(b) Add 5 drops of 25 per cent salicylsulphonic acid to about 5 ml urine in a test tube.

(c) Shake the tube and look for cloudiness in the urine. Cloudiness indicates protein, and the degree of cloudiness gives some idea of the relative protein concentration.

4. Esbach test

(a) All the urine passed by the subject over a period, say 6 hours, is collected in a clean stoppered bottle and mixed. Measure its sp. gr.; if this exceeds 1.010, dilute a portion with an equal volume of water. If the urine is alkaline, acidify it with a few drops of 10 per cent acetic acid.

(b) Add urine to an Esbach tube (see diagram) to the level marked U. Add Esbach's reagent up to the level marked R. Cork the tube and invert it gently several times to mix the contents.

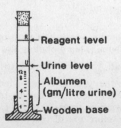

R ← Reagent level

U ← Urine level

Albumen (gm/litre urine)

Wooden base

(c) Stand the tube upright and leave it in a constant temperature for 24 hours. Then read the level of the precipitate of protein on the tube's scale, with the eye on a level with the top of the sediment. This gives the protein concentration of the urine in parts per 1000 (g/l).

Reducing sugars

Although glucose is the commonest reducing sugar found in urine, more rarely galactose, lactose, fructose, pentose and maltose may be found. Because of these possibilities, routine urine screening, especially for infants, should not rely on the enzymic tests specific for glucose but should include a test for reducing sugars.

Such tests are based on the reduction of hot alkaline copper sulphate to give cuprous oxide. They can react with other moderately strong reducing substances besides the abovementioned sugars, e.g. metabolites of aspirin, nalidixic acid, metaxalone, cephalothin and with ascorbic acid, etc. The precise composition of the reagent will determine the degree of non-specificity of various tests based on copper reduction. The result will represent the sum of the effects of whatever substances that can affect the test are present in the urine. If the urine gives a positive result for reducing sugars but a negative result to a test specific for glucose, further investigation may be needed to find what the non-glucose reducing substance is, or possibly whether the specific enzyme test for glucose has been inhibited.

1. Clinitest reagent tablets. (Caution: these tablets are caustic)

Always use the Ames test tubes and droppers provided for the test; other equipment may give incorrect results.

(a) Holding dropper upright, put 5 drops of urine into a clean dry test tube. Rinse dropper.
(b) Using the same dropper, add 10 drops of water.
(c) Drop in one Clinitest tablet. Watch the test carefully until boiling stops and for 15 seconds longer. Do not shake the tube during this period.
(d) Now shake the tube gently and compare the colour of the contents with the colour chart. If during the test a bright orange colour appears (even for a moment) and then changes to a brownish colour, more than 2 per cent sugar is present.

To estimate sugar concentrations above 2 per cent, dilute the urine being tested with normal urine (negative to Clinitest) and repeat the test. Multiply the result obtained by the dilution to give the percentage of sugar.

The sensitivity of Clinitest to glucose is about 150 mg/dl. It will react with reducing sugars, ascorbic acid, nalidixic acid, metaxalone, cephalothin, probenecid and salicylate metabolites if present in sufficient quantity, but not with uric acid, creatinine, penicillin, streptomycin, isoniazid, or chloral hydrate in the quantities in which these are likely to be found in urine; (these lists are not exhaustive).

2. Benedict's qualitative test

(a) To 5 ml of Benedict's qualitative reagent in a boiling tube add 8 drops of urine.

(b) Boil the mixture virorously for 2 minutes over a flame, or place the tube in a boiling waterbath for 5 minutes.

(c) In the presence of reducing substances the mixture will turn bluish-green, green, yellow, orange or brick red, depending on the nature and quantity of reducing substances present.

3. Benedict's quantitative test

This is a more elaborate version of the foregoing test using Benedict's quantitative reagent designed to give semiquantitative results by titration.

Glucose

Tests for glucose based on glucose oxidase involve two reactions, firstly the oxidation of glucose by atmospheric oxygen, catalysed by glucose oxidase, to gluconic acid and hydrogen peroxide, and secondly the oxidation by hydrogen peroxide, catalysed by peroxidase, of a chromogen system such as *o*-tolidine or potassium iodide. The first reaction is specific for glucose and is not given by other sugars. The second is not; positive results can be given by strong oxidizing agents such as sodium hypochlorite or bleaches containing hydrogen peroxide. The second can be inhibited by strong reducing substances which compete with the chromogen for oxygen from the hydrogen peroxide. This inhibition, e.g. from ascorbic acid, will vary with different chromogens according to the reducing power of the chromogen relative to that of the inhibitor.

It should be noted that strong reducing agents like ascorbic acid *inhibit* enzymic tests for glucose but *enhance* the results of copper reduction tests. Thus they are a common cause of discrepant results between the two types of test for glucose, the reduction test being positive and the enzymic test negative.

The enzymic tests are generally more sensitive than copper reduction tests. Thus it is possible in certain urines whose glucose concentration lies between the sensitivities of the two tests to get a positive result with the enzymic, more sensitive one and a negative with the copper reduction, less sensitive one.

1. Clinistix strips

This test uses glucose oxidase and peroxidase, with *o*-tolidine plus a red dye as its chromogen system. It is qualitative only. When the colour developed at 10 seconds resembles any of the positive colour blocks, presence of glucose is indicated. 'Light' generally indicates $\frac{1}{4}$ per cent or less. 'Dark' generally indicates $\frac{1}{2}$ per cent or more. 'Medium' indicates that glucose is present but does not denote amount. On average, the strips will detect about 0.1 per cent glucose in urine (100 mg/dl, 5.5 mmol/l).

2. Diastix strips (and glucose portions of Ames 'improved' multiple test strips)

This test uses glucose oxidase and peroxidase, with potassium iodide plus a blue dye as its chromogen system. It is less affected by strong reducing substances like ascorbic acid and by sp. gr. of the urine than is Clinistix, and so can give semiquantitative results over the range 0.1 to 2 per cent if read at 30 seconds.

Large concentrations of ketones (80 mg/dl or greater) may decrease the colour development of this glucose test. It is unlikely that the presence of ketones simultaneously with glucose in the urine is sufficient to produce false-negative glucose results. However, when the Ames ketones test shows a 'medium' or 'large' result, the amount of glucose present may be greater than the amount shown by this test, and Clinitest tablets should be used to estimate the glucose. Diastix strips should not be used when ketonuria is likely to be present; in that circumstance Keto-Diastix strips would be preferred.

The strips will detect approximately 0.1 per cent glucose in urine (100 mg/dl, 5.5 mmol/l).

Ketones

The abnormal metabolites present in the urine as a result of ketoacidosis are ß-hydroxybutyric acid, acetoacetic acid and acetone. They are related chemically by oxidation, the first being the reduced form which can be oxidized to the second and on to the third. Of these three, ß-hydroxybutyric acid is not a ketone and no test for ketones detects it or includes it in its estimate of ketones.

Ketones in urine are unstable; chilling the specimen is the best way to preserve ketones if there must be a delay before testing for them.

Tests for ketones are based either on their reaction with sodium nitroprusside to give a purple colour (Ames tests and Rothera's test) or with ferric chloride to give a deep red colour (Gerhardt's test). The colour given with sodium nitroprusside by acetoacetic acid is stronger than that by acetone; the reaction is specific for ketones. Ferric chloride does not react with acetone, but can give reddish colours with several chemicals other than acetoacetic acid, and other colours with various other substances.

1. Ketostix strips (and ketones portions of Keto-Diastix, Labstix, Bili-Labstix, N-Labstix, Multistix and N-Multistix strips)

The reagent portion of Ketostix is impregnated with sodium nitroprusside, glycine and buffers.

This test reacts with acetoacetic acid and acetone but not ß-hydroxybutyric acid. It should be read at 15 seconds. It detects 5 to 10 mg acetoacetate per dl of urine (0.5 to 1 mmol/l), and is less sensitive to acetone. The results may be interpreted as small, moderate or large. Colours which are sufficiently similar to that produced by ketones can be confusing and may be obtained from urine specimens containing bromosulphthalein or large amounts of phenylketones or metabolites of L-dopa.

2. Acetest reagent tablets

Acetest tablets contain sodium nitroprusside, glycine and buffers.

(a) Place an Acetest tablet on clean, dry, white paper.
(b) Put 1 drop of urine on the tablet.
(c) Compare colour of the tablet with the colour chart exactly 30 seconds later.

This test resembles Ketostix strips in chemistry, sensitivity and specificity.

3. Rothera's test

(a) Saturate a portion of urine with ammonium sulphate by shaking about 5 ml of urine in a test tube with about the same volume of crystals of this salt.
(b) Add 10 drops of a freshly prepared 2 per cent solution of sodium nitroprusside.
(c) Add 10 drops of strong ammonia solution (sp. gr. 0.880).
(d) Allow to stand for 15 minutes. The development of a purple colour indicates ketones.

This test is generally considered to be too sensitive, as it often gives a positive on a well subject who has not eaten for several hours.

4. Gerhardt's test

(a) Put 2 ml urine in a test tube.
(b) Add 10 per cent ferric chloride solution drop by drop. A precipitate may form if phosphates are present but will redissolve on addition of more ferric chloride.
(c) A reddish-brown colour indicates acetoacetic acid.

This test is generally considered too insensitive, as clinically significant ketonuria can be present when the test is negative.

Gerhardt's test will not react with acetone or ß-hydroxybutyric acid, but will give a similar colour to that produced by acetoacetic acid with the urinary metabolites of a number of drugs including salicylates.

Blood

Chemical tests for blood in urine are based on the peroxidase-like activity of haemoglobin, myoglobin and some of their degradation products, which can catalyse the oxidation of a chromogen system by hydrogen peroxide to give a colour. They will react with free haemoglobin and with erythrocytes, which are lysed by the reagents used in the test, but are usually a little less sensitive to the latter.

The alternative test for blood in urine is microscopy, looking for and counting the erythrocytes in a known volume, in which the sediment has been concentrated by centrifugation. This test does not detect free haemoglobin, whether excreted as such (haemoglobinuria resulting from *in vivo* haemolysis) or lysed from excreted erythrocytes in urine left to stand (haematuria followed by *in vitro* haemolysis). As it may be more sensitive to intact erythrocytes than a chemical test, the two complement each other.

Thus the presence of free haemoglobin in the absence of intact erythrocytes in the urine is a cause of a positive result from a chemical test and a negative result by microscopy. Urine for testing for blood should be stirred immediately before testing (or withdrawing a portion for testing) and microscopy should be carried out on fresh urine.

It should be noted that a negative result to a test for protein does not preclude a positive result for blood in the same urine, although haemoglobin is a protein. This is because urine normally contains up to about 5 mg per dl of protein (mainly as albumin), and a test for proteinuria must have its sensitivity adjusted to give a negative at this physiological level. Concentrations of haemoglobin that are pathological are much lower than this, about 150 μg per dl, and therefore tests for haemoglobin must give positives with concentrations of this order which would be negative to a protein test. Urine should be tested for both protein and blood, regardless of the result of either.

1. Hemastix strips (and the blood portion of Hema-Combistix, Labstix, Bili-Labstix, N-Labstix, Multistix and N-Multistix strips)

The reagent portion of Hemastix contains a peroxide, buffers and o-tolidine.

This test gives results which can be graded as 'small', 'moderate' or 'large'. Any blue spots or blue colour developing on the reagent area within 30 seconds is significant. Its sensitivity is 0.015 mg per dl for free haemoglobin, or 5–10 intact erythrocytes per μl at the time of manufacture for urines with low specific gravity and ascorbic acid concentrations of less than 5 mg per dl (0.28 mmol/l). The sensitivity may be expected to be less in urines of high specific gravity and ascorbic acid content. The test is slightly more sensitive to free haemoglobin and myoglobin that to intact erythrocytes.

Certain oxidizing contaminants such as hypochlorite may produce falsely positive results, as also may microbial peroxidase, associated with urinary tract infection.

2. Guaiac test

(a) Ensure that no flame is near when this test is carried out.

(b) Put about 5 ml of urine in a test tube and add 1 or 2 drops of freshly prepared tincture of guaiacum.

(c) Carefully overlay this with about half the volume of ozonic ether (*which is highly inflammable*).

(d) Hold the tube in the hand for a few minutes to warm it a little. The appearance of a blue line at the junction of the fluids indicates blood.

3. Microscopy

Techniques for this test vary in detail from laboratory to laboratory. Essentially, one takes a known volume of fresh well-stirred urine (usually 10 ml), centrifuges it, pours off most of the supernatant liquid and resuspends the sediment in a known volume of the liquid. A known quantity of this suspension is then put on a microscope slide, covered with a cover slip and examined under th high power of a microscope.

The number of erythrocytes visible are counted, the slide moved slightly and the erythrocytes in the new field counted. This is repeated for, say, 10 fields and the numbers averaged.

The result is commonly expressed as the number of erythrocytes 'per high-power field'. With constant use of the same technique, this gives comparative results which are meaningful within that laboratory and can be interpreted in the light of what is 'normal' for it. But results obtained from even a slightly different technique will be numerically different for the same urine and probably the 'normal' range will be different. It is only possible to compare results between different techniques and laboratories if each arbitrary unit 'per high-power field' is related to a scientific unit. e.g., 'per mm³'.

Bilirubin

Many tests for bilirubin in urine have been devised; the two main groups depend on coupling with a diazotized compound and on oxidation respectively. Diazotization methods can be specific for bilirubin, whereas oxidation methods are not and can give positive results on urine in which bilirubin was present initially but has oxidized to biliverdin on standing. Tests for bilirubin should be made on fresh urine.

1. Ictostix strips (and the bilirubin portions of Bili-Labstix, Multistix and N-Multistix strips)

This test depends on the reaction of bilirubin with diazotized dichloroaniline. It should be read at 20 seconds, and gives readings which can be graded as 'negative', 'small', 'moderate' or 'large'. Its sensitivity is 0.2–0.4 mg per dl (3.4–6.8 mmol/l) of bilirubin as assayed by the procedure of Golden and Snavely (*J. Clin. Lab. Med.* 1948, **33**, 890). This is 2 to 4 times less sensitive than Ictotest tablets (see below), which may be preferred when very small concentrations of bilirubin are sought.

The test is considered specific for bilirubin if the colour developed at 20 seconds matches one of those shown on the chart. Different colours may indicate that other bile pigments, derived from bilirubin, are present in the sample, and they may mask the reaction to bilirubin. Large doses of chlorpromazine may give rise to reactions which could be confused with those for bilirubin. Metabolites of drugs which give a colour at low pH, such as pyridium and serenium, may give a red or other colour on this test portion. If atypical colours are seen on the bilirubin test portion, the urine should be tested further (e.g. with Ictotest tablets).

2. Ictotest reagent tablets

(a) Place 5 drops of urine on one square of the absorbent test mat provided.
(b) Place an Ictotest tablet in the middle of the moist area.
(c) Flow 2 drops of water onto the tablet so that the water runs off onto the mat.
(d) Observe the colour of the *mat* around the tablet after 30 seconds. A bluish-purple colour indicates bilirubin.

Ictotest tablets employ a similar reaction to that of Ictostix strips but a different diazonium salt. The use of an absorbent mat has a chromatographic effect of concentrating the bilirubin, and so Icotest tablets are 2 to 4 times more sensitive than Ictostix strips. Because even trace amounts of bilirubin in urine are abnormal, the tablets should be preferred to the strips when seeking very low concentrations, e.g. in the earliest phase of viral hepatitis.

Urobilinogen

Urobilnogen is even less stable than bilirubin in urine which has been left to stand; it oxidizes to urobilin, which does not react with some tests for urobilinogen, i.e. those based on p-dimethylaminobenzaldehyde, such as Ames Urobilistix and most of the laboratory methods. Another test (Schlesinger's), however, first oxidizes urobilinogen to urobilin and then estimates the latter by its ability to produce a fluorescent compound with a zinc salt. This would give a positive even after urobilinogen initially present had disappeared on standing.

1. Urobilistix strips (and the urobilinogen portion of Multistix and N-Multistix strips)

This test is based on the development of an orange colour from the reaction of urobilinogen with p-dimethylaminobenzaldehyde. It must be performed on fresh urine.

The colour scale permits assessment of the urobilinogen content as 0.1, 1, 4, 8 or 12 Ehrlich units per dl, when read at 60 seconds. The normal range of urobilinogen in urine is 0.1–1 Ehrlich unit per dl, and the absence of urobilinogen from the specimen being tested cannot be detected with the strip.

The test is not completely specific for urobilinogen, and will react with some other substances known to interfere with its reagent, e.g. porphobilinogen and p aminosalicylic acid, but the test is not a reliable method for the detection of porphobilinogen. Drugs containing an azo dye (e.g. azo gantrisin) may give a masking golden colour.

Nitrite

The production of nitrite from nitrate ion in urine is brought about by the activity of many of the common species of bacteria, but not all. Those species that do produce nitrite do so at different rates for different species. The production of nitrite depends also on the amount of nitrate available (from dietary sources) in the urine and on the time that the bacteria have had to work in that specimen of urine since the bladder was last emptied.

Thus, while the presence of nitrite in a urine specimen implies bacterial infection, it does not indicate the degree of infection, and the absence of nitrite from the specimen does not imply that there is no bacterial infection.

1. Ames nitrite test (on N-Labstix and N-Multistix strips but not available singly)

This test converts the nitrite ion to nitrous acid, diazotizes that and then converts the product to an azo dye. It is sensitive to 0.075 mg per dl (0.007 mmol/l) of sodium nitrite at the time of manufacture, in urines having low specific gravity and less than 5 mg per dl (0.28 mmol/l) ascorbic acid; the sensitivity will be reduced in urines of high specific gravity and ascorbic acid content. It assesses the concentration of nitrite as 'negative', or 'positive'. Any shade of pink is positive and suggestive of the presence of 10^5 or more organisms per ml, but the degree of the reaction cannot be correlated with the degree of bacteriuria. A 'negative' result indicates that the nitrite concentration is below the test's sensitivity, but does not indicate that bacteriuria is absent, as explained above. Where there is bacterial infection the test is more likely to give a positive result if the urine has been in the baldder for about 4 hours at least. Comparison of the reagent area with a white background may help to detect very pale pink reactions. The test is specific for nitrite and will not react with any other substance normally excreted in urine.

This test has the advantages that its result is available in one minute and that it does not require the specimen to have been obtained using 'clean-catch' teahniques.

Phenylketones (and metabolites of salicylates and phenothiazines)
Testing of infants' urine for phenylketones is carried out less commonly now that many Health Authorities test infant's blood for phenylalaninaemia (and other abnormalities) instead, as this sign is more reliable than phenylketonuria as an indication of the disorder. However, Phenistix reagent strips, which were developed to screen for plenylketonuria, still have a use for this, and additional ones for checking on the ingestion of prescribed doses of paraaminosalicylic acid (PAS) or for detecting over-doses of salicylates or phenothiazines.

1. Phenistix strips

The reagent area of Phenistix is impregnated with ferric ammonium sulphate, magnesium sulphate and cyclohexylsulphamic acid. Ferric ions give various colours with a number of substances in acidic conditions.

(a) As a test for phenylketonuria

The strip is dipped in urine, or pressed against a freshly wet napkin (not merely damp), and removed immediately. If the test end turns a greenish-grey similar to the shades on the colour chart within 30 seconds, the test is positive for phenylketonuria. If it turns off-white or cream within 30 seconds the test is negative. The sensitivity of the strip to phenylpyruvic acid is 8 mg per dl.

(b) As a test for the ingestion of prescribed PAS

The strip is dipped in urine and removed immediately. A brownish-red colour appearing at once indicates that the subject has taken PAS within 12–18 hours (or possibly some other salicylate). The sensitivity of Phenistix strips to PAS is 5–10 mg per dl.

(c) As a test for overdoses of salicylates or phenothiazines

The test is dipped in urine and removed immediately. If the test end turns brownish red or a shade within dull pink–red–purple colour range, the ingestion of salicylates or phenothiazines is indicated.

To ascertain which of these classes of drug was responsible, add a small volume (about 1 ml) of concentrated sulphuric acid slowly and with stirring to an equal volume of water and cool it. Put one drop of the mixture on the reagent pad of the used strip. If the colour is bleached, it was caused by a salicylate; if it is enhanced, it was caused by a phenothiazine.

The test gives a light brownish-red colour with 50 mg per dl of 'free' salicylate. The colours given by metabolites of phenothiazines are not usually sufficiently intense to be used as a check on whether a patient has taken the prescribed dose of one of this group of drugs, but the colour in the case of an overdose would be more definite.

Chlorides
1. Fantus test

(a) Rinse a test tube and pipette with distilled water and put 10 drops of urine in the tube.

(b) Rinse the pipette with distilled water and add 1 drop of 20 per cent potassium chromate solution.

(c) Rinse the pipette with distilled water and add 2.9 per cent silver nitrate solution drop by drop, counting the drops and shaking the tube after each addition, until the mixture changes colour sharply from yellow to reddish-brown.

The number of drops denotes the chloride in the urine, in g per l of sodium chloride; a normal result is 3 to 5 drops.

B. BLOOD, SERUM AND PLASMA TESTING

Quick tests are available in the form of Ames strips or tablets for glucose, ketones and urea in blood (Dextrostix strips, Acetest tablets and Azostix strips respectively) and for ketones in serum or plasma (Ketostix strips and Acetest tablets). They are intended for immediate use on one drop of fresh specimen, e.g. blood from a fingertip or ear prick, or from the tip of a syringe used to withdraw a larger specimen for laboratory testing. Thus there is no occasion to add preservatives to the blood used for these 'on the spot' tests, even if the rest of the specimen may require it. In particular, Dextrostix strips should not be used on blood to which a fluoride has been added because this will inhibit the test to some degree, depending on its concentration, and Azostix strips should not be used on blood containing a fluoride or an ammonium salt.

These quick tests give semiquantitative results. They are not intended to replace quantitative laboratory analyses but to give a guide to the patient's condition in circumstances where speed is of more importance than exactitude.

Glucose
1. Dextrostix strips

The chemistry of Dextrostix is similar to that of Clinistix (see under Glucose in Urine testing) but the chromogen system is slightly different, and the reagent area is covered with a semipermeable membrane to hold back erythrocytes, etc.

For reliable results these directions must be followed exactly:

(a) Compare Dextrostix reagent area against 'O' block on colour chart. Do not use if colour of unreacted strip does not closely match that of 'O' colour block.

(b) Freely apply a large drop of capillary or venous blood sufficient to cover *entire* reagent area on *printed side* of strip.

(c) *Wait exactly 60 seconds.* (Use sweep seconds hand or stopwatch for timing.)
(d) Quickly wash off blood (in 1 or 2 seconds) with a sharp stream of water, *using a wash bottle*, directed just above reagent area.
(e) Read immediately after washing (within 1 or 2 seconds). Hold the strip close to the colour chart.
(f) Interpolate if necessary.

The colour blocks are labelled 0, 25, 45, 90, 130, 175 and 250 mg per dl or more respectively. The test cannot give numerical values for concentrations above 250 mg per dl (unless read instrumentally, see the following item). It is specific for glucose in blood and does not react with other reducing substances as do methods depending on, for example, potassium ferricyanide. Glucose concentrations are lower in whole blood than in the serum or plasma from that blood. In blood of unusually high haematocrit (e.g. from some neonates) the strip may give a slight underestimate.

Dextrostix strips should not be used on blood to which a fluoride has been added; however, no anticoagulant is needed for the application of this test to one drop of fresh blood from a prick. A Tek-Chek synthetic control set is available for Dextrostix, similar to those described previously for the Ames urine tests.

This test will not give numerically correct results on serum or plasma.

2. Dextrostix Eyetone system

It has been found that a major factor in the overall error of estimating blood glucose with Dextrostix is the visual comparison of the strip's reagent area with the colour chart. To improve this factor, instrumental reading was introduced, first with the Ames reflectance meter and then with the Eyetone instrument.

Eyetone is a small mains-operated instrument which provides a more objective and precise interpretation of the colour developed on Dextrostix strips. It has a range of reading from 10 to 400 mg per dl (0.55 to 22.2 mmol/l glucose in whole blood). It gives a better degree of quantitation than the visual test, but makes even more important the correct technique for using the strip. A calibration and control set is available to standardize the Dextrostix Eyetone or Dextrostix reflectance meter systems.

Full details and instructions accompany the instruments and their calibration and control set or are available from Ames Company.

Ketones
1. Acetest tablets

This test has been described under Ketones in Urine Testing.

(a) Place an Acetest tablet on clean dry white paper.
(b) Put 1 drop of whole blood on top of the tablet.
(c) About 10 minutes later, remove the blood clot and compare the colour of the tablet below it to the colour chart.

The test reacts with acetoacetic acid and acetone (more strongly to the former) but not to ß-hydroxybutyric acid. It is sensitive to about 10 mg acetoacetic acid per dl.

The tablet may be used with serum or plasma, substituting one drop of either for one drop of blood in instruction (b) above and substituting for (c) above:

(d) Two minutes later compare colour of the tablet with the colour chart.

2. Ketostix strips

This test has been described under Ketones in Urine Testing. It is not suitable for use on whole blood, but may be used on serum or plasma thus:

(a) Dip test area in fresh serum or plasma and remove it immediately.
(b) Gently tap edge of strip against the side of the specimen container, to remove excess specimen.
(c) Compare test area with colour chart, exactly 15 seconds later.

This test is sensitive to 5–10 mg/dl of acetoacetic acid; it is less sensitive to acetone, and does not react with ß-hydroxybutric acid.

Urea
1. Azostix strips

The reagent area of Azostix is impregnated with a mixture of urease, buffers and bromothymol blue, under a semi-permeable membrane to hold back erythrocytes etc. Urea is hydrolysed by urease and produces ammonium ions which cause a colour change in the indicator.

(a) Freely apply a large drop of capillary or venous blood sufficient to cover entire reagent area on printed side of strip.
(b) Wait exactly 60 seconds. (Use sweep seconds hand or stopwatch for timing.)
(c) Quickly wash off blood (in 1 or 2 seconds) with a sharp stream of water using a wash bottle and directing the stream just above the reagent area.
(d) Read the result within 1 or 2 seconds after washing. Hold the strip close to the colour chart. Interpolate if colour produced falls between colour blocks. Any delay in reading will give erroneously low results due to rapid fading of the colour reaction.

The colour blocks are marked 20, 45, 85 and 130 mg per dl of urea. To convert from blood urea to blood urea nitrogen, divide by 2.14.

Fluoride preservatives may cause erroneously low results, and ammonium salts from anticoagulants will give false elevation of the result. As with Dextrostix strips, no preservative is needed for this 'on the spot' test. In a minor proportion of patients in severe alkalosis, the pH and buffers of the blood may be sufficiently extreme to cause a slight overestimate of blood urea concentration by Azostix. In a minor proportion of patients in severe acidosis, an underestimate may be caused.

C. FAECES TESTING

Faeces are more difficult to analyse than blood or urine because they are very non-homogeneous and one cannot mix them adequately by merely stirring, as one can a liquid. Thus when a small portion is taken for testing it is unlikely to be representative of the whole, i.e. there is a large sampling error. This can be decreased either by blending the whole specimen (usually with water to make an emulsion) in a homogenizer or by replicate testing of several portions withdrawn from different parts of the specimen. The latter is probably somewhat less effective, but quicker and simpler. If three tests are made on different portions and the results agree, one can have more confidence in the finding than if it is based on one test only, and if the results disagree one can either consider the specimen to be 'borderline' or make, say, two more tests and accept the majority finding, (see Ross and Gray, *Br. med. J.* 1964, i, 1351).

On account both of the sampling error and of the wide variation in composition of faeces, and hence in factors which may interfere with various analyses, tests on faeces are inherently less reliable than tests on urine or blood.

Blood

By far the most commonly requested test on faeces is that for occult blood. This is an extremely difficult analysis, because faecal samples are not very suitable for microscopy for intact red cells (which in any case would probably be disrupted unless they had come from low down in the gastrointestinal tract), and chemical tests for haemoglobin, such as are used on urine, are liable to much interference. They can be inhibited to a variable degree by the specimen (faecal material generally has mildly reducing properties) and enhanced by several factors, e.g.

> Haemoglobin from dietary sources such as rare steaks, liver, black puddings
> Peroxidases of bacterial origin
> Peroxidases of vegetable origin, e.g. from lettuce, turnips, bananas
> Blood from the patient not originating from gastrointestinal bleeding but from, for example, vigorous brushing of the teeth and gums.

Thus it is not surprising that a large number of tests for blood in faeces has been proposed and that there is no consensus of opinion as to the desirable sensitivity for the test. A test of low sensitivity will miss some specimens containing a little blood, whereas a test of higher sensitivity will give many positive results from the causes listed above in patients who may or may not have gastrointestinal bleeding.

To decrease the number of such 'false' positives, it is helpful to put the patient on a diet free from, or very low in, items which might contribute to a positive result, and possibly to prohibit toothbrushing, for a few days before the test. For more information see Illingworth, D.G., 'Influence of diet on occult blood tests, *Gut* 1965, **6**, 595.

Interference by peroxidases of vegetable and bacterial origin can be removed, wholly or partially, by emulsifying a portion (or preferably several portions from different parts of the specimen) with water and boiling it. However, this obviously lowers the concentration of blood to be detected.

1. Hematest reagent tablets

The chemistry of Hematest tablets is similar to that of Hemastix strips (see under Blood in Urine Testing).

(a) Make *thin* smear of faeces on filter paper square provided. Do not use emulsion.
(b) Place Hematest tablet across edge of smear.
(c) Flow one drop of water on top of tablet, wait 5 to 10 seconds, and flow second drop on tablet so that it runs down sides onto filter paper.
(d) Observe colour of filter paper around tablet exactly 2 minutes later.

A positive is indicated by the appearance within 2 minutes of a blue colour. The concentration of blood is roughly proportional to the intensity of blue colour and the speed with which it develops. Ignore any colour appearing on tablet or smear, and colour appearing in filter paper after 2 minutes.

This test is relatively insensitive and is intended for use on undieted patients.

2. Occultest reagent tablets

The chemistry of Occultest tablets is similar to that of Hemastix strips (see under Blood in Urine Testing).

These tablets, although developed originally for testing urine for blood, may be used on faeces in the same way as Hematest reagent tablets. They are about 5 times more sensitive than Hematest and are suitable for use on patients who have been dieted suitably for the previous 3–5 days. If used on the faeces of undieted patients they must be expected to give positive results from other causes besides gastrointestinal bleeding, as indicated above.

3. Hemastix strips

This test has been described under Blood in Urine Testing. It is intended for the detection of blood in urine, and the manufacturers do not recommend its use on faeces, in which it is less reliable than in urine. However, various workers have tried it in this application using various techniques and have found it at least as reliable as some routine quick tests for occult blood (e.g. Lehmann and Kitchin, *Lancet* 1971, ii, 258).

Techniques vary in detail, but substantially consist of either putting a dry strip into an emulsion, if used, or applying a piece of the dry specimen to the reagent area of the strip, previously wetted briefly with distilled water. In both cases the reagent pad should be only half-covered with the specimen, so that the test can be read by observing the colour developing on the unsoiled remainder of the reagent area. A blue colour is positive; no change from cream colour is negative.

The sensitivity of the test can be varied by altering the time at which the reading is made, e.g. 15, 20 or 30 seconds, or by altering the dilution of the emulsion if used. Hemastix strips are more liable to inhibition from reducing substances in the faeces than are Hematest or Occultest, because more of the reagents can be put in a tablet than in a reagent pad.

4. Tests using solutions, not commercial products

There are too many of these to give in detail. They are all based on the peroxidase-like activity of haemoglobin to catalyse the oxidation of a chromogen by hydrogen peroxide. The preferred chromogen was benzidine until its carcinogenicity became known, since when a number of other chromogens has been tried. Some methods employ the faecal sample as it is, others use an emulsion, others an emulsion which has been boiled and cooled.

The following papers describe tests for occult blood in faeces, the chromogen being given in brackets after the reference.

Kohn and Kelly (1955), *J. clin. Path.* **8**, 249 (*o*-tolidine)

Ross and Gray (1964), *Br. med. J.* i, 1351 (*o*-tolidine)

Benson (1968), *Proc. Ass. clin. Biochem,* **5**, 31 (phenolphthalein)

Wilkinson and Penfold (1969), *Lancet* ii, 847 (guaiac)

Deadman and Timms (1969, *Clin. chim. acta* **20**, 396 (2, 6-dichlorophenol indophenol)

Woodman (1970), *Clin. chim. acta* **29**, 249 (diphenylamine)

Crossley (1970), *J. med. lab. Techn.* **27**, 340 (aminopyridine)

Clarke (1971), *Med. lab. Techn.,* **28**, 187 (reduced thymolphthalein)

SUGARS

Disorders of sugar metabolism may result in the presence of reducing sugars such as lactose in the patient's faeces, for which a simple quick test would be useful routinely.

1. Clinitest tablets. (Caution: these tablets are caustic).

This test has been described under Reducing Sugars in Urine Testing.

Kerry and Anderson (*Lancet* 1964, i, 981) proposed the use of Clinitest tablets as a qualitative test for sugars in faeces. Their technique was to mix thoroughly 1 volume of the faecal specimen with 2 volumes of water (these can be measured easily using a measuring cylinder), and then to perform the CLINITEST test on 15 drops of the resulting suspension, using the AMES dropper and tube without additional water. The result was read by matching the colour blocks of the chart provided for urine and interpreted as follows:

Up to and including ¼% — negative

Over ¼% to ½% — suspect

Over ½% — positive

(These percentages should not be taken as numerically correct for sugars in faeces).

Clinitest tablets will react with glucose, fructose, lactose, galactose, pentose and maltose, but not with sucrose (unless this is previously hydrolysed to glucose and fructose). Their results will include a contribution from other reducing substances present in faeces, which accounts for the interpretation, in this context, being negative up to a match to the colour block that indicates ¼ per cent glucose in urine. Other references to this application of the tablets are:

Anderson *et al.* (1966), *Lancet* i, 1322
Townley (1966), *Pediatrics* **38**, 127
Davidson and Mullinger (1970), *Pediatrics* **46**, 632
Soeparto *et al.* (1972), *Archs. Dis. Childh.* **47**, 56.

Body Fluids Tests

Blood tests

Normal ranges vary between laboratories. These ranges should be taken as a guide only

Test	Trad	SI
Albumin (see Protein)	—	—
Alkali reserve	55–70 ml CO_2/100ml (23.8–34.6 mEq/l)	—
Amino acid nitrogen	3.5–5.5mg/ 100ml	2.5–4.0 mmol/l
Aminotransferases (see Transaminases)	—	—
Ammonia	20–100µg/ 100ml	12–60 µmol/l
Amylase	50–160 Somogyi units/100ml	90–300iu/l
Antistreptolysin 'O' titre	Up to 200U/ml	—
Ascorbic acid	0.7–1.4mg/ 100ml	—
Bicarbonate	24–30mEq/l	24–30mmol/l
Bilirubin—total	0.3–1.0mg/ 100ml	0.5–1.7 µmol/l
-conjugated	Up to 0.2 mg/ 100ml	Up to 0.3 µmol/l
Bleeding time	1–6min	—
Blood volume	Approx 1/12 or 8% body weight	—
Bromsulphthalein	Less than 15% after 25 min	—
Caeruloplasmin (copper oxidase)	30–60mg/ 100ml	0.3–0.6g/l

Test	Trad	SI
Calcium	8.5–10.5mg/ 100ml (4.3–5.3mEq/l)	2.1–2.6 mmol/l
Carbon dioxide (whole blood)	35–46mmHg	4.5–6.0kPa
Carbonic acid	1.1–1.4mEq/l	1.1–1.4mmol/l
Carbon monoxide	Less than 0.8 vol %	—
Carotenoids	50–300μg/ 100ml	1.0–5.5 μmol/l
Cephalin-cholesterol reaction	0–1+	0–1+
Chloride	95–105mEq/l	95–105mmol/l
Cholesterol	140–270mg/ 100ml	3.5–7.0 mmol/l
Cholinesterase	2–5iu/l	2–5iu/l
Clotting time	4–10min	—
Factor V assay (AcG)	75–125%	—
Factor VIII assay (AHG)	50–200%	—
Factor IX assay (PTC, Christmas factor)	75–125%	—
Factor X assay (Stuart factor)	75–125%	—
Clot retraction	Starts 1h Complete 24h	—
CO_2 combining power (see Alkali reserve)	—	—
Colloidal gold	0–1 units	0–1 units
Colour index	0.85–1.15	—
Congo red	60–100% retained in bloodstream	—
Copper	75–140μg/ 100ml	—
Corticosteroids (cortisol)	10–25μg/ 100ml	0.3–0.7 μmol/l

Test	Trad	SI
Creatine	0.2–0.8mg/100ml	15–60μmol/l
Creatine kinase	4–60iu/l	4–60iu/l
Creatinine	0.7–1.4mg/100ml	60–120 μmol/l
Copper	80–150μg/100ml	13–24μmol/l
Enzymes (see individual enzymes)	—	—
Erythrocyte sedimentation rate (ESR)		
Men	3–5mm/1h; 7–15mm/2h (Westergren)	
Women	7–12mm/1h; 12–17/2h (Westergren)	
Fasting blood sugar (see Glucose)	—	—
Fatty acids (free)	0.3–0.6mEq/l	0.3–0.6mmol/l
Fibrinogen (see Protein)	—	—
Flocculation tests (see under individual tests)	—	
Folic acid	greater than 3ng/ml	—
Gammaglobulin (see Protein)—		—
Gamma-glutamyl-transpeptidase	5–30iu/l	5–30iu/l
Globulin (see Protein)	—	—
Glucose (whole blood, fasting)		
venous	55–90mg/100ml	3.0–5.0mmol/l
capillary (arterial)	60–95mg/100ml	3.3–5.3mmol/l
Glucose tolerance	max. 180mg/100ml returns fasting 1½–2h	—
Glutamic oxalacetic transaminase (GOT) (see also Transaminases)	5–40units/ml	—

Test	Trad	SI
Glutamic pyruvic transaminase (GPT) (see also Transaminases)	5-35units/ml	—
Glycerol (see Triglyceride)	—	—
Haematocrit (see PCV)	—	—
Haemoglobin	12-18g/100ml (14.6g=100%)	12-18g/dl
Haptoglobins	30-180mg/100ml	20-110 μmol/l
Hydrogen ion activity exponent (pH)	7.36-7.42	7.36-7.42
Hydrogen ion concentration	35-44nEq/l	35-44nmol/l
Icteric index	4-6U	—
Iron Men	70-180μg/100ml	13-32 μmol/l
Women	Approx. 20μg/100ml less	
Iron-binding capacity (total)	250-400μg/100ml	45-70μmol/l
Kahn	negative	—
Ketones	0.06-0.2 mEq/l	0.06-0.2 mmol/l
Lactate	0.75-2.0 mEq/l	0.75-2.0 mmol/l
Lactate dehydrogenase total	60-250iu/l	60-250iu/l
'heart specific'	50-150iu/l	50-150iu/l
Lead (whole blood)	10-35μg/100ml	0.5-1.7 μmol/l
LE cells	None	—
Leucine aminopeptidase	1-3μmol/h/ml	—
Lipase	0-1.5 Cherry-Crandall units	18-280iu/l
Lipids (total)	450-1000mg/100ml	4.5-10g/l

Test	Trad	SI
ß-Lipoproteins	350–650mg/100ml	3.5–6.5g/l
Liver function (see individual tests)	—	—
Magnesium	1.8–2.4mg/100ml	0.7–1.0mmol
Methaemoglobin	None	—
5'-Nucleotidase	1–15iu/l	2 15iu/l
Osmolality	275–295 mosmol/kg	275, 295 mosmol/kg
Oxygen (whole blood)	85–105mmHg	11–15kPa
Oxygen capacity	14.4–24.7ml	—
Oxygen combining power Men Women	17.8–22.2ml 16.1–18.9ml	— —
Paul-Bunnell	Agglutination up to 1:20	—
CO_2	35–46mmHg	4.5–6.0kPa
pH	7.36–7.42	7.36–7.42
Phosphatase Acid-total	0.5–3.0KA units/100ml	3.5–20iu/l
Acid-prostatic	0–0.5 KA units/100ml	0–3.5iu/l
Alkaline-total	3–13 KA units/100ml	20–90iu/l
Phosphate (inorganic)	2.5–4.5mg/100ml	0.8–1.4mmol/l
Phospholipids (as fatty acids)	150–250mg/100ml	5.0–9.0mmol/l
(as phosphorus)	6–10mg/100ml	1.9–3.2mmol/l
Phosphorus (see Phosphate, inorganic)		
Platelets	200 000–500 000/mm^3	200–500 × 10^9/l

Test	Trad	SI
P_{O_2} (whole blood)	85-105mmHg	11-15kPa
Potassium	3.8-5.0mEq/l	3.8-5.0mmol/l
Protein		
—total	6.2-8.0g/ 100ml	62-80g/l
—Albumin	3.6-5.0g/ 100ml	35-50g/l
—Globulin (total)	1.8-3.2g/ 100ml	18-32g/l
—Gammaglobulin	0.7-1.5g/ 100ml	7-15g/l
—Fibrinogen	0.2-0.4g/ 100ml	2-4g/l
—A–G ratio	1.5:1-2.5:1	—
Protein-bound iodine	4.0-7.5μg/ 100ml	0.3-0.6 μmol/l
Prothrombin time	11-18s	—
Pseudocholinesterase (see also Cholinesterase)	60-90 Warburg units	—
Pyruvate (fasting)	0.4-0.7mg/ 100ml	0.05-0.08 mmol/l
Red cell count Total:	4 000 000- 6 000 000/ mm³	4.0-6.0 × 10¹²/l
Reticulocytes	0.1-2.0/ 100 RBCs	—
Packed cell volume (PCV) Men:	40-54%	—
Women:	36-47%	—
Mean cell volume (MCV)	78-94 μm³	78-94fl
Mean corpuscular haemoglobin concentration (MCHC)	32-36%	—
Mean corpuscular haemoglobin (MCH)	27-32μμg	27-32pg
Mean cell diameter	6.7-7.7μm	6.7-7.7μm
Red cell fragility	Haemolysis slight 0.44% NaCl	—
	Haemolysis complete 0.3% NaCl	—

Test	Trad	SI
Sodium	136-148 mEq/l	136-148 mmol/l
Sulphaemoglobin	None	—
Thymol flocculation turbidity	0-± 0-4 units	0-± 0-4 units
Thyroxine	3.0-6.5μg/ 100ml	0.04-0.085 μmol/l
Transaminase alanine (at 25° C) aspartate (at 25° C)	4-12iu/l 5-15iu/l	4-12iu/l 5-15iu/l
Transferrin	120-200mg/ 100ml	0.12-0.2g/l
Triglyceride	2.5-15mg/ 100ml	0.3-1.8mmol/l
Urea	18-40mg/ 100ml	3.0-6.5mmol/l
Uric acid	2.0-7.0mg/ 100ml	0.1-0.45 mmol/l
Vitamin A	30-90μg/ 100ml	1.0-3.0 μmol/l
Vitamin B_{12}	150-800pg/ml	—
Vitamin C (see Ascorbic acid)	—	—
Wasserman reaction (WR)	Negative	—
White cell count *Total:*	4000-10 000/ mm^3	4.0-10.0 × 10^9/l
Differential Neutrophils	2500-7 500/ mm^3	2 500-7 500 × 10^6/l
Eosinophils	200-400/ mm^3	200-400 × 10^6/l
Basophils	0-50/ mm^3	0-50 × 10^6/l
Lymphocytes	1500-3 500/ mm^3	1 500-3 500 × 10^6/l
Monocytes	400-800/ mm^3	400-800 × 10^6/l
Zinc sulphate reaction	2-8 units	2.8 units

Normal characteristics of body fluids

Cerebrospinal fluid

Pressure (adult)	50 to 200 mm water
Cells	0 to 5 lymphocytes/mm^3
Glucose	3.3–4.4 mmol/l
Protein	100–400 mg/l

Urine

Total quantity per 24 hours	1000 to 1500 ml
Specific gravity	1.012 to 1.030
Reaction	pH 4 to 8

Average amounts of inorganic and organic solids in urine each 24 hours

Calcium	2.5–7.5 mmol
Creatinine	9–17 mmol
5HIAA	15–75 μmol
HMMA*	10–35 μmol
Hydroxyproline	0.08–0.25 mmol
Magnesium	3.3–5.0 mmol
Oestriol	varies widely during pregnancy—μmol
Phosphate	15–50 mmol
Urea	250–500 mmol
17-ketosteroids:	
Men	8 to 15 mg/24 hours
Women	5 to 12 mg/24 hours

Faeces, normal fat content

Daily output on normal diet	less than 7 g
Fat (as stearic acid)	11–18 mmol/24h

*4-Hydroxy-3-methoxy mandelic acid.

Vitamins Table

Vitamin	Functions	Properties	Deficiency	Sources	Daily Requirements
A	Anti-infective. Essential for healthy skin and mucous membranes. Aids night vision	Within the body vit. A can be synthesized from carotene, a yellow pigment (provitamin) present in food. Can be stored in the liver	Poor growth. Rough dry skin and mucous membrane. Liability to infection of skin and mucous membranes. Lessened ability to see in the dark. In severe deficiency xerophthalmia which can lead to blindness	All animal fats Carrots Apricots Tomatoes Spinnach Water cress	3000 5000 iu
D D₂Calciferol D₁7-dehydrotacysterol	Antirachitic. Assists absorption and metabolism of calcium and phosphorus	Produced in the body by action of sunlight on the ergosterol in the skin	Rickets in children. Osteomalacia and osteoporosis in adults	Oily fish Prepared from the livers of cod and halibut Dairy produce	400 800 iu This level essential for children and nursing mothers
E Alpha-tocopherol	Necessary for the reproduction of rats; not proven that this is so in human beings		Thought to interfere with reproduction: also thought to cause certain degenerative diseases of the nervous system and damage to the liver	Wheat germ Milk Cereals Egg yolk Liver	
K Menadione K₁ Phytomenadione	Antihaemorrhagic. Essential for the production of prothrombin.	Only absorbed in the presence of bile	Delayed clotting time. Liver damage	Vegetables with green leaves Peas	

FAT - SOLUBLE

WATER - SOLUBLE

B complex					
B_1 Aneurine or Thiamine	Antineuritic. Antiberi-beri. Health of nervous system.	Destroyed by excessive heat and baking soda	Poor growth. Neuritis. Beri-beri	Brewer's yeast, Cereals, Vegetables, Eggs, Fruit, Liver, Meat	1 15 mg
B_2 Riboflavine	Steady and continuous release of energy from carbohydrates. Antipellagra	Can withstand normal cooking	Fissures at corners of mouth and on tongue. Corneal opacities. Skin manifestations (dermatitis). Diarrhoea.		1.5 2.5 mg
Nicotinic acid			Mental symptoms, possibly dementia. Pellagra		10 17 mg
B_6 Pyridoxine	Protein metabolism	Relieves postradiotherapy nausea and vomiting	Nervousness and insomnia		
Folic acid	Assists production of red blood cells		Some forms of macrocytic anaemia	Green vegetables, Liver	
B_{12} Cyanocobalamin	Essential for red blood cell formation	Can only be absorbed in the presence of the intrinsic factor secreted by gastric cells. Stored in the liver. Maintenance therapy for patients with pernicious anaemia	Pernicious anaemia	Liver and all other foods containing B complex	
Cytamen	—			Prepared from growth of Streptomyces	

Vitamins Table (cont.)

Vitamin	Functions	Properties	Deficiency	Sources	Daily Requirements
C Ascorbic acid	Formation of bones, teeth and collagen	Destroyed by cooking in the presence of air and by plant enzymes released when cutting and grating raw food. Lost by long storage	Sore mouth and gums. Capillary bleeding. Scurvy. Delayed healing of wounds	Fresh fruits Fresh vegetables Rose-hip and blackcurrant syrups	30–50 mg

Weights and heights

Weights for Age, birth to 5 years, sexes combined (Jelliffe, 1966)

Age (Months)	Weight (kg) Standard*	80% Standard	60% Standard	Age (months)	Weight (kg) Standard*	80% Standard	60%
0	3.4	2.7	2.0	31	13.7	11.0	8.2
				32	13.8	11.1	8.3
1	4.3	3.4	2.5	33	14.0	11.2	8.4
2	5.0	4.0	2.9				
3	5.7	4.5	3.4	34	14.2	11.3	8.5
				35	14.4	11.5	8.6
4	6.3	5.0	3.8	36	14.5	11.6	8.7
5	6.9	5.5	4.2				
6	7.4	5.9	4.5	37	14.7	11.8	8.8
				38	14.85	11.9	8.9
7	8.0	6.3	4.9	39	15.0	12.05	9.0
8	8.4	6.7	5.1				
9	8.9	7.1	5.3	40	15.2	12.2	9.1
				41	15.35	12.3	9.2
10	9.3	7.4	5.5	42	15.5	12.4	9.3
11	9.6	7.7	5.8				
12	9.9	7.9	6.0	43	15.7	12.6	9.4
				44	15.85	12.7	9.5
13	10.2	8.1	6.2	45	16.0	12.9	9.6
14	10.4	8.3	6.3				
15	10.6	8.5	6.4	46	16.2	12.95	9.7
				47	16.35	13.1	9.8
16	10.8	8.7	6.6	48	16.5	13.2	9.9
17	11.0	8.9	6.7				
18	11.3	9.0	6.8	49	16.65	13.35	10.0
				50	16.8	13.5	10.1
19	11.5	9.2	7.0	51	16.95	13.65	10.2
20	11.7	9.4	7.1				
21	11.9	9.6	7.2	52	17.1	13.8	10.3
				53	17.25	13.9	10.4
22	12.05	9.7	7.3	54	17.4	14.0	10.5
23	12.2	9.8	7.4				
24	12.4	9.9	7.5	55	17.6	14.2	10.6
				56	17.7	14.3	10.7
25	12.6	10.1	7.6	57	17.9	14.4	10.75
26	12.7	10.3	7.7				
27	12.9	10.5	7.8	58	18.05	14.5	10.8
				59	18.25	14.6	10.9
28	13.1	10.6	7.9	60	18.4	14.7	11.0
29	13.3	10.7	8.0				
30	13.5	10.8	8.1				

*Means of the Boston standards for boys and girls (Stuart and Stevenson, 1959). Means for boys are 0.05 to 0.15 kg heavier and for girls 0.05 to 0.15 kg lighter.

Standard heights and weights of boys and girls, 5–18 years old

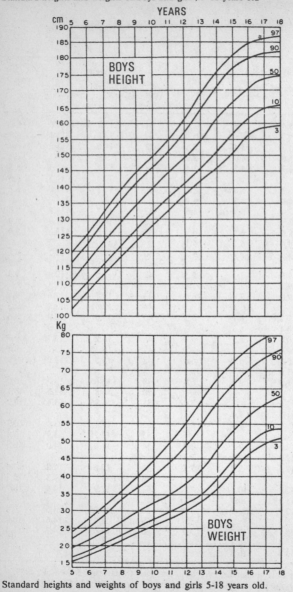

Standard heights and weights of boys and girls 5-18 years old.

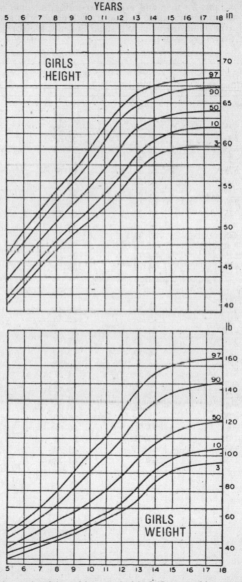

YEARS

GIRLS
HEIGHT

97
90
50
10
3

GIRLS
WEIGHT

97
90
50
10
3

Standard heights and weights of boys and girls 5-18 years old.

Desirable weights for men and women according to height and frame, based on measurements made in indoor clothing without shoes. Age 25 years and over (modified from Statistical Bulletin, Metropolitan Life Insurance Company (1959))

Height (metres)	Small frame	Weight in kg Medium frame	Large frame
Men			
1.550	51–54	54–59	57–64
1.575	52–56	55–60	59–65
1.600	53–57	56–62	60–67
1.625	55–58	58–63	61–69
1.650	56–60	59–65	63–71
1.675	58–62	61–67	64–73
1.700	60–64	63–69	67–75
1.725	62–66	64–71	68–77
1.750	64–68	66–73	70–79
1.775	65–70	68–75	72–81
1.800	67–72	70–77	74–84
1.825	69–74	72–79	76–86
1.850	71–76	74–82	78–88
1.875	73–78	76–84	81–90
1.900	74–79	78–86	83–93
Women			
1.425	42–44	44–49	47–54
1.450	43–46	45–50	48–55
1.475	44–48	46–51	49–57
1.500	45–49	47–53	51–58
1.525	46–50	49–54	52–59
1.550	48–51	50–55	53–61
1.575	49–53	51–57	55–63
1.600	50–54	53–59	57–64
1.625	52–56	54–61	59–66
1.650	54–58	56–63	60–68
1.675	55–59	58–65	62–70
1.700	57–61	60–67	64–72
1.725	59–63	62–69	66–74
1.750	61–65	63–70	68–76
1.775	63–67	65–72	69–79

SI—International System of Units

Base units which have multiples and submultiples

	$\dfrac{1}{1\,000\,000}$	$\dfrac{1}{1\,000}$	Base unit	1 000
Length	μm	mm	m	km
Mass	mg	g	kg	
Time		ms	s	
Electric current*		mA	A	
Amount of substance	μmol	mmol	mol	

Remember these base units and their multiples and submultiples. There are others, but these are the ones you are likely to meet in your work. Don't forget that the kilogram, kg, is the base unit of mass, not the gram, g.

Multiples and their prefixes

Name	Multiplies by		Symbol	Examples
kilo	x 1 000	x 10^3	k	kilometre km, kilonewton kN
mega	x 1 000 000	x 10^6	M	megawatt MW, megajoule MJ
milli	x $\dfrac{1}{1\,000}$	x 10^{-3}	m	millimetre mm, milliamp mA
micro	x $\dfrac{1}{1\,000\,000}$	x 10^{-6}	μ	micromole μmol, micrometre μm

With a few specified units these prefixes can be used, but if in doubt use one of the four above.

deca	x 10	x 10	da	
hecto	x 100	x 10^2	h	hectobar hbar
deci	x $\dfrac{1}{10}$	x 10^{-1}	d	decimetre dm
centi	x $\dfrac{1}{100}$	x 10^{-2}	c	centimetre cm

Conversion scales for certain chemical pathology tests and units of measurement

(*From* D. Goodsell, (1975) Coming to terms with SI metric. *Nursing Mirror,* **141**, 55-59. Reproduced by kind permission of the author and the *Nursing Mirror.*)

Chemical pathology Blood plasma

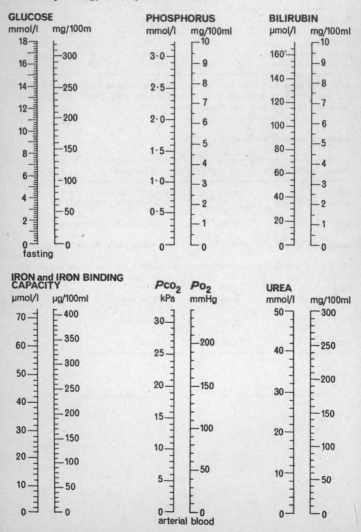

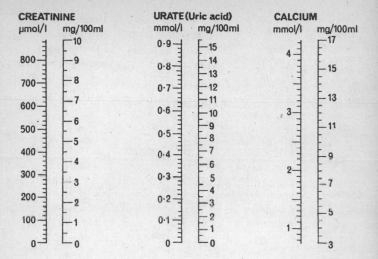

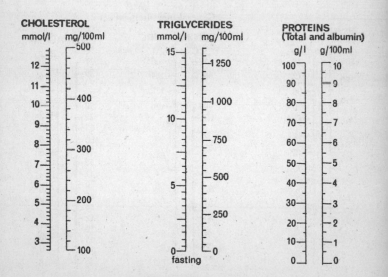

384

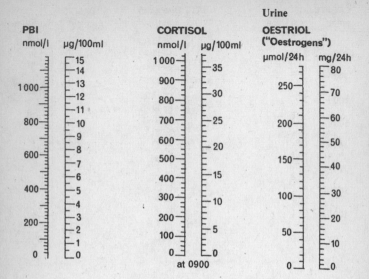

PBI
nmol/l   µg/100ml

1000 —
800 —
600 —
400 —
200 —
0 —

15
14
13
12
11
10
9
8
7
6
5
4
3
2
1
0

CORTISOL
nmol/l   µg/100ml

1000 —
900 —
800 —
700 —
600 —
500 —
400 —
300 —
200 —
100 —
0 —

35
30
25
20
15
10
5
0

at 0900

Urine

OESTRIOL
("Oestrogens")
µmol/24h   mg/24h

250 —
200 —
150 —
100 —
50 —
0 —

80
70
60
50
40
30
20
10
0

General measurements

HEIGHT
cm   inches

200 —
180 —
160 —
140 —
120 —
100 —
80 —
60 —
40 —
20 —
0 —

78
72
66
60
54
48
42
36
30
24
18
12
6
0

TEMPERATURE
°C   °F

41 —
40 —
39 —
38 —
37 —
36 —
35 —
34 —
33 —
32 —
31 —
30 —
29 —
28 —
27 —

106
104
102
100
98
96
94
92
90
88
86
84
82
80

ROOM
TEMPERATURE
°C   °F

27 —
26 —
25 —
24 —
23 —
22 —
21 —
20 —
19 —
18 —
17 —
16 —
15 —
14 —
13 —
12 —
11 —
10 —
9 —

80
78
76
74
72
70
68
66
64
62
60
58
56
54
52
50
48

385

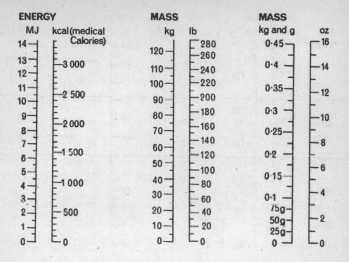

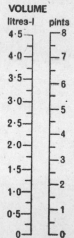

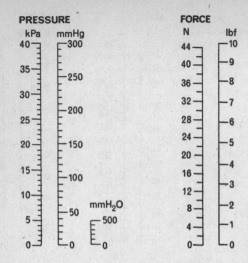

PRESSURE

kPa	mmHg
40	300
35	250
30	200
25	
20	150
15	100
10	50
5	
0	0

mmH₂O

500

0

FORCE

N	lbf
44	10
40	9
36	8
32	7
28	6
24	5
20	4
16	3
12	
8	2
4	1
0	0

List of abbreviations

ADMS	Assistant Director Medical Services.
AHA	Area Health Authority.
AMS	Army Medical Service.
ARRC	Associate of the Royal Red Cross.
ARSH	Associate of the Royal Society of Health.
ARSanA(Scot.)	Associate of the Royal Sanitary Association.
BA	Bachelor of Arts.
BAO	Bachelor of the Art of Obstetrics.
BC, BCh	Bachelor of Surgery.
BChD, BDS	Bachelor of Dental Surgery.
BDA	British Dental Association.
BDS	Bachelor of Dental Surgery.
BDSc	Bachelor of Dental Science.
BHyg	Bachelor of Hygiene.
BM	Bachelor of Medicine.
BMA	British Medical Association.
BPharm	Bachelor of Pharmacy.
BRC	British Red Cross.
BS, BCh	Bachelor of Surgery.
BSc	Bachelor of Science.
ChB	Bachelor of Surgery.
ChD	Doctor of Surgery.
CM, ChM	Master in Surgery.
COHSE	Confederation of Health Service Employees.
CPH	Certificate of the Society of Public Health.
CStJ	Commander of the Order of St John of Jerusalem.
CSP	Chartered Society of Physiotherapy.
DA	Diploma in Anaesthetics.
DBO	Diploma of the British Orthoptic Board.
DCh	Doctor of Surgery.
DCH	Diploma in Child Health.
DCP	Diploma in Clinical Pathology.
DDM	Diploma in Dermatological Medicine.
DDMS	Deputy Director Medical Services.
DDO	Diploma in Dental Orthopaedics
DDR	Diploma in Diagnostic Radiology.
DDS	Doctor of Dental Surgery.
DGMS	Director-General Medical Services.
DGO	Diploma in Gynaecology and Obstetrics.
DHSS	Department of Health and Social Security.
DHyg	Doctor of Hygiene.
DIH	Diploma in Industrial Health.
DLO	Diploma in Laryngology and Otology.

DM	Doctor of Medicine.
DMD	Director of Dental Medicine.
DMHS	Director Medical and Health Services.
DMJ	Diploma in Medical Jurisprudence.
DMR	Diploma in Medical Radiology.
DMRD	Diploma in Medical Radio-Diagnosis.
DMRE	Diploma of Medical Radiology and Electrology.
DMRT	Diploma in Medical Radio-Therapy.
DMS	Director of Medical Services.
DMSS	Director of Medical and Sanitary Services.
DMT	District Management Team.
DMV	Doctor of Veterinary Medicine.
DN	Diploma in Nursing.
DO	Diploma in Ophthalmology.
DOrth	Diploma in Orthodontics.
DOMS	Diploma in Ophthalmic Medicine and Surgery.
DPA	Diploma in Public Administration.
DPH	Diploma in Public Health.
DPM	Diploma in Psychological Medicine.
DPhysMed	Diploma in Physical Medicine
DR	Diploma in Radiology.
DRCOG	Diploma of the Royal College of Obstetricians and Gynaecologists.
DSc	Doctor of Science.
DTCD	Diploma in Tuberculosis and Chest Diseases.
DTH	Diploma in Tropical Hygiene.
DTM	Diploma in Tropical Medicine.
DTMH	Diploma Tropical Medicine and hygiene.
ENT	Ear, Nose and throat.
FACA	Fellow of the American College of Anesthetists.
FACC	Fellow of the American College of Cardiology.
FACD	Fellow of the American College of Dentists.
FACOG	Fellow of the American College of Obstetricians and Gynecologists.
FACP	Fellow of the American College of Physicians.
FACR	Fellow of the American College of Radiologists.
FACS	Fellow of the American College of Surgeons.
FBPsS	Fellow of the British Psychological Society.
FCAP	Fellow of the College of American Pathologists.
FCPS	Fellow of the College of Physicians and Surgeons.
FCPSA	Fellow of the College of Physicians and Surgeons of S. Africa.
FCRA	Fellow of the College of Radiologists of Australasia.
FCS	Fellow of the Chemical Society.
FDS	Fellow in Dental Surgery
FFARCS	Fellow of the Faculty of Anaesthetists of the Royal College of Surgeons.

FFCM	Fellow of the Faculty of Community Medicine.
FFD	Fellow of the Faculty of Dental Surgeons.
FFHom	Fellow of theFaculty of Homeopathy.
FFR	Fellow of the Faculty of Radiologists.
FGS	Fellow of the Geological Society.
FICS	Fellow of the International College of Surgeons.
FPA	Family Planning Association.
FPC	Family Practitioner Committee.
FPS	Fellow of the Pharmaceutical Society.
FRACGP	Fellow of the Royal Australian College GP.
FRACP	Fellow of the Australasian College of Physicians.
FRACS	Fellow of the Australasian College of Surgeons.
FRCOG	Fellow of the Royal College of Obstetricians and Gynaecologists.
FRCGP	Fellow of the Royal College GP.
FRCP	Fellow of the Royal College of Physicians.
FRCPath	Fellow of the Royal College Pathologists.
FRCPC	Fellow of the Royal College of Physicians of Canada.
FRCPE	Fellow of the Royal College of Physicians, Edinburgh.
FRCPI	Fellow of the Royal College of Physicians, Ireland.
FRCS	Fellow of the Royal College of Surgeons.
FRCSC	Fellow of the Royal College of Surgeons of Canada.
FRCSE	Fellow of the Royal College of Surgeons, Edinburgh.
FRCSI	Fellow of the Royal College of Surgeons, Ireland.
FRFPS	Fellow of the Royal Faculty of Physicians and Surgeons.
FRIC	Fellow of the Royal Institute of Chemistry.
FRIPHH	Fellow of the Royal Institute of Public Health and Hygiene.
FRMS	Fellow of the Royal Microscopical Society.
FRS	Fellow of the Royal Society.
FRSC	Fellow of the Royal Society of Canada.
FRSE	Fellow of the Royal Society of Edinburgh.
FRSH	Fellow of the Royal Society of Health.
FSS	Fellow of the Statistical Society.
GMC	General Medical Council.
GP	General practitioner.
HDD	Higher Dental Diploma.
HV	Health Visitor.
ICN	International Council of Nurses.
IMA	Irish Medical Association.
IMS	Indian Medical Service.
LAH	Licentiate of the Apothecaries Hall, Dublin.

LAO	Licentiate in the Art of Obstetrics.
LCh	Licentiate in Surgery.
LCPS	Licentiate of the College of Physicians and Surgeons.
LDS	Licentiate in Dental Surgery.
LDSc	Licentiate in Dental Science.
LM	Licentiate in Midwifery.
LMRCP	Licentiate in Midwifery of the Royal College of Physicians.
LMS	Licentiate in Medicine and Surgery.
LMSSA	Licentiate in Medicine and Surgery of the Society of Apothecaries of London.
LRCP	Licentiate of the Royal College of Physicians.
LRCPE	Licentiate of the Royal College of Physicians of Edinburgh.
LRCPI	Licentiate of the Royal College of Physicians of Ireland.
LRCS	Licentiate of the Royal College of Surgeons.
LRCSE	Licentiate of the Royal College of Surgeons of Edinburgh.
LRCSI	Licentiate of the Royal College of Surgeons of Ireland.
LRFPS	Licentiate of the Royal Faculty of Physicians and Surgeons.
LSA	Licentiate of the Society of Apothecaries of London.
MA	Master of Arts.
MAO	Master of the Art of Obstetrics.
MB	Bachelor of Medicine.
MC, MS, MCh	Master of Surgery.
MChD	Master of Dental Surgery.
MCh(Orth)	Master of Orthopaedic Surgery.
MCPath	Member of the College of Pathologists.
MCPA	Member of the College of Pathologists of Australia.
MCPS	Member of the College of Physicians and Surgeons.
MCRA	Member of the College of Radiologists of Australasia.
MCSP	Member of the Chartered Society of Physiotherapists.
MD	Doctor of Medicine.
MDD	Doctor of Dental Medicine.
MDentSc	Master of Dental Science.
MDS	Master of Dental Surgery.
MFCM	Member Faculty Community Medicine.
MFHom	Member of the Faculty of Homeopathy.
MHyg	Master of Hygiene.
MMed	Master of Medicine.
MMF	Member of the Medical Faculty.
MO	Medical Officer.
MO&G	Master of Obstetrics and Gynaecology.

MOH	Medical Officer of Health.
MORC	Medical Officers Reserve Corps.
MPH	Master of Public Health.
MPS	Member of the Pharmaceutical Society.
MRACGP	Member of the Royal Australian College GP.
MRad	Master of Radiology.
MRC	Medical Research Council
MRCGP	Member of the Royal College GP.
MRCOG	Member of the Royal College of Obstetricians and Gynaecologists.
MRCPath	Member of the Royal College of Pathologists.
MRCP	Member of the Royal College of Physicians.
MRCPE	Member of the Royal College of Physicians of Edinburgh.
MRCPI	Member of the Royal College of Physicians of Ireland.
MRCS	Member of the Royal College of Surgeons.
MRCSE	Member of the Royal College of Surgeons of Edinburgh.
MRCSI	Member of the Royal College of Surgeons of Ireland.
MRCVS	Member of the Royal College of Veterinary Surgeons.
MRSanA(Scot)	Member of the Royal Sanitary Association.
MRSH	Member of the Royal Society of Health.
MS	Master of Surgery.
MSc	Master of Science.
MSR	Member of the Society of Radiographers.
NHI	National Health Insurance.
NHS	National Health Service.
NUPE	National Union of Public Employees (a Health Service Union)
ONC	Orthopaedic Nursing Certificate.
OStJ	Officer of the Order of St John of Jerusalem.
PhC	Pharmaceutical Chemist.
PhD	Doctor of Philosophy.
PHI	Public Health Inspector.
PMO	Principal Medical Officer.
PMRAFNS	Princess Mary's Royal Air Force Nursing Service.
QAIMNS	Queen Alexandra's Imperial Military Nursing Service (now QARANC).
QARANC	Queen Alexandra's Royal Army Nursing Corps (formerly QAIMNS).
QARNNS	Queen Alexandra's Royal Naval Nursing Service.
QIDN	Queen's Institute of District Nursing.

RADC	Royal Army Dental Corps.
RAMC	Royal Army Medical Corps.
Rcn	Royal College of Nursing and National Council of Nurses of the United Kingdom.
RCT	Registered Clinical Teacher
RFN	Registered Fever Nurse.
RGN	Registered General Nurse (Scotland).
RHB	Regional Hospital Board.
RMN	Registered Mental Nurse.
RMO	Resident Medical Officer.
RMPA	Royal Medico-Psychological Association.
RN	Registered Nurse (USA).
RNMS	Registered Nurse for the Mentally Subnormal.
RNT	Registered Nurse Teacher
RRC	Royal Red Cross.
RSCN	Registered Sick Children's Nurse.
SBStJ	Serving Brother of the Order of St John of Jerusalem.
SCM	State Certified Midwife.
SEN	State Enrolled Nurse.
SHO	Senior House Officer.
SMO	Senior Medical Officer.
SRN	State Registered Nurse (England and Wales).
SSStJ	Serving Sister of the Order of St John of Jerusalem.
TANS	Territorial Army Nursing Service.
TANS(R)	Territorial Army Nursing Service (Reserve).
TDD	Tuberculous Diseases Diploma.
TFNS	Territorial Force Nursing Service.
WHO	World Health Organization.

Surgical instruments

Artery forceps (Chas. F. Thackray Ltd.)

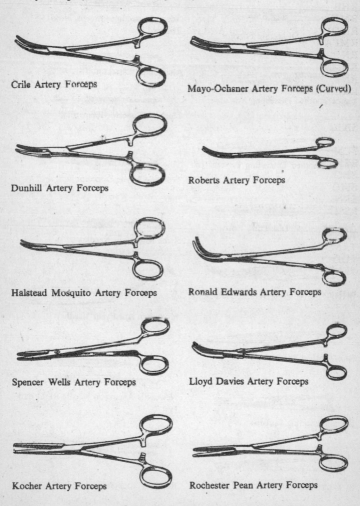

Crile Artery Forceps

Mayo-Ochsner Artery Forceps (Curved)

Dunhill Artery Forceps

Roberts Artery Forceps

Halstead Mosquito Artery Forceps

Ronald Edwards Artery Forceps

Spencer Wells Artery Forceps

Lloyd Davies Artery Forceps

Kocher Artery Forceps

Rochester Pean Artery Forceps

Dissecting forceps (Chas. F. Thackray Ltd.)

Bonney Toothed Dissecting Forceps

Adson Dissecting Forceps, Toothed

Lane Toothed Dissecting Forceps

Adson Dissecting Forceps, Non-Toothed

Treves Toothed Dissecting Forceps

Macdonald Dissector

Waugh Toothed Dissecting Forceps

Durham Dissector-Raspatory

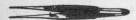

Gillies Toothed Dissecting Forceps

Watson-Cheyne Dissector

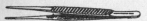

McIndoe Non-Toothed Dissecting Forceps

Syme Aneurysm Needle

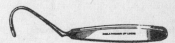

Non-Toothed Dissecting Forceps

Moynihan Aneurysm Needle

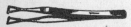

Duval Dissecting Forceps

Newcastle Aneurysm Needle Right and Left

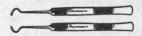

St Marks Dissecting Forceps

Rampley Sponge-Holding Forceps

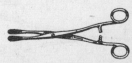

Needle holders (Chas. F. Thackray Ltd.)

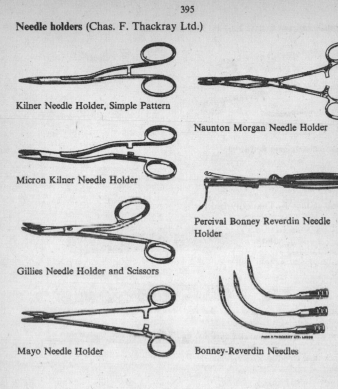

Kilner Needle Holder, Simple Pattern

Naunton Morgan Needle Holder

Micron Kilner Needle Holder

Percival Bonney Reverdin Needle
Holder

Gillies Needle Holder and Scissors

Mayo Needle Holder

Bonney-Reverdin Needles

Retractors (Chas. F. Thackray Ltd.)

Single Hook Retractor

Kilner Skin Retractor

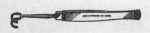

Double Hook Retractor

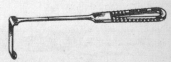

Langenbeck Retractor

Self retaining retractor (Chas. F. Thackray Ltd.)

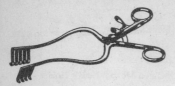

Travers Self-Retaining Retractor

Scalpels (Chas. F. Thackray Ltd.)

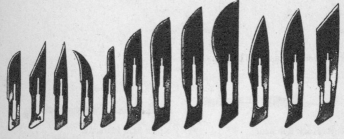

Duray Scalpel Handles Sizes 3, 4 and 5

Disposable Scalpel Blades Sizes 10–25

Major Scalpel Handle

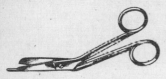
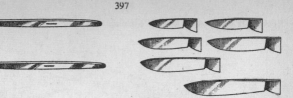

Robert Jones Tenotomy Knives

Solid Scalpels

Scissors (Chas. F. Thackray Ltd.)

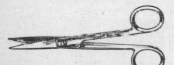

Sheffield Pattern Bandage Scissors

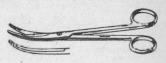

Mayo Scissors (Curved)

Stitch Scissors

Metzenbaum Dissecting Scissors (Curved)

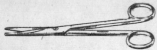

Mayo Scissors (Straight)

Tissue forceps (Chas. F. Thackray Ltd.)

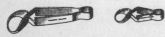

Shardle Towel Forceps

E.N.T. aural instruments (Down Surgical Ltd.)

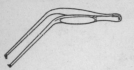

Wilde Aural Forceps

Yearsley Aural Specula

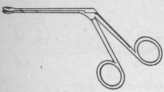

Henckel Aural Forceps

E.N.T. nasal instruments (Down Surgical Ltd.)

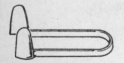

Thudichum Nasal Speculum

E.N.T. tracheal instruments (Down Surgical Ltd.)

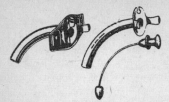

Chevalier Jackson Tracheostomy Tubes

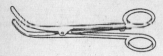

Trousseau Tracheal Dilating Forceps